M. R. Pinsky · L. Brochard · J. Mancebo· M. Antonelli (Eds.)

Applied Physiology in Intensive Care Medicine 2

M. R. Pinsky · L. Brochard · J. Mancebo
M. Antonelli (Eds.)

Applied Physiology in Intensive Care Medicine 2

Physiological Reviews and Editorials

Third Edition

Springer

Editors
MICHAEL R. PINSKY, MD
Dept. of Critical Care Medicine
University of Pittsburgh Medical Center
Scaife Hall 606
3550 Terrace Street
Pittsburgh, PA 15261
USA

LAURENT BROCHARD, MD
Dept. Intensive Care Medicine
Hôpital Henri Mondor
51 av. Maréchal Lattre de Tassigny
94010 Créteil CX
France

JORDI MANCEBO, MD
Dept. Intensive Care Medicine
Hospital de Sant Pau
Avda. S. Antonio M. Claret 167
08025 Barcelona
Spain

MASSIMO ANTONELLI
General Intensive Care Unit
Università Cattolica des Sacro Cuore
Largo A. Gemelli 8
00168 Rome
Italy

The articles in this book appeared in the journal "Intensive Care Medicine" between 2002 and 2011.

ISBN 978-3-662-50102-3 ISBN 978-3-642-28233-1 (eBook)
DOI 10.1007/978-3-642-28233-1
Springer Heidelberg New York Dordrecht London

Printed on acid-free paper

Springer is part of Springer Science+Business Media (www.springer.com)

Preface

Perhaps no field of medicine witnesses such dynamic change in practice over similar time intervals as the practice of intensive care medicine. Thus, the practice of intensive care medicine is at the very forefront of treatment and monitoring response innovation and discovery. The challenge for the healthcare practitioner facing the critically ill is daunting because the critically ill patient is by definition at the limits of his or her physiologic reserve. Such patients need immediate, aggressive but balanced life-altering interventions to minimize the detrimental aspects of acute illness and hasten recovery. Treatment decisions and response to therapy are usually assessed by measures of physiologic function but also require an understanding of a myriad of new information. However, how one uses such information is often unclear and rarely supported by prospective clinical trials and if clinical trials are available, rarely do they address the specific needs of the specific patient being treated. Thus, the bedside clinician is forced to rely primarily on physiologic principals in determining the best treatments and response to therapy. However, the physiologic foundation present in practicing physicians is uneven and occasionally supported more by habit or prior training than science. Furthermore, although excellent textbooks are available as background information, they are by necessity unable to present the latest changes or place specific novel aspects of applied physiology into perspectives based on new information.

To address this issue we have collected in this volume a series of review articles published in Intensive Care Medicine from 2002 until July 2011. This present volume combines these selected review articles, specifically included for their ability to address central critical care issues and published in the same time interval. This collection of review articles, written by some of the most respected experts in the field, represent an up-to-date and invaluable compendium of practical bedside knowledge essential to the effective delivery of acute care medicine. Although this text could be read from cover to cover, the reader is encouraged to use this text as a reference source, referring to individual review articles that pertain to specific clinical issues. In that way the relevant information will have immediate practical meaning and hopefully become incorporated into routine practice.

We hope that the reader finds these reviews useful in their practice and enjoys reading them as much as we enjoyed editing the original articles.

Michael R. Pinsky, MD, Dr hc
Laurent Brochard, MD, PhD
Jordi Mancebo, MD, PhD
Massimo Antonelli, MD, PhD

Contents

Contributors

H. Ait-Oufella
Inserm U970,
Paris Research Cardiovascular Center (PARCC),
Paris, France
and
Service de Réanimation Médicale,
Hôpital Saint-Antoine,
AP-HP, Paris, France
and
Service de Réanimation Médicale,
Hôpital Saint-Antoine,
rue du Faubourg Saint-Antoine,
Paris Cedex, France

Lars Algotsson
Department of Anaesthesiology–
Heart-Lung Division,
University Hospital of Lund,
Lund, Sweden

Peter J. D. Andrews
Department of Anaesthetics, Intensive
Care and Pain Medicine
University of Edinburgh, Western General Hospital
Edinburgh, Scotland, UK

P. Asfar
Laboratoire HIFIH UPRES EA 3859,
Université d'Angers,
Angers, France
and
Laboratoire HIFIH, IFR 132,
Universitéd' Angers et service
de réanimation médicale
et médecine hyperbare,
CHU Angers,
rue Larrey,
Angers Cedex, France

J.-F. Augusto
Laboratoire HIFIH,
IFR 132,
Universitéd' Angers et service de réanimation médicale
et médecine hyperbare,
CHU Angers,
rue Larrey,
Angers Cedex, France

Elie Azoulay
Department of Clinical Immunology,
and Hôpital Saint-Louis, Medical ICU, AP–HP,
University Paris-7 Diderot, UFR de Médecine,
Paris, France

Jan Bakker
Department of Intensive Care, Erasmus MC,
University Medical Center Rotterdam,
Rotterdam, The Netherlands

Karim Bendjelid
Surgical Intensive Care Division,
Geneva University Hospitals,
Geneva, Switzerland

Willem Boer
Intensive Care Unit, Nephrology Unit
and Internal Medicine Department,
Atrium Medical Center,
Heerlen, The Netherlands

E. Christiaan Boerma
Department of Translational Physiology,
Academic Medical Center Amsterdam,
Amsterdam, The Netherlands
and
Department of Intensive Care,
Medical Center Leeuwarden,
BR Leeuwarden,
The Netherlands

Chiara Bonetto
Dipartimento di Anestesia e Rianimazione,
Ospedale S. Giovanni Battista-Molinette,
Universita di Torino,
Corso Dogliotti,
Turin, Italy

Sophie Buyse
Department of Clinical Immunology,
and Hôpital Saint-Louis, Medical ICU,
AP–HP, University Paris-7 Diderot,
UFR de Médecine,
Paris, France

Enrico Calzia
Sektion Anästhesiologische Pathophysiologie und Verfahrensentwicklung Universitätsklinik für Anästhesiologie, Universität Ulm,
Ulm, Germany

René Chiolero
Department of Intensive Care,
Centre Hospitalo-universitaire de Liege,
Domaine du Sart Tilman B35,
Liege, Belgium

S. Collin
Groupe Choc,
Contrat Avenir INSERM 2006,
Faculté de Médecine,
Nancy Université,
Avenue de la Forêt de Haye, BP,
Vandoeuvre-lès-Nancy Cedex, France

Caroline Créput
Department of Clinical Immunology,
and Hôpital Saint-Louis,
Medical ICU,
AP–HP,
University Paris-7 Diderot,
UFR de Médecine,
Paris, France

Jacques Creteur
Department of Intensive Care,
Erasme University Hospital,
Free University of Brussels,
Brussels, Belgium

Daniel De Backer
Department of Intensive Care,
Erasme University Hospital,
Free University of Brussels,
Brussels, Belgium

B. L. De Keulenaer
Intensive Care Unit,
Fremantle Hospital,
Alma Street,
Fremantle,
WA, Australia

J. J. De Waele
Intensive Care Unit,
Ghent University Hospital,
Ghent, Belgium

Ioanna Dimopoulou
Second Department of Critical Care Medicine,
Attikon Hospital, Medical School National
and Kapodistrian University of Athens,
Athens, Greece

N. Ducrocq
Groupe Choc,
Contrat Avenir INSERM 2006,
Faculté de Médecine,
Nancy Université,
Avenue de la Forêt de Haye,
BP 184,
Vandoeuvre-lès-Nancy Cedex, France
and
Service de Réanimation Médicale,
Institut du Coeur et des Vaisseaux,
Hôpitaux de Brabois,
CHU de Nancy,
Rue du Morvan,
Vandoeuvre-lès-Nancy, France

Andrew Durward
Evelina Children's Hospital, Guy's and
Saint Thomas' NHS Trust,
Paediatric Intensive Care Unit,
London, UK

M.W. Elliott
St James's University Hospital,
Leeds, UK

Raphaël Favory
Department of Intensive Care,
Erasme University Hospital,
Université Libre de Bruxelles,
Route de Lennik,
Brussels, Belgium

Oliver Flower
National Hospital for Neurology and Neurosurgery,
University College London
Hospitals' NHS Foundation Trust,
Queen Square,
London, UK

Lionel Galicier
Department of Clinical Immunology,
and Hôpital Saint-Louis, Medical ICU, AP–HP,
University Paris-7 Diderot, UFR de Médecine,
Paris, France

Robb W. Glenny
Division of Pulmonary and Critical Care Medicine,
Departments of Medicine
and of Physiology and Biophysics,
University of Washington,
Seattle, USA

Ian S. Grant
Department of Anaesthesia,
University of Edinburgh,
Western General Hospital, Edinburgh,
Scotland, UK

Richard Griffiths
Department of Intensive Care,
Centre Hospitalo-universitaire de Liege,
Domaine du Sart Tilman B35,
Liege, Belgium

B. Guidet
Service de Réanimation Médicale,
Hôpital Saint-Antoine,
AP-HP,
Paris, France
and
Université Pierre et Marie Curie-Paris 6,
UMR S707,
Paris, France
and
Inserm U707,
Paris, France

Göran Hedenstierna
Clinical Physiology, Department of
Medical Sciences, University Hospital,
Uppsala, Sweden

Patrick M. Honore
Intensive Care Unit,
St-Pierre Para-Universitary Hospital,
Ottignies-Louvain-La-Neuve, Belgium

Yumiko Imai
St. Michael's Hospital,
Toronto,
Ontario, Canada

Can Ince
Department of Translational Physiology,
Academic Medical Center Amsterdam,
Amsterdam, The Netherlands

S.M. Jakob
Department of Intensive Care Medicine,
University Hospital Bern,
Bern, Switzerland

François Jardin
Hôpital Ambroise Paré,
Service de Réanimation Médicale,
Boulogne, France

Olivier Joannes-Boyau
Anaesthesia and Intensive Care Department II,
University Hospital of Bordeaux,
University of Bordeaux II,
Pessac, France

Peter Karpati
Department of Anaesthesiology
and Critical Care Medicine,
Hopital Lariboisière,
Paris Cedex, France

Brian P. Kavanagh
Department of Critical Care Medicine,
Hospital for Sick Children,
Toronto,
ON, Canada

A. Kimmoun
Groupe Choc, Contrat Avenir INSERM 2006,
Faculté de Médecine,
Nancy Université,
Avenue de la Forêt de Haye, BP,
Vandoeuvre-lès-Nancy Cedex, France
and
Service de Réanimation Médicale,
Institut du Coeur et des Vaisseaux,
Hôpitaux de Brabois,
CHU de Nancy,
Rue du Morvan,
Vandoeuvre-lès-Nancy, France

Ioanna Korovesi
Department of Critical Care & Pulmonary
Medicine and "M. Simou" Laboratory
Medical School, University of
Athens, Evangelismos Hospital,
Athens, Greece

John G. Laffey
Department of Anaesthesia,
University College Hospital,
Galway and Clinical Sciences Institute,
National University of Ireland, Galway, Ireland

S. Lehoux
Lady Davis Institute for Medical Research,
McGill University,
Montreal, Canada

Xavier Leverve
Laboratoire de Bioenergetique Fondamentale
et Appliquee,
Universite Joseph Fourier,
rue de la piscine,
Grenoble Cedex, France
and
Department of Intensive Care,
Centre Hospitalo-universitaire de Liege,
Domaine du Sart Tilman B35,
Liege, Belgium

B. Levy
Groupe Choc, Contrat Avenir INSERM 2006,
Faculté de Médecine,
Nancy Université,
Avenue de la Forêt de Haye, BP,
Vandoeuvre-lès-Nancy Cedex, France
and
Service de Réanimation Médicale,
Institut du Coeur et des Vaisseaux,
Hôpitaux de Brabois,
CHU de Nancy,
Rue du Morvan,
Vandoeuvre-lès-Nancy, France

Alexandre Lima
Department of Intensive Care, Erasmus MC
University Medical Center Rotterdam,
Rotterdam, The Netherlands

Alexandre Toledo Maciel
Department of Intensive Care,
Erasme University Hospital, Free
University of Brussels,
Brussels, Belgium

Carol S. A. Macmillan
University of Dundee, Department of Anaesthesia,
Ninewells Hospital, Dundee, UK

Manu L. N. G. Malbrain
Medical Intensive Care Unit,
ACZA Campus Stuivenberg,
Antwerpen, Belgium
and
Department of Intensive Care Medicine,
Ziekenhuis Netwerk Antwerpen (ZNA),
Stuivenberg,
Antwerp, Belgium

Paul E. Marik
Department of Critical Care Medicine,
University of Pittsburgh Medical Center,
Pittsburgh, PA, USA

John J. Marini
University of Minnesota,
Department of Medicine,
Regions Hospital,
Pulmonary and Critical Care Medicine,
Jackson St,
Rm 3571, St Paul 55101-2595,
MN, USA
and
University of Minnesota,
Minneapolis/St. Paul, USA

George M. Matuschak
Division of Pulmonary, Critical Care
and Occupational Medicine,
Departments of Internal Medicine and
Pharmacological and Physiological Science
School of Medicine,
Saint Louis University,
Saint Louis, MO, USA

E. Maury
Service de Réanimation Médicale,
Hôpital Saint-Antoine,
AP-HP, Paris, France
and
Université Pierre et Marie Curie-Paris 6,
UMR S707,
Paris, France
and
Inserm U707,
Paris, France

Irene Mavrommati
Department of Critical Care & Pulmonary Medicine and "M. Simou" Laboratory
Medical School, University of Athens, Evangelismos Hospital,
Athens, Greece

Paul McLoughlin
Department of Physiology,
University College Dublin,
Dublin, Ireland

Alexandre Mebazaa
Department of Anaesthesiology and Critical Care Medicine,
Hopital Lariboisière,
Paris Cedex, France

Sangeeta Mehta
Medical-Surgical ICU,
Mount Sinai Hospital,
Toronto,
Ont., Canada

L. Joanne Meyer
Department of Medicine,
St. Joseph's Hospital,
Toronto, Canada

F. Meziani
Laboratoire de Biophotonique et Pharmacologie,
UMR 7213 CNRS,
Faculté de Pharmacie,
Université de Strasbourg,
Illkirch,
Strasbourg, France

Xavier Monnet
Hôpital de Bicêtre, AP-HP,
Service de réanimation médicale,
Le Kremlin-Bicêtre, France
and
Université Paris-Sud, Equipe d'accueil EA 4046,
Faculté de Médecine Paris-Sud,
Le Kremlin-Bicêtre, France

Christian Mueller
University Hospital,
Department of Internal Medicine,
Petersgraben,
Basel, Switzerland

Stefano Nava
Respiratory Intensive Care Unit,
Fondazione S. Maugeri,
IRCCS,
Istituto Scientifico di Pavia,
Via Ferrata,
Pavia, Italia

A. Nitenberg
Service de Physiologie et d'Explorations Fonctionnelles,
CHU Jean Verdier,
Bondy, France

Gérard Nitenberg
Department of Intensive Care,
Centre Hospitalo-universitaire de Liege,
Domaine du Sart Tilman B35,
Liege, Belgium
and
Service de Physiologie
et d'Explorations Fonctionnelles,
CHU Jean Verdier,
Avenue du 14 Juillet,
Bondy, France

Luis J. Noronha
Division of Pulmonary, Critical Care and Occupational Medicine,
Departments of Internal Medicine and Pharmacological and Physiological Science
School of Medicine,
Saint Louis University,
Saint Louis, MO, USA

Donall O'Croinin
Department of Physiology,
University College Dublin
Dublin, Ireland

G. Offenstadt
Service de Réanimation Médicale,
Hôpital Saint-Antoine,
AP-HP, Paris, France
and
Université Pierre et Marie Curie-Paris 6,
UMR S707,
Paris, France
and
Inserm U707,
Paris, France

Stylianos E. Orfanos
2nd Department of Critical Care,
University of Athens Medical
School, Attikon Hospital,
Haidari (Athens), Greece

Gustavo Ospina-Tascon
Department of Intensive Care,
Erasme University Hospital,
Université Libre de Bruxelles,
Route de Lennik 808,
Brussels, Belgium

Sairam Parthasarathy
Division of Pulmonary and Critical
Care, Medicine Edward Hines Jr.
Veterans Administrative Hospital, Loyola
University of Chicago Stritch School of Medicine,
Hines, IL, USA

P. Perez
Groupe Choc, Contrat Avenir INSERM 2006,
Faculté de Médecine,
Nancy Université,
Avenue de la Forêt de Haye, BP,
Vandoeuvre-lès-Nancy
Cedex, France

Marek Pertkiewicz
Department of Intensive Care,
Centre Hospitalo-universitaire de Liege,
Domaine du Sart Tilman B35,
Liege, Belgium

Michael Piagnerelli
Department of intensive care,
Erasme University Hospital,
Free University of Brussels,
Brussels, Belgium

Claude Pichard
Department of Intensive Care,
Centre Hospitalo-universitaire de Liege,
Domaine du Sart Tilman B35,
Liege, Belgium

Michael R. Pinsky
Department of Critical Care Medicine,
University of Pittsburgh Medical Center,
Pittsburgh, PA, USA

B. Powell
Intensive Care Unit,
Fremantle Hospital,
Alma Street,
Fremantle,
WA, Australia

Jean-Charles Preiser
Department of Intensive Care,
Centre Hospitalo-universitaire de Liege,
Domaine du Sart Tilman B35,
Liege, Belgium

Peter Radermacher
Sektion Anästhesiologische Pathophysiologie
und Verfahrensentwicklung Universitätsklinik
für Anästhesiologie, Universität Ulm,
Ulm, Germany
and
Laboratoire de Bioenergetique
Fondamentale et Appliquee,
Universite Joseph Fourier,
rue de la piscine,
Grenoble Cedex, France

Murugan Raghavan
Conemaugh Memorial Medical Center,
Johnstown, PA, USA

V. Marco Ranieri
Dipartimento di Anestesia e Rianimazione,
Ospedale S. Giovanni Battista-Molinette,
Universita di Torino,
Corso Dogliotti,
Turin, Italy

Estelle Renaud
Department of Anaesthesiology
and Critical Care Medicine,
Hopital Lariboisière,
Paris Cedex 10, France

Christian Richard
Reanimation medicale,
Hopital de Bicetre,
AP-HP, Universite Paris XI,
Paris, France

Jacques-André Romand
Surgical Intensive Care Division,
Geneva University Hospitals,
Geneva, Switzerland

Erich Roth
Department of Intensive Care,
Centre Hospitalo-universitaire de Liege,
Domaine du Sart Tilman B35,
Liege, Belgium

Charis Roussos
Department of Critical Care & Pulmonary
Medicine and "M. Simou" Laboratory
Medical School, University of
Athens, Evangelismos Hospital,
Ipsilandou St., Athens, Greece

Diamantino Salgado
Department of Intensive Care,
Erasme University Hospital,
Université Libre de Bruxelles,
Route de Lennik,
Brussels, Belgium

N. Sennoun
Groupe Choc, Contrat Avenir INSERM 2006,
Faculté de Médecine,
Nancy Université,
Avenue de la Forét de Haye, BP,
Vandoeuvre-lès-Nancy Cedex, France

Pratik Sinha
Magill Department of Anaesthesia,
Intensive Care Medicine and Pain Management,
Chelsea and Westminster NHS Foundation Trust,
Imperial College London,
London, UK

Arthur S. Slutsky
Queen Wing, St. Michael's Hospital,
Toronto, ON, Canada

Neil Soni
Magill Department of Anaesthesia,
Intensive Care Medicine and Pain Management,
Chelsea and Westminster NHS Foundation Trust,
Imperial College London,
London, UK

Pierre Squara
CERIC Clinique Ambroise Pare,
Neuilly-sur-Seine, France

Jukka Takala
Department of Intensive Care Medicine,
University Hospital Bern (Inselspital),
University of Bern, Bern, Switzerland

Jean-Louis Teboul
Hôpital de Bicêtre, AP-HP,
Service de réanimation médicale,
Kremlin-Bicêtre, France
and
Université Paris-Sud, Equipe d'accueil EA 4046,
Faculté de Médecine Paris-Sud,
Le Kremlin-Bicêtre, France
and
Reanimation medicale,
Hopital de Bicetre,
AP-HP, Université Paris XI,
Paris, France
and
Service de réanimation médicale,
CHU de Bicêtre,
Le Kremlin-Bicêtre
Cedex, France

Pierpaolo Terragni
Dipartimento di Anestesia e Rianimazione,
Ospedale S. Giovanni Battista-Molinette,
Universita di Torino,
Corso Dogliotti,
Turin, Italy

Shane M. Tibby
Paediatric Intensive Care Unit,
Evelina Children's Hospital,
Guy's and Saint Thomas' NHS Trust,
London, UK

Martin J. Tobin
Division of Pulmonary and Critical Care Medicine,
Edward Hines Jr. VA Hospital,
Hines, IL, USA

Karl Träger
Sektion Anasthesiologische Pathophysiologie
und Verfahrensentwicklung,
Universitätsklinik für Anasthesiologie,
Universität Ulm,
Parkstrasse,
Ulm, Germany

Stylianos Tsagarakis
Department of Endocrinology,
Athens Polyclinic,
Athens, Greece

Michel Vanhaeverbeek
Experimental Medicine Laboratory,
André Vésale Hospital,
Montigny-le-Tilleul, Belgium

Peter Varga
Department of Intensive Care,
Centre Hospitalo-universitaire de Liege,
Domaine du Sart Tilman B35,
Liege, Belgium

Theodoros Vassilakopoulos
Department of Critical Care and Pulmonary Services,
University of Athens Medical School,
Evangelismos Hospital,
Athens, Greece

Antoine Vieillard-Baron
Intensive Care Unit,
Assistance Publique des Hôpitaux de Paris,
University Hospital Ambroise Paré,
Avenue Charles-de-Gaulle,
Boulogne, France
and
Faculté de Paris Ile-de-France Ouest,
Université de Versailles Saint Quentin en Yvelines,
Versailles, France

Philippe Vignon
Medical-surgical Intensive Care Unit,
Dupuytren Teaching Hospital,
Avenue Martin Luther King,
Limoges, France

Jean-Louis Vincent
Department of Intensive Care,
Erasme University Hospital,
Université Libre de Bruxelles,
Route de Lennik,
Brussels, Belgium

Jan Wernerman
Department of Intensive Care,
Centre Hospitalo-universitaire de Liege,
Domaine du Sart Tilman B35,
Liege, Belgium

Karim Zouaoui-Boudjeltia
Experimental Medicine Laboratory,
André Vésale Hospital,
Montigny-le-Tilleul, Belgium

Physiological Reviews 1

1.1. Measurement Techniques

1.2. Physiological Processes

Karim Bendjelid
Jacques-A. Romand

Fluid responsiveness in mechanically ventilated patients: a review of indices used in intensive care

Abstract *Objective:* In mechanically ventilated patients the indices which assess preload are used with increasing frequency to predict the hemodynamic response to volume expansion. We discuss the clinical utility and accuracy of some indices which were tested as bedside indicators of preload reserve and fluid responsiveness in hypotensive patients under positive pressure ventilation. *Results and conclusions:* Although preload assessment can be obtained with fair accuracy, the clinical utility of volume responsiveness-guided fluid therapy still needs to be demonstrated. Indeed, it is still not clear whether any form of monitoring-guided fluid therapy improves survival.

Keywords Positive pressure ventilation · Hypotension · Volume expansion · Cardiac index

Prediction is very difficult, especially about the future.

Niels Bohr

Introduction

Hypotension is one of the most frequent clinical signs observed in critically ill patients. To restore normal blood pressure, the cardiovascular filling (preload-defined as end-diastolic volume of both ventricular chambers), cardiac function (inotropism), and vascular resistance (afterload) must be assessed. Hemodynamic instability secondary to effective or relative intravascular volume depletion are very common, and intravascular fluid resuscitation or volume expansion (VE) allows restoration of ventricular filling, cardiac output and ultimately arterial blood pressure [1, 2]. However, in the Frank-Starling curve (stroke volume as a function of preload) the slope presents on its early phase a steep portion which is followed by a plateau (Fig. 1). As a consequence, when the plateau is reached, vigorous fluid resuscitation carries out the risk of generating volume overload and pulmonary edema and/or right-ventricular dysfunction. Thus in hypotensive patients methods able to unmask decreased preload and to predict whether cardiac output will increase or not with VE have been sought after for many years. Presently, as few methods are able to assess ventricular volumes continuously and directly, static pressure measurements and echocardiographically measured ventricular end-diastolic areas are used as tools to monitor cardiovascular filling. Replacing static measurements, dynamic monitoring consisting in assessment of fluid responsiveness using changes in systolic arterial pressure, and pulse pressure induced by positive pressure ventilation have been proposed. The present review analyses the current roles and limitations of the most frequently used methods in clinical practice to predict fluid responsiveness in patients undergoing mechanical ventilation (MV) (Table 1).

One method routinely used to evaluate intravascular volume in hypotensive patients uses hemodynamic response to a fluid challenge [3]. This method consists in infusing a defined amount of fluid over a brief period of time. The response to the intravascular volume loading can be monitored clinically by heart rate, blood pressure, pulse pressure (systolic minus diastolic blood pressure), and urine output or by invasive monitoring with the measurements of the right atrial pressure (RAP), pulmonary artery occlusion pressure (Ppao), and cardiac output. Such a fluid management protocol assumes that the in-

M.R. Pinsky et al. (eds.), *Applied Physiology in Intensive Care Medicine 2: Physiological Reviews and Editorials*,
DOI 10.1007/978-3-642-28233-1_1, © Springer-Verlag Berlin Heidelberg 2012

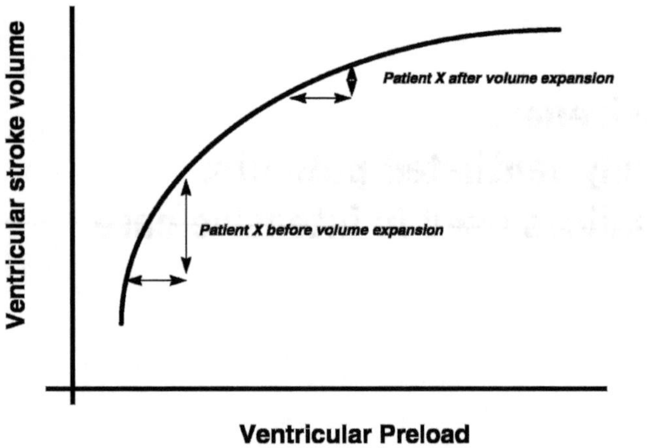

Fig. 1 Representation of Frank-Starling curve with relationship between ventricular preload and ventricular stroke volume in patient X. After volume expansion the same magnitude of change in preload recruit less stroke volume, because the plateau of the curve is reached which characterize a condition of preload independency

travascular volume of the critically ill patients can be defined by the relationship between preload and cardiac output, and that changing preload with volume infusion affects cardiac output. Thus an increase in cardiac output following VE (patient responder) unmasks an hypovolemic state or preload dependency. On the other hand, lack of change or a decrease in cardiac output following VE (nonresponding patient) is attributed to a normovolemic, to an overloaded, or to cardiac failure state. Therefore, as the fluid responsiveness defines the response of cardiac output to volume challenge, indices which can predict the latter are necessary.

Static measurements for preload assessment

Measures of intracardiac pressures

According to the Frank-Starling law, left-ventricular preload is defined as the myocardial fiber length at the end

Table 1 Studies of indices used as bedside indicators of preload reserve and fluid responsiveness in hypotensive patients under positive-pressure ventilation (*BMI* body mass index, *CO* cardiac output, *CI* cardiac index, *SV* stroke volume, *SVI* stroke volume index, *IAC* invasive arterial catheter, *MV* proportion of patients mechanically ventilated, ↑ increase, ↓ decrease, *PAC* pulmonary artery catheter, *R* responders, *NR* nonresponders, *FC* fluid challenge, *HES* hydroxyethyl starch, *RL* Ringer's lactate, *Alb* albumin, *Δdown* delta down, *ΔPP* respiratory variation in pulse pressure, *LVEDV* left-ventricular end diastolic volume, *SPV* systolic pressure variation, *SVV* stroke volume variation, *TEE* transesophageal echocardiography, *Ppao* pulmonary artery occlusion pressure, *RAP* right atrial pressure, *RVEDV* right-ventricular-end diastolic volume, *FC* fluid challenge)

Variable measured	Technique	*n*	MV (%)	Volume (ml) and type of plasma substitute	Duration of FC (min)	Definition of R	Definition of NR	*p*: difference in baseline values R vs. NR	Reference
Rap	PAC	28	46	250 Alb 5%	20–30	↑ SVI	↓ SVI or unchanged	NS	37
Rap	PAC	41	76	300 Alb 4.5%	30	↑ CI	CI ↓ or unchanged	NS	18
Rap	PAC	25	94.4	NaCl 9‰ + Alb 5% to ↑ Ppao	Until ↑Ppao	↑ SV ≥10%	↑ SV <10%	0.04	31
Rap	PAC	40	100	500 HES 6%	30	↑ CI >15%	↑ CI <15%	NS	36
Ppao	PAC	28	46	250 Alb 5%	20–30	↑ SVI	↓ SVI or unchanged	NS	37
Ppao	PAC	41	76	300 Alb 4.5%	30	↑ CI	CI ↓ or unchanged	NS	18
Ppao	PAC	29	69	300–500 RL	? bolus	↑ CO>10%	CO ↓ or unchanged	<0.01	40
Ppao	PAC	32	84	300–500 RL	?	↑ CI >20%	↑ CI <20%	NS	41
Ppao	PAC	16	100	500 HES 6%	30	↑ CI >15%	↑ CI <15%	0.1	42
Ppao	PAC	41	100	500 pPentastarch	15	↑ SV ≥20%	↑ SV <20%	0.003	25
Ppao	PAC	25	94.4	NaCl 9‰, Alb 5% to ↑ Ppao	Until ↑Ppao	↑ SV ≥10%	↑ SV <10%	0.001	31
Ppao	PAC	40	100	500 HES 6%	30	↑ CI >15%	↑ CI <15%	NS	36
Ppao	PAC	19	100	500–750 HES 6%	10	↑ CO>10%	↑ SV <10%	0.0085	39
RVEDV	PAC	29	69	300–500 RL	? bolus	↑ CO>10%	CO ↓ or unchanged	<0.001	40
RVEDV	PAC	32	84	300–500 RL	?	↑ CI >20%	↑ CI <20%	<0.002	41
RVEDV	PAC	25	94.4	NaCl 9‰, Alb 5% to ↑ Ppao	Until ↑Ppao	↑ SV ≥10%	↑ SV <10%	0.22	31
LVEDV	TEE	16	100	500 HES 6%	30	↑ CI >15%	↑ CI <15%	0.005	42
LVEDV	TEE	41	100	500 Pentastarch	15	↑ SV ≥20%	↑ SV <20%	0.012	25
LVEDV	TEE	19	100	8 ml/kg HES 6%	30	↑ CI >15%	↑ CI <15%	NS	79
LVEDV	TEE	19	100	500–750 HES 6%	10	↑ CO>10%	↑ SV <10%	NS	39
SPV	IAC	16	100	500 HES 6%	30	↑ CI >15%	↑ CI <15%	0.0001	42
SPV	IAC	40	100	500 HES 6%	30	↑ CI >15%	↑ CI <15%	<0.001	36
SPV	IAC	19	100	500–750 HES 6%	10	↑ CO>10%	↑ SV <10%	0.017	39
Δdown	IAC	16	100	500 HES 6%	30	↑ CI >15%	↑ CI <15%	0.0001	42
Δdown	IAC	19	100	500–750 HES 6%	10	↑ CO>10%	↑ SV <10%	0.025	39
ΔPP	IAC	40	100	500 HES 6%	30	↑ CI >15%	↑ CI <15%	<0.001	36

of the diastole. In clinical practice, the left-ventricular end-diastolic volume is used as a surrogate to define left-ventricular preload [4]. However, this volumetric parameter is not easily assessed in critically ill patients. In normal conditions, a fairly good correlation exists between ventricular end-diastolic volumes and mean atrial pressures, and ventricular preloads are approximated by RAP and/or Ppao in patients breathing spontaneously [5, 6]. Critically ill patients often require positive pressure ventilation, which modifies the pressure regimen in the thorax in comparison to spontaneous breathing. Indeed, during MV RAP and Ppao rise secondary to an increase in intrathoracic pressure which rises pericardial pressure. This pressure increase induces a decrease in venous return [7, 8] with first a decrease in right and few heart beats later in left-ventricular end-diastolic volumes, respectively [9, 10]. Under extreme conditions such as acute severe pulmonary emboli and/or marked hyperinflation, RAP may also rise secondary to an increase afterload of the right ventricle. Moreover, under positive pressure ventilation not only ventricular but also thoracopulmonary compliances and abdominal pressure variations are observed over time. Thus a variable relationship between cardiac pressures and cardiac volumes is often observed [11, 12, 13, 14]. It has also been demonstrated that changes in intracardiac pressure (RAP, Ppao) no longer directly reflect changes in intravascular volume [15]. Pinsky et al. [16, 17] have demonstrated that changes in RAP do not follow changes in right ventricular end-diastolic volume in postoperative cardiac surgery patients under positive pressure ventilation. Reuse et al. [18] observed no correlation between RAP and right-ventricular end-diastolic volume calculated from a thermodilution technique in hypovolemic patients before and after fluid resuscitation. The discordance between RAP and right-ventricular end-diastolic volume measurements may result from a systematic underestimation of the effect of positive-pressure ventilation on the right heart [16, 17]. Nevertheless, the RAP value measured either with a central venous catheter or a pulmonary artery catheter is still used to estimate preload and to guide intravascular volume therapy in patient under positive pressure ventilation [19, 20].

On the left side, the MV-induced intrathoracic pressure changes, compared to spontaneously breathing, only minimally alters the relationship between left atrial pressure and left-ventricular end-diastolic volume measurement in postoperative cardiac surgery patients [21]. However, several other studies show no relationship between Ppao and left-ventricular end-diastolic volume measured by either radionuclide angiography [12, 22], transthoracic echocardiography (TTE) [23], or transesophageal echocardiography (TEE) [24, 25, 26]. The latter findings may be related to the indirect pulmonary artery catheter method for assessing left atrial pressure [27, 28], although several studies have demonstrated that Ppao using PAC is a reliable indirect measurement of left atrial pressure [29, 30] in positive-pressure MV patients.

Right atrial pressure used to predict fluid responsiveness

Wagner et al. [31] reported that RAP was significantly lower before volume challenge in responders than in nonresponders (p=0.04) when patients were under positive pressure ventilation. Jellinek et al. [32] found that a RAP lower than 10 mmHg predicts a decrease in cardiac index higher than 20% when a transient 30 cm H_2O increase in intrathoracic pressure is administrated. Presuming that the principle cause of decrease in cardiac output in the latter study was due to a reduction in venous return [9, 33, 34, 35], RAP predicts reverse VE hemodynamic effect. Nevertheless, some clinical investigations studying fluid responsiveness in MV patients have reported that RAP poorly predicts increased cardiac output after volume expansion [18, 36, 37]. Indeed, in these studies RAP did not differentiate patients whose cardiac output did or did not increase after VE (responders and nonresponders, respectively).

Ppao used to predict fluid responsiveness

Some studies have demonstrated that Ppao is a good predictor of fluid responsiveness [13, 31, 38]. Recently Bennett-Guerrero et al. [39] also found that Ppao was a better predictor of response to VE than systolic pressure variation (SPV) and left-ventricular end-diastolic area measured by TEE. However, several other studies noted that Ppao is unable to predict fluid responsiveness and to differentiate between VE-responders and VE-nonresponders [18, 25, 36, 37, 40, 41, 42]. The discrepancy between the results of these studies may partly reflect differences in patients' baseline characteristics (e.g., demographic differences, medical history, chest and lung compliances) at study entry. Furthermore, differences in location of the pulmonary artery catheter extremity relative to the left atrium may be present [43]. Indeed, according to its position, pulmonary artery catheter may display alveolar pressure instead of left atrial pressure (West zone I or II) [44]. The value of Ppao is also influenced by juxtacardiac pressure [45, 46] particularly if positive end-expiratory pressure (PEEP) is used [28]. To overcome the latter difficulty in MV patients when PEEP is used, nadir Ppao (Ppao measured after airway disconnection) may be used [46]. However, as nadir Ppao requires temporary disconnection from the ventilator, it might be deleterious to severely hypoxemic patients. No study has yet evaluated the predictive value of nadir Ppao for estimating fluid responsiveness in MV patients.

In brief, although static intracardiac pressure measurements such as RAP and Ppao have been studied and used for many years for hemodynamic monitoring, their low predictive value in estimating fluid responsiveness in MV patients must be underlined. Thus using only intravascular static pressures to guide fluid therapy can lead to inappropriate therapeutic decisions [47].

Measures of ventricular end-diastolic volumes

Radionuclide angiography [48], cineangiocardiography [49], and thermodilution [50] have been used to estimate ventricular volumes for one-half a century. In intensive care units, various methods have been used to measure ventricular end-diastolic volume at the bedside, such as radionuclide angiography [51, 52], TTE [23, 53, 54], TEE [55], and a modified flow-directed pulmonary artery catheter which allows the measurement of cardiac output and right-ventricular ejection fraction (and the calculation of right-ventricular end-systolic and end-diastolic volume) [31, 41].

Right-ventricular end-diastolic volume measured by pulmonary artery catheter used to predict fluid responsiveness

During MV right-ventricular end-diastolic volume measured with a pulmonary artery catheter is decreased by PEEP [56] but is still well correlated with cardiac index [57, 58] and is a more reliable predictor of fluid responsiveness than Ppao [40, 41]. On the other hand, other studies have found no relationship between change in right-ventricular end-diastolic volume measured by pulmonary artery catheter and change in stroke volume in two series of cardiac surgery patients [16, 18]. Similarly, Wagner et al. [31] found that right-ventricular end-diastolic volume measured by pulmonary artery catheter was not a reliable predictor of fluid responsiveness in patients under MV, and that Ppao and RAP were superior to right-ventricular end-diastolic volume. The discrepancy between the results of these studies may partly reflect the measurement errors of cardiac output due to the cyclic change induced by positive pressure ventilation [59, 60, 61, 62], the inaccuracy of cardiac output measurement obtained by pulmonary artery catheter when the flux is low [63], and the influence of tricuspid regurgitation on the measurement of cardiac output [64]. Moreover, as right-ventricular end-diastolic volume is calculated (stroke volume divided by right ejection fraction), cardiac output becomes a shared variable in the calculation of both stroke volume and right-ventricular end-diastolic volume, and a mathematical coupling may have contributed to the close correlation observed between these two variables. Nevertheless, right-ventricular end-diastolic volume compared to Ppao may be useful in a small group of patients with high intra-abdominal pressure or when clinicians are reluctant to obtain off-PEEP nadir Ppao measurements [65].

Right-ventricular end-diastolic volume measured by echocardiography used to predict fluid responsiveness

TTE has been shown to be a reliable method to assess right-ventricular dimensions in patients ventilated with continuous positive airway pressure or positive-pressure ventilation [66, 67]. Using this approach, right-ventricular end-diastolic area is obtained on the apical four chambers view [68]. When no right-ventricular window is available, TEE is preferred to monitor right-ventricular end-volume in MV patients [53, 55, 69, 70, 71]. The latter method has become more popular in recent years due to technical improvements [72]. Nevertheless, no study has evaluated right-ventricular size measurements by TTE or TEE as a predictor of fluid responsiveness in MV patients.

Left-ventricular end-diastolic volume measured by echocardiography used to predict fluid responsiveness

TTE has been used in the past to measure left-ventricular end-diastolic volume and/or area [23, 67, 73, 74] in MV patients. However, no study has evaluated the left-ventricular end-diastolic volume and/or area measured by TTE as predictors of fluid responsiveness in MV patients. Due to its greater resolving power, TEE easily and accurately assesses left-ventricular end-diastolic volume and/or area in clinical practice [53, 75] except in patients undergoing coronary artery bypass grafting [76]. However, different studies have reported conflicting results about the usefulness of left-ventricular end-diastolic volume and/or area measured by TEE to predict fluid responsiveness in MV patients. Cheung et al. [26] have shown that left-ventricular end-diastolic area measured by TEE is an accurate method to predict the hemodynamic effects of acute blood loss. Other studies have reported either a modest [25, 42, 77] or a poor [78, 79] predictive value of left-ventricular end-diastolic volume and area to predict the cardiac output response to fluid loading. Recent studies have also produced conflicting results. Bennett-Guerrero et al. [39] measuring left-ventricular end-diastolic area with TEE before VE found no significant difference between responders and nonresponders. Paradoxically, Reuter et al. [80] found that left-ventricular end-diastolic area index assessed by TEE before VE predicts fluid responsiveness more accurately than RAP, Ppao, and stroke volume variation (SVV). In the future three-dimensional echocardiography could supplant other methods for measuring left-ventricular end-diastolic volume and their predictive value of fluid responsiveness. In a word, although measurements of ventricular volumes should theoretically reflect preload dependence more accurately than other indices, conflicting results have been reported so far. These negative findings may be related to the method used to estimate end-diastolic ventricular volumes which do not reflect the geometric complexity of the right ventricle and to the influences of the positive intrathoracic pressure on left-ventricular preload, afterload and myocardial contractility [81].

Dynamic measurements for preload assessment

Measure of respiratory changes in systolic pressure, pulse pressure, and stroke volume

Positive pressure breath decreases temporary right-ventricular end-diastolic volume secondary to a reduction in venous return [7, 82]. A decrease in right-ventricular stroke volume ensues which become minimal at end positive pressure breath. This inspiratory reduction in right-ventricular stroke volume induces a decrease in left-ventricular end-diastolic volume after a phase lag of few heart beats (due to the pulmonary vascular transit time [83]), which becomes evident during the expiratory phase. This expiratory reduction in left-ventricular end-diastolic volume induces a decrease in left-ventricular stroke volume, determining the minimal value of systolic blood pressure observed during expiration. Conversely, the inspiratory increase in left-ventricular end-diastolic volume determining the maximal value of systolic blood pressure is observed secondary to the rise in left-ventricular preload reflecting the few heart beats earlier increased in right-ventricular preload during expiration. Furthermore, increasing lung volume during positive pressure ventilation may also contribute to the increased pulmonary venous blood flow (related to the compression of pulmonary blood vessels [84]) and/or to a decrease in left-ventricular afterload [85, 86, 87], which together induce an increase in left-ventricular preload. Finally, a decrease in right-ventricular end-diastolic volume during a positive pressure breath may increase left-ventricular compliance and then left-ventricular preload [88]. Thus due to heart-lung interaction during positive pressure ventilation the left-ventricular stroke volume varies cyclically (maximal during inspiration and minimal during expiration).

These variations have been used clinically to assess preload status and predict fluid responsiveness in deeply sedated patients under positive pressure ventilation. In 1983 Coyle et al. [89] in a preliminary study demonstrated that the SPV following one mechanical breath is increased in hypovolemic sedated patients and decreased after fluid resuscitation. This study defined SPV as the difference between maximal and minimal values of systolic blood pressure during one positive pressure mechanical breath. Using the systolic pressure at end expiration as a reference point or baseline the SPV was further divided into two components: an increase (Δup) and a decrease (Δdown) in systolic pressure vs. baseline (Fig. 2). These authors concluded that in hypovolemic patients Δdown was the main component of SPV. These preliminary conclusions were confirmed in 1987 by Perel et al. [90] who demonstrated that SPV following a positive pressure breath is a sensitive indicator of hypovolemia in ventilated dogs. Thereafter Coriat et al. [91] demonstrated that SPV and Δdown predict the response of cardiac index to VE in a group of sedated MV patients after vascular surgery. Exploring another pathophysiological concept, Jardin et al. [92] found that pulse pressure (PP; defined as the difference between the systolic and the diastolic pressure) is related to left-ventricular stroke volume in MV patients. Using these findings, Michard et al. [35, 36,] have shown that respiratory changes in PP [ΔPP=maximal PP at inspiration (PPmax) minus minimal PP at expiration (PPmin); (Fig. 2) and calculated as: ΔPP (%)=100 (PPmax-PPmin)/(Ppmax+PPmin)/2] predict the effect of VE on cardiac index in patients with acute lung injury [35] or septic shock [36]. The same team proposed another approach to assess SVV in MV patients and to predict cardiac responsiveness to VE [79]. Using Doppler measurement of beat-to-beat aortic blood flow, they found that respiratory change in aortic blood flow maximal velocity predicts fluid responsiveness in septic MV patients. Measuring SVV during positive pressure ventilation by continuous arterial pulse contour analysis, Reuter et al. [80] have recently demonstrated that SVV accurately predicts fluid responsiveness following volume infusion in ventilated patients after cardiac surgery.

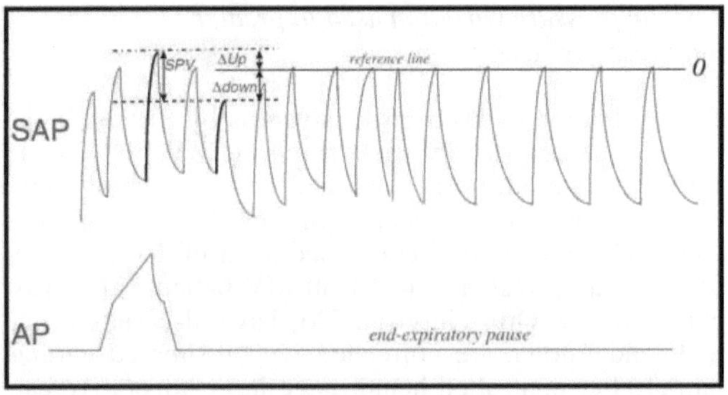

Fig. 2 Systolic pressure variation (*SPV*) after one mechanical breath followed by an end-expiratory pause. Reference line permits the measurement of Δup and Δdown. *Bold* Maximal and minimal pulse pressure. *AP* Airway pressure; *SAP* systolic arterial pressure

Systolic pressure variation used to predict fluid responsiveness

The evaluation of fluid responsiveness by SPV is based on cardiopulmonary interaction during MV [93, 94]. In 1995 Rooke et al. [95] found that SPV is a useful monitor of volume status in healthy MV patients during anesthesia. Coriat et al. [91] confirmed the usefulness of SPV for estimating response to VE in MV patients after vascular surgery. Ornstein et al. [96] have also shown that SPV and Δdown are correlated with decreased cardiac output after controlled hemorrhage in postoperative cardiac surgical patients. Furthermore, Tavernier et al. [42] found Δdown before VE to be an accurate index of the fluid responsiveness in septic patients, and that a Δdown value of 5 mmHg is the cutoff point for distinguishing responders from nonresponders to VE. Finally, in septic patients Michard et al. [36] found that SPV is correlated with volume expansion-induced change in cardiac output. However, Denault et al. [81] have demonstrated that SPV is not correlated with changes in left-ventricular end-diastolic volume measured by TEE in cardiac surgery patients. Indeed, in this study, SPV was observed despite no variation in left-ventricular stroke volume, suggesting that SPV involves processes independent of changes in the left-ventricular preload (airway pressure, pleural pressure, and its resultant afterload) [81].

Pulse pressure variation used to predict fluid responsiveness

Extending the concept elaborated by Jardin et al. [92], Michard et al. [36] found that ΔPP predicted the effect of VE on cardiac output in 40 septic shock hypotensive patients. These authors demonstrated that both ΔPP and SPV, when greater than 15%, are superior to RAP and Ppao, for predicting fluid responsiveness. Moreover, ΔPP was more accurate and with less bias than SPV. These authors proposed ΔPP as a surrogate for stroke volume variation concept [93], which has not been validated yet. In another study these authors [35] included VE in six MV patients with acute lung injury and found that ΔPP is a useful guide to predict fluid responsiveness.

Stroke volume variation to predict fluid responsiveness

Using Doppler TEE, Feissel et al. [79] studied changes in left-ventricular stroke volume induced by the cyclic positive pressure breathing. By measuring the respiratory variation in maximal aortic blood flow velocity these authors predicted fluid responsiveness in septic MV patients. Left-ventricular stroke volume was obtained by multiplying flow velocity time integral over aortic valve by valve opening area during expiration. However, this finding may be biased, as expiratory flow velocity time integral is a shared variable in the calculation of both cardiac output and expiratory maximal aortic blood flow velocity and a mathematical coupling may contribute to the observed correlation between changes in cardiac output and variation in maximal aortic blood flow velocity. Finally, Reuter et al. [80] used continuous arterial pulse contour analysis and found that SVV during positive pressure breath accurately predicts fluid responsiveness following VE in ventilated cardiac surgery patients [80]. Using the receiver operating characteristics curve, these authors demonstrated that the area under the curve is statistically greater for SVV (0.82; confidence interval: 0.64–1) and SPV (0.81; confidence interval: 0.62–1) than for RAP (0.45; confidence interval: 0.17–0.74) ($p<0.001$) [97]. Concisely, dynamic indices have been explored to evaluate fluid responsiveness in critically ill patients. All of them have been validated in deeply sedated patients under positive-pressure MV. Thus such indices are useless in spontaneously breathing intubated patients, a MV mode often used in ICU. Moreover, regular cardiac rhythm is an obligatory condition to allow their use.

Conclusion

Positive pressure ventilation cyclically increases intrathoracic pressure and lung volume, both of which decrease venous return and alter stroke volume. Thus VE which rapidly restore cardiac output and arterial blood pressure is an often used therapy in hypotensive MV patients and indices which would predict fluid responsiveness are necessary. RAP, Ppao, and right-ventricular end-diastolic volume, which are static measurements, have been studied but produced conflicting data in estimating preload and fluid responsiveness. On the other hand, SPV and ΔPP, which are dynamic measurements, have been shown to identify hypotension related to decrease in preload, to distinguish between responders and nonresponders to fluid challenge (Table 1), and to permit titration of VE in various patient populations.

Although there is substantial literature on indices of hypovolemia, only few studies have evaluated the cardiac output changes induced by VE in MV patients. Moreover, therapeutic recommendations regarding unmasked preload dependency states without hypotension need further studies. Finally, another unanswered question is related to patients outcome: does therapy guided by fluid responsiveness indices improve patients survival?

Acknowledgements The authors thank Dr. M.R. Pinsky, University of Pittsburgh Medical Center, for his helpful advice in the preparation of this manuscript. The authors are also grateful for the translation support provided by Angela Frei.

References

1. Guyton AC, Richardson TQ, Langston JB (1964) Regulation of cardiac output and venous return. Clin Anesth 3:1–34
2. Guyton AC (1967) Regulation of cardiac output. N Engl J Med 277:805–812
3. Horst HM, Obeid FN (1986) Hemodynamic response to fluid challenge: a means of assessing volume status in the critically ill. Henry Ford Hosp Med J 34:90–94
4. Suga H, Sagawa K (1974) Instantaneous pressure-volume relationships and their ratio in the excised, supported canine left ventricle. Circ Res 35:117–126
5. Crexells C, Chatterjee K, Forrester JS, Dikshit K, Swan HJ (1973) Optimal level of filling pressure in the left side of the heart in acute myocardial infarction. N Engl J Med 289:1263–1266
6. Buchbinder N, Ganz W (1976) Hemodynamic monitoring: invasive techniques. Anesthesiology 45:146–155
7. Cournand A, Motley H, Werko L, Richards D (1948) Physiological studies of the effect of intermittent positive pressure breathing on cardiac output in man. Am J Physiol 152:162–174
8. Fessler HE, Brower RG, Wise RA, Permutt S (1992) Effects of positive end-expiratory pressure on the canine venous return curve. Am Rev Respir Dis 146:4–10
9. Potkin RT, Hudson LD, Weaver LJ, Trobaugh G (1987) Effect of positive end-expiratory pressure on right and left ventricular function in patients with the adult respiratory distress syndrome. Am Rev Respir Dis 135:307–311
10. Fewell JE, Abendschein DR, Carlson CJ, Murray JF, Rapaport E (1980) Continuous positive-pressure ventilation decreases right and left ventricular end-diastolic volumes in the dog. Circ Res 46:125–132
11. McKenney PA, Apstein CS, Mendes LA, Connelly GP, Aldea GS, Shemin RJ, Davidoff R (1994) Increased left ventricular diastolic chamber stiffness immediately after coronary artery bypass surgery. J Am Coll Cardiol 24:1189–1194
12. Calvin JE, Driedger AA, Sibbald WJ (1981) Does the pulmonary capillary wedge pressure predict left ventricular preload in critically ill patients? Crit Care Med 9:437–443
13. Packman MI, Rackow EC (1983) Optimum left heart filling pressure during fluid resuscitation of patients with hypovolemic and septic shock. Crit Care Med 11:165–169
14. Jardin F, Gueret P, Dubourg O, Farcot JC, Margairaz A, Bourdarias JP (1985) Right ventricular volumes by thermodilution in the adult respiratory distress syndrome. A comparative study using two-dimensional echocardiography as a reference method. Chest 88:34–39
15. Lichtwarck-Aschoff M, Zeravik J, Pfeiffer UJ (1992) Intrathoracic blood volume accurately reflects circulatory volume status in critically ill patients with mechanical ventilation. Intensive Care Med 18:142–147
16. Pinsky MR, Desmet JM, Vincent JL (1992) Effect of positive end-expiratory pressure on right ventricular function in humans. Am Rev Respir Dis 146:681–687
17. Pinsky MR (1994) Cardiovascular effects of ventilatory support and withdrawal. Anesth Analg 79:567–576
18. Reuse C, Vincent JL, Pinsky MR (1990) Measurements of right ventricular volumes during fluid challenge. Chest 98:1450–1454
19. Saarela E, Kari A, Nikki P, Rauhala V, Iisalo E, Kaukinen L (1991) Current practice regarding invasive monitoring in intensive care units in Finland. A nationwide study of the uses of arterial, pulmonary artery and central venous catheters and their effect on outcome. The Finnish Intensive Care Study Group. Intensive Care Med 17:264–271
20. Boldt J, Lenz M, Kumle B, Papsdorf M (1998) Volume replacement strategies on intensive care units: results from a postal survey. Intensive Care Med 24:147–151
21. Guyton RA, Chiavarelli M, Padgett CA, Cheung EH, Staton GW, Hatcher CR (1987) The influence of positive end-expiratory pressure on intrapericardial pressure and cardiac function after coronary artery bypass surgery. J Cardiothorac Anesth 1:98–107
22. Lemaire F, Teboul JL, Cinotti L, Giotto G, Abrouk F, Steg G, Macquin-Mavier I, Zapol WM (1988) Acute left ventricular dysfunction during unsuccessful weaning from mechanical ventilation. Anesthesiology 69:171–179
23. Jardin F, Valtier B, Beauchet A, Dubourg O, Bourdarias JP (1994) Invasive monitoring combined with two-dimensional echocardiographic study in septic shock. Intensive Care Med 20:550–554
24. Hinder F, Poelaert JI, Schmidt C, Hoeft A, Mollhoff T, Loick HM, Van Aken H (1998) Assessment of cardiovascular volume status by transoesophageal echocardiography and dye dilution during cardiac surgery. Eur J Anaesthesiol 15:633–640
25. Tousignant CP, Walsh F, Mazer CD (2000) The use of transoesophageal echocardiography for preload assessment in critically ill patients. Anesth Analg 90:351–355
26. Cheung AT, Savino JS, Weiss SJ, Aukburg SJ, Berlin JA (1994) Echocardiographic and hemodynamic indexes of left ventricular preload in patients with normal and abnormal ventricular function. Anesthesiology 81:376–387
27. Swan HJ, Ganz W, Forrester J, Marcus H, Diamond G, Chonette D (1970) Catheterization of the heart in man with use of a flow-directed balloon-tipped catheter. N Engl J Med 283:447–451
28. Berryhill RE, Benumof JL (1979) PEEP-induced discrepancy between pulmonary arterial wedge pressure and left atrial pressure: the effects of controlled vs. spontaneous ventilation and compliant vs. noncompliant lungs in the dog. Anesthesiology 51:303–308
29. Humphrey CB, Gibbons JA, Folkerth TL, Shapiro AR, Fosburg RG (1976) An analysis of direct and indirect measurements of left atrial filling pressure. J Thorac Cardiovasc Surg 71:643–647
30. Lozman J, Powers SR Jr, Older T, Dutton RE, Roy RJ, English M, Marco D, Eckert C (1974) Correlation of pulmonary wedge and left atrial pressures. A study in the patient receiving positive end expiratory pressure ventilation. Arch Surg 109:270–277
31. Wagner JG, Leatherman JW (1998) Right ventricular end-diastolic volume as a predictor of the hemodynamic response to a fluid challenge. Chest 113:1048–1054
32. Jellinek H, Krafft P, Fitzgerald RD, Schwarz S, Pinsky MR (2000) Right atrial pressure predicts hemodynamic response to apneic positive airway pressure. Crit Care Med 28:672–688
33. Van Trigt P, Spray TL, Pasque MK, Peyton RB, Pellom GL, Christian CM, Fagraeus L, Wechsler AS (1982) The effect of PEEP on left ventricular diastolic dimensions and systolic performance following myocardial revascularization. Ann Thorac Surg 33:585–5892
34. Johnston WE, Vinten-Johansen J, Santamore WP, Case LD, Little WC (1989) Mechanism of reduced cardiac output during positive end-expiratory pressure in the dog. Am Rev Respir Dis 140:1257–1264

35. Michard F, Chemla D, Richard C, Wysocki M, Pinsky MR, Lecarpentier Y, Teboul JL (1999) Clinical use of respiratory changes in arterial pulse pressure to monitor the hemodynamic effects of PEEP. Am J Respir Crit Care Med 159:935–939
36. Michard F, Boussat S, Chemla D, Anguel N, Mercat A, Lecarpentier Y, Richard C, Pinsky, MR, Teboul JL (2000) Relation between respiratory changes in arterial pulse pressure and fluid responsiveness in septic patients with acute circulatory failure. Am J Respir Crit Care Med 162:134–138
37. Calvin JE, Driedger AA, Sibbald WJ (1981) The hemodynamic effect of rapid fluid infusion in critically ill patients. Surgery 90:61–76
38. Krausz MM, Perel A, Eimerl D, Cotev S (1977) Cardiopulmonary effects of volume loading in patients in septic shock. Ann Surg 185:429–434
39. Bennett-Guerrero E, Kahn RA, Moskowitz DM, Falcucci O, Bodian CA (2002) Comparison of arterial systolic pressure variation with other clinical parameters to predict the response to fluid challenges during cardiac surgery. Mt Sinai J Med 69:96–100
40. Diebel LN, Wilson RF, Tagett MG, Kline RA (1992) End-diastolic volume. A better indicator of preload in the critically ill. Arch Surg 127:817–821
41. Diebel L, Wilson RF, Heins J, Larky H, Warsow K, Wilson S (1994) End-diastolic volume versus pulmonary artery wedge pressure in evaluating cardiac preload in trauma patients. J Trauma 37:950–955
42. Tavernier B, Makhotine O, Lebuffe G, Dupont J, Scherpereel P (1998) Systolic pressure variation as a guide to fluid therapy in patients with sepsis-induced hypotension. Anesthesiology 89:1313–1321
43. Rajacich N, Burchard KW, Hasan FM, Singh AK (1989) Central venous pressure and pulmonary capillary wedge pressure as estimates of left atrial pressure: effects of positive end-expiratory pressure and catheter tip malposition. Crit Care Med 17:7–11
44. Shasby DM, Dauber IM, Pfister S (1981) Swan-Ganz catheter location and left atrial pressure determine the accuracy of the wedge pressure when positive end-expiratory pressure is used. Chest 80:666–670
45. Raper R, Sibbald WJ (1986) Misled by the wedge? The Swan-Ganz catheter and left ventricular preload. Chest 89:427–434
46. Pinsky M, Vincent JL, De Smet JM (1991) Estimating left ventricular filling pressure during positive end-expiratory pressure in humans. Am Rev Respir Dis 143:25–31
47. Swenson JD, Bull D, Stringham J (2001) Subjective assessment of left ventricular preload using transesophageal echocardiography: corresponding pulmonary artery occlusion pressures. J Cardiothorac Vasc Anesth 15:580–583
48. Mullins CB, Mason DT, Ashburn WL, Ross J (1969) Determination of ventricular volume by radioisotope-angiography. Am J Cardiol 24:72–78
49. Kasser IS, Kennedy JW (1969) Measurement of left ventricular volumes in man by single-plane cineangiocardiography. Invest Radiol 4:83–90
50. Balcon R, Oram S (1968) Measurement of right ventricular end-systolic and end-diastolic volumes by the thermodilution technique. Br Heart J 30:690–695
51. Viquerat CE, Righetti A, Suter PM (1983) Biventricular volumes and function in patients with adult respiratory distress syndrome ventilated with PEEP. Chest 83:509–514
52. Dhainaut JF, Devaux JY, Monsallier JF, Brunet F, Villemant D, Huyghebaert MF (1986) Mechanisms of decreased left ventricular preload during continuous positive pressure ventilation in ARDS. Chest 90:74–80
53. Terai C, Uenishi M, Sugimoto H, Shimazu T, Yoshioka T, Sugimoto T (1985) Transesophageal echocardiographic dimensional analysis of four cardiac chambers during positive end-expiratory pressure. Anesthesiology 63:640–646
54. Jardin F, Brun-Ney D, Hardy A, Aegerter P, Beauchet A, Bourdarias JP (1991) Combined thermodilution and two-dimensional echocardiographic evaluation of right ventricular function during respiratory support with PEEP. Chest 99:162–168
55. Vieillard A, Schmitt JM, Beauchet A, Augarde R, Prin S, Page B, Jardin F (2001) Early preload adaptation in septic shock? A transesophageal echocardiographic study. Anesthesiology 94:400–406
56. Jellinek H, Krafft P, Hiesmayr M, Steltzer H (1997) Measurement of right ventricular performance during apnea in patients with acute lung injury. J Trauma 42:1062–1067
57. Diebel LN, Myers T, Dulchavsky S (1997) Effects of increasing airway pressure and PEEP on the assessment of cardiac preload. J Trauma 42:585–590
58. Cheatham ML, Nelson LD, Chang MC, Safcsak K (1998) Right ventricular end-diastolic volume index as a predictor of preload status in patients on positive end-expiratory pressure. Crit Care Med 26:1801–186
59. Jansen JR, Schreuder JJ, Bogaard JM, van Rooyen W, Versprille A (1981) Thermodilution technique for measurement of cardiac output during artificial ventilation. J Appl Physiol 51:584–591
60. Stevens JH, Raffin TA, Mihm FG, Rosenthal MH, Stetz CW (1985) Thermodilution cardiac output measurement. Effects of the respiratory cycle on its reproducibility. JAMA 253:2240–2242
61. Okamoto K, Komatsu T, Kumar V, Sanchala V, Kubal K, Bhalodia R, Shibutani K (1986) Effects of intermittent positive-pressure ventilation on cardiac output measurements by thermodilution. Crit Care Med 14:977–980
62. Jansen JR, Schreuder JJ, Settels JJ, Kloek JJ, Versprille A (1990) An adequate strategy for the thermodilution technique in patients during mechanical ventilation. Intensive Care Med 16:422–425
63. Siniorakis EE, Nikolaou NI, Sarantopoulos CD, Sotirelos KT, Iliopoulos NE, Bonoris PE (1994) Volume loading in predominant right ventricular infarction: bedside haemodynamics using rapid response thermistors. Eur Heart J 15:1340–1347
64. Spinale FG, Mukherjee R, Tanaka R, Zile MR (1992) The effects of valvular regurgitation on thermodilution ejection fraction measurements. Chest 101:723–731
65. Yu M, Takiguchi S, Takanishi D, Myers S, McNamara JJ (1995) Evaluation of the clinical usefulness of thermodilution volumetric catheters. Crit Care Med 23:681–686
66. Jardin F, Farcot JC, Gueret P, Prost JF, Ozier Y, Bourdarias JP (1984) Echocardiographic evaluation of ventricles during continuous positive airway pressure breathing. J Appl Physiol 56:619–627
67. Huemer G, Kolev N, Kurz A, Zimpfer M (1994) Influence of positive end-expiratory pressure on right and left ventricular performance assessed by Doppler two-dimensional echocardiography. Chest 106:67–73
68. Jardin F, Dubourg O, Bourdarias JP (1997) Echocardiographic pattern of acute cor pulmonale. Chest 111:209–217
69. Mathru M, Kleinman B, Dries DJ, Rao T, Calandra D (1990) Effect of opening the pericardium on right ventricular hemodynamics during cardiac surgery. Chest 98:120–123

70. Schuster S, Erbel R, Weilemann LS, Lu WY, Henkel B, Wellek S, Schinzel H, Meyer J (1990) Hemodynamics during PEEP ventilation in patients with severe left ventricular failure studied by transesophageal echocardiography. Chest 97:1181–1189
71. Le Tulzo Y, Seguin P, Gacouin A, Camus C, Suprin E, Jouannic I, Thomas R (1997) Effects of epinephrine on right ventricular function in patients with severe septic shock and right ventricular failure: a preliminary descriptive study. Intensive Care Med 23:664–670
72. Vignon P, Mentec H, Terre S, Gastinne H, Gueret P, Lemaire F (1994) Diagnostic accuracy and therapeutic impact of transthoracic and transesophageal echocardiography in mechanically ventilated patients in the ICU. Chest 106:1829–1834
73. Jardin F, Brun-Ney D, Auvert B, Beauchet A, Bourdarias JP (1990) Sepsis-related cardiogenic shock. Crit Care Med 18:1055–1060
74. Jardin F, Fourme T, Page B, Loubieres Y, Vieillard-Baron A, Beauchet A, Bourdarias JP (1999) Persistent preload defect in severe sepsis despite fluid loading: a longitudinal echocardiographic study in patients with septic shock. Chest 116:1354–1359
75. Clements FM, Harpole DH, Quill T, Jones RH, McCann RL (1990) Estimation of left ventricular volume and ejection fraction by two-dimensional transoesophageal echocardiography: comparison of short axis imaging and simultaneous radionuclide angiography. Br J Anaesth 64:331–336
76. Urbanowicz JH, Shaaban MJ, Cohen NH, Cahalan MK, Botvinick EH, Chatterjee K, Schiller NB, Dae MW, Matthay MA (1990) Comparison of transesophageal echocardiographic and scintigraphic estimates of left ventricular end-diastolic volume index and ejection fraction in patients following coronary artery bypass grafting. Anesthesiology 72:607–612
77. van Daele ME, Trouwborst A, van Woerkens LC, Tenbrinck R, Fraser AG, Roelandt JR (1994) Transesophageal echocardiographic monitoring of preoperative acute hypervolemic hemodilution. Anesthesiology 81:602–609
78. Greim CA, Roewer N, Apfel C, Laux G, Schulte am Esch J (1997) Relation of echocardiographic preload indices to stroke volume in critically ill patients with normal and low cardiac index. Intensive Care Med 23:411–416
79. Feissel M, Michard F, Mangin I, Ruyer O, Faller JP, Teboul JL (2001) Respiratory changes in aortic blood velocity as an indicator of fluid responsiveness in ventilated patients with septic shock. Chest 119:867–873
80. Reuter DA, Felbinger TW, Schmidt C, Kilger E, Goedje O, Lamm P, Goetz AE (2002) Stroke volume variations for assessment of cardiac responsiveness to volume loading in mechanically ventilated patients after cardiac surgery. Intensive Care Med 28:392
81. Denault AY, Gasior TA, Gorcsan J, 3rd, Mandarino WA, Deneault LG, Pinsky MR (1999) Determinants of aortic pressure variation during positive-pressure ventilation in man. Chest 116:176–186
82. Morgan BC, Martin WE, Hornbein TF, Crawford EW, Guntheroth WG (1966) Hemodynamic effects of intermittent positive pressure respiration. Anesthesiology 27:584–590
83. Scharf SM, Brown R, Saunders N, Green LH (1980) Hemodynamic effects of positive-pressure inflation. J Appl Physiol 49:124–131
84. Brower R, Wise RA, Hassapoyannes C, Bromberger-Barnea B, Permutt S (1985) Effect of lung inflation on lung blood volume and pulmonary venous flow. J Appl Physiol 58:954–963
85. Abel JG, Salerno TA, Panos A, Greyson ND, Rice TW, Teoh K, Lichtenstein SV (1987) Cardiovascular effects of positive pressure ventilation in humans. Ann Thorac Surg 43:198–206
86. Fessler HE, Brower RG, Wise RA, Permutt S (1988) Mechanism of reduced LV afterload by systolic and diastolic positive pleural pressure. J Appl Physiol 65:1244–1250
87. Pinsky MR, Matuschak GM, Klain M (1985) Determinants of cardiac augmentation by elevations in intrathoracic pressure. J Appl Physiol 58:1189–1198
88. Taylor RR, Covell JW, Sonnenblick EH, Ross J (1967) Dependence of ventricular distensibility on filling of the opposite ventricle. Am J Physiol 213:711–718
89. Coyle JP, Teplick RS, Michael CL, Davison JK (1983) Respiratory variations in systemic arterial pressure as an indicator of volume status. Anesthesiology 59:A53
90. Perel A, Pizov R, Cotev S (1987) Systolic blood pressure variation is a sensitive indicator of hypovolemia in ventilated dogs subjected to graded hemorrhage. Anesthesiology 67:498–502
91. Coriat P, Vrillon M, Perel A, Baron JF, Le Bret F, Saada M, Viars P (1994) A comparison of systolic blood pressure variations and echocardiographic estimates of end-diastolic left ventricular size in patients after aortic surgery. Anesth Analg 78:46–53
92. Jardin F, Farcot JC, Gueret P, Prost JF, Ozier Y, Bourdarias JP (1983) Cyclic changes in arterial pulse during respiratory support. Circulation 68:266–274
93. Michard F, Teboul JL (2000) Using heart-lung interactions to assess fluid responsiveness during mechanical ventilation. Crit Care 4:282–289
94. Gunn SR, Pinsky MR (2001) Implications of arterial pressure variation in patients in the intensive care unit. Curr Opin Crit Care 7:212–217
95. Rooke GA, Schwid HA, Shapira Y (1995) The effect of graded hemorrhage and intravascular volume replacement on systolic pressure variation in humans during mechanical and spontaneous ventilation. Anesth Analg 80:925–932
96. Ornstein E, Eidelman LA, Drenger B, Elami A, Pizov R (1998) Systolic pressure variation predicts the response to acute blood loss. J Clin Anesth 10:137–140
97. Reuter DA, Felbinger TW, Kilger E, Schmidt C, Lamm P, Goetz AE (2002) Optimising fluid therapy in mechanically ventilated patients after cardiac surgery by on-line monitoring of left ventricular stroke volume variations. Comparison with aortic systolic pressure variations. Br J Anaesth 88:124–126

Manu L. N. G. Malbrain

Different techniques to measure intra-abdominal pressure (IAP): time for a critical re-appraisal

Abstract The diagnosis of intra-abdominal hypertension (IAH) or abdominal compartment syndrome (ACS) is heavily dependant on the reproducibility of the intra-abdominal pressure (IAP) measurement technique. Recent studies have shown that a clinical estimation of IAP by abdominal girth or by examiner's feel of the tenseness of the abdomen is far from accurate, with a sensitivity of around 40%. Consequently, the IAP needs to be measured with a more accurate, reproducible and reliable tool. The role of the intra-vesical pressure (IVP) as the gold standard for IAP has become a matter of debate. This review will focus on the previously described indirect IAP measurement techniques and will suggest new revised methods of IVP measurement less prone to error. Cost-effective manometry screening techniques will be discussed, as well as some options for the future with microchip transducers.

Keywords Intra-abdominal pressure · Intra-abdominal hypertension · Abdominal compartment syndrome · Intra-vesical pressure

Introduction

There is an exponential increase in studies on intra-abdominal hypertension (IAH) and abdominal compartment syndrome (ACS) in the literature. There is still controversy about the ideal method for measuring intra-abdominal pressure (IAP) [1, 2]. The intra-vesical route evolved as the gold standard. It, however, has considerable variability in the measurement technique, not only between individuals but also institutions. Common pitfalls are air bubbles in the system and wrong transducer positions. Variations in IAP from −6 to +30 mmHg have been reported previously [3]. A recent multicentre snapshot study showed that the coefficient of variation was around 25%, even up to 66% in some centres, raising questions on the reproducibility of the measurement itself. This makes it, difficult to compare literature data [4].

The volumes reported in the literature for bladder priming before the IAP measurement are not uniform (ranging from 50 to 250 ml). Injecting over 50 ml in a noncompliant bladder will raise intrinsic vesical pressure (IVP) and thus overestimate IAP [5, 6] (Fig. 1). By constructing bladder pressure volume curves we found that IVP was not raised when the volume instilled was limited to 50–100 ml [7] (Fig. 2). This is in accordance with others who found that baseline IAP alters the amount of volume in the bladder needed to increase IAP: the lower the baseline IAP, the higher the extra bladder volume needed for the same IAP increase [6].

The purpose of this report is: (1) to review the most commonly used indirect techniques for IAP measurement; (2) to provide the reader with a full description and important (dis)advantages of each technique; (3) to describe some new or revised techniques; and (4) to highlight the cost-effectiveness of each method.

Panel A

Panel B

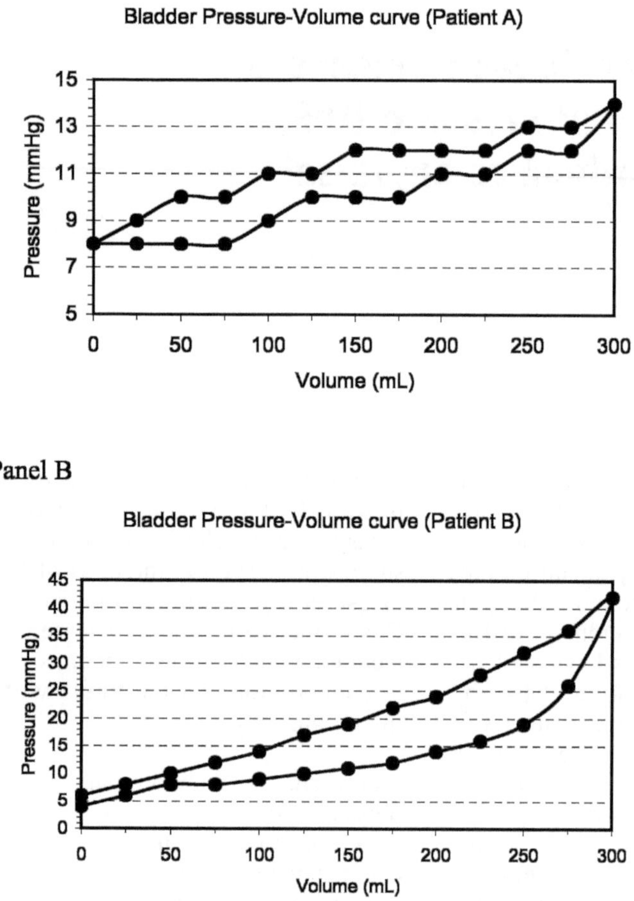

Fig. 1 A Bladder PV curve in a patient with a compliant bladder. Note that pressures are higher during insufflation than during deflation. Note that regardless of the amount of saline instilled in the bladder the pressures are comparable: 10 mmHg at 50 ml, 11 mmHg at 100 ml and 12 mmHg at 200 ml. **B** Bladder PV curve in a septic patient with a poor bladder compliance. Note that pressures are higher during insufflation than deflation. Note the significant difference in IAP value with regard to the amount of saline instilled in the bladder: 10 mmHg at 50 ml, 14 mmHg at 100 ml and 24 mmHg at 200 ml

IAP assessment

In analogy with the paradigm "if you don't take a temperature you can't find a fever" (in Samuel Shem, *The house of god*, Dell Publishing, ISBN: 0-440-13368-8), one can state that "if you don't measure IAP you cannot make a diagnosis of IAH or ACS". Abdominal perimeter cannot be used as an alternative method for IAP. In a recent study of 132 paired measurements in 12 ICU patients, we found a poor correlation between IAP and abdominal perimeter (R^2=0.12, P=0.04) [8]. Clinically significant IAH may be present in the absence of abdominal distension [9]. Chronic abdominal distension with sufficient time for adaptation, as seen with pregnancy, obesity, cirrhosis, or ovarian tumours, is an example of increased abdominal perimeter that is not necessarily accompanied by an increase in IAP. Other studies have shown that clinical IAP estimation by putting one or two hands on the abdomen is also far from accurate, with a sensitivity of only around 40%. So, one needs to measure it [10–12]. The question then arises: how? Since the abdomen and its contents can be considered as relatively non-compressive and primarily fluid in character, subject to Pascal's law, the IAP can be measured in nearly every part of the abdomen. Different direct and indirect measurement methods have been reported.

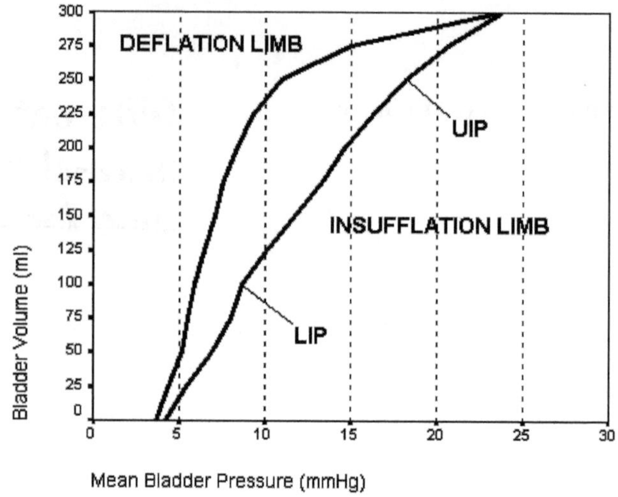

Fig. 2 Plot of the "insufflation" and "deflation" PV curve as a curve fit of the means of 13 measurements in six mechanically ventilated patients. The bladder PV curves were obtained by instilling sterile saline into the bladder with 25-ml increments. A lower inflection point can be seen at a bladder volume of 50–100 ml and an upper inflection point (UIP) at a bladder volume of 250 ml. The difference in bladder pressure was 2.7±3.3 mmHg between 0 and 50 ml volume, 1.7±1.2 mmHg between 50 and 100 ml, 7.7±5.7 mmHg between 50 and 200 ml and 16.8±13.4 mmHg between 50 and 300 ml. See text for explanation

Table 1 lists the different techniques and their major advantages and disadvantages, with an overall score calculated by dividing twice the number of advantages by the total number of (dis)advantages reported. Table 2 lists the cost estimate in Euros for the different techniques, with the cost of the initial set-up as well as the cost per measurement. Cost estimations were based on the number of measurements per day as well as the duration of the measurement period.

Table 1 Overview of the advantages (-) and disadvantages (+) of the different techniques for indirect IAP measurement. The overall score was calculated as the fraction of twice the number of advantages and the total number of (dis)advantages

General information	**Bladder techniques**				**Manometry**		
Author	Kron	Iberti	Cheatham	Malbrain	Harrahil	Lee	Malbrain
Reference	[13]	[16, 17]	[18]	Current	[26]	[27]	[28]
Publication year	1984	1987, 1989	1998	2003	1998	2002	2002
Properties	Fluid	Fluid	Fluid	Fluid	Fluid	Fluid	Fluid
General — Volume	50 ml	250 ml	50 ml	50 ml	?	?	50 ml
Manipulation	+++	++	+	+	-	-	-
Difficult	+	-	+	-	-	-	-
Time consuming initial set-up	+++	++	+	+	-	-	-
Time consuming next measurement	+++	++	-	-	-	-	-
Cost of device initial set-up	+	+	+	+	-	-	-
Cost per measurement	++	++	+	+	-	-	-
Interference urine output	+	+	+	+	-	-	-
Glass syringe	-	-	-	-	-	-	-
Technique							
No repeated measurements	+	+	-	-	-	-	-
No continuous trend	+	+	+	+	+	+	+
Not automated	+	+	+	+	+	+	+
Recalibration	+	+	+	+	-	-	-
Volume not standardised	+	+	+	+	+	+	-
Not accurate or reproducible	+	+	+	+	+	+	+
Not well validated	-	-	-	-	+	+	+
Air-bubbles	+	+	+	+	+	+	+
Multiple menisci	-	-	-	-	+	+	+
Bio-filter blocking	-	-	-	-	-	-	+
MMC interference	-	-	-	-	-	-	-
Hydrostatic fluid column							
Zero-reference problem	+	+	+	+	-	-	-
Over-under damping	+	+	+	+	+	+	+
Body position dependent	++	++	++	++	++	++	++
Risks							
Needle stick injury	+	+	+	-	-	-	-
Urinary infection	+	+	+	+	-	-	-
Sepsis	-	-	-	-	-	-	-
Contra-indications							
Bladder trauma	+	+	+	+	+	+	+
Neurogenic bladder	+	+	+	+	+	+	+
Hematuria	+	+	+	+	+	+	+
Gastric trauma	-	-	-	-	-	-	-
Other abdominal trauma	-	-	-	-	-	-	-
Overall conclusion							
Disadvantages	30	26	21	19	13	13	13
Advantages	8	9	10	12	18	18	18
Overall score	34.8%	0.9%	48.8%	55.8%	73.5%	73.5%	73.5%
Clinical indications	None	None	Screening	Intermittent monitoring	None	?	Quick screening

Bladder

The original open system single measurement technique [13]

Description

Traditionally the bladder has been used as the method of choice for measuring IAP. The technique was originally described by Kron and co-workers [13] and disrupts for each IAP measurement what is normally a closed sterile system. Thus, IAP measurement involves disconnecting the patient's Foley catheter and instilling 50–100 ml of saline using a sterile field. After reconnection, the urinary drainage bag is clamped distal to the culture aspiration port. For each individual IAP measurement a 16-gauche needle is then used to Y-connect a manometer or pressure

Table 1 (continued)

General Information	**IVC**	**Uterus**	**Rectum**	**Stomach**			
Author	Lacey	Dowdle	Shafik	Collee	Sugrue	Malbrain	Malbrain
Reference	[29]	[31]	[30]	[20]	[21, 22]	Current	Current
Publication	1987	1997	1997	1993	1994, 2000	2003	2003
Properties	Fluid	Microchip	Fluid-filled balloon	Fluid	Air-filled balloon	Air-filled balloon	Air-filled balloon
General-Volume			?	50 ml	2 ml	1–2 ml	0.1 ml
Manipulation	++	+++	+++	++	+	+	-
Difficult	+	++	++	+	+	+	-
Time taken for initial set-up	++	++	++	++	++	+	+
Time taken for next measurement	-	++	++	++	+	-	-
Cost of device initial set-up	++	++++	++	+	+++	++	++
Cost per measurement	-	-	-	++	-	-	-
Interference urine output	-	-	-	-	-	-	-
Glass syringe	-	-	-	-	+	+	-
Technique							
No Repeated measurements	-	+	+	+	-	-	-
No continuous trend	-	+	+	+	-	-	-
Not automated	+	+	+	+	+	+	-
Recalibration	+	+	+	+	+	+	-
Volume not standardised	-	+	+	+	+	+	-
Not accurate or reproducible	+	+	+	+	-	-	-
Not well validated	+++	+++	++	+	+	+	+
Air-bubbles	+	+	+	+	-	-	-
Multiple menisci	-	-	-	-	-	-	-
Bio-filter blocking	-	-	-	-	-	-	-
MMC interference	-	-	-	+	+	+	-
Hydrostatic fluid column							
Zero-reference problem	+	+	+	+	-	-	-
Over-under damping	+	+	+	+	-	-	-
Body position dependent	+	++	++	++	-	-	-
Risks							
Needle stick injury	+	-	-	-	-	-	-
Urinary infection	-	-	-	-	-	-	-
Sepsis	+++	-	-	-	-	-	-
Contra-indications							
Bladder trauma	-	-	-	-	-	-	-
Neurogenic bladder	-	-	-	-	-	-	-
Hematuria	-	-	-	-	-	-	-
Gastric trauma	-	-	-	+	+	+	+
Other abdominal trauma	-	+	+	-	-	-	-
Overall conclusion							
Disadvantages	21	28	25	24	15	12	5
Advantages	16	13	13	11	18	19	26
Overall score	60.4%	48%	50.1%	47.8%	70.6%	76%	91.2%
Clinical implications	?	None	?	Screening	Research	Research	APP trend, Research

transducer. The symphysis pubis is used as reference line. (See ESM addendum 1.)

Advantages and disadvantage (Table 1)

This technique implicates a lot of time-consuming manipulations that disrupt a closed sterile system at every measurement. It has all the problems that come along with the hydrostatic convective fluid column. Even though zero-reference at the symphysis pubis poses no problem, the problems come when the same pressure transducer is used for IAP and CVP, with zero-reference at the midaxillary line. Putting the patient upright with concomitant rise in the transducer may lead to underestimation of IAP, while putting the patient in the Trendelenburg position can lead to overestimation. The fact that recalibration needs to be done before every measurement augments the risk for errors. We have all seen the "magic" drop or rise in CVP at changes of nurse shifts, the same

Table 2 Cost estimation (in Euros) of the different IAP measurement techniques: cost of initial set-up and next measurement, as well as cost projection based on number of IAP measurements per day and duration of measurement period. The cost evaluation was based on the following estimates: transducer: €24.75; 50 ml of saline: €0.3; syringe: €0.36; needle: €0.023; Foley catheter: € 0.53; nasogastric tube: €0.53; oesophageal catheter (Ackrad): €55; tonometer (Datex): €175; IAP catheter (Spiegelberg): €100; Foleymanometer (Holtech): €17.5; rectal/uterinel probe: €34.8; microchip transducer (Rehau): €1,250; conical connector: €2.2; male-male connector: €0.4; stopcock: €0.31; sterile drapings: €1.36; nursing costs: €25 per hour

Technique	Author	Reference	Set-up cost	Cost per measurement	2 times per day				6 times per day				12 times per day			
					1week	2weeks	3weeks	4weeks	1week	2weeks	3weeks	4weeks	1week	2weeks	3weeks	4weeks
Bladder	Kron.	[13]	30.6	3.7	5.9	4.8	4.4	4.3	4.4	4.1	3.9	3.9	4.1	3.9	3.8	3.8
	Iberti	[17]	30.2	2.7	4.8	3.8	3.4	3.2	3.4	3.0	2.9	2.9	3.0	2.9	2.8	2.8
	Cheatham	[18]	31.3	1.3	3.7	2.6	2.3	2.1	2.1	1.7	1.6	1.6	1.7	1.5	1.5	1.4
	Malbrain	Current	34.7	1.0	3.6	2.3	1.9	1.7	1.8	1.4	1.3	1.2	1.4	1.2	1.1	1.1
Stomach	Collee	[20]	29.9	2.3	4.5	3.4	3.1	2.9	3.1	2.7	2.6	2.5	2.7	2.5	2.5	2.4
	Malbrain	Current	101.7	0.1	7.4	3.7	2.5	1.9	2.5	1.3	0.9	0.7	1.3	0.7	0.5	0.4
	Sugrue	[21]	202.7	0.3	14.7	7.5	5.1	3.9	5.1	2.7	1.9	1.5	2.7	1.5	1.1	0.9
	Malbrain	Current	83.7	0.3	6.2	3.2	2.2	1.8	2.2	1.3	0.9	0.8	1.3	0.8	0.6	0.5
Rectal	Shafik	[30]	70.1	0.2	5.2	2.7	1.8	1.4	1.8	1.0	0.7	0.6	1.0	0.6	0.4	0.4
Manometry	Lee	[27]	1.2	0.3	0.4	0.4	0.4	0.4	0.4	0.3	0.3	0.3	0.3	0.3	0.3	0.3
	Malbrain	[28]	18.2	0.3	1.6	1.0	0.8	0.7	0.8	0.6	0.5	0.4	0.6	0.4	0.4	0.4
Vena cava	Lacey	[29]	66.3	0.2	4.9	2.5	1.8	1.4	1.8	1.0	0.7	0.6	1.0	0.6	0.4	0.4
Microchip	Dowdle	[31]	1278.1	0.1	91.4	45.7	30.5	22.9	30.5	15.3	10.2	7.7	15.3	7.7	5.2	3.9

can happen with IAP. Furthermore, a fluid-filled system can produce artefacts that further distort the IAP pressure waveform. Failure to recognise these recording system artefacts can lead to interpretation errors [14]. It can oscillate spontaneously, and these oscillations can distort the IAP pressure curve. The performance of a resonant system is defined by the resonant frequency (this is the inherent oscillatory frequency) and the damping factor (this is a measure of the tendency of the system to attenuate the pressure signal). Therefore, any fluid-filled system is prone to changes in body-position and over- or underdamping due to the presence of air-bubbles, a tubing that is too compliant or too long, etc. A rapid flush test should, therefore, always be performed before an IAP reading in order to obtain an idea of the dynamic response properties and to minimise these distortions and artefacts [16]. Confirmation of correct measurement can be done by inspection of respiratory variations and by gently applying oscillations to the abdomen that should be immediately transmitted and seen on the monitor with a quick return to baseline (Fig. 3). In case of a damped signal the flush test should be repeated.

Other disadvantages are: it is an intermittent technique that interferes with urine output without the possibility of obtaining a continuous trend, it places the patient at increased risk of urinary tract infection or sepsis, and subjects healthcare providers to the risk of needle stick injuries and exposure to blood and body fluids [13]. In conclusion, the Kron technique has at the present time no clinical implications.

The closed system single measurement technique [16, 17]

Description

Iberti and co-workers reported the use of a closed system drain and transurethral bladder pressure monitoring method [16, 17]. Using a sterile technique they infused an average of 250 ml of normal saline through the urinary catheter to purge catheter tubing and bladder. The bladder catheter is clamped and a 20-gauche needle is inserted through the culture aspiration port for each IAP measurement. The transducer is zeroed at the symphysis and mean IAP is read after a 2-min equilibration period. (See ESM addendum 2)

Advantages and disadvantages (Table 1)

It has the same disadvantages related to the hydrostatic fluid column as the Kron technique, and since it is not needle-free it also subjects health care workers to needle-stick injuries [10, 11].

The advantage compared with the Kron technique is that it is simpler, less time-consuming, and there are fewer manipulations. In conclusion, the Iberti technique

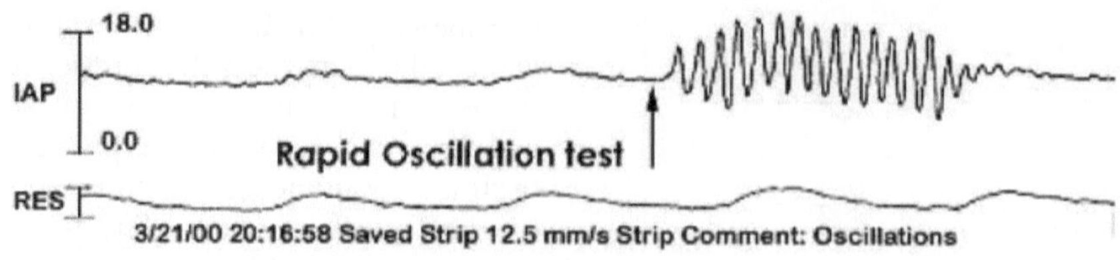

Fig. 3 Confirmation of correct IAP measurement can be done by inspection of respiratory variations and by gently applying oscillations to the abdomen that should be immediately transmitted and seen on the monitor with a quick return to the baseline

has at the present time limited clinical implications (e.g. screening for IAH).

The closed system repeated measurement technique [18]

Description

Cheatham and Safcsak reported a revision of Kron's original technique [18]. A standard intravenous infusion set is connected to 1,000 ml of normal saline, two stopcocks, a 60-ml Luer-lock syringe and a disposable pressure transducer. An 18-gauche plastic intravenous infusion catheter is inserted into the culture aspiration port of the Foley catheter and the needle is removed. The infusion catheter is attached to the pressure tubing and the system flushed with saline. (See ESM addendum 3.)

Advantages and disadvantages (Table 1)

It has the same inconveniencies related to any fluid-filled system as described with the Kron and Iberti techniques. It can pose problems after a couple of days because the culture aspiration port membrane can become leaky or the catheter kinky, leading to false IAP measurement. The fact that the infusion catheter needs to be replaced after a couple of days could increase the infection risk and needle-stick injuries.

This technique has minimal side effects and complications, e.g. without an increased risk for urinary tract infection [19]. It is safer and less invasive, takes less than 1 min, is more efficient with repeated measurements possible and thus is more cost-effective [18]. This technique is ideal for screening and monitoring for a short period of time (a couple of days) because of leakage.

The revised closed system repeated measurement technique

Description

The technique of Cheatham and Safcsak was modified (Fig. 4), as follows. A ramp with three stopcocks is inserted in the drainage tubing connected to a Foley catheter (Fig. 4A). A standard infusion set is connected to a bag of 1,000 ml of normal saline and attached to the first stopcock. A 60-ml syringe is connected to the second stopcock and the third stopcock is connected to a pressure transducer via rigid pressure tubing. The system is flushed with normal saline and the pressure transducer is zeroed at the symphysis pubis (or the midaxillary line when the patient is in complete supine position). Figure 4B shows a picture of the device in a patient with a close-up of the manifold set with conical connectors. (See ESM addendum 4.)

Advantages and disadvantages (Table 1)

It has the same inconveniencies related to a fluid-filled system as described with the Kron, Iberti or Cheatham technique. This technique has the same advantages as the Cheatham technique, with a required nursing time less than 2 min per measurement, a minimized risk of urinary tract infection and sepsis since it is a closed sterile system, the possibility of repeated measurements and reduced cost. Since it is a needle-free system it does not interfere with the culture aspiration port and the risk of injuries is absent. This technique can be used for screening or for monitoring for a longer period of time (2–3 weeks).

The revised closed system repeated measurement technique

In an anuric patient, continuous IAP recordings are possible via the bladder using a closed system connected to the Foley catheter after the culture aspiration port or directly to the Foley catheter using a conical connection piece connected to a standard pressure transducer via pressure tubing (Fig. 5). After initial "calibration" of the system with 50 ml of saline and zeroing at the sypmhysis pubis, the transducer is taped at the symphysis or thigh and a continuous IAP reading can be obtained. Daily calibration can be done in oliguric patients after voiding of rest diuresis.

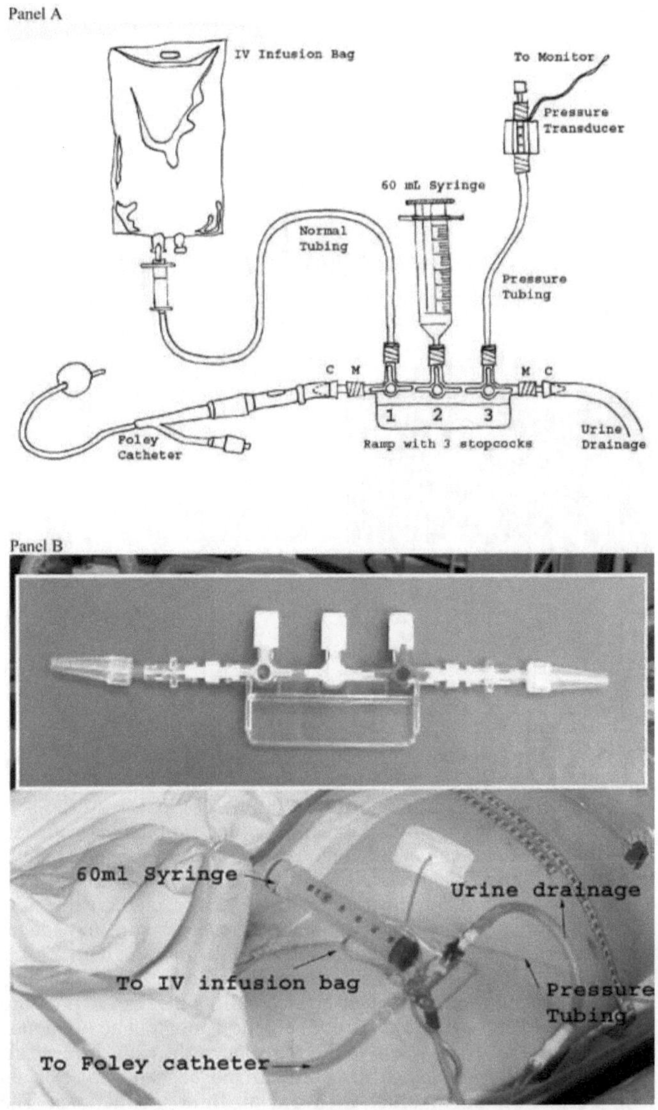

Fig. 4 A A closed needle-free revised method for measurement of intra-abdominal pressure. A standard intravenous infusion set is connected to a bag of 1,000 ml of normal saline and attached to the first stopcock. A 60-ml syringe is connected to the second stopcock and the third stopcock is connected to a pressure transducer via rigid pressure tubing. The system is flushed with normal saline and the pressure transducer is zeroed at the symphysis pubis. To measure IAP, the urinary drainage tubing is clamped distal to the ramp-device, 50 ml of normal saline is aspirated from the IV bag into the syringe and then instilled in the bladder. After opening the stopcocks to the pressure transducer mean IAP can be read from the bedside monitor. See ESM addendum 4 for explanation. **B** Mounted patient view of the device and close up of manifold and conical connection pieces

Conclusion

In conclusion, if one wants to use IVP as estimate for IAP the Cheatham or revised technique is preferred over the Kron or Iberti technique. The revised methods for IAP

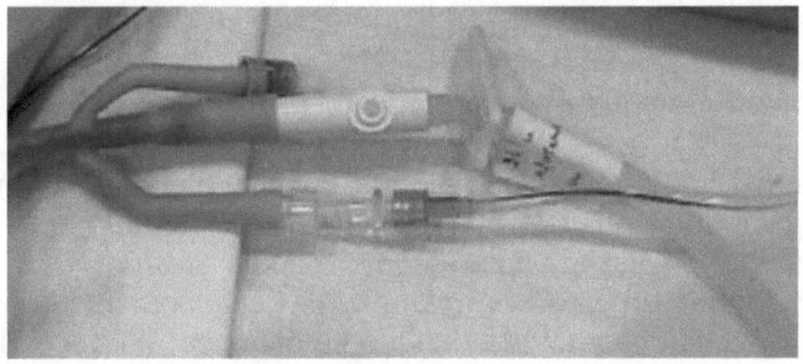

Fig. 5 Close up view of a closed needle-free system for continuous intra-abdominal pressure measurement in an anuric patients, using a conic connection piece (conical connector with female or male lock fitting; B Braun, Melsungen, Germany — Ref. 4896629 or 4438450) connected to a standard pressure transducer via pressure tubing

measurement via the bladder maintain the patient's Foley catheter as a closed system, limiting the risk of infection. Since these are needle-free systems they also avoid the risks of needle-stick injury and overcome the problems of leakage and catheter knick in the method described by Cheatham. They are more cost-effective, and facilitate repeated measurements of IAP.

Stomach

The classic intermittent technique [20]

Background and description

The IAP can also be measured by means of a nasogastric or gastrostomy tube and this method can be used when the patient has no Foley catheter in place, or when accurate bladder pressures are not possible due to the absence of free movement of the bladder wall. In case of bladder trauma, peritoneal adhesions, pelvic haematomas or fractures, abdominal packing, or a neurogenic bladder, IVP may overestimate IAP, and the procedure used for the bladder can then be applied via the stomach [20]. (See ESM addendum 5.)

Advantages and disadvantages (Table 1)

The same inconveniences as with every fluid-filled system apply. Another disadvantage is that gastric pressures might interfere with the migrating motor complex or with nasogastric feeding. Furthermore all air needs to be aspirated from the stomach before measuring IAP, something that is difficult to verify.

The advantages are that it is cheap, does not interfere with urine output, and the risks of infection and needle-stick injuries are absent. This cost-effective technique is ideal for screening.

The semi-continuous technique [21, 22]

Background and description

Sugrue and co-workers assessed the accuracy of measuring simultaneous IVP and IAP via the balloon of a gastric tonometer during laparoscopic cholecystectomy [21]. They found a good correlation between both methods. This technique allows a trend to be obtained. We recently validated these results and found good correlation between the classic gastric method, the tonometer method and IVP [22]. Simultaneous IAPtono and PrCO2 measurement was also possible. (See ESM addendum 6.)

Advantages and disadvantages (Table 1)

Measurement via the tonometer balloon limits the risks and has major advantages over the standard intravesical method: no infection risk and no interference with estimation of urine output. Simultaneous measurement of IAP and PrCO2 is possible; however, only in an intermittent way. Since it is air-filled it has none of the disadvantages associated with fluid-filled systems: no problem with zero-reference, over- or underdamping or body position. A possible disadvantage is the effect on interpretation of IAP values by the migrating motor complex. Recording the "diastolic" value of IAP at end-expiration can solve this problem. Other problems are that a 5-ml glass syringe is needed and that no data are available on effects of enteral feedings on these IAP measurements. This technique could be used for study purposes and clinicians interested in simultaneous CO2 gap and IAP monitoring.

The revised semi-continuous technique

Description

An oesophageal balloon catheter is inserted into the stomach. When the balloon is in the stomach, the whole respiratory IAP pressure wave will be positive and increasing upon inspiration in case of a functional diaphragm. If the balloon is too high in the thorax the pressure will flip from positive to negative on inspiration measuring oesophageal or pleural pressure instead. A standard three-way stopcock is connected to a pressure transducer (Fig. 6A). All air is evacuated from the balloon with a glass syringe and 1–2 ml of air reintroduced to the balloon. The balloon is connected via a "dry" system to the transducer, the transducer itself is NOT classically connected to a pressurized bag and *not* flushed with normal saline in order to avoid air/fluid interactions. The transducer is zeroed to atmosphere and IAP is read end-expiratory. Figure 6B shows a close-up of the oesophageal balloon catheter. (See ESM addendum 7.)

Panel A

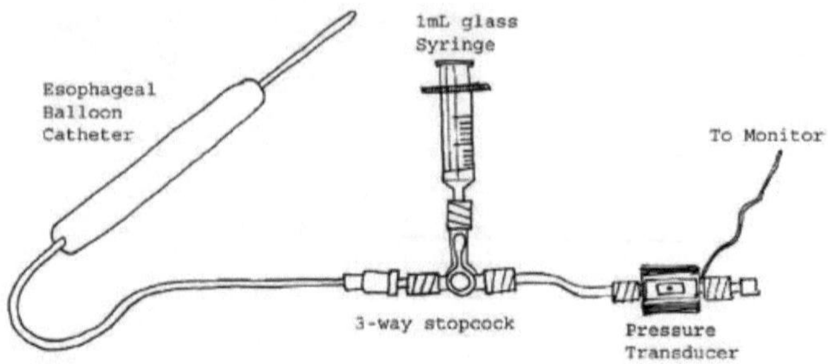

Panel B

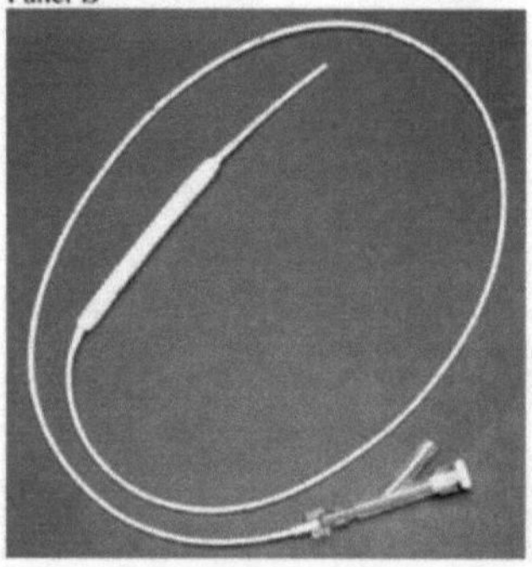

Fig. 6 A An oesophageal balloon catheter is inserted into the stomach (Oesophageal balloon catheter set, adult size with PTFE coated stylet; Ackrad Laboratories, Cranford, N.J., USA — Ref. 47-9005, see at http://www.ackrad.com/products/c-balloon_catheter.cfm or compliance catheter female or male, International Medical Products, Zuthpen, Netherlands, distributed by Allegiance — Ref. 84310). A standard three-way stopcock is connected to the now "nasogastric" tube; one end is connected to a pressure transducer via arterial tubing. All air is evacuated from the balloon with a glass syringe and 1 ml of air reintroduced to the balloon. A glass syringe is recommended to minimize the risk of pulling a negative pressure inside the catheter prior to reintroducing the 1 ml air. The balloon is connected via a "dry" system to the transducer, the transducer itself is *not* classically connected to a pressurized bag and *not* flushed with normal saline in order to avoid air/fluid interactions. The transducer is zeroed to atmosphere and IAP is read end-expiratory. See text for explanation. **B** Close-up view of the oesophageal balloon catheter

Advantages and disadvantages (Table 1)

A disadvantage is that the air in the balloon gets resorbed after a couple of hours (Fig. 7), so that "recalibration" of the balloon is necessary with a 2–5 ml glass syringe for continuous measurement, this might cause inaccurate measurement if the nurse waits too long for recalibration or if the re-instilled volume is not exactly the same as the previous one. It is less time-consuming and has all the advantages of an air-filled system (cfr tonometer). By

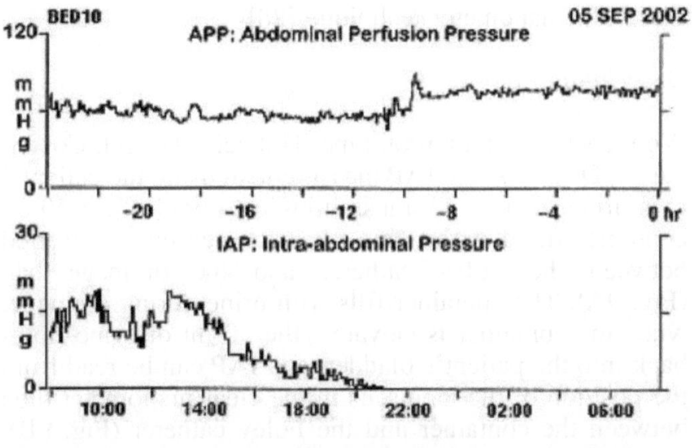

Fig. 7 A trend of 24-h IAP and APP recordings obtained with an oesophageal balloon placed in the stomach (Ackrad). Note the resorption of air after a couple of hours, with loss of IAP signal, confirming the need for recalibration

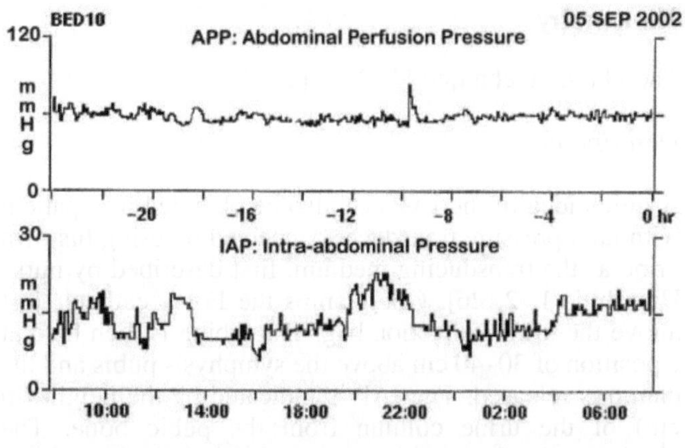

Fig. 8 A continuous trend of 24-h IAP and APP recordings obtained with the Spiegelberg balloon-tipped IAP catheter placed in the stomach. Note the absence of resorption of air due to automated recalibration every hour. Note also the effect of CAPD fluid inflow on IAP. If IAP was measured only twice a day the fluctuations and peak pressures would have been missed

using this technique the cost of IAP is further reduced depending on the catheter used. Moreover, a semi-continuous measurement of IAP as a trend over time is possible. The oesophageal balloon catheter price ranges from €15 (International Medical Systems, The Netherlands) to €55 (Ackrad, USA). This technique is ideal for monitoring for a longer period of time; however, when using multiple tubes the risk of sinusitis or infection needs to be evaluated in the future.

The continuous fully-automated technique

Description: IAP measurement with the air-pouch system

The IAP-catheter is introduced like a nasogastric tube; it is equipped with an air pouch at the tip. The catheter has one lumen that connects the air-pouch with the IAP-monitor and one lumen that takes the guide wire for introduction. The pressure transducer, the electronic hardware, and the device for filling the air-pouch are integrated in the IAP-monitor. Once every hour the IAP-monitor opens the pressure transducer to atmospheric pressure for automatic zero adjustment. The air-pouch is then filled with a volume of 0.1 ml required for accurate pressure transmission. Initial validation in ICU patients and laparoscopic surgery showed good correlation with the standard IVP method [23]. Recently Schachtrupp and co-authors used the same technique to directly measure IAP in a porcine model and found a very good correlation between the air pouch system and direct insufflator pressure (R^2=0.99) with a mean bias of 0.5±2.5 mmHg and small limits of agreement (–4.5 to 5.4 mmHg) [24]. (See ESM addendum 8.)

Advantages and disadvantages (Table 1)

This technique has no major disadvantage except that validation in humans is still in its infant stage. The advantages are those related to other gastric and air-filled methods. In summary, it is simple, fast, accurate, reproducible, and fully automated, so that a real continuous 24-h trend can be obtained (Fig. 8). This technique is not suited for screening, but is best for continuous fully automated monitoring for a long period of time. Since it is less prone to errors and most cost-effective if in place for a longer period of time, this technique has a lot of potential in becoming the future standard for multicentre research purposes.

Conclusion

The revised methods via the stomach have the advantage of being free from interference caused by wrong transducer positions, since the creation of a conductive fluid column is not needed as air is used as the transmitting medium. The last described fully automated technique also gives a continuous tracing of IAP together with abdominal perfusion pressure (APP) in analogy with intracranial pressure and cerebral perfusion pressure, allowing both parameters to be monitored as a trend over time. The APP is calculated by subtracting IAP from the mean arterial blood pressure. Recent data showed the importance of APP as a superior marker for IAH to titrate better the resuscitation of patients with IAH and ACS, hence avoiding end-organ failure and associated morbidity and mortality [2, 25].

Manometry

The classic technique [1, 2, 26]

Description

A quick idea of the IAP can also be obtained in a patient without a pressure transducer connected by using his own urine as the transducing medium, first described by nurse Harrahill [1, 2, 26]. One clamps the Foley catheter just above the urine collection bag. The tubing is then held at a position of 30–40 cm above the symphysis pubis and the clamp is released. The IAP is indicated by the height (in cm) of the urine column from the pubic bone. The meniscus should show respiratory variations. This rapid estimation of IAP can only be done in case of sufficient urine output. In an oliguric patient 50 ml saline can be injected as priming. (See ESM addendum 9.)

Advantages and disadvantages (Table 1)

It has all the inconveniencies that come along with a fluid-filled system as described before. However, since it is needle-free it poses no risks for injuries. It allows repeated measurements, is very inexpensive and fast with minimal manipulation. Since the volume re-instilled into the bladder is not constant raising questions on accuracy and reproducibility, it has limited clinical implications.

The U-tube technique [27]

Description

In a recent animal study, Lee and co-workers compared direct insufflated abdominal pressure with indirect bladder, gastric and inferior vena cava pressures [27]. IVP was measured by both the standard and U-tube technique. With the U-tube technique, the catheter tubing was raised approximately 60 cm above the animal to form a U-tube manometer, and IVP was measured as the height of the meniscus of urine from the pubic symphysis. The authors found a good correlation between the U-tube pressure and other direct and indirect techniques. (See ESM addendum 10.)

Advantages and disadvantages (Table 1)

It has the same advantages and inconveniences as the classic "Harrahill" technique, as with the previous technique the clinical validation is poor. The major advantage of this technique is that the volume re-instilled into the bladder is more stable (but still not well defined), so it can be used as a quick screening method.

The Foleymanometer technique [28]

Description

We recently tested a prototype (Holtech Medical, Copenhagen, Denmark) for IAP measurement using the patients' own urine as pressure transmitting medium [28]. A 50 ml container fitted with a bio-filter for venting is inserted between the Foley catheter and the drainage bag (Fig. 9A). The container fills with urine during drainage; when the container is elevated, the 50 ml of urine flows back into the patient's bladder, and IAP can be read from the position of the meniscus in the clear manometer tube between the container and the Foley catheter (Fig. 9B). We found a good correlation between the IAP obtained via the Foleymanometer and the "gold standard" in 119 paired measurements (R^2=0.71, P<0.0001). The analysis according to Bland and Altman showed that both measurements were almost identical with a mean bias of 0.17±0.8(SD) mmHg (95% CI 0.03–0.3). (See ESM addendum 11.)

Advantages and disadvantages (Table 1)

It has the same inconveniencies and advantages as the other manometry techniques. It allows repeated measurements, is very cost-effective and fast, with minimal manipulation. The great advantage with the Foleymanometer is that the volume re-instilled into the bladder is standardised at 50 ml; therefore, it is preferred over the other manometry techniques. A major drawback is the possibility of occasional blocking of the bio-filter, leading to overestimation of IAP in some cases and the presence of air-bubbles in the manometer tube, producing multiple menisci leading to misinterpretation of IAP. Further refinement and multicentric validation needs to be done before being used in a clinical setting.

Conclusion

The manometry techniques give a rapid and cost-effective idea of the magnitude of IAP and may be as accurate as other direct and indirect techniques. They can easily be done two-hourly together with and without interfering with urine output measurements. Moreover, the risk of infection and needle stick injury is absent. Since they need to be validated in a multicentre setting they are not ready for general clinical usage at the present moment.

Panel A

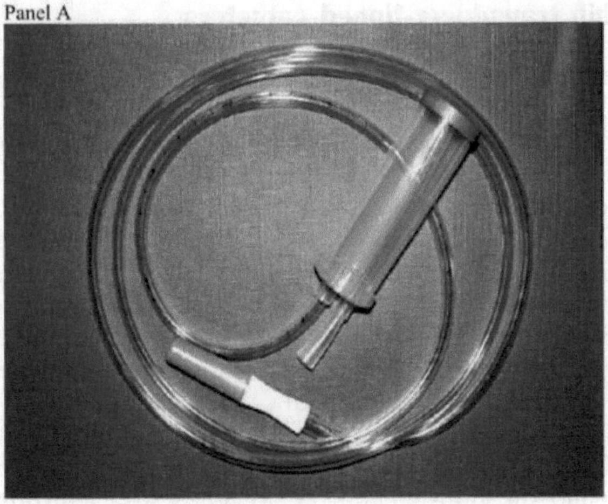

Panel B

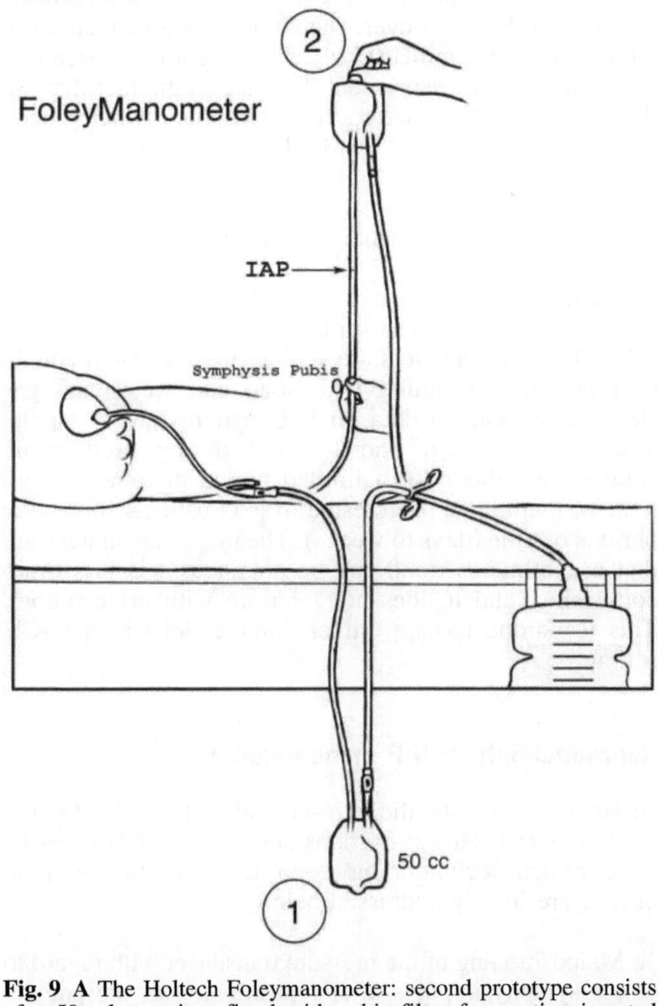

Fig. 9 **A** The Holtech Foleymanometer: second prototype consists of a 50 ml container fitted with a bio-filter for venting inserted between the Foley catheter and the drainage bag. **B** The use of the Holtech Foleymanometer: schematic drawing. The container fills with urine during drainage (position 1); when the container is elevated (position 2), the 50 ml of urine flows back into the patient's bladder, and IAP can be read from the position of the meniscus in the clear manometer tube between the container and the Foley catheter

Rectal pressure

Description

Rectal pressures are used routinely as estimate for IAP during urodynamic studies to calculate the transmural detrusor muscle pressure as IVP minus IAP [29, 30]. Rectal pressures can be obtained by means of an open rectal catheter with a continuous slow irrigation (1 ml/min), but special fluid-filled balloon catheters are used more routinely, although are more expensive. (See ESM addendum 12.)

Advantages and disadvantages (Table 1)

The major problem with the open catheter is that residual faecal mass can block the catheter-tip opening leading to overestimation of IAP. Other disadvantages of this technique are that it is more difficult, implicates more manipulation, is intermittent, and cannot be used in patients with lower gastro-intestinal bleeding or profound diarrhoea. There is also a great reluctance among nurses to use it. Since it is fluid-filled, it has all the problems associated with a hydrostatic fluid column, but since it is needle-free it decreases patient and healthcare worker infections or injuries. The fluid-filled balloon catheters are more expensive and, even though could theoretically stay in place for a longer period of time, interfere with gastro-intestinal transit and can cause erosions and even necrosis of the anal sphincter and rectal ampulla. Finally these techniques have not been validated in the ICU setting. This technique has no clinical implications in the ICU setting.

Uterine pressure

Description

Basically this technique is mostly done with the same catheters as for the rectal route. Uterine pressures are used routinely by gynaecologists during pregnancy and labour. Most classically a standard so-called "intra-uterine pressure catheter" (IUPC) is used for this purpose [31]. Uterine pressures are mostly obtained by means of a closed special fluid-filled balloon catheter (as for rectal pressure). (See ESM addendum 12.)

Advantages and disadvantages (Table 1)

The major disadvantages of this technique are the same as for rectal pressures: i.e. it is more difficult, implicates more manipulation, is intermittent, and cannot be used on patients with gynaecological bleeding or infection. Since it is also fluid-filled it has all the problems associated with a hydrostatic fluid column, but is needle-free. Finally, this technique has not been validated in specific ICU patient populations. This technique has no clinical implications in the ICU setting.

Inferior vena cava pressure

Description

The inferior vena cava pressure (IVCP) has been suggested as an estimation for IAP. Basically it uses the same techniques as described previously but applied to an IVC catheter. A normal central venous line is inserted into the inferior vena cava via the left or right femoral vein. The intra-abdominal position of the catheter is confirmed by portable lower abdomen X-ray, and confirmation of a rise in IAP following external abdominal pressure. A three-way stopcock is connected to the distal lumen, one end is connected to a pressure transducer via arterial tubing and the other end is connected to a pressurized infusion bag of 1,000 ml saline. The transducer is zeroed at the midaxillary line with the patient in the supine position and IAP is read end-expiratory as with CVP.

Advantages and disadvantages (Table 1)

The major disadvantage of this technique is the risk of (possible catheter-related) bloodstream infections and septic shock. The initial placement is more time-consuming. It has also the problems inherent to fluid-filled systems and poses potential injury to the patient and healthcare workers. The major advantages are that a continuous trend can be obtained, it does not interfere with urine output, and it could be used in bladder-trauma patients. Finally this technique has not been validated in specific ICU patient populations. In an animal study comparing different methods of indirect IAP measurement, Lacey and co-workers found a good correlation between bladder and inferior vena cava pressure with direct intraperitoneal IAP measurement, but not with gastric, femoral or rectal pressure [29]. Lee and co-workers also found a good correlation in 30 patients during laparoscopy [27]. A recent study in man, comparing superior vena cava pressure (SVCP) with common iliac venous pressure (CIVP) in various conditions of IAP and PEEP showed that the difference between CIVP and SVCP was not affected by the IAP, which implies that CIVP does not reflect IAP correctly [32]. The most likely explanation is the differing anatomy and experimental model used to induce increased IAP in canine studies. In humans both CVIP and SVCP increase as IAP increases [32]. Recently, Joynt and co-workers also found a good correlation between SVCP and IVCP regardless of IAH [33]. This technique has limited implications in the ICU setting.

Microchip transducer-tipped catheters

Description

Different types of catheters tipped with microchip transducers are nowadays available on the market. They can either be placed via the rectal, uterine, vesical or gastric route. These catheters can either have a 360° membrane pressor sensor in the organ (rectum, uterus, bladder, stomach) connected to an external transducer in a reusable cable or they can have a fibre-optic in vivo pressure transducer in the tip of the catheter itself. These catheters provide true zero in-situ calibration. By disconnecting and checking for zero on the monitor, clinicians can instantly validate and check the zero status of the monitor and the transducer [31]. Recently, Schachtrupp and co-workers found a good correlation between IAP calculated be a piezoresistive pressure measurement and direct insufflator pressure (R^2=0.92), with a difference of 1.6±4.8 mmHg; however, the limits of agreement were large (−8 to 11.2 mmHg) [24]. This might have been due to an unknown measurement drift due to the fact that the device cannot be zeroed to the environment when placed intra-abdominally. (See ESM addendum 13.)

Advantages and disadvantages (Table 1)

The major disadvantages of this technique is that it is very expensive, with catheter-price ranging from €1,000 to €1,500. These catheters are said to be re-usable a couple of times after cleaning with soap and water and gas sterilisation, but no data on ICU patients are available. These catheters are mostly used during urodynamic studies and labour for a limited period of time (hours); none of them have been tested in ICU patients for longer periods of time (days to weeks). The major advantages are that a continuous trend can be obtained, it is less time-consuming, and it does not interfere with urine output. This technique has no clinical implications in the ICU setting.

Reproducibility of IAP measurement

As stated previously, the intra-vesical route evolved as the gold standard. However, considerable variability in the measurement technique has been noted and the common pitfalls are briefly addressed below.

1. Malpositioning of the pressure transducer with regard to the symphysis pubis after repositioning of the patient. This may lead to over- and underestimation of IAP, which is commonly seen at changes of nurse shifts.
2. All fluid-filled systems connected to a pressure transducer have their own dynamic response properties

that can create distortions or artefacts in the IAP pressure waveform, leading to signal over- or underdamping [14, 15].

3. It is the most used and validated technique, but with inadequate accuracy and reproducibility. The inaccuracy can come from the presence of air-bubbles in any fluid-filled system leading to over- or underestimation. If the measurement itself is inaccurate, this also implies that it is not reproducible. However, when the pressure transducer position is consistently too high or too low with a fully compliant transducer system of high intrinsic resonant frequency the IAP value obtained will be too low or too high, respectively, but may be reproducible. In order to get an idea of these reproducibility problems with bladder pressure we performed a multicentre snapshot study (four IAP measurements each every 6 h) on a given day [4]. The mean IAP was 10.2±2.7 mmHg, (range 7.6±4 to 12.7±5.7). Analysis according to Bland and Altman showed a global bias of IAP within 24 h (difference between minimum and maximum value) of 5.1±3.8 (SD) mmHg (95% CI 4.3–5.9); the limits of agreement were −2.5 to 12.7 mmHg. The bias differed from centre to centre between 2.4 and 6.2 mmHg, with one outlier bias value as high as 11 mmHg, raising questions as to the reproducibility of the measurement technique used in that centre and making it difficult to compare literature data [4]. The mean coefficient of variation (defined as the standard deviation divided by the mean IAP) was 25%, which is comparable to daily fluctuations in other pressures, like central venous pressure or pulmonary artery occlusion pressure. However, this coefficient ranged from 4% to 66% between centres. Since the literature provides no data on 24-h continuous IAP-measurement in the ICU, it is not possible to determine whether these variations or fluctuations in IAP during one study day were normal or related to the measurement technique used.
4. The bladder "gold standard" measurement techniques reported are not uniform; most authors recommend to inject 50 ml [1, 2], others 0 ml [16], 100 ml [13, 23], 200 ml (data from internet: Brenda Morgan, Clinical Educator, CCTC on http://critcare.lhsc.on.ca/education/abdcompt.html, last revised 2001) or even 250 ml [17] of saline into the bladder. In fact, in the initial article from Iberti and co-workers, data are presented from a canine model without stating the volume instilled in the bladder. The only statement was that "the bladder was continuously emptied between measurements" [16]. In a following study, Iberti and co-workers presented human data stating, "using a sterile technique an average of 250 ml of normal saline was infused through the urinary catheter to gently fill the bladder and eliminate air in the drainage catheter" [17].
5. Conflicting results are reported in the literature regarding the validation of IVP versus directly measured IAP during laparoscopy. In a recent study, Yol and co-workers compared bladder pressure with direct insufflation pressure during laparoscopic cholecystectomy in 40 patients and he found a very good correlation between the two measurements (R=0.973, P<0.0001) [32]. This was also shown by Fusco and co-workers, who compared direct laparoscopic insufflation pressure with bladder pressures measured with bladder volumes of 0, 50, 150 and 200 ml [5]. He found that there was a good correlation across the IAP range from 0 to 25 mmHg between direct and indirect methods with all tested volumes. A bladder volume of 0 ml demonstrated the lowest bias, but when considering only elevated IAPs (25 mmHg) a bladder volume of 50 ml revealed the lowest bias. He concluded that intravesicular pressure closely approximates IAP and that instilling 50 ml of saline improved the accuracy of the bladder pressure in measuring elevated IAPs. However Johna and co-workers recently found that intravesicular pressure did not reflect actual intra-abdominal insufflation pressure (limited up to 15 mmHg) during laparoscopy [34]. He concluded that further research is needed to identify possible variables that may play a role in the relationship between the urinary bladder and abdominal cavity pressures, providing better means for diagnosing ACS. Further reading shows that the methodology of this study was poor.
6. Although many articles have validated IVP against direct insufflation pressures, it is difficult to extrapolate these single observer comparisons in patients undergoing general anesthesia and paralysis to a mixed ICU population of patients not under muscle relaxation as well as subject to other confounding factors (nurse shifts, position, zero reference, etc.). Direct IAP measurement via a laparoscopic insufflator is prone to errors by flow dynamics, resulting in rapid increases in pressure during insufflation. The Verres needle opening can be blocked by tissue or fluid leading to over- or underestimation of IAP and pressures can be influenced by muscle relaxation. Laparoscopy remains an artificial environment, this makes it even more difficult to validate indirect IAP measurement methods.
7. Baseline IAP and the volume instilled in the bladder are important. Gudmundsson and co-workers found recently in an animal study that the IAP increase by instilling Ringer's solution into the abdominal cavity correlated well with intra-vesical pressures [6]. It was also found that IVP as an estimation for IAP is affected by the amount of fluid in the bladder that should not exceed 10–15 ml. If the baseline IAP is lower than 8 mmHg, a 131-ml extra bladder volume is needed to increase IAP by 2 mmHg; however, if baseline IAP is 20 mmHg, only 39-ml extra bladder volume is needed for the same IAP increase [6]. We recently came to the same conclusions: by analysing bladder pressure

volume curves we found that IVP significantly increased depending on the volume instilled. The IVP rose from 4.2±3.2 mmHg at the baseline to 6.9±5 mm Hg with 50 ml and 23.7±16.1 at 300 ml ($P<0.0001$, ANOVA) [7]. If IVP is used as an estimate for IAP, the volume instilled in the bladder should be between 50 and 100 ml; however, in some patients with a low bladder compliance IVP can be raised at low bladder volumes. Ideally a bladder PV curve should be constructed for each individual patient before using IVP as an estimation for IAP. This study makes it difficult to compare the literature data. It raises not only questions with regard to the previously published definitions and IAP cut-offs, but it also puts the IVP in question as the so-called gold standard. Ideally the bladder should be fully emptied before an IAP measurement, but how can you be really sure?

8. Body position is important. Putting a patient in different body positions has significant effects on IAP (Fig. 10). This is in contradiction with the hypothesis that the abdominal compartment is primarily fluid in character and should follow the law of Pascal, since IAP would then remain constant regardless of body position as fluid is not compressible. The abdomen should in fact be looked at as a "fluidlike" compartment with different components that may influence IVP (the intrinsic weight of the organs, the presence of ascites, the air in the bowel, etc.). Assessment of IAP should, therefore, always be done in the complete supine position. The upright position significantly increases IAP compared with the supine. The effects on IAP being more pronounced in obese patients [35].

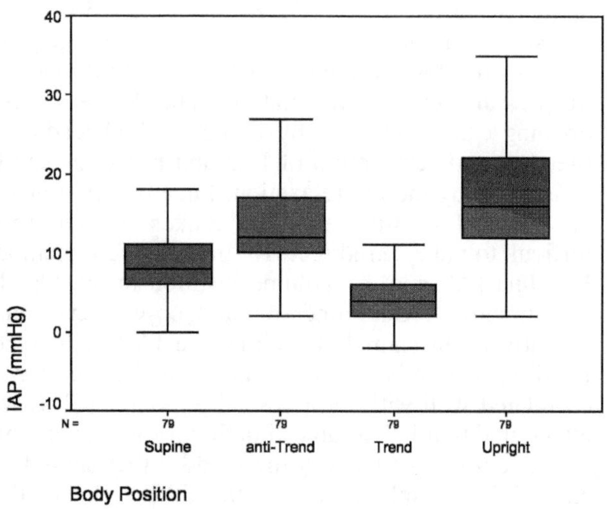

Fig. 10 Boxplot of mean IAP values in different body positions. The IAP was significantly higher in the anti-Trendelenburg and upright position versus the supine, and significantly lower in the Trendelenburg position versus the supine ($P<0.0001$, one-way Anova)

Many of these drawbacks are not only true for the bladder but are also present when IAP is estimated via other routes. Not much has been studied on the effects of spontaneous breathing, mechanical ventilation, the presence of expiratory muscle activity, auto-PEEP, and curarisation on IAP measurement via the different routes.

Definitions for IAH and ACS stand or fall by the correct measurement of IAP and its reproducibility. Recent literature data put the bladder pressure in question as the so-called gold standard for abdominal pressure [5, 6, 34–36].

Conclusion

This review has undertaken an analysis of the advantages and disadvantages, as well as a cost projection, for each IAP measurement technique and supports the view that: (1) there is no gold standard; (2) it is difficult to compare the different techniques; (3) cost-effectiveness is an issue; (4) IVP can be used as an estimation for IAP as a screening method to identify patients at risk via manometry; (5) IVP can be used as an estimation for IAP for initial follow-up either with the Cheatham or revised bladder technique; (6) for (multicentre) study purposes, surgical patients, trauma patients, patients at risk for IAH and difficult ICU patients, like mechanically ventilated patients with one or more other organ failures (assessed by SOFA score), it is preferable to switch to a continuous method for IAP monitoring via the stomach and focus therapy on optimising IAP and APP.

Acknowledgements I am indebted to my wife, Ms. Bieke Depré, for her patience, advice and technical assistance with the preparation of this manuscript, and to my three sons for providing a quiet writing environment. I also thank Dr. Rao Ivatury and Julia Wendon for their English editing of the manuscript. Part of this work was presented at: the 14th Annual Congress of the European Society of Intensive Care Medicine, Geneva, Switzerland, 30 September–3 October 2001; the 22nd International Symposium on Intensive Care and Emergency Medicine, Brussels, Belgium, 19–22 March 2002; the 13th Symposium Intensivmedizin and Intensivpflege, Bremen, Germany, 19–21 February 2003; the 23rd International Symposium on Intensive Care and Emergency Medicine, Brussels, Belgium, 18–21 March 2003; the 16th Annual Congress of the European Society of Intensive Care Medicine, Amsterdam, The Netherlands, 5–8 October 2003. This study was supported by Holtech Medical, Denmark (contact Bo Holte at holtech@email.dk). There was no financial support from Holtech other than making the product (Foleymanometer) available, free of charge. This study was supported by Ackrad Medical, USA (contact Charles Noto at cnoto@ackrad.com). There was no financial support from Ackrad other than making five oesophageal balloon catheters available, free of charge. This study was supported by Spiegelberg, Germany (contact Andreas Spiegelberg at info@spiegelberg.de). There was no financial support from Spiegelberg other than making the gastric balloon IAP-catheters and IAP-monitors available for study purposes, free of charge.

References

1. Malbrain MLNG (2001) Intra-abdominal pressure in the Intensive Care Unit: clinical tool or toy? In: Vincent JL (ed) Yearbook of Intensive Care and Emergency Medicine. Springer, Berlin Heidelberg New York, pp 547–585
2. Malbrain MLNG (2002) Abdominal perfusion pressure as a prognostic marker in intra-abdominal hypertension. In: Vincent JL (ed) Yearbook of Intensive Care and Emergency Medicine. Springer, Berlin Heidelberg New York, pp 792–814
3. Pouliart N, Huyghens L (2002) An observational study on intraabdominal pressure in 125 critically ill patients. Crit Care 6 (Suppl 1):S3
4. Malbrain MLNG, for the CIAH study group (2001) Prevalence of intra-abdominal hypertension in the ICU. Intensive Care Med 27 (Suppl 2):S176
5. Fusco MA, Martin RS, Chang MC (2001) Estimation of intra-abdominal pressure by bladder pressure measurement: validity and methodology. J Trauma 50:297–302
6. Gudmundsson FF, Viste A, Gislason H, Svanes K (2002) Comparison of different methods for measuring intra-abdominal pressure. Intensive Care Med 28:509–514
7. Verbrugghe W, Van Mieghem N, Daelemans R, Lins R, Malbrain MLNG (2003) Estimating the optimal bladder volume for intra-abdominal pressure measurement by bladder pressure-volume curves. Critical Care 7(Suppl 2):P184
8. Van Mieghem N, Verbrugghe W, Daelemans R, Lins R, Malbrain MLNG (2003) Can abdominal perimeter be used as an accurate estimation of intra-abdominal pressure? Critical Care 7 (Suppl 2):P183
9. Kirkpatrick AW, Brenneman FD, McLean RF, Rapanos T (2000) Is clinical examination an accurate indicator of raised intra-abdominal pressure in critically injured patients? Can J Surg 43:207–211
10. Sugrue M, Bauman A, Jones F, Bishop G, Flabouris A, Parr M, Stewart A, Hillman K, Deane SA (2002) Clinical examination is an inaccurate predictor of intraabdominal pressure. World J Surg 26:1428–1431
11. Castillo M, Lis RJ, Ulrich H, Rivera G, Hanf C, Kvetan V (1998) Clinical estimate compared to intra-abdominal pressure measurement. Crit Care Med 26 (Suppl 1):78A
12. Platell CF, Hall J, Clarke G, Lawrence-Brown (1990) Intra-abdominal pressure and renal function after surgery to the abdominal aorta. Aust N Z J Surg 60:213–216
13. Kron JL, Harman PK, Nolan SP (1984) The measurement of intra-abdominal pressure as a criterion for abdominal re-exploration. Ann Surg 199:28–30
14. Darovic GO, Vanriper S, Vanriper J (1995) In: Darovic GO (Ed) Hemodynamic monitoring, 2nd edn. WB Saunders, Philadelphia, pp 149–175
15. Kleinman B, Powell S, Kumar P, Gardner RM (1992) The fast flush test measures the dynamic response of the entire blood pressure monitoring system. Anesthesiology 77:1215–1220
16. Iberti TJ, Kelly KM, Gentil DR, Hirsch S, Benjamin E (1987) A simple technique to accurately determine intra-abdominal pressure. Crit Care Med 15:1140–1142
17. Iberti TJ, Lieber CE, Benjamin E (1989) Determination of intra-abdominal pressure using a transurethral bladder catheter: clinical validation of the technique. Anesthesiology 70:47–50
18. Cheatham ML, Safcsak K (1998) Intraabdominal pressure : a revised method for measurement. J Am Coll Surg 186:594–595
19. Sagraves SG; Cheatham ML; Johnson JL; White M; Block EF; Nelson LD (1997) Intravesicular pressure monitoring does not increase the risk of urinary tract or systemic infection. Crit Care Med 27:A48
20. Collee GG, Lomax DM, Ferguson C, Hanson GC (1993) Bedside measurement of intra-abdominal pressure (IAP) via an indwelling naso-gastric tube: clinical validation of the technique. Intensive Care Med 19:478–480
21. Sugrue M, Buist MD, Lee A, Sanchez DJ, Hillman KM (1994) Intra-abdominal pressure measurement using a modified nasogastric tube: description and validation of a new technique. Intensive Care Med 20:588–590
22. Debaveye Y, Bertieaux S, Malbrain M (2000) Simultaneous measurement of intra-abdominal pressure and regional CO2 via a gastric tonometer. Intensive Care Med 26 (Suppl 3):S324
23. Malbrain MLNG (2003) Validation of a novel fully automated continuous method to measure intra-abdominal pressure (IAP). Intensive Care Med 29 (Suppl 1):S73
24. Schachtrupp A, Tons C, Fackeldey V, Hoer J, Reinges M, Schumpelick V (2003) Evaluation of two novel methods for the direct and continuous measurement of intra-abdominal pressure in a porcine model. Intensive Care Med 29:1605–1608
25. Cheatham ML, White MW, Sagraves SG, Johnson JL, Block EFJ (2000) Abdominal perfusion pressure: a superior parameter in the assessment of intra-abdominal hypertension. J Trauma 49:621–627
26. Harrahill M (1998) Intra-abdominal pressure monitoring. J Emerg Nurs 24:465–466
27. Lee SL, Anderson JT, Kraut EJ, Wisner DH, Wolfe BM (2002) A simplified approach to the diagnosis of elevated intra-abdominal pressure. J Trauma 52:1169–1172
28. Malbrain MLNG, Leonard M, Delmarcelle D (2002) A novel technique of intra-abdominal pressure measurement: validation of two prototypes. Crit Care 6 (Suppl 1):S2–S3
29. Lacey SR, Bruce J, Brooks SP, Griswald J, Ferguson W, Allen JE, Jewett TC, Karp MP, Cooney DR (1987) The relative merits of various methods of indirect measurement of intra-abdominal pressure as a guide to closure of abdominal wall defects. J Ped Surg 22:1207–1211
30. Shafik A, El-Sharkawy A, Sharaf WM (1997) Direct measurement of intra-abdominal pressure in various conditions. Eur J Surg 163:883–887
31. Dowdle M (1997) Evaluating a new intrauterine pressure catheter. J Reprod Med 42:506–513
32. Yol S, Kartal A, Tavli S, Tatkan Y (1998) Is urinary bladder pressure a sensitive indicator of intra-abdominal pressure? Endoscopy 30:778–780
33. Joynt GM, Gomersall CD, Buckley TA, Oh TE, Young RJ, Freebairn RC (1996) Comparison of intrathoracic and intra-abdominal measurements of central venous pressure. Lancet 347:1155–1157
34. Johna S, Taylor E, Brown C, Zimmerman G (1999) Abdominal compartment syndrome: does intra-cystic pressure reflect actual intra-abdominal pressure? A prospective study in surgical patients. Crit Care 3:135–138
35. Malbrain MLNG, Van Mieghem BN, Verbrugghe W, Daelemans R, Lins R (2003) Effects of different body positions on intra-abdominal pressure and dynamic respiratory compliance. Crit Care 7 (Suppl 2):P179
36. Malbrain MLNG (1999) Abdominal pressure in the critically ill: measurement and clinical relevance. Intensive Care Med 25:1453–1458

Alexandre Toledo Maciel
Jacques Creteur
Jean-Louis Vincent

Tissue capnometry: does the answer lie under the tongue?

Abstract Increases in tissue partial pressure of carbon dioxide (PCO_2) can reflect an abnormal oxygen supply to the cells, so that monitoring tissue PCO_2 may help identify circulatory abnormalities and guide their correction. Gastric tonometry aims at monitoring regional PCO_2 in the stomach, an easily accessible organ that becomes ischemic quite early when the circulatory status is jeopardized. Despite substantial initial enthusiasm, this technique has never been widely implemented due to various technical problems and artifacts during measurement. Experimental studies have suggested that sublingual PCO_2 ($P_{sl}CO_2$) is a reliable marker of tissue perfusion. Clinical studies have demonstrated that high $P_{sl}CO_2$ values and, especially, high gradients between $P_{sl}CO_2$ and arterial PCO_2 ($\Delta P_{sl\text{-}a}CO_2$) are associated with impaired microcirculatory blood flow and a worse prognosis in critically ill patients. Although some questions remain to be answered about sublingual capnometry and its utility, this technique could offer new hope for tissue PCO_2 monitoring in clinical practice.

Keywords Sublingual capnometry · Gastric tonometry · Tissue PCO_2 · Microvascular blood flow · Outcome · Critically ill patients

Introduction

Tissue hypoperfusion is a common pathophysiological process leading to multiple organ dysfunction and death [1–4]. The major objectives in the management of acutely ill patients are to prevent, detect and correct tissue dysoxia as soon as possible to minimize organ damage [5]. Unfortunately, none of the currently available monitoring systems are very reliable at the bedside. Systemic hemodynamic and oxygenation parameters lack sensibility and specificity [5–7], especially in sepsis [8, 9].

The possibility of detecting early signs of tissue hypoperfusion by regional monitoring led to a great interest in gastric tonometry. However, much of the enthusiasm was tempered by technical or artifactual problems and difficulties in demonstrating the utility of gastric tonometry-derived variables as therapeutic guides. Sublingual capnometry has emerged in recent years as a potential alternative to monitoring tissue perfusion without some of the shortcomings that preclude the widespread use of gastric tonometry.

Here we review current knowledge about sublingual capnometry, its applicability and its limitations, as a technique to evaluate organ perfusion in acutely ill patients.

The saga of gastric tonometry

Current hemodynamic monitoring techniques, including the pulmonary artery catheter, are quite invasive and carry a risk of complications [10, 11] and higher costs [12], with controversial benefit [13, 14]. The measurement of arterial lactate concentrations may not reflect early alterations and have their own limitations [7, 15, 16].

Gastric tonometry has raised a lot of interest [17, 18] based on three important concepts: (a) tissue hypercarbia is a marker of mismatch between blood flow and oxygen demand [19]; (b) introduction of a gastric tube is a

M.R. Pinsky et al. (eds.), *Applied Physiology in Intensive Care Medicine 2: Physiological Reviews and Editorials*,
DOI 10.1007/978-3-642-28233-1_3, © Springer-Verlag Berlin Heidelberg 2012

common procedure in acutely ill patients and (c) the gut mucosa is exquisitely susceptible to hypoperfusion [20]. A number of studies have indicated that gastric tonometry-derived variables have prognostic value [9, 21, 22]. Changes in gastric mucosal PCO_2 (P_gCO_2) may precede alterations in systemic variables [23–25] and the PCO_2 gap (the difference between P_gCO_2 and arterial PCO_2) may represent a valuable monitoring system [21, 22, 26].

Unfortunately, gastric tonometry has serious limitations, even after the advent of gas tonometry [27, 28], including interruption of enteral feeding and concomitant use of H_2-blockers [28]. All these drawbacks reduce the clinical utility of the stomach as a practical place for routine tissue PCO_2 measurement.

Physiological concepts to interpret tissue partial pressure of carbon dioxide

Blood flow as the main determinant of tissue carbon dioxide content (CCO_2)

Tissue CCO_2 is determined by three variables: arterial CCO_2 (C_aCO_2), regional blood flow and tissue CO_2 production (aerobic or anaerobic). In stable respiratory conditions when C_aCO_2 is constant, tissue CCO_2 reflects the balance between tissue blood flow and local CO_2 production. In low flow states, CCO_2 increases as a result of the "CO_2 stagnation phenomenon" [29], even in the absence of dysoxia. Studies comparing ischemic and hypoxic hypoxia in animal models [30, 31] have demonstrated that the reduction in blood flow is the main determinant of tissue CO_2 accumulation, since even in severe dysoxic conditions induced by pure hypoxic hypoxia (a condition in which blood flow is maintained), CO_2 accumulation has not occurred [31]. However, while mechanistically interesting, the hypoxic hypoxia model is not clinically relevant.

Aerobic and anaerobic production of carbon dioxide

Carbon dioxide production occurs in both aerobic and anaerobic situations [32–35]. Increases in aerobic metabolism are associated with higher CO_2 production by the cells, which is generally associated with parallel increases in blood flow, so that tissue PCO_2 does not increase ("washout phenomenon"). When oxygen delivery decreases and reaches a critical value, aerobiosis can no longer be sustained and anaerobic production of CO_2 by the cells increases as a result of buffering of excess protons by bicarbonate ions and decarboxylation of metabolic intermediates [36]. However, during tissue dysoxia, total CO_2 production may be decreased [37–39] because the fall in aerobic CO_2 production can be greater than the increase in anaerobic CO_2 production. In fact, a distinction between aerobic and anaerobic production of CO_2 in the body is quite difficult [32].

Carbon dioxide content-partial pressure of carbon dioxide relationship

The relation between CCO_2 and PCO_2 follows a curvilinear shape so that changes in PCO_2 are not always associated with similar changes in CCO_2. Some physiological variables can also interfere with this relationship, such as hemoglobin concentration and its oxygen saturation [40], pH and temperature: none of which are of established clinical significance [41, 42].

Monitoring tissue partial pressure of carbon dioxide in sites other than the stomach

Tissue hypercapnia is ubiquitous in shock states. The methodological limitations of gastric tonometry prompted a search for alternative sites of tissue PCO_2 monitoring. Walley et al. [43] proposed, in an experimental model of hemorrhagic shock in pigs, that small bowel (jejunum) tonometry is more accurate than gastric tonometry in detecting gut ischemia, and sigmoid tonometry has been studied as a surrogate monitor of gastrointestinal ischemia, especially useful in aorto-iliac surgery—in which left ischemic colitis is a well known complication [44–46]. Sato et al. [47] demonstrated, in a rodent model of hemorrhagic shock, that the esophagus luminal PCO_2 (P_eCO_2) was a reliable surrogate for the P_gCO_2.

In addition to the gastrointestinal tract, experimental studies have used tonometry to detect hypoperfusion in other places in the body including the brain [48], bladder [49], muscle [50] and peritoneum [51]. However, these sites are not practical for routine use and, in the search for a place in the body where tissue PCO_2 could be easily and rapidly measured in a non-invasive and more practical way, Nakagawa et al. [52] suggested that the sublingual mucosa could be a valuable site.

Relevant aspects of sublingual anatomy and physiology

The sublingual mucosa is a highly vascularized surface supplied by the sublingual arteries, which stem from the lingual arteries, branches of the external carotid arteries. Indeed, in addition to the esophagus, the sublingual region is not part of the splanchnic area. However, alterations in sublingual blood flow may occur in response to feeding, with increased production of saliva by sublingual glands. This process is mediated mainly by the parasympathetic nervous system in response to many factors, including direct tactile stimulus and as a reflex response to the presence of food in the stomach or proximal intestine.

Sublingual partial pressure of carbon dioxide measurement

Experimental and clinical studies regarding sublingual capnometry have used essentially two different devices: MI-720 CO_2 electrode (Microelectrodes; Londonderry, NH, USA) and CapnoProbe SL Monitoring System (Nellcor; Pleasanton, CA, USA).

MI-720 is a CO_2 electrode that needs to be calibrated in standard gases with known percent values of CO_2 before use. Although not originally designed to be used under the tongue, it is the device that has been used in most relevant experimental studies regarding $P_{sl}CO_2$ measurement [52–54] and also in the first clinical study reported [55]. Weil et al. [55] made some modifications to the device in such a way that it fits better in the human sublingual space and avoids contact with room air, which can interfere badly with measurements.

The CapnoProbe was specially designed for the measurement of $P_{sl}CO_2$ and has been used in most of the clinical studies on this subject [7, 56, 57]. It consists of a disposable $P_{sl}CO_2$ sensor, which is actually a CO_2-sensing optode. The optode comprises a CO_2-permeable silicone capsule filled with a fluorescent dye in a buffer solution, at the distal end of an optical fiber. The fluorescent indicator is excited by light conducted through the optical fiber and changes in the projected light caused by changes in fluorescent emission are monitored by the optical fiber. These changes occur as a consequence of parallel changes in the pH of the solution, which is a result of the presence of CO_2 and formation of carbonic acid (H_2CO_3). Light signals are then transferred via the optical fiber to an instrument where they are converted to a numerical value of PCO_2. If properly placed under the tongue with the mouth shut, exposure to the environmental air and light is minimal. A few minutes are necessary for calibration and equilibration, which are made in a liquid solution with a known concentration of CO_2. The capability range of measurement with this device is from 30 to 150 mmHg.

Current experience with sublingual partial pressure of carbon dioxide measurement

Experimental studies

The first evidence that sublingual capnometry may be useful in the diagnosis and quantitation of circulatory shock came from the work of Nakagawa et al. [52]. These investigators observed, during hemorrhagic and septic shock in rats, that changes in $P_{sl}CO_2$ were parallel to changes in P_gCO_2 and systemic markers of hypoperfusion, such as mean arterial pressure, cardiac index and arterial lactate concentration. It is important to note that the septic shock model used in this study was characterized by a hypodynamic status.

Povoas et al. [53] demonstrated similar phenomena in pigs during bleeding and re-infusion, with a close correlation between P_gCO_2 and $P_{sl}CO_2$ values. In another study in rats [58], hemorrhage resulted in a decrease in blood flow in several organs, including the sublingual region, and these decreases were associated with simultaneous increases in $P_{sl}CO_2$.

As with gut mucosal PCO_2 [59–62], arterial PCO_2 (P_aCO_2) also influences $P_{sl}CO_2$. Pernat et al. [54] showed that acute changes in P_aCO_2 induced by hypo- and hyperventilation in rats influence $P_{sl}CO_2$ under physiological conditions and during hemorrhagic shock. Hence, changes in $P_{sl}CO_2$ should be interpreted in relation to the concurrent P_aCO_2; the gradient ($\Delta P_{sl-a}CO_2$) rather than $P_{sl}CO_2$ per se must be considered.

Clinical studies

Four clinical studies using sublingual capnometry in critically ill patients have been reported [7, 55–57] (Table 1). Weil et al. [55] reported the first clinical, prospective investigation on sublingual capnometry. These authors measured $P_{sl}CO_2$ and simultaneous values of arterial blood pressure, heart rate and arterial lactate concentrations in 46 patients admitted to the emergency room, intensive care unit (ICU) or trauma service with life-threatening illness or injuries, 26 of whom were considered to be in shock on the basis of a systolic pressure less than 100 mmHg and physical signs of circulatory failure at the time of admission. The authors found higher $P_{sl}CO_2$ values in the shock group and suggested that a $P_{sl}CO_2$ threshold value of 70 mmHg was predictive of the severity of the circulatory failure and the likelihood of hospital survival. Initial $P_{sl}CO_2$ values were highly correlated with arterial lactate concentrations but decreased more promptly during effective treatment, suggesting that decreases in $P_{sl}CO_2$ occur faster and closer to the real time of hemodynamic improvement than arterial lactate concentrations. They concluded that sublingual capnometry was a reliable method for diagnosis and quantitation of severity of circulatory failure in humans.

Marik [56] also measured $P_{sl}CO_2$ in hemodynamically unstable patients during the first 24 h of ICU admission. Initial $\Delta P_{sl-a}CO_2$ values were statistically higher in non-survivors than in survivors but the $P_{sl}CO_2$ values were not, suggesting that $\Delta P_{sl-a}CO_2$ is a better prognostic factor than $P_{sl}CO_2$. In a similar study design, Rackow and coworkers [57] also found higher $\Delta P_{sl-a}CO_2$ in non-survivors than in survivors, but this time measured at 24 h after the start of the study. These authors observed that the correlation between $P_{sl}CO_2$ and the other indexes of tissue

Table 1 Summary of clinical studies using sublingual capnometry

Author(s)/year	Number of patients	Diagnosis	Time of $P_{sl}CO_2$ measurement	$P_{sl}CO_2/\Delta P_{sl-a}CO_2$ survivors, non-survivors	*p* value
Weil et al, 1999 [55]	46	21 trauma 14 infection 6 cardiac emergency 5 miscellaneous	ICU, ER or TS admission, every 30 min, (total 6 h)	$P_{sl}CO_2$ (admission), 58.4±11.3, 92.6±26.6	<0.001
Marik, 2001 [56]	22	15 severe sepsis/septic shock 7 cardiogenic shock	ICU admission, every 4–6 h, (total 24 h)	$\Delta P_{sl-a}CO_2$ (admission), 9.2±5.0, 17.8±11.5	0.04
Rackow et al, 2001 [57]	25	19 sepsis 6 cardiac failure	0, 1, 3, 6, 12, 24 h after Swan-Ganz insertion	$\Delta P_{sl-a}CO_2$ (at 24 h), 14±3, 29±4	<0.05
Marik and Bankov, 2003 [7]	54	21 severe sepsis/septic shock 9 cardiogenic shock 8 major abdominal surgery 8 polytrauma 5 hypovolemic shock 3 severe pancreatitis	0, 4, 8 h after Swan-Ganz insertion	$\Delta P_{sl-a}CO_2$ (at the time of Swan-Ganz insertion), 19.0±12.8, 35.3±18.3	0.0004

$P_{sl}CO_2$ sublingual partial pressure of carbon dioxide, *$\Delta P_{sl-a}CO_2$* sublingual-arterial partial pressure of carbon dioxide gradient, *ICU* intensive care unit, *ER* emergency room, *TS* trauma service

Table 2 Well-established facts, limitations and unanswered questions about sublingual capnometry

Well-established facts	1. $P_{sl}CO_2$ depends on P_aCO_2, sublingual tissue CO_2 production and regional blood flow 2. Low blood flow is the main determinant of CO_2 accumulation in tissues 3. Measurement of $P_{sl}CO_2$ is non-invasive and easily obtained in cooperative or sedated patients 4. High $\Delta P_{sl-a}CO_2$ values in critically ill patients predict a poor prognosis
Limitations and questions to be answered	1. Current physiological concepts preclude $\Delta P_{sl-a}CO_2$ as a sensitive and specific marker of dysoxia 2. Possible differences in $\Delta P_{sl-a}CO_2$ patterns in hypodynamic and hyperdynamic shock 3. Cut-off values between normal and pathological values are hard to define 4. $\Delta P_{sl-a}CO_2$-guided therapy has not yet been shown to be beneficial

$P_{sl}CO_2$ sublingual partial pressure of carbon dioxide, *P_aCO_2* arterial partial pressure of carbon dioxide, *CO_2* carbon dioxide, *$\Delta P_{sl-a}CO_2$* gradient between $P_{sl}CO_2$ and P_aCO_2

perfusion was greater in patients with cardiac failure than with sepsis. Marik and Bankov [7] recently confirmed that $\Delta P_{sl-a}CO_2$ is a good outcome predictor. They observed that patients with an initial $\Delta P_{sl-a}CO_2$ higher than 25 mmHg have a high mortality rate. In their study, despite optimization of traditional hemodynamic end points, the $\Delta P_{sl-a}CO_2$ decreased but remained higher in the non-survivors than in the survivors. When they excluded $\Delta P_{sl-a}CO_2$ from the analysis, $P_{sl}CO_2$ became the most significant predictor of outcome by multivariate analysis. Based on this, they concluded that, in their study, $P_{sl}CO_2$ alone might be suitable for management, obviating the need for blood gas analysis to calculate $\Delta P_{sl-a}CO_2$.

By simultaneously monitoring $P_{sl}CO_2$ with CapnoProbe and sublingual microcirculation with the use of the Orthogonal Polarization Spectral imaging technique (Cytoscan, Cytometrics, Philadelphia, PA, USA), our group was able to demonstrate a significant correlation between $P_{sl}CO_2$ and the percentage of perfused sublingual capillaries in 12 septic shock patients [63, 64]. Hence, $\Delta P_{sl-a}CO_2$ seems to be mainly determined by sublingual microcirculatory blood flow.

Limitations, controversies and unanswered questions

With the currently available data on sublingual capnometry, some questions (Table 2) remain and need proper evaluation and consideration.

Drawbacks of tissue partial pressure of carbon dioxide measurement in the sublingual mucosa

Although more practical than the stomach for measurement of tissue PCO_2, some potential disadvantages need to be discussed. First, since tactile stimuli can increase sublingual blood flow and production of saliva, the presence of the device itself under the tongue can increase sublingual blood flow. Most acutely ill patients are not

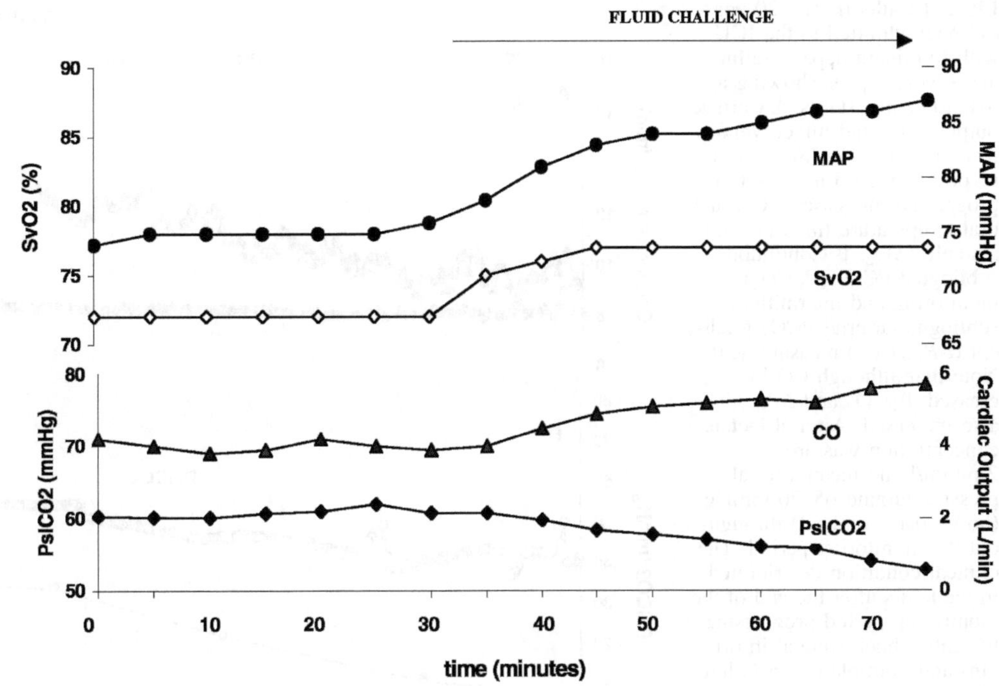

Fig. 1 Results from a 73-year-old woman admitted to the ICU with subarachnoid hemorrhage. Cardiac output was felt to be inadequate in the presence of an increased arterial lactate concentration and a high $P_{sl}CO_2$ (around 60 mmHg). Mean arterial pressure (*MAP*), cardiac output (*CO*), mixed venous oxygen saturation (*SvO_2*) and sublingual PCO_2 (*$P_{sl}CO_2$*) were continuously monitored. A fluid challenge resulted in increases in MAP, CO, and SvO_2 and decreases in $P_{sl}CO_2$. Since arterial PCO_2 remained constant (38 mmHg), decreases in the sublingual-arterial PCO_2 gradient ($\Delta P_{sl\text{-}a}CO_2$) were equally significant. Arterial lactate concentration normalized in the subsequent hours

fed orally so that the direct interference of food on sublingual measurement is not a major problem, as it is for gastric tonometry. However, enteral feeding could theoretically interfere indirectly with sublingual blood flow through reflex mechanisms, as previously mentioned. It is important to remember that the sublingual mucosa is sometimes used for drug administration but this should be avoided during sublingual PCO_2 monitoring. In addition, CO_2 production by bacteria of the oral flora and interference of saliva and its composition as well as vomitus in the measurement of the $P_{sl}CO_2$ value are potential areas of concern, but their effects are probably negligible.

The devices clinically available for $P_{sl}CO_2$ measurement measure the value intermittently. However, since $P_{sl}CO_2$ seems to respond fast to changes in hemodynamic conditions, intermittent measurements are not very practical for use in critically ill patients. For this reason, a system that measures $P_{sl}CO_2$ continuously would be more appropriate. This system has already been developed (CapnoProbe SL Model 2000 Sensor; Optical Sensor, MN, USA) but is still not clinically available. Fig. 1 shows an example of the use of this device in a single patient.

Another important aspect of the measurement of tissue PCO_2 in the sublingual mucosa is that, since it is not part of the splanchnic area, elevations in $P_{sl}CO_2$ may not occur as fast as in the stomach in progressive shock states. Hence, it may not serve as a "canary of the body" [65]. In addition, $P_{sl}CO_2$ should always be interpreted in relation to the arterial PCO_2. This latter measurement is subject to bias and imprecisions related to blood gas sampling and analysis, including the pitfalls of the temperature correction of blood gases. Since sublingual and arterial PCO_2 are measured by different equipment and at different temperatures, a methodological error may be introduced [66].

Normal values of sublingual partial pressure of carbon dioxide

There is no large study evaluating the normal value of $P_{sl}CO_2$. Weil et al. [55] measured $P_{sl}CO_2$ in five healthy human volunteers with the MI-720 CO_2 electrode and the range was from 43 to 47 mmHg.

Sublingual partial pressure of carbon dioxide measurement in different types of shock

Most experimental studies on sublingual capnometry have included hypodynamic types of circulatory shock. Even in models of septic shock, the cardiac index started to fall at the beginning of the experiment [52]. This has been a limitation of models using a bolus intravenous injection of bacteria (or endotoxin) [67]. Most of the clinical studies did not evaluate different types of shock separately [7, 55, 56], yet it is possible that different types of shock modify $P_{sl}CO_2$ values in different ways. This may also contribute to the variability in the correlations between $P_{sl}CO_2$ and other markers of tissue perfusion in the various studies, as suggested by Rackow et al. [57].

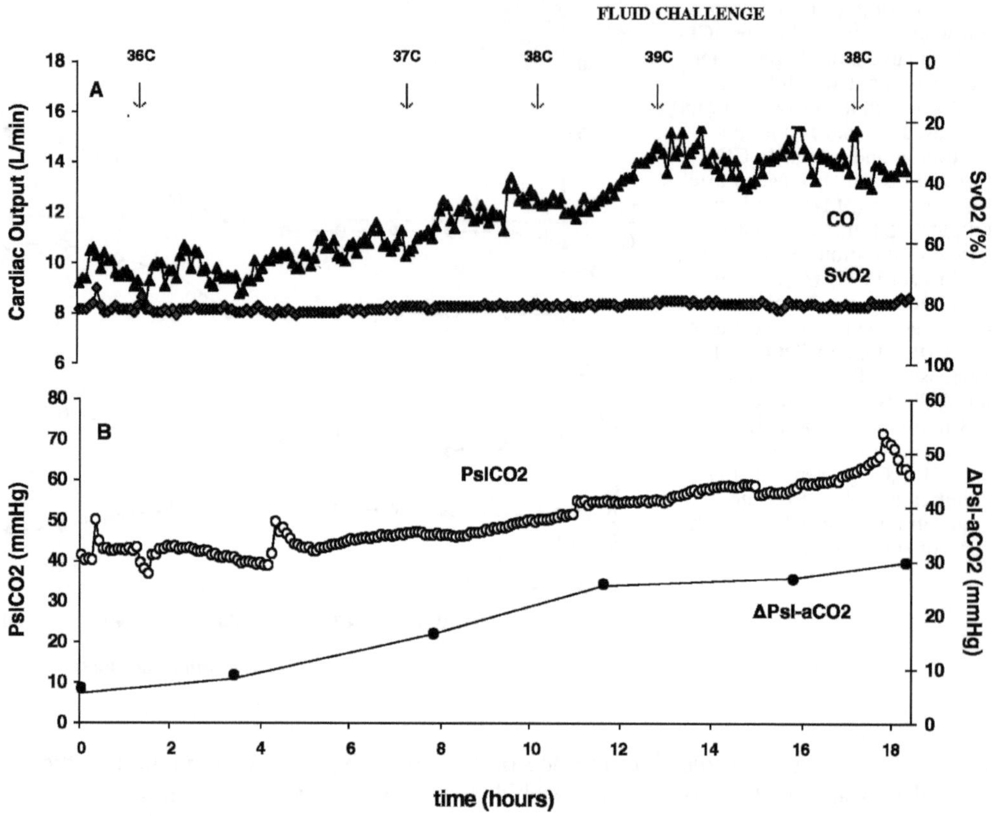

Fig. 2 Results from a 20-year-old man admitted to the ICU with fulminant hepatic failure and severe sepsis, showing a hyperdynamic status. **A** Cardiac output (*CO*) and mixed venous oxygen saturation (*SvO_2*) were recorded every 5 min. Note the progressive increase in CO and oral temperature (*arrows*) with a stable SvO_2. **B** Continuous sublingual PCO_2 ($P_{sl}CO_2$) monitoring and intermittent sublingual-arterial PCO_2 gradient ($\Delta P_{sl\text{-}a}CO_2$) measurement. Note that although CO increased, $P_{sl}CO_2$ and $\Delta P_{sl\text{-}a}CO_2$ also increased. Arterial lactate concentration was around 2 mmol/l and mean arterial pressure around 65–70 mmHg (no vasoactive agent) throughout the monitoring period. The clinical condition deteriorated in the hours after the end of the monitoring period progressing to septic shock (fungal in origin) and multiple organ failure. The patient died 2 days later

What is the behavior of sublingual partial pressure of carbon dioxide in hyperdynamic sepsis?

We have reported high values of $P_{sl}CO_2$ in hemodynamically stabilized septic shock patients [63, 64], even when cardiac output increased (Fig. 2). The most feasible explanation for increases in $\Delta P_{sl\text{-}a}CO_2$ despite increases in systemic blood flow is compromised microvascular blood flow in patients with sepsis [68–71], including in the sublingual mucosa [63, 72]. Low microvascular blood flow may occur despite high systemic blood flow due to shunts in "weak microcirculatory units" [73, 74] and this is mainly responsible for CO_2 accumulation and increases in $P_{sl}CO_2$ despite the presence of a high cardiac index. Distributive abnormalities of macrocirculatory and microcirculatory blood flow play a key role in the impairment of sepsis-related oxygen extraction [75] and, probably, also in tissue CO_2 accumulation. $P_{sl}CO_2$ seems to correlate well with the microcirculatory alterations reported in sepsis [63, 64], so it could be used as a reliable marker to quantify these alterations.

It is reasonable to speculate that in all types of shock, even in hyperdynamic sepsis, compromised blood flow and impairment in tissue perfusion are a common end point. Hence, tissue PCO_2 is expected to increase in all these situations, whatever the etiology or mechanism. However, dysoxia may occur despite maintained blood flow; adequate perfusion, although essential, is not always a guarantee of normal aerobic cell metabolism, especially in sepsis.

Should treatment be guided by gradients between sublingual partial pressure of carbon dioxide and arterial partial pressure of carbon dioxide?

No study exists on the efficacy of $\Delta P_{sl\text{-}a}CO_2$-guided therapy. A high value for $\Delta P_{sl\text{-}a}CO_2$ suggests a mismatch between blood flow (especially in the microcirculation) and oxygen demand in all types of shock, a situation that usually precedes the occurrence of dysoxia itself and multiple organ failure. However, care must be taken since the literature already has good examples of very promising monitoring techniques, such as pHi measurement, which, although useful as a prognostic index [76, 77], is still controversial as a therapeutic guide, having been shown to be beneficial in some studies [18, 78, 79], but not in others [80, 81]. Since interpretation of $\Delta P_{sl\text{-}a}CO_2$ is not always easy to achieve, the best approach at this moment is to analyze its value in conjunction with the traditional hemodynamic parameters in current use.

Conclusion

Sublingual capnometry has emerged in recent years as a promising technique for non-invasive monitoring of hemodynamic disturbances. Experimental and clinical studies have indicated that: (a) acute and severe reductions in blood flow are associated with significant PCO_2 elevation in virtually all tissues; (b) sublingual tissue is a potential site for measurement of PCO_2 non-invasively, which is the great advantage of this method; (c) P_aCO_2 must be taken into account when interpreting $P_{sl}CO_2$; (d) higher $P_{sl}CO_2$ values and, more specifically, higher $\Delta P_{sl\text{-}a}CO_2$ values correlate with altered sublingual microcirculatory blood flow and an increased risk of death in critically ill patients.

With our current knowledge, some questions and limitations are still present: (a) correct tissue PCO_2 interpretation is not always easy to achieve since some variables can potentially interfere with the measurement, even when it is made in the sublingual mucosa; (b) the sublingual mucosa may not be as susceptible to ischemia as the gastrointestinal tract, so that it may not be compromised so early in progressive shock states; (c) there may be differences in $P_{sl}CO_2$ kinetics in different types of shock; (d) the absence of a "gold standard" monitor of dysoxia to compare with; (e) no well-established normal and pathological $\Delta P_{sl\text{-}a}CO_2$ values; and (f) it is still uncertain if correction of $\Delta P_{sl\text{-}a}CO_2$ improves prognosis. Nevertheless, since $P_{sl}CO_2$ measurement is technically simple and non-invasive, new studies should be encouraged to define the precise role of sublingual PCO_2 measurement in the management of critically ill patients.

References

1. Walley KR, Wood LDH (1992) Shock. In: Hall JB, Schmidt GA, Wood LDH (eds) Principals of critical care. McGraw-Hill, New York, pp 1393–1416
2. Shoemaker WC, Appel PL, Kram HB (1988) Tissue oxygen debt as a determinant of lethal and nonlethal postoperative organ failure. Crit Care Med 16:1117–1120
3. Beal AL, Cerra FB (1994) Multiple organ failure in the 1990s. JAMA 271:226–233
4. Deitch EA (1992) Multiple organ failure: pathophysiology and potential future therapy. Ann Surg 216:117–134
5. Consensus conference (1996) Tissue hypoxia: how to detect, how to correct, how to prevent. Am J Respir Crit Care Med 154:1573–1578
6. Russell JA, Phang PT (1994) The oxygen delivery/consumption controversy: approaches to management of the critically ill. Am J Respir Crit Care Med 149:533–537
7. Marik PE, Bankov A (2003) Sublingual capnometry versus traditional markers of tissue oxygenation in critically ill patients. Crit Care Med 31:818–822
8. Marik PE, Varon J (1998) The hemodynamic derangements in sepsis: implications for treatment strategies. Chest 114:854–860
9. Marik PE (1993) Gastric intramucosal pH. A better predictor of multiorgan dysfunction syndrome and death than oxygen-derived variables in patients with sepsis. Chest 104:225–229
10. Boyd KD, Thomas SJ, Gold J, Boyd AD (1983) A prospective study of complications of pulmonary artery catheterizations in 500 consecutive patients. Chest 84:245–249
11. Rello J, Coll P, Net A, Prats G (1993) Infection of pulmonary artery catheters. Epidemiologic characteristics and multivariate analysis of risk factors. Chest 103:132–136
12. Ramsey SD, Saint S, Sullivan SD, Dey L, Kelley K, Bowdle A (2000) Clinical and economic effects of pulmonary artery catheterization in nonemergent coronary artery bypass graft surgery. J Cardiothorac Vasc Anesth 14:113–118
13. Dalen JE, Bone RC (1996) Is it time to pull the pulmonary catheter? JAMA 276:916–918
14. Williams G, Grounds M, Rhodes A (2002) Pulmonary artery catheter. Curr Opin Crit Care 8:251–256
15. De Backer D (2003) Lactic acidosis. Intensive Care Med 29:699–702
16. Hotchkiss RS, Karl IE (1992) Reevaluation of the role of cellular hypoxia and bioenergetic failure in sepsis. JAMA 267:1503–1510
17. Fiddian-Green RG, Baker S (1987) Predictive value of the stomach wall pH for complications after cardiac operations: comparison with other monitoring. Crit Care Med 15:153–156
18. Gutierrez G, Palizas F, Doglio G, Wainsztein N, Gallesio A, Pacin J, Dubin A, Schiavi E, Jorge M, Pusajo J, Klein F, San Roman E, Dorfman B, Shottlender J, Giniger R (1992) Gastric intramucosal pH as a therapeutic index of tissue oxygenation in critically ill patients. Lancet 339:195–199
19. Johnson BA, Weil MH (1991) Redefining ischemia due to circulatory failure as dual defects of oxygen deficits and of carbon dioxide excesses. Crit Care Med 19:1432–1438
20. Kivilaakso E, Ahonen J, Aronsen KF, Hockerstedt K, Kalima T, Lempinen M, Suoranta H, Vernerson E (1982) Gastric blood flow, tissue gas tension and microvascular changes during hemorrhage-induced stress ulceration in the pig. Am J Surg 143:322–330
21. Hurley R, Chapman MV, Mythen MG (2000) Current status of gastrointestinal tonometry. Curr Opin Crit Care 6:130–135
22. Levy B, Gawalkiewicz P, Vallet B, Briancon S, Nace L, Bollaert PE (2003) Gastric capnometry with air-automated tonometry predicts outcome in critically ill patients. Crit Care Med 31:474–480
23. Pastores SM, Katz DP, Kvetan V (1996) Splanchnic ischemia and gut mucosal injury in sepsis and the multiple organ dysfunction syndrome. Am J Gastroenterol 91:1697–1710
24. Fink MP (1993) Adequacy of gut oxygenation in endotoxemia and sepsis. Crit Care Med 21:S4–S8
25. Antonsson JB, Boyle CC, Kruithoff KL, Wang HL, Sacristan E, Rothschild HR, Fink MP (1990) Validation of tonometric measurement of gut intramural pH during endotoxemia and mesenteric occlusion in pigs. Am J Physiol 259:G519–G523
26. Schlichtig R, Mehta N, Gayowski TJ (1996) Tissue-arterial PCO_2 difference is a better marker of ischemia than intramural pH (pHi) or arterial pH-pHi difference. J Crit Care 11:51–56

27. Salzman AL, Strong KE, Wang H, Wollert PS, VanderMeer TJ, Fink MP (1994) Intraluminal balloonless air tonometry: a new method for determination of gastrointestinal mucosal carbon dioxide tension. Crit Care Med 1:126–134
28. Guzman JA, Kruse JA (1996) Development and validation of a technique for continuous monitoring of gastric intramucosal pH. Am J Respir Crit Care Med 153:694–700
29. Teboul JL, Michard F, Richard C (1996) Critical analysis of venoarterial CO_2 gradient as a marker of tissue hypoxia. In: Vincent JL, (ed) Yearbook of intensive care and emergency medicine. Springer, Heidelberg, pp 296–307
30. Neviere R, Chagnon JL, Teboul JL, Vallet B, Wattel F (2002) Small intestine intramucosal $PCO_{(2)}$ and microvascular blood flow during hypoxic and ischemic hypoxia. Crit Care Med 30:379–384
31. Vallet B, Teboul JL, Cain S, Curtis S (2000) Venoarterial $CO_{(2)}$ difference during regional ischemic or hypoxic hypoxia. J Appl Physiol 89:1317–1321
32. Schlichtig R, Heard SO (1999) Sublingual PCO_2 measurement: the nitroglycerin of monitoring? Crit Care Med 27:1380–1381
33. Schlichtig R, Bowles SA (1994) Distinguishing between aerobic and anaerobic appearance of dissolved CO_2 in intestine during low flow. J Appl Physiol 76:2443–2451
34. Rozenfeld RA, Dishart MK, Tonnessen TI, Schlichtig R (1996) Methods for detecting local intestinal ischemic anaerobic metabolic acidosis by PCO_2. J Appl Physiol 81:1834–1842
35. Raza O, Schlichtig R (2000) Metabolic component of intestinal $PCO_{(2)}$ during dysoxia. J Appl Physiol 89:2422–2429
36. Randall HM, Cohen JJ (1966) Anaerobic CO_2 production by dog kidney in vitro. Am J Physiol 211:493–505
37. Mathias DW, Clifford PS, Klopfenstein HS (1988) Mixed venous blood gases are superior to arterial blood gases in assessing acid-base status and oxygenation during acute cardiac tamponade in dogs. J Clin Invest 82:833–838
38. Groeneveld AB, Vermeij CG, Thijs LG (1991) Arterial and mixed venous blood acid-base balance during hypoperfusion with incremental positive end-expiratory pressure in the pig. Anesth Analg 73:576–582
39. Zhang H, Vincent JL (1993) Arteriovenous differences in PCO_2 and pH are good indicators of critical hypoperfusion. Am Rev Respir Dis 148:867–871
40. Jakob SM, Kosonen P, Ruokonen E, Parviainen I, Takala J (1999) The Haldane effect—an alternative explanation for increasing gastric mucosal PCO_2 gradients? Br J Anaesth 83:740–746
41. Hurley R, Mythen MG (2000) The Haldane effect—an explanation for increasing gastric mucosal PCO_2 gradients? Br J Anaesth 85:167–169
42. De Backer D, Creteur J, Vincent JL (2000) The Haldane effect—an explanation for increasing gastric mucosal PCO_2 gradients? Br J Anaesth 85:169
43. Walley KR, Friesen BP, Humer MF, Phang PT (1998) Small bowel tonometry is more accurate than gastric tonometry in detecting gut ischemia. J Appl Physiol 85:1770–1777
44. Fiddian-Green RG, Amelin PM, Herrmann JB, Arous E, Cutler BS, Schiedler M, Wheeler HB, Baker S (1986) Prediction of the development of sigmoid ischemia on the day of aortic operations. Indirect measurements of intramural pH in the colon. Arch Surg 121:654–660
45. Schiedler MG, Cutler BS, Fiddian-Green RG (1987) Sigmoid intramural pH for prediction of ischemic colitis during aortic surgery. A comparison with risk factors and inferior mesenteric artery stump pressures. Arch Surg 122:881–886
46. Klok T, Moll FL, Leusink JA, Theunissen DJ, Gerrits CM, Keijer C, J (1996) The relationship between sigmoidal intramucosal pH and intestinal arterial occlusion during aortic reconstructive surgery. Eur J Vasc Endovasc Surg 11:304–307
47. Sato Y, Weil MH, Tang W, Sun S, Xie J, Bisera J, Hosaka H (1997) Esophageal PCO_2 as a monitor of perfusion failure during hemorrhagic shock. J Appl Physiol 82:558–562
48. Van Hulst RA, Hasan D, Lachmann B (2002) Intracranial pressure, brain PCO_2, PO_2 and pH during hypo- and hyperventilation at constant mean airway pressure in pigs. Intensive Care Med 28:68–73
49. Lang JD Jr, Evans DJ, deFigueiredo LP, Hays S, Mathru M, Kramer GC (1999) A novel approach to monitor tissue perfusion: bladder mucosal PCO_2, PO_2 and pHi during ischemia and reperfusion. J Crit Care 14:93–98
50. Kvarstein G, Mirtaheri P, Tonnessen TI (2004) Detection of ischemia by PCO_2 before adenosine triphosphate declines in skeletal muscle. Crit Care Med 32:232–237
51. Koga I, Stiernstrom H, Christiansson L, Wiklund L (2000) Intraperitoneal tonometry for detection of regional enteric ischaemia. Acta Anaesthesiol Scand 44:985–990
52. Nakagawa Y, Weil MH, Tang W, Sun S, Yamaguchi H, Jin X, Bisera J (1998) Sublingual capnometry for diagnosis and quantitation of circulatory shock. Am J Respir Crit Care Med 157:1838–1843
53. Povoas HP, Weil MH, Tang W, Moran B, Kamohara T, Bisera J (2000) Comparisons between sublingual and gastric tonometry during hemorrhagic shock. Chest 118:1127–1132
54. Pernat A, Weil MH, Tang W, Yamaguchi H, Pernat AM, Sun S, Bisera J (1999) Effects of hyper- and hypoventilation on gastric and sublingual $PCO_{(2)}$. J Appl Physiol 87:933–937
55. Weil MH, Nakagawa Y, Tang W, Sato Y, Ercoli F, Finegan R, Grayman G, Bisera J (1999) Sublingual capnometry: a new noninvasive measurement for diagnosis and quantitation of severity of circulatory shock. Crit Care Med 27:1225–1229
56. Marik PE (2001) Sublingual capnography: a clinical validation study. Chest 120:923–927
57. Rackow EC, O'Neil P, Astiz ME, Carpati CM (2001) Sublingual capnometry and indexes of tissue perfusion in patients with circulatory failure. Chest 120:1633–1638
58. Jin X, Weil MH, Sun S, Tang W, Bisera J, Mason EJ (1998) Decreases in organ blood flows associated with increases in sublingual PCO_2 during hemorrhagic shock. J Appl Physiol 85:2360–2364
59. Creteur J, De Backer D, Vincent JL (1997) Monitoring of gastric mucosal PCO_2 by gas tonometry: in vitro and in vivo validation studies. Anesthesiology 87:504–510
60. Grum CM, Fiddian Green RG, Pittenger GL, Grant BJ, Rothman ED, Dantzker DR (1984) Adequacy of tissue oxygenation in intact dog intestine. J Appl Physiol 56:1065–1069
61. VanderMeer TJ, Wang H, Fink MP (1995) Endotoxemia causes ileal mucosal acidosis in the absence of mucosal hypoxia in a normodynamic porcine model of septic shock. Crit Care Med 23:1217–1226
62. Bernardin G, Lucas P, Hyvernat H, Deloffre P, Mattei M (1999) Influence of alveolar ventilation changes on calculated gastric intramucosal pH and gastric-arterial PCO_2 difference. Intensive Care Med 25:269–273
63. De Backer D, Creteur J, Dubois MJ (2003) Microvascular alterations in patients with circulatory failure. In: Vincent JL (ed) Yearbook of intensive care and emergency medicine. Springer, Heidelberg, pp 535–544

64. Creteur J, De Backer D, Sakr Y, Koch M, Vincent JL (2003) Determinant of sublingual PCO_2 in patients with septic shock (abstract). Crit Care Med 31:A116
65. Dantzker DR (1993) The gastrointestinal tract: the canary of the body? JAMA 270:1247–1248
66. Ackland G, Grocott MP, Mythen MG (2000) Understanding gastrointestinal perfusion in critical care: so near and yet so far. Crit Care 4:269–281
67. Deitch EA (1998) Animal models of sepsis and shock: a review and lessons learned. Shock 9:1–11
68. Cryer HM, Garrison RN, Kaebnick HW, Harris PD, Flint LM (1987) Skeletal microcirculatory responses to hyperdynamic Escherichia coli sepsis in unanesthetized rats. Arch Surg 122:86–92
69. Lam C, Tyml K, Martin C, Sibbald W (1994) Microvascular perfusion is impaired in a rat model of normotensive sepsis. J Clin Invest 94:2077–2083
70. Piper RD, Pitt-Hyde M, Li F, Sibbald WJ, Potter RF (1996) Microcirculatory changes in rat skeletal muscle in sepsis. Am J Respir Crit Care Med 154:931–937
71. Farquhar I, Martin CM, Lam C, Potter R, Ellis CG, Sibbald WJ (1996) Decreased capillary density in vivo in bowel mucosa of rats with normotensive sepsis. J Surg Res 61:190–196
72. De Backer D, Creteur J, Preiser JC, Dubois MJ, Vincent JL (2002) Microvascular blood flow is altered in patients with sepsis. Am J Respir Crit Care Med 166:98–104
73. Ince C, Sinaasappel M (1999) Microcirculatory oxygenation and shunting in sepsis and shock. Crit Care Med 27:1369–1377
74. Zuurbier CJ, van Iterson M, Ince C (1999) Functional heterogeneity of oxygen supply-consumption ratio in the heart. Cardiovasc Res 44:488–497
75. Astiz ME, Rackow EC, Weil MH (1986) Oxygen delivery and utilization during rapidly fatal septic shock in rats. Circ Shock 20:281–290
76. Gutierrez G, Oksenholt RL (1996) Prognostic value of gastric mucosal pH. Réan Urg 5:238–242
77. Doglio GR, Pusajo JF, Egurrola MA, Bonfigli GC, Parra C, Vetere L, Hernandez MS, Fernandez S, Palizas F, Gutierrez G (1991) Gastric mucosal pH as a prognostic index of mortality in critically ill patients. Crit Care Med 19:1037–1040
78. Ivatury RR, Simon RJ, Islam S, Fueg A, Rohman M, Stahl WM (1996) A prospective randomized study of end points of resuscitation after major trauma: global oxygen transport indices versus organ-specific gastric mucosal pH. J Am Coll Surg 183:145–154
79. Ivatury RR, Simon RJ, Havriliak D, Garcia C, Greenbarg J, Stahl WM (1995) Gastric mucosal pH and oxygen delivery and oxygen consumption indices in the assessment of adequacy of resuscitation after trauma: a prospective, randomized study. J Trauma 39:128–134
80. Pargger H, Hampl KF, Christen P, Staender S, Scheidegger D (1998) Gastric intramucosal pH-guided therapy in patients after elective repair of infrarenal abdominal aneurysms: is it beneficial? Intensive Care Med 24:769–776
81. Gomersall CD, Joynt GM, Freebairn RC, Hung V, Buckley TA, Oh TE (2000) Resuscitation of critically ill patients based on the results of gastric tonometry: a prospective, randomized, controlled trial. Crit Care Med 28:607–614

Alexandre Lima
Jan Bakker

Noninvasive monitoring of peripheral perfusion

Abstract *Background:* Early hemodynamic assessment of global parameters in critically ill patients fails to provide adequate information on tissue perfusion. It requires invasive monitoring and may represent a late intervention initiated mainly in the intensive care unit. Noninvasive monitoring of peripheral perfusion can be a complementary approach that allows very early application throughout the hospital. In addition, as peripheral tissues are sensitive to alterations in perfusion, monitoring of the periphery could be an early marker of tissue hypoperfusion. This review discusses noninvasive methods for monitoring perfusion in peripheral tissues based on clinical signs, body temperature gradient, optical monitoring, transcutaneous oximetry, and sublingual capnometry. *Discussion:* Clinical signs of poor peripheral perfusion consist of a cold, pale, clammy, and mottled skin, associated with an increase in capillary refill time. The temperature gradients peripheral-to-ambient, central-to-peripheral and forearm-to-fingertip skin are validated methods to estimate dynamic variations in skin blood flow. Commonly used optical methods for peripheral monitoring are perfusion index, near-infrared spectroscopy, laser Doppler flowmetry and orthogonal polarization spectroscopy. Continuous noninvasive transcutaneous measurement of oxygen and carbon dioxide tensions can be used to estimate cutaneous blood flow. Sublingual capnometry is a noninvasive alternative for gastric tonometry.

Keywords Body temperature gradient · Hemodynamic assessment · Noninvasive monitoring · Peripheral tissue perfusion · Sublingual capnometry · Transcutaneous oximetry

This study was in part supported by materials provided by Hutchinson Technology and a grant from Philips USA. Both authors received a grant US $12,000 from Philips USA and $10,000 from Hutchinson Technology.

Introduction

An important goal of hemodynamic monitoring is the early detection of inadequate tissue perfusion and oxygenation to institute prompt therapy and guide resuscitation, avoiding organ damage. In clinical practice tissue oxygenation is frequently assessed by using conventional global measurements such as blood pressure, oxygen derived variables, and blood lactate levels. However, the assessment of global hemodynamic parameters fails to reflect increased blood lactate levels, the imbalance between oxygen demand and oxygen supply, or the status of the microcirculation [1, 2, 3]. In addition, it often requires invasive monitoring techniques that usually limit early initiation, typically after the patient has been admitted to the intensive care unit (ICU).

To address these limitations there have been many attempts to perform measurements of blood flow and oxygenation in peripheral tissues [4, 5]. In circulatory failure blood flow is diverted from the less important tissues (skin, subcutaneous, muscle, gastrointestinal tract) to vital organs (heart, brain, kidneys). Thus monitoring perfusion in these less vital tissues could be an early marker of vital tissue hypoperfusion. Second, the assess-

M.R. Pinsky et al. (eds.), *Applied Physiology in Intensive Care Medicine 2: Physiological Reviews and Editorials*,
DOI 10.1007/978-3-642-28233-1_4, © Springer-Verlag Berlin Heidelberg 2012

ment of perfusion in peripheral tissues is more easily obtainable using noninvasive monitoring techniques, thus facilitating earlier initiation.

Monitoring of peripheral perfusion and oxygenation does not need any intravascular catheter, transesophageal probe insertion, blood component analysis or penetration of the skin. Also, it can be performed directly (clinical evaluation and body temperature gradient) or by signal processing (optical monitoring; transcutaneous oximetry; sublingual capnometry). This review discusses several available noninvasive methods to monitor peripheral perfusion and oxygenation (Table 1).

Clinical assessment

During circulatory failure the global decrease in oxygen supply and redistribution of blood flow caused by increased vasoconstriction results in decreased perfusion in organ systems. Some organs, including the brain, heart, and kidney, have vasomotor autoregulation that maintains blood flow in low blood pressure states. However, the cutaneous circulation is deprived of autoregulation, and the sympathetic neurohumoral response predominates, resulting in a decrease in skin perfusion and temperature in these conditions. Skin temperature is measured using the dorsal surface of the examiner hands or fingers because these areas are most sensitive to temperature perception. Patients are considered to have cool extremities if all examined extremities are cool to the examiner, or only the lower extremities are cool despite warm upper extremities, in the absence of peripheral vascular occlusive disease. Clinical signs of poor peripheral perfusion consist of a cold, pale, clammy, and mottled skin, associated with an increase in capillary refill time. In particular, skin temperature and capillary refill time have been advocated as a measure of peripheral perfusion [6, 7, 8, 9, 10, 11].

Capillary refill time (CRT) has been introduced into the assessment of trauma, and a value less than 2 s is considered normal [12]. This is based on the assumption that a delayed return of a normal color after emptying the capillary bed by compression is due to decreased peripheral perfusion. CRT has been validated as a measure of peripheral perfusion with significant variation in children and adults. Schriger and Baraff [8] in a study on a normal population reported that CRT varied with age and sex. It was found that a CRT of 2 s was a normal value for most young children and young adults, but the lowest CRT was substantially higher in healthy women (2.9 s) and in the elderly (4.5 s). Using these normal variations it was further shown that a prolonged CRT did not predict a 450-ml blood loss in adult blood donors or hypovolemic states in patients admitted to the emergency room [10]. Several clinical studies have reported a poor correlation between CRT, heart rate, blood pressure, and cardiac output [6, 7, 10]. However, prolonged CRT in pediatric

Table 1 Measurement methods to study peripheral perfusion (*CRT* capillary refill time, *dTc-p* temperature gradient central-to-peripheral, *dTp-a* temperature gradient peripheral-to-ambient, *Tskin-diff* forearm-to-fingertip skin-temperature gradient, *PFI* peripheral perfusion index, *NIRS* Near-infrared spectroscopy, *Hb* deoxygenated hemoglobin, *HbO₂* oxygenated hemoglobin, *HbT* total hemoglobin, *StO₂* tissue oxygen saturation, *Cytaa₃* cytochrome *aa₃*, *OPS* orthogonal polarization spectroscopy, *FCD* functional capillary density, *LDF* Laser Doppler flowmetry, *PtcO₂* oxygen partial pressure in the skin, *PtcCO₂* carbon dioxide partial pressure in the skin, *Tc-index* transcutaneous oxygen index, *PslCO₂* sublingual tissue PCO_2, *Psl-aCO₂* gradient between $PslCO_2$ and arterial PCO_2)

Method	Variable	Advantage	Limitations
Clinical assessment	Warmth and coolness skin CRT	Depends only on physical examination; valuable adjunct for hemodynamic monitoring in circulatory shock	Difficult interpretation in distributive shock
Body temperature gradient	dTc-p dTp-a Tskin-diff	Validated method to estimate dynamic variations in skin blood flow	At least two temperature probes required; does not reflect the variations in real time
Pulse oximetry	PFI	Easily obtainable; reflect real time changes in peripheral blood flow	Not accurate during patient motion
NIRS	Hb, HbO_2, and HbT variations StO_2 $Cytaa_3$	Assessment of oxygenation in all vascular compartments; can be applied to measure regional blood flow and oxygen consumption	Requires specific software to display the variables
OPS	FCD	Direct visualization of the microcirculation	Observer-related bias; semiquantitative measure of perfusion
LDF	Microvascular blood flow	Useful method to evaluate endothelium-dependent vascular responses	Small sampling volume for cutaneous blood flow measurement; does not reflect heterogeneity of blood flow
Transcutaneous oximetry	$PtcO_2/PtcCO_2$ Tc-index	Direct measurement of $PtcO_2/PtcCO_2$; early detection of peripheral hypoperfusion	Necessity to frequently change the sensor position; requires blood gas analysis
Sublingual capnometry	$PslCO_2$ $Psl\text{-}aCO_2$	Direct measurement of tissue PCO_2 noninvasively	Requires blood gas analysis to obtain $PaCO_2$; normal and pathological values not yet defined

patients has been found to be a good predictor of dehydration, reduced stroke volume, and increased blood lactate levels [6, 11]. In adult patients following cardiac surgery no significant relationship between cardiac index and CRT was found during the first 8 h following ICU admission [7].

Distal extremity skin temperature has also been related to the adequacy of the circulation. Kaplan et al. [9] compared distal extremity skin temperature (evaluated by subjective physical examination) with biochemical and hemodynamic markers of hypoperfusion in adult ICU patients. This study found that patients with cold periphery (including septic patients) had lower cardiac output and higher blood lactate levels as a marker of more severe tissue hypoxia. In another study Hasdai et al. [13] showed the importance of the physical examination in determining the prognosis of patients with cardiogenic shock. This study reported the presence of a cold and clammy skin to be an independent predictor of 30-day mortality in patients with cardiogenic shock complicating acute myocardial infarction.

The findings of these studies show that skin temperature together with CRT are a valuable adjunct in hemodynamic monitoring during circulatory shock, and should be the first approach to assess critically ill patient. Not much is known about the clinical applicability of these variables after the patient has been admitted to the intensive care unit [14].

Temperature gradients

Since Joly and Weil [15] and Ibsen [16] studied the toe temperature as an indicator of the circulatory shock, body temperature gradients have been used as a parameter of peripheral perfusion. In the presence of a constant environmental temperature a change in the skin temperature is the result of a change in skin blood flow [17]. The temperature gradients peripheral-to-ambient (dTp-a) and central-to-peripheral (dTc-p) can better reflect cutaneous blood flow than the skin temperature itself. Considering a constant environment condition, dTp-a decreases and dTc-p increases during vasoconstriction. The peripheral skin temperature is measured using a regular temperature probe attached to the ventral face of the great toe. This site is more convenient for peripheral temperature measurement because of the negligible local heat production and the distal location from other monitoring devices [18]. The concept of the dTc-p is based on the transfer of heat from the body core to the skin. The heat conduction to the skin by the blood is also controlled by the degree of vasoconstriction of the arterioles and arteriovenous anastomoses. High blood flow causes heat to be conducted from the core to the skin, whereas reduction in blood flow decreases the heat conduction from the core. During vasoconstriction the temperature of the skin falls and the heat conduction from the core decreases, and therefore the central temperature rises and the dTc-p increases. A gradient of 3–7°C occurs in patients with stable hemodynamics [19]. Hypothermia, cold ambient temperature (<20°C) [20], and vasodilatory shock limits the use of dTc-p as an estimate of peripheral perfusion. Forearm-to-fingertip skin-temperature gradient (Tskin-diff) has also been used as an index of peripheral circulation to identify the initiation of thermoregulatory vasoconstriction in patients following surgery [21]. Fingertip temperature is measured with the temperature probe attached to the ventral face of the finger. The use of Tskin-diff is based on assumption that the reference temperature is a skin site exposed to the same ambient temperature as the fingertip. It has been applied in conditions where an ambient temperature is not stable, such as in patients undergoing surgery [21, 22, 23]. A change in ambient temperature therefore affects similarly forearm and fingertip temperature, producing little influence in the gradient. Basically, when vasoconstriction decreases fingertip blood flow, finger skin temperature decreases, and Tskin-diff increases. Experimental studies have suggested a Tskin-diff threshold of 0°C for the initiation of vasoconstriction, and a threshold of 4°C for severe vasoconstriction in anesthetized patients [22, 23].

The body temperature gradient was first applied to assess patients with circulatory shock and to differentiate central heat retention caused by fever from peripheral vasoconstriction [15, 16, 24]. A number of studies have examined the correlation between body temperature gradient and global hemodynamic variables in hypovolemic, septic and cardiogenic shock, but these have produced conflicting results [15, 25, 26, 27, 28, 29, 30, 31]. Henning et al. [28] studied dTp-a in patients with circulatory failure associated with hypovolemia and low cardiac output. An increase in dTp-a to more than 4–6°C over 12 h was observed in survivors, and a good relationship between the lowest dTp-a and the highest blood lactate levels was found in hypovolemic patients at time of admission. In assessing the potential value of dopamine as a therapeutic agent to treat circulatory shock Ruiz et al. [25] showed that survival is associated with an increase in dTp-a of more than 2°C, and that dTp-a is correlated to increases in cardiac output and a reduction in blood lactate levels. In examining the value of dTp-a for assessing peripheral perfusion in cardiogenic shock Vincent et al. [27] found that a cardiac index below 1.8 l/min^{-1} m^{-2} is associated with a decrease in dTp-a below 5°C, and that the increase in dTp-a occurs earlier than the increase in skin oxygen partial pressure during recovery; this correlation was not found in septic shock. No relationship has been observed between dTc-p and cardiac output in adults with diverse causes of shock [31] or in children after open heart surgery [26, 29, 30]. One reason for the inaccurate relationship between body temperature gradient and global hemodynamic parameters could be related to an unstable environment, as skin temperature depends also on ambient temperature, and the thermoregulatory response is suppressed in anesthetized patients [32]. In addition, global hemodynamic parameters may not be sensitive enough to reflect changes in peripheral blood flow in critically ill patients [33, 34]. Tskin-diff may be an alternative, but its use in these conditions has not yet been defined.

Optical monitoring

Optical methods apply light with different wave lengths directly to tissue components using the scattering characteristics of tissue to assess various states of these tissues [35]. At physiological concentrations the molecules that absorb most light are hemoglobin, myoglobin, cytochrome, melanins, carotenes, and bilirrubin. These substances can be quantified and measured in intact tissues using simple optical methods. The assessment of tissue oxygenation is based on the specific absorption spectrum of oxygenated hemoglobin (HbO_2), deoxygenated hemoglobin (Hb) and cytochrome *aa₃* (cytaa₃). Commonly used optical methods for peripheral monitoring are perfusion index, near-infrared spectroscopy, laser-Doppler flowmetry, and orthogonal polarization spectral.

Peripheral perfusion index

The peripheral perfusion index (PFI) is derived from the photoeletric plesthysmographic signal of pulse oximetry and has been used as a noninvasive measure of peripheral perfusion in critically ill patients [36]. Pulse oximetry is a monitoring technique used in probably every trauma, critically ill and surgical patient. The principle of pulse oximetry is based on two light sources with different wavelengths (660 nm and 940 nm) emitted through the cutaneous vascular bed of a finger or earlobe. The Hb absorbs more light at 660 nm and HbO_2 absorbs more light at 940 nm. A detector at the far side measures the intensity of the transmitted light at each wavelength, and the oxygen saturation is derived by the ratio between the red light (660 nm) and the infrared light (940 nm) absorbed. As other tissues also absorb light, such as connective tissue, bone, and venous blood, the pulse oximetry distinguishes the pulsatile component of arterial blood from the nonpulsatile component of other tissues. Using a two-wavelength system the nonpulsatile component is then discarded, and the pulsatile component is used to calculate the arterial oxygen saturation. The overall hemoglobin concentration can be determined by a third wavelength at 800 nm, with a spectrum that resembles that of both Hb and HbO_2. The resulting variation in intensity of this light can be used to determine the variation in arterial blood volume (pulsatile component). The PFI is calculated as the ratio between the pulsatile component (arterial compartment) and the nonpulsatile component (other tissues) of the light reaching the detector of the pulse oximetry, and it is calculated independently of the patient's oxygen saturation (Fig. 1). A peripheral perfusion alteration is accompanied by variation in the pulsatile component, and because the nonpulsatile component does not change, the ratio changes. As a result the value displayed on the monitor reflects changes in peripheral perfusion.

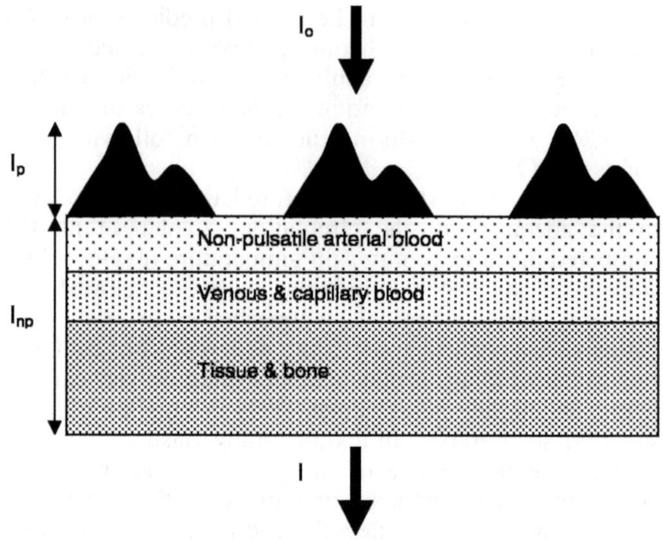

Fig. 1 The pulsation of arterial blood causes a pulsating volume variation. Peripheral perfusion index (*PFI*) is calculated as the ratio between the arterial pulsatile component (I_P) and the nonpulsatile component (I_{NP}). I_O Source light intensity; *I* light intensity at the detector

Studies with body temperature gradient suggest that PFI can be a direct indicator of peripheral perfusion. A PFI of 1.4 has been found to be correlated best with hypoperfusion in critically ill patients using normal values in healthy adults [36]. A good relationship between Tskin-diff and PFI is observed in anesthetized patients to identify the initiation of thermoregulatory vasoconstriction [37]. The PFI reflects changes in dTc-p and Tskin-diff and therefore vascular reactivity in adult critically ill patients [36, 38]. Another study has shown that PFI can be used to predict severity of illness in neonates, with a cutoff value of1.24 [39]. The inclusion of PFI into the pulse oximetry signal is a recent advance in clinical monitoring. However, more studies are needed to define its clinical utility.

Near-infrared spectroscopy

Near-infrared spectroscopy (NIRS) offers a technique for continuous, noninvasive, bedside monitoring of tissue

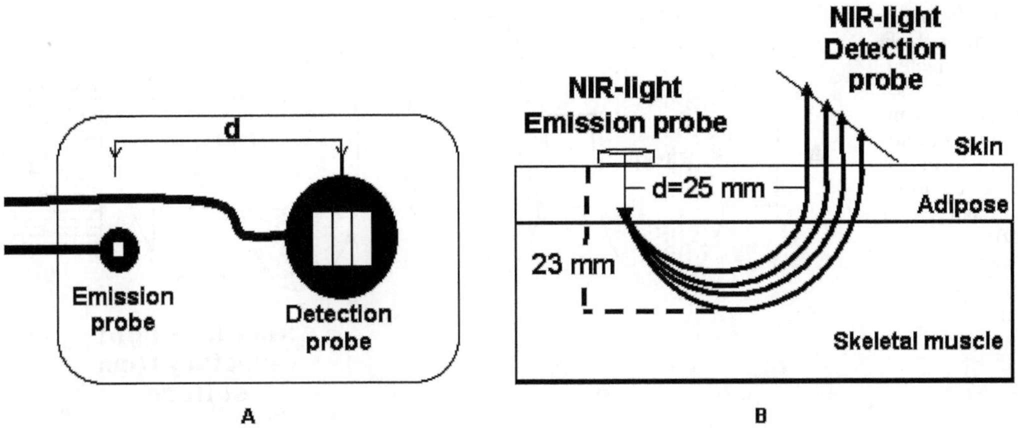

Fig. 2 **A** Diagram of a distal tip of the NIRS optical cable. **B** With 25 mm spacing (*d*) between emission and detection probes, approx. 95% of the detected optical signal is from 23 mm of tissue penetration

oxygenation. As with pulse oximetry, NIRS uses the principles of light transmission and absorption to measure the concentrations of hemoglobin, oxygen saturation (StO_2), and cytaa$_3$ noninvasively in tissues. NIRS has a greater tissue penetration than pulse oximetry and provides a global assessment of oxygenation in all vascular compartments (arterial, venous, and capillary). Tissue penetration is directly related to the spacing between illumination and detection fibers. At 25 mm spacing approx. 95% of the detected optical signal is from a depth of 0 to 23 mm (Fig. 2). NIRS has been used to assess forearm skeletal muscle oxygenation during induced reactive hyperemia in healthy adults and produces reproducible measurements of tissue oxygenation during both arterial and venous occlusive events [40]. Using the venous and arterial occlusion methods NIRS can be applied to measure regional blood flow and oxygen consumption by following the rate of HbO_2 and Hb changes [40, 41, 42]. In the venous occlusion method a pneumatic cuff is inflated to a pressure of approx. 50 mmHg. Such a pressure blocks venous occlusion but does not impede arterial inflow. As a result venous blood volume and pressure increase. NIRS can reflect this change by an increase in HbO_2, Hb, and total hemoglobin. In arterial occlusion method, the pneumatic cuff is inflated to a pressure of approx. 30 mmHg greater than systolic pressure. Such a pressure blocks both venous outflow and arterial inflow. Depletion of local available O_2 is monitored by NIRS as a decrease in HbO_2 and a simultaneous increase in Hb, whereas total Hb remains constant. After release of the occluding cuff a hyperemic response is observed (Fig. 3). Blood volume increases rapidly, resulting in an increase in HbO_2 and a quick washout of Hb. In addition to blood flow and evaluation of HbO_2 and Hb changes, NIRS can assess cytaa$_3$ redox state. Cytaa$_3$ is the final receptor in the oxygen transport chain that reacts with oxygen to form water, and approx. 90% of cellular energy is derived from this reaction. Cytaa$_3$ remains in a reduced state

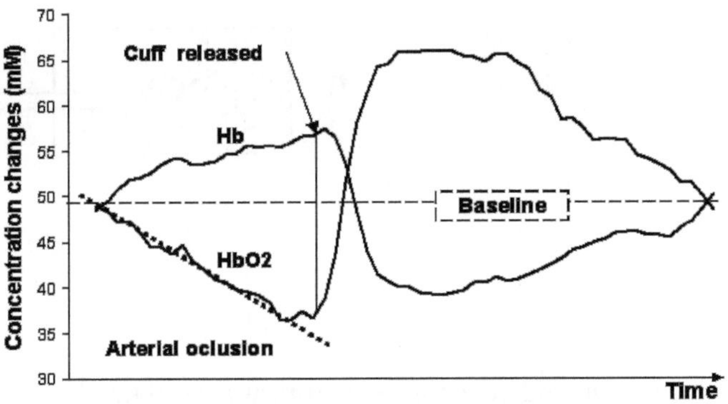

Fig. 3 Quantitative NIRS measurements during arterial occlusion. After release of the occluding cuff blood volume increases rapidly, resulting in an increase in HbO_2 and a quick washout of Hb, followed by a hyperemic response. Oxygen consumption is calculated as the rate of decrease in HbO_2 (*dotted line*)

during hypoxemia. The absorption spectrum of cytaa$_3$ in its reduced state shows a weak peak at 70 nm, whereas the oxygenated form does not. Therefore monitoring changes in its redox state can provide a measure of the adequacy of oxidative metabolism. Despite the potential clinical applications of NIRS, some limitations still exist. The contribution of the cytaa$_3$ signal is small, and its interpretation remains controversial, requiring more rigorous development [43]. There is no a gold standard to which NIRS data can be directly compared, and one of the reasons is that a variety of NIRS equipment is commercially available with different working systems.

In both small- and large-animal models of hemorrhagic shock and resuscitation NIRS has demonstrated sensitivity in detecting skeletal muscle and visceral ischemia [44, 45, 46, 47]. As a noninvasive measure of peripheral perfusion NIRS has been applied in superficial muscles (brachioradialis muscle, deltoid muscle, tibialis anterior) of trauma ICU patients to monitor the adequacy of tissue

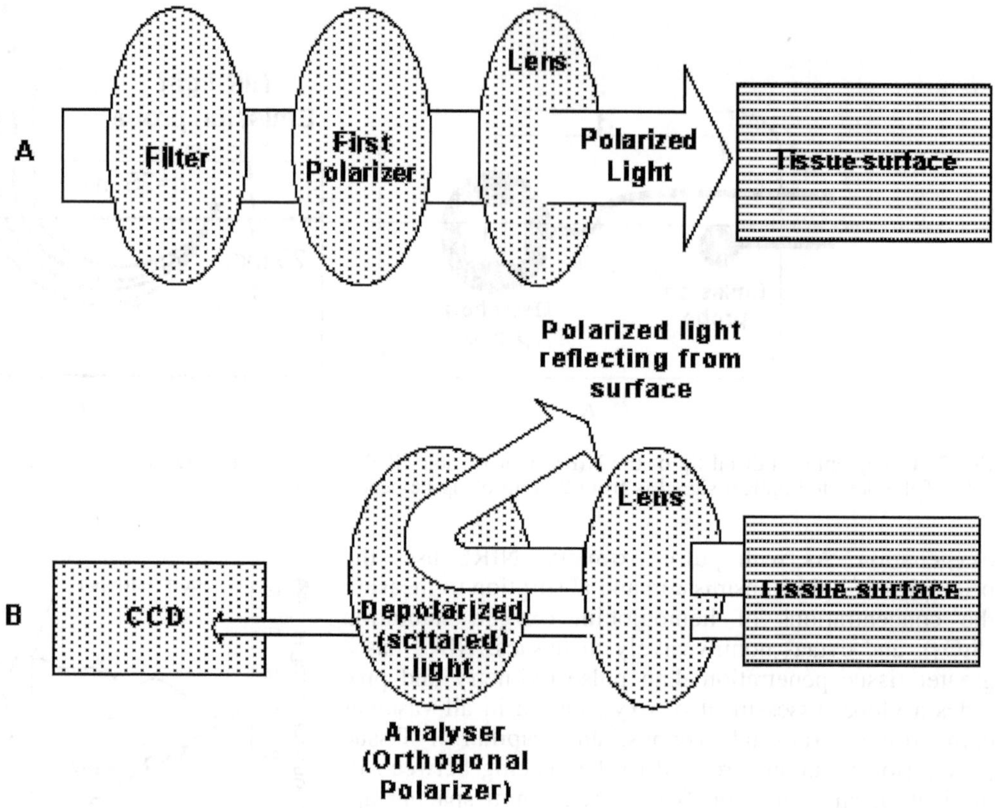

Fig. 4 OPS optical schematic. **A** The light passes through the first polarizer and is reflected back through the lens. **B** The polarized light reflecting from the surface is eliminated, and the depolarized light forms an image of the microcirculation on a videocamera (charge-coupled device, *CCD*)

oxygenation and detect a compartment syndrome [48, 49, 50, 51, 52]. The use of NIRS in deltoid muscle during resuscitation of severe trauma patients has recently been reported [48, 49]. Cairns et al. [49] studied trauma ICU patients and reported a strong association between elevated serum lactate levels and elevated cytaa$_3$ redox state during 12 h of shock resuscitation and development of multiple organ failure. More recently Mckinley et al. [48] showed a good relationship between StO_2, systemic oxygen delivery and lactate in severely trauma patients during and after resuscitation over a period of 24 h. A recent study with septic and nonseptic patients used NIRS to measure both regional blood flow and oxygen consumption after venous occlusion [53]. In this study septic patients had muscular oxygen consumption twice that of nonseptic patients, but oxygen extraction was similar in both groups, emphasizing oxygen extraction dysfunction in sepsis. Another study observed no relationship between forearm blood flow, measured by NIRS, and systemic vascular resistance in septic shock patients [41]. These findings demonstrate the ability of NIRS to reflect microcirculatory dysfunction in skeletal muscle in septic shock. The potential to monitor regional perfusion and oxygenation noninvasively at the bedside makes clinical application of NIRS technology of particular interest in intensive care.

Orthogonal polarization spectral

Orthogonal polarization spectral (OPS) is a noninvasive technique that uses reflected light to produce real-time images of the microcirculation. The technical characteristics of the device have been described elsewhere [54]. Light from a source passes through the first polarizer, and it is directed towards the tissue by a set of lens. As the light reaches the tissue, the depolarized light is reflected back through the lenses to a second polarizer or analyzer and forms an image of the microcirculation on the charge-coupled device, which can be captured through a single videotape (Fig. 4). The technology has been incorporated into a small hand-held video-microscope which can be used in both research and clinical settings. OPS can assess tissue perfusion using the functional capillary density (FCD), i.e., the length of perfused capillaries per observation area (measured as cm/cm^2). FCD is a very sensitive parameter for determining the status of nutritive perfusion to the tissue and it is an indirect measure of oxygen delivery. One of the most easily accessible sites in humans for peripheral perfusion monitoring is the mouth. OPS produces excellent images of the sublingual microcirculation by placing the probe under the tongue. Movement artifacts, semiquantitative measure of perfusion, the presence of various secretions such as saliva and blood, observer-related bias, and inadequacy of sedation to prevent patients from damaging the device are some of the limitations of the technique.

The use of sublingual tissues with OPS provides information about the dynamics of microcirculatory blood flow, and therefore it can monitor the perfusion during clinical treatment of circulatory shock. It has been used to monitor the effects of improvements in microcirculatory blood flow with dobutamine and nitroglycerin in volume resuscitated septic patients [55, 56]. OPS has been applied in the ICU to study the properties of sublingual microcirculation in both septic shock and cardiogenic shock [2, 56, 57, 58]. In septic patients it has been shown with OPS that microvascular alterations are more severe in patients with a worse outcome, and that these microvascular alterations can be reversed using vasodilators [2]. In patients with cardiac failure and cardiogenic shock the number of small vessels and the density of perfused vessels are lower than in controls, and the proportion of perfused vessels is higher in patients who survived than in patients who did not survive [57]. Using OPS during the time course of treatment of patients with septic shock, Sakr et al. [58] demonstrated that the behavior of the sublingual microcirculation differs between survivors and nonsurvivors. Although alterations in the sublingual microcirculation may not be representative of other microvascular beds, changes in the sublingual circulation evaluated by capnometry during hemorrhagic shock have been related to changes in perfusion of internal organs such as the liver and intestine [59]. Thus OPS could be of use in the monitoring of tissue perfusion.

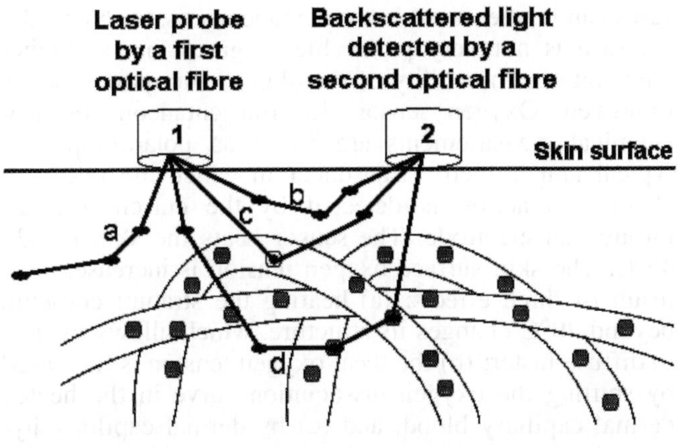

Fig. 5 Schematic diagram of laser Doppler flowmetry. When the tissue is illuminated by a laser source (*1*), 93–97% of the light is either absorbed by various structures or undergoes scattering (*a*, *b*). The remaining 3–7% is reflected by moving red blood cells (*c*, *d*) and returns to the second optical fiber (*2*). Microvascular perfusion is defined as the product of mean red blood cells (*RBC*) velocity and mean RBC concentration in the volume of tissue under illumination from the probe

Laser Doppler flowmetry

Laser Doppler flowmetry (LDF) is a noninvasive, continuous measure of microcirculatory blood flow, and it has been used to measure microcirculatory blood flow in many tissues including neural, muscle, skin, bone, and intestine. The principle of this method is to measure the Doppler shift—the frequency change that light undergoes when reflected by moving objects, such as red blood cells. LDF works by illuminating the tissue under observation with a monochromatic laser from a probe. When the tissue is illuminated, only 3–7% is reflected. The remaining 93–97% of the light is either absorbed by various structures or undergoes scattering. Another optical fiber collects the backscattered light from the tissue and returns it to the monitor (Fig. 5). As a result LDF produces an output signal that is proportional to the microvascular perfusion [60]. Depending on the device and the degree of invasiveness it can be used to assess blood flow in muscle, gastric, rectal, and vagina mucosae. As a noninvasive measure of peripheral blood flow, however, its use is limited to the skin [60]. LDF has been applied to obtain information on the functional state of the skin microcirculation during reactive hyperemia in several conditions, such as diabetes mellitus, essential hypertension, atherosclerosis, and sepsis [61]. A major limitation of this technique is that it does not take into account the heterogeneity of blood flow as the velocity measurements represent the average of velocities in all vessels of the window studied. In addition, skin blood flow signal varies markedly depending on probe position. No current laser Doppler instrument can present absolute perfusion values (e.g., ml/min per 100 g tissue) and measurements are expressed as perfusion units, which are arbitrary.

LDF is useful in evaluating endothelium-dependent vascular responses in the skin microcirculation during either reactive hyperemia [61, 62] or the noninvasive local application of acetylcholine or sodium nitroprusside [63, 64, 65]. This characteristic of LDF was used in critically ill patients to evaluate endothelial dysfunction in sepsis. Observational studies have shown that the hyperemic response in septic patients is decreased, and a relationship between changes in vasculature tone and severity of sepsis has been described [66, 67, 68]. In addition, restored vasomotion in patients with sepsis evaluated by LDF seems to be associated with a favorable prognosis [67]. The ability of LDF to assess abnormalities of skin blood flow control in sepsis could be of clinical use for early detection of microcirculatory derangements in high-risk patients.

PO_2 and PCO_2 transcutaneous measurements

Continuous noninvasive measurement of oxygen and carbon dioxide tensions is possible because both gases can diffuse through the skin, and thus their partial pressures can be measured in transcutaneous tissue. Normally the skin is not very permeable to gases, but at higher temperatures the ability of the skin to transport gases is improved. Oxygen sensors for transcutaneous electrochemical measurements are based on polarography: a typical amperometric transducer in which the rate of a chemical reaction is detected by the current drained through an electrode. The sensor heats the skin to 43–45°C. The skin surface oxygen tension is increased as a result of three effects: (a) heating the stratum corneum beyond 40°C changes its structure, which allows oxygen to diffuse faster; (b) the local oxygen tension is increased by shifting the oxygen dissociation curve in the heated dermal capillary blood; and (c) by dermal capillary hyperemia. These transcutaneous sensors enable us directly to estimate arterial oxygen pressure (PaO_2) and arterial carbon dioxide pressure ($PaCO_2$), and it has been successfully used for monitoring PaO_2 and $PaCO_2$ in both neonates and in adults [69, 70, 71]. Newborn infant is suitable because of its thin epidermal layer. However, in adults the skin is thicker, and differences in the skin cause the transcutaneous oxygen partial pressure ($PtcO_2$) to be lower than PaO_2. The correlation between $PtcO_2$ and PaO_2 also depends on the adequacy of blood flow. The low blood flow caused by vasoconstriction during shock overcomes the vasodilatory effect of $PtcO_2$ sensor. This causes a mild tissue hypoxia beneath the $PtcO_2$ sensor. The lack of the $PtcO_2$ ability to accurately reflect the PaO_2 in low flow shock enables us to estimate cutaneous blood flow through the relationship between the two variables. Some studies have suggested the use of a transcutaneous oxygen index (tc-index), i.e., the changes in $PtcO_2$ relative to changes in PaO_2 [69, 72, 73, 74, 75]. When blood flow is adequate, $PtcO_2$ and PaO_2 values are almost equal, and the tc-index is close to 1. During low flow shock the $PtcO_2$ drops and becomes dependent on the PaO_2 value, and tc-index decreases. A tc-index greater than 0.7 has been reported to be associated with hemodynamic stability [69, 72, 74, 75]. Transcutaneous carbon dioxide partial pressure ($PtcCO_2$) has been also used as an index of cutaneous blood flow. Differences between $PaCO_2$ and $PtcCO_2$ have been explained by local accumulation of CO_2 in the skin due to hypoperfusion. Because of the diffusion constant of CO_2 is about 20 times greater than O_2, $PtcCO_2$ has been showed to be less sensitive to changes in hemodynamics than $PtcO_2$ [76]. One of the main limitations of this technique is the necessity of blood gas analysis to obtain the tc-index and $PaCO_2$. In addition, the sensor position must be changed every 1–2 h to avoid burns. After each repositioning a period of 15–20 min is required for the next readings, which limits its use in emergency situations.

The ability of $PtcO_2$ to reflect tissue perfusion in critically ill adult patients has been applied using the tc-index. Tremper and Shoemaker [72] found a good correlation (r=0.86) between tc-index and cardiac index in patients with shock. These authors reported that at cardiac index values higher than 2.2 $l\ min^{-1}\ m^{-2}$ the tc-index averages 0.79, at 1.5–2.2 $l\ min^{-1}\ m^{-2}$ it is 0.48, and at values lower than 1.5 $l\ min^{-1}\ m^{-2}$ it is 0.12. However, the relationship between tc-index and cardiac index may not exist in hyperdynamic shock. Reed et al. [75] studied $PtcO_2$ at different cardiac indices. In this study 71 measurements were made in 19 patients, and a low tc-index was seen in 71% of the patients with a cardiac index higher than 4.2l $min^{-1}\ m^{-2}$. $PtcO_2$ and $PtcCO_2$ monitoring has been used as an early indicator of tissue hypoxia and subclinical hypovolemia in acutely ill patients [77, 78]. Tatevossian et al. [78] studied 48 severely injured patients during early resuscitation in the emergency department and operating room. The sequential patterns of $PtcO_2$ and $PtcCO_2$ were described throughout initial resuscitation. Nonsurvivors had lower $PtcO_2$ values and higher $PtcCO_2$ values than survivors. These differences were evident even early after the patient's arrival. The authors reported a critical tissue perfusion threshold of $PtcO_2$ 50 mmHg for more than 60 min and $PtcCO_2$ 60 mmHg for more than 30 min. Patients who failed to avoid these critical thresholds had 89% to 100% mortality. This technology has not gained widespread acceptance in clinical practice as the time needed for calibration limits its early use in the emergency department, and critical $PtcO_2$ and $PtcCO_2$ values have not been established.

Sublingual capnometry

Measurement of the tissue-arterial CO_2 tension gradient has been used to reflect the adequacy of tissue perfusion. The gastric and ileal mucosal CO_2 clearance is been the primary reference for measurements of regional PCO_2 gradient during circulatory shock [79]. The regional PCO_2 gradient represents the balance between regional CO_2 production and clearance. During tissue hypoxia CO_2 is produced by hydrogen anions buffered by tissue bicarbonate, which adds to the amount of CO_2 produced by normal oxidative metabolism. The amount of CO_2 produced, either aerobically or because of tissue hypoxia, will be cleared if blood flow is maintained. In low flow states CO_2 increases as a result of stagnation phenomenon [80]. Gastric tonometry is a technique that can be used to assess the adequacy of gut mucosal blood flow to metabolism. The methodological limitations of gastric tonometry required a search for a tissue in which PCO_2 can be measured easily in a noninvasive approach. Comparable decreases in blood flow during circulatory shock have been also demonstrated in the sublingual tissue PCO_2 ($PslCO_2$) [81, 82]. The currently available system for measuring $PslCO_2$ consists of a disposable PCO_2 sensor and a battery powered handheld instrument. The instrument uses fiberoptic technology to transmit light through the sensor placed between the tongue and the sublingual mucosa. Carbon dioxide diffuses across a semipermeable membrane of the sensor and into a fluorescent dye solution. The dye emits light that is proportional to the amount of CO_2 present. This light intensity is analyzed by the instrument and displayed as a numeric $PslCO_2$ value.

Clinical studies have suggested that $PslCO_2$ is a reliable marker of tissue hypoperfusion [83, 84, 85, 86]. Weil et al. [86] applied $PslCO_2$ in 46 patients with acutely life threatening illness or injuries admitted to the emergency department or ICU. In this study 26 patients with physical signs of circulatory shock and high blood lactate levels had higher $PslCO_2$ values, and a $PslCO_2$ threshold value of 70 mmHg was predictive for the severity of the circulatory failure. Similarly as PCO_2 in the gut mucosal, $PslCO_2$ is also influenced by $PaCO_2$ [87]. Hence the gradient between $PslCO_2$ and $PaCO_2$ (Psl-aCO_2) is more specific for tissue hypoperfusion. This was shown in the study by Marik and Bankov [85] who determined the prognostic value of sublingual capnometry in 54 hemodynamic unstable critically ill patients. In this study Psl-aCO_2 was a sensitive marker for tissue perfusion and a useful endpoint for the titration of goal-directed therapy. Psl-aCO_2 differentiated better than $PslCO_2$ alone between survivors and nonsurvivors, and a difference of more than 25 mmHg indicated a poor prognosis. One limitation of this technique includes the necessity of blood gas analysis to obtain $PaCO_2$. In addition, normal vs. pathological Psl-aCO_2 values are not well defined.

Conclusion

The conventional systemic hemodynamic and oxygenation parameters are neither specific nor sensitive enough to detect regional hypoperfusion. In clinical practice a more complete evaluation of tissue oxygenation can be achieved by adding noninvasive assessment of perfusion in peripheral tissues to global parameters. Noninvasive monitoring of peripheral perfusion could be a complementary approach that allows very early application throughout the hospital, including the emergency department, operating room, and hospital wards. Such approach can be applied using both simple physical examination and new current technologies, as discussed above. Although these methods may reflect variations in peripheral perfusion with certain accuracy, more studies are needed to define the precise role of such methods in the management of the critically ill patients. Finally, evidence for clinical and cost effectiveness of these methods is an important aspect that needs a formal technology assessment.

References

1. Bakker J, Coffernils M, Leon M, Gris P, Vincent J-L (1991) Blood lactate levels are superior to oxygen-derived variables in predicting outcome in human septic shock. Chest 99:956–962
2. De Backer D, Creteur J, Preiser JC, Dubois MJ, Vincent JL (2002) Microvascular blood flow is altered in patients with sepsis. Am J Respir Crit Care Med 166:98–104
3. Rady MY, Rivers EP, Nowak RM (1996) Resuscitation of the critically ill in the ED: responses of blood pressure, heart rate, shock index, central venous oxygen saturation, and lactate. Am J Emerg Med 14:218–225
4. Shoemaker WC, Appel PL, Kram HB, Nathan RC, Thompson JL (1988) Multicomponent noninvasive physiologic monitoring of circulatory function. Crit Care Med 16:482–490
5. Siegemund M, van Bommel J, Ince C (1999) Assessment of regional tissue oxygenation. Intensive Care Med 25:1044–1060
6. Tibby SM, Hatherill M, Murdoch IA (1999) Capillary refill and core-peripheral temperature gap as indicators of haemodynamic status in paediatric intensive care patients. Arch Dis Child 80:163–166
7. Bailey JM, Levy JH, Kopel MA, Tobia V, Grabenkort WR (1990) Relationship between clinical evaluation of peripheral perfusion and global hemodynamics in adults after cardiac surgery. Crit Care Med 18:1353–1356
8. Schriger DL, Baraff L (1988) Defining normal capillary refill: variation with age, sex, and temperature. Ann Emerg Med 17:932–935
9. Kaplan LJ, McPartland K, Santora TA, Trooskin SZ (2001) Start with a subjective assessment of skin temperature to identify hypoperfusion in intensive care unit patients. J Trauma 50:620–627
10. Schriger DL, Baraff L (1991) Capillary refill: is it a useful predictor of hypovolemic states? Ann Emerg Med 20:601–605
11. Steiner MJ, DeWalt DA, Byerley JS (2004) Is this child dehydrated? JAMA 291:2746–2754
12. Champion HR, Sacco WJ, Carnazzo AJ, Copes W, Fouty WJ (1981) Trauma score. Crit Care Med 9:672–676
13. Hasdai D, Holmes DR Jr, Califf RM, Thompson TD, Hochman JS, Pfisterer M, Topol EJ (1999) Cardiogenic shock complicating acute myocardial infarction: predictors of death. GUSTO Investigators. Global Utilization of Streptokinase and Tissue-Plasminogen Activator for Occluded Coronary Arteries. Am Heart J 138:21–31
14. McGee S, Abernethy WB, III, Simel DL (1999) Is this patient hypovolemic? JAMA 281:1022–1029
15. Joly HR, Weil MH (1969) Temperature of the great toe as an indication of the severity of shock. Circulation 39:131–138
16. Ibsen B (1967) Treatment of shock with vasodilators measuring temperature of the great toe: ten years experience in 150 cases. Dis Chest 52:425
17. Guyton AC (1996) Body temperature, temperature regulation, and fever. In: Guyton AC, Hall JE (eds) Textbook of medical physiology. Saunders, Philadelphia, pp 911–922
18. Ross BA, Brock L, Aynsley-Green A (1969) Observations on central and peripheral temperatures in the understanding and management of shock. Br J Surg 56:877–882

19. Curley FJ, Smyrnios NA (2003) Routine monitoring of critically ill patients. In: Irwin RS, Cerra FB, Rippe JM (eds) Intensive care medicine. Lippincott Williams & Wilkins, New York, pp 250–270
20. Ibsen B (1966) Further observations in the use of air-conditioned rooms in the treatment of hyperthermia and shock. Acta Anaesthesiol Scand Suppl 23:565–570
21. Rubinstein EH, Sessler DI (1990) Skin-surface temperature gradients correlate with fingertip blood flow in humans. Anesthesiology 73:541–545
22. Sessler DI (2003) Skin-temperature gradients are a validated measure of fingertip perfusion. Eur J Appl Physiol 89:401–402
23. House JR, Tipton MJ (2002) Using skin temperature gradients or skin heat flux measurements to determine thresholds of vasoconstriction and vasodilatation. Eur J Appl Physiol 88:141–145
24. Brock L, Skinner JM, Manders JT (1975) Observations on peripheral and central temperatures with particular reference to the occurrence of vasoconstriction. Br J Surg 62:589–595
25. Ruiz CE, Weil MH, Carlson RW (1979) Treatment of circulatory shock with dopamine. Studies on survival. JAMA 242:165–168
26. Ryan CA, Soder CM (1989) Relationship between core/peripheral temperature gradient and central hemodynamics in children after open heart surgery. Crit Care Med 17:638–640
27. Vincent JL, Moraine JJ, van der LP (1988) Toe temperature versus transcutaneous oxygen tension monitoring during acute circulatory failure. Intensive Care Med 14:64–68
28. Henning RJ, Wiener F, Valdes S, Weil MH (1979) Measurement of toe temperature for assessing the severity of acute circulatory failure. Surg Gynecol Obstet 149:1–7
29. Murdoch IA, Qureshi SA, Mitchell A, Huggon IC (1993) Core-peripheral temperature gradient in children: does it reflect clinically important changes in circulatory haemodynamics? Acta Paediatr 82:773–776
30. Butt W, Shann F (1991) Core-peripheral temperature gradient does not predict cardiac output or systemic vascular resistance in children. Anaesth Intensive Care 19:84–87
31. Woods I, Wilkins RG, Edwards JD, Martin PD, Faragher EB (1987) Danger of using core/peripheral temperature gradient as a guide to therapy in shock. Crit Care Med 15:850–852
32. Sessler DI (2000) Perioperative heat balance. Anesthesiology 92:578–596
33. Rivers E, Nguyen B, Havstad S, Ressler J, Muzzin A, Knoblich B, Peterson E, Tomlanovich M (2001) Early goal-directed therapy in the treatment of severe sepsis and septic shock. N Engl J Med 345:1368–1377
34. Vincent JL (1996) End-points of resuscitation: arterial blood pressure, oxygen delivery, blood lactate, or..? Intensive Care Med 22:3–5
35. Flewelling R (2000) Noninvasive optical monitoring. In: Bronzino JD (ed) The biomedical engineering handbook. Springer, Berlin Heidelberg New York, pp 1–10
36. Lima AP, Beelen P, Bakker J (2002) Use of a peripheral perfusion index derived from the pulse oximetry signal as a noninvasive indicator of perfusion. Crit Care Med 30:1210–1213
37. Kurz A, Xiong J, Sessler DI, Dechert M, Noyes K, Belani K (1995) Desflurane reduces the gain of thermoregulatory arteriovenous shunt vasoconstriction in humans. Anesthesiology 83:1212–1219
38. Lima A, Bakker J (2004) The peripheral perfusion index in reactive hyperemia in critically ill patients. Crit Care 8:S27–P53
39. De Felice C, Latini G, Vacca P, Kopotic RJ (2002) The pulse oximeter perfusion index as a predictor for high illness severity in neonates. Eur J Pediatr 161:561–562
40. Van Beekvelt MC, Colier WN, Wevers RA, Van Engelen BG (2001) Performance of near-infrared spectroscopy in measuring local O (2) consumption and blood flow in skeletal muscle. J Appl Physiol 90:511–519
41. De Blasi RA, Ferrari M, Natali A, Conti G, Mega A, Gasparetto A (1994) Noninvasive measurement of forearm blood flow and oxygen consumption by near-infrared spectroscopy. J Appl Physiol 76:1388–1393
42. Edwards AD, Richardson C, van der ZP, Elwell C, Wyatt JS, Cope M, Delpy DT, Reynolds EO (1993) Measurement of hemoglobin flow and blood flow by near-infrared spectroscopy. J Appl Physiol 75:1884–1889
43. Taylor DE, Simonson SG (1996) Use of near-infrared spectroscopy to monitor tissue oxygenation. New Horiz 4:420–425
44. Rhee P, Langdale L, Mock C, Gentilello LM (1997) Near-infrared spectroscopy: continuous measurement of cytochrome oxidation during hemorrhagic shock. Crit Care Med 25:166–170
45. Puyana JC, Soller BR, Zhang S, Heard SO (1999) Continuous measurement of gut pH with near-infrared spectroscopy during hemorrhagic shock. J Trauma 46:9–15
46. Beilman GJ, Myers D, Cerra FB, Lazaron V, Dahms RA, Conroy MJ, Hammer BE (2001) Near-infrared and nuclear magnetic resonance spectroscopic assessment of tissue energetics in an isolated, perfused canine hind limb model of dysoxia. Shock 15:392–397
47. Crookes BA, Cohn SM, Burton EA, Nelson J, Proctor KG (2004) Noninvasive muscle oxygenation to guide fluid resuscitation after traumatic shock. Surgery 135:662–670
48. McKinley BA, Marvin RG, Cocanour CS, Moore FA (2000) Tissue hemoglobin O2 saturation during resuscitation of traumatic shock monitored using near infrared spectrometry. J Trauma 48:637–642
49. Cairns CB, Moore FA, Haenel JB, Gallea BL, Ortner JP, Rose SJ, Moore EE (1997) Evidence for early supply independent mitochondrial dysfunction in patients developing multiple organ failure after trauma. J Trauma 42:532–536
50. Muellner T, Nikolic A, Schramm W, Vecsei V (1999) New instrument that uses near-infrared spectroscopy for the monitoring of human muscle oxygenation. J Trauma 46:1082–1084
51. Arbabi S, Brundage SI, Gentilello LM (1999) Near-infrared spectroscopy: a potential method for continuous, transcutaneous monitoring for compartmental syndrome in critically injured patients. J Trauma 47:829–833
52. Giannotti G, Cohn SM, Brown M, Varela JE, McKenney MG, Wiseberg JA (2000) Utility of near-infrared spectroscopy in the diagnosis of lower extremity compartment syndrome. J Trauma 48:396–399
53. Girardis M, Rinaldi L, Busani S, Flore I, Mauro S, Pasetto A (2003) Muscle perfusion and oxygen consumption by near-infrared spectroscopy in septic-shock and non-septic-shock patients. Intensive Care Med 29:1173–1176
54. Groner W, Winkelman JW, Harris AG, Ince C, Bouma GJ, Messmer K, Nadeau RG (1999) Orthogonal polarization spectral imaging: a new method for study of the microcirculation. Nat Med 5:1209–1212
55. De Backer D, Dubois MJ, Creteur J, Vincent J-L (2001) Effects of dobutamine on microcirculatory alterations in patients with septic shock. Intensive Care Med 27:S237
56. Spronk PE, Ince C, Gardien MJ, Mathura KR, Oudemans-van Straaten HM, Zandstra DF (2002) Nitroglycerin in septic shock after intravascular volume resuscitation. Lancet 360:1395–1396

57. De Backer D, Creteur J, Dubois MJ, Sakr Y, Vincent JL (2004) Microvascular alterations in patients with acute severe heart failure and cardiogenic shock. Am Heart J 147:91–99
58. Sakr Y, Dubois MJ, De Backer D, Creteur J, Vincent JL (2004) Persistent microcirculatory alterations are associated with organ failure and death in patients with septic shock. Crit Care Med 32:1825–1831
59. Jin X, Weil MH, Sun S, Tang W, Bisera J, Mason EJ (1998) Decreases in organ blood flows associated with increases in sublingual PCO2 during hemorrhagic shock. J Appl Physiol 85:2360–2364
60. Schabauer AM, Rooke TW (1994) Cutaneous laser Doppler flowmetry: applications and findings. Mayo Clin Proc 69:564–574
61. Farkas K, Fabian E, Kolossvary E, Jarai Z, Farsang C (2003) Noninvasive assessment of endothelial dysfunction in essential hypertension: comparison of the forearm microvascular reactivity with flow-mediated dilatation of the brachial artery. Int J Angiol 12:224–228
62. Koller A, Kaley G (1990) Role of endothelium in reactive dilation of skeletal muscle arterioles. Am J Physiol 259:H1313–H1316
63. Morris SJ, Shore AC, Tooke JE (1995) Responses of the skin microcirculation to acetylcholine and sodium nitroprusside in patients with NIDDM. Diabetologia 38:1337–1344
64. Warren JB (1994) Nitric oxide and human skin blood flow responses to acetylcholine and ultraviolet light. FASEB J 8:247–251
65. Blaauw J, Graaff R, van Pampus MG, van Doormaal JJ, Smit AJ, Rakhorst G, Aarnoudse JG (2005) Abnormal endothelium-dependent microvascular reactivity in recently preeclamptic women. Obstet Gynecol 105:626–632
66. Hartl WH, Gunther B, Inthorn D, Heberer G (1988) Reactive hyperemia in patients with septic conditions. Surgery 103:440–444
67. Young JD, Cameron EM (1995) Dynamics of skin blood flow in human sepsis. Intensive Care Med 21:669–674
68. Sair M, Etherington PJ, Peter WC, Evans TW (2001) Tissue oxygenation and perfusion in patients with systemic sepsis. Crit Care Med 29:1343–1349
69. Hasibeder W, Haisjackl M, Sparr H, Klaunzer S, Horman C, Salak N, Germann R, Stronegger WJ, Hackl JM (1991) Factors influencing transcutaneous oxygen and carbon dioxide measurements in adult intensive care patients. Intensive Care Med 17:272–275
70. Carter B, Hochmann M, Osborne A, Nisbet A, Campbell N (1995) A comparison of two transcutaneous monitors for the measurement of arterial PO2 and PCO2 in neonates. Anaesth Intensive Care 23:708–714
71. Phan CQ, Tremper KK, Lee SE, Barker SJ (1987) Noninvasive monitoring of carbon dioxide: a comparison of the partial pressure of transcutaneous and end-tidal carbon dioxide with the partial pressure of arterial carbon dioxide. J Clin Monit 3:149–154
72. Tremper KK, Shoemaker WC (1981) Transcutaneous oxygen monitoring of critically ill adults, with and without low flow shock. Crit Care Med 9:706–709
73. Shoemaker WC, Wo CC, Bishop MH, Thangathurai D, Patil RS (1996) Noninvasive hemodynamic monitoring of critical patients in the emergency department. Acad Emerg Med 3:675–681
74. Tremper KK, Barker SJ (1987) Transcutaneous oxygen measurement: experimental studies and adult applications. Int Anesthesiol Clin 25:67–96
75. Reed RL, Maier RV, Landicho D, Kenny MA, Carrico CJ (1985) Correlation of hemodynamic variables with transcutaneous PO2 measurements in critically ill adult patients. J Trauma 25:1045–1053
76. Tremper KK, Shoemaker WC, Shippy CR, Nolan LS (1981) Transcutaneous PCO2 monitoring on adult patients in the ICU and the operating room. Crit Care Med 9:752–755
77. Waxman K, Sadler R, Eisner ME, Applebaum R, Tremper KK, Mason GR (1983) Transcutaneous oxygen monitoring of emergency department patients. Am J Surg 146:35–38
78. Tatevossian RG, Wo CC, Velmahos GC, Demetriades D, Shoemaker WC (2000) Transcutaneous oxygen and CO2 as early warning of tissue hypoxia and hemodynamic shock in critically ill emergency patients. Crit Care Med 28:2248–2253
79. Fiddian-Green RG, Baker S (1987) Predictive value of the stomach wall pH for complications after cardiac operations: comparison with other monitoring. Crit Care Med 15:153–156
80. De Backer D, Creteur J (2003) Regional hypoxia and partial pressure of carbon dioxide gradients: what is the link? Intensive Care Med 29:2116–2118
81. Nakagawa Y, Weil MH, Tang W, Sun S, Yamaguchi H, Jin X, Bisera J (1998) Sublingual capnometry for diagnosis and quantitation of circulatory shock. Am J Respir Crit Care Med 157:1838–1843
82. Povoas HP, Weil MH, Tang W, Moran B, Kamohara T, Bisera J (2000) Comparisons between sublingual and gastric tonometry during hemorrhagic shock. Chest 118:1127–1132
83. Rackow EC, O'Neil P, Astiz ME, Carpati CM (2001) Sublingual capnometry and indexes of tissue perfusion in patients with circulatory failure. Chest 120:1633–1638
84. Marik PE (2001) Sublingual capnography: a clinical validation study. Chest 120:923–927
85. Marik PE, Bankov A (2003) Sublingual capnometry versus traditional markers of tissue oxygenation in critically ill patients. Crit Care Med 31:818–822
86. Weil MH, Nakagawa Y, Tang W, Sato Y, Ercoli F, Finegan R, Grayman G, Bisera J (1999) Sublingual capnometry: a new noninvasive measurement for diagnosis and quantitation of severity of circulatory shock. Crit Care Med 27:1225–1229
87. Pernat A, Weil MH, Tang W, Yamaguchi H, Pernat AM, Sun S, Bisera J (1999) Effects of hyper- and hypoventilation on gastric and sublingual PCO (2). J Appl Physiol 87:933–937

François Jardin
Antoine Vieillard-Baron

Ultrasonographic examination of the venae cavae

There are two venae cavae in humans. The superior vena cava (SVC) comprises the connection of the left and right brachiocephalic veins and ends on the top of the right atrium, after entering the pericardium. The inferior vena cava (IVC) comprises the connection of the left and right iliac veins and ends on the floor of right atrium, after crossing the diaphragm. Whereas the SVC is an intrathoracic vessel, the IVC is an intraabdominal one, its short intrathoracic part being purely virtual. Both venae cavae provide venous return to the right heart, approx. 25% via the SVC and 75% via IVC [1, 2].

Ultrasonographic examination of the SVC can be performed by a transesophageal approach [3]. To remain open this collapsible vessel requires a distending pressure greater than the critical pressure producing collapse, i.e. its closing pressure. Because lung inflation increases pleural pressure more than right atrial pressure, the distending pressure of the SVC, i.e. right atrial pressure minus pleural pressure, is reduced by lung inflation, and may become insufficient to maintain the vessel open in a hypovolemic patient (Fig. 1). This collapsible vessel can be compared to a "Starling resistor." The influence of SVC zone conditions on respiratory changes in SVC diameter is illustrated with clinical examples in Fig. 2.

We have thus proposed to use the SVC collapsibility index, calculated as maximal expiratory diameter minus minimal inspiratory diameter, divided by maximal expiratory diameter, as an index of fluid responsiveness in mechanically ventilated patients exhibiting circulatory failure [4]. This requires recording of a long-axis view of the vessel using a multiplane transesophageal probe, by coupling motion mode with two-dimensional mode. Our measurements in a group of 66 patients with septic shock as reported in a previous issue, demonstrated that a SVC collapsibility index higher than 36% predicts a positive response to volume expansion, marked by a significant increase in Doppler cardiac output, with 90% sensitivity and 100% specificity [4]. We also found a bimodal distribution for the SVC collapsibility index: most patients exhibited either a partial or complete collapse of the vessel or the absence of significant change in its diameter during inflation. This confirms our hypothesis that the SVC can be compared to a "Starling resistor" which obeys the all-or-nothing law.

Ultrasonographic examination of the IVC can be performed by a transthoracic, subcostal approach [5, 6]. Mea-

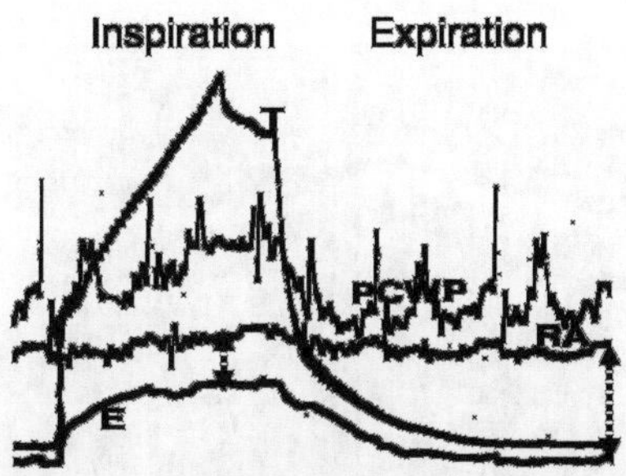

Fig. 1 Simultaneous recordings of tracheal pressure (*T*), pulmonary capillary wedge pressure (*PCWP*), right atrial pressure (*RA*), and esophageal pressure (*E*, as a surrogate for pleural pressure). During lung inflation (inspiration) pleural pressure increases more than right atrial (or central venous) pressure, leading to an inspiratory decrease in venous distending pressure (*arrows*)

M.R. Pinsky et al. (eds.), *Applied Physiology in Intensive Care Medicine 2: Physiological Reviews and Editorials*,
DOI 10.1007/978-3-642-28233-1_5,

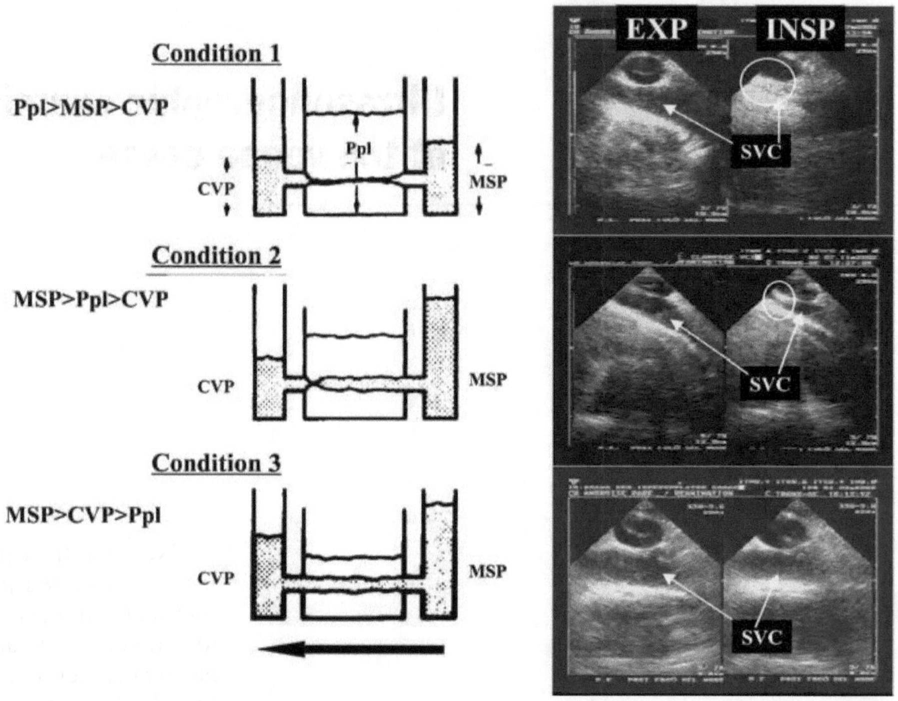

Fig. 2 *Left* Schematic representation of the superior vena cava (*SVC*) as a Starling resistor, with an inflow pressure (the upper body mean systemic pressure, *MSP*), an outflow pressure (the central venous pressure, itCVP), and an external pressure (the pleural pressure, *Ppl*). *Right panel* Cli nical examples illustrating the three zone conditions. *Top panel* (condition 1) Inflow pressure becomes lower than the pleural pressure during lung inflation, which produces a complete collapse of the whole vessel. This setting is illustrated by ultrasonographic examination of the venae cavae in a hypovolemic patient exhibiting low MSP. *Middle panel* (condition 2) the outflow pressure is reduced, and lung inflation produces a localized collapse at entry into the right atrium. This setting is illustrated (*right*) by ultrasonographic examination after clamping of the inferior vena cava during a surgical procedure, a maneuver which suddenly decreases CVP but does not change MSP. *Bottom panel* (condition 3) Outflow pressure is much greater than the external pressure, and the SVC remains fully open during lung inflation. This setting is illustrated (*right*) by ultrasonographic examination of the venae cavae after volume expansion

surement of IVC diameter in different positions has proven useful in separating normal subjects from patients with elevated right atrial pressure [7]. In their famous study of venous return Guyton et al. [8] observed in dogs that negative right atrial pressure from 0 down to –4 mm Hg increases venous return, but then beyond –4mm Hg, further increase in the negative pressure causes no more increase in the venous return. Guyton et al. explained this failure by the collapse of the IVC when entering the thoracic cavity, illustrating the inability of a collapsible vessel to transmit a negative pressure. To our knowledge, the first demonstration of the reality of this phenomenon in humans was provided by our group in asthmatic patients [9] (Fig. 3).

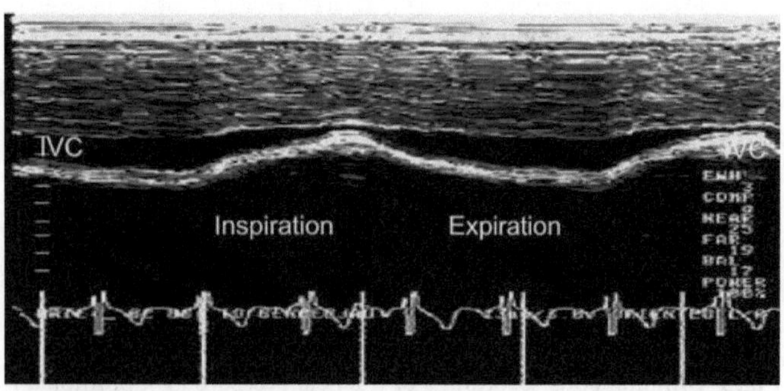

Fig. 3 An example of M mode echocardiography of the inferior vena cava (*IVC*) in spontaneously breathing asthmatic patients. Note the short duration of inspiration, accompanied by a collapse of the vessel, and the increased duration of the expiration (compare Fig. 4, above)

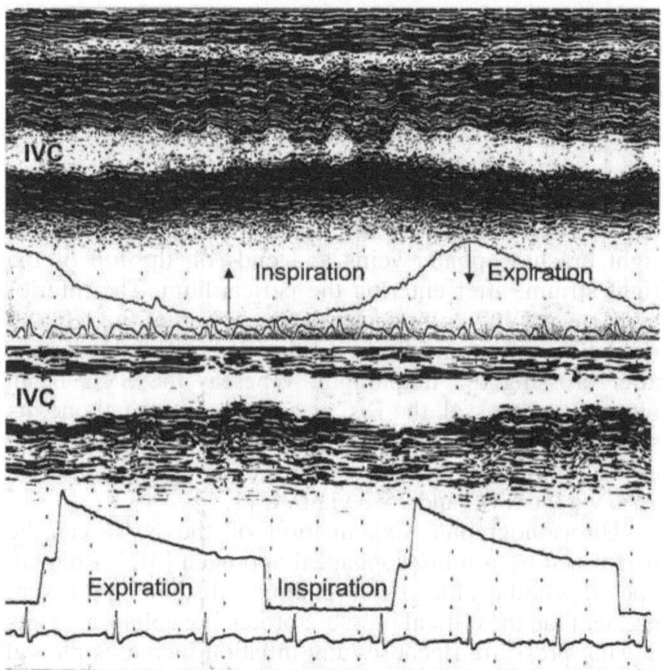

Fig. 4 M mode echocardiography of the inferior vena cava (*IVC*) in a spontaneously breathing healthy volunteer (*above*) and in a mechanically ventilated patient (*below*). Cyclic changes in IVC diameters are opposite, the largest value being observed during expiration in spontaneous breathing, and during inspiration in positive pressure breathing

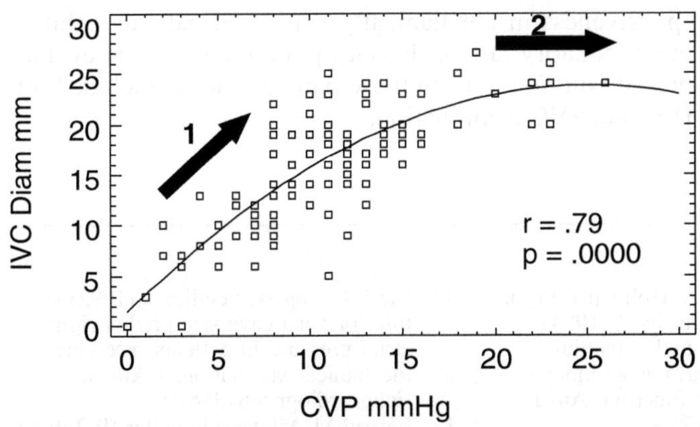

Fig. 5 Simultaneous measurement of central venous pressure (*CVP*) and inferior vena cava diameter (*IVC diam*) recorded at end-expiration in 108 mechanically ventilated patients. The pressure/diameter relationship for the vessel is characterized by an initial ascending part (*arrow 1*), where the index of compliance (slope of diameter/pressure curve) does not change, and a final horizontal part (*arrow 2*), where the index of compliance progressively decreases, reflecting distension

In a healthy subject breathing spontaneously, cyclic changes in pleural pressure, which are transmitted to the right atrial pressure, produce cyclic changes in venous return, with an inspiratory acceleration, inducing an inspiratory decrease in IVC diameter of approx. 50% (Fig. 4, *above*) [5]. This cyclic change in vena cava diameter is abolished, however, when the vessel is dilated because, although some inspiratory increase in venous return persists, the vessel actually stays on the horizontal part of its pressure-diameter relationship (Fig. 5). This is the case when cardiac tamponade [10] or severe right ventricular failure is present [6].

In a mechanically ventilated patient, the inspiratory phase produces an increase in pleural pressure, which is transmitted to the right atrial pressure, thus reducing the venous return. As a result respiratory changes in IVC diameter are reversed, compared with those observed during spontaneous breathing, with an inspiratory increase, and an expiratory decrease (Fig. 4, *below*). However, regarding spontaneous breathing these changes are abolished by vena cava dilatation produced by a high volume status, and/or a high right atrial pressure, the inferior vena cava staying on the horizontal part of its pressure-diameter relationship (Fig. 5). Cyclic respiratory changes in IVC diameter can thus be observed only with a normal or low volume status in a mechanically ventilated patient. In the past, these changes were poorly correlated with atrial pressure during mechanical ventilation [11]. Lack of IVC diameter variation in a mechanically ventilated patient exhibiting circulatory failure rules out the patient's ability to respond fluid in more than 90% of cases [12].

Feissel et al. [12] first proposed the use of cyclic respiratory changes in IVC diameter to detect fluid responsiveness in a mechanically ventilated patient, and their original findings are reported in a recent issue. Expressing respiratory variability in IVC diameter as maximal inspiratory diameter minus minimal expiratory diameter, divided by the average value of the two diameters, they found that a 12% increase in inferior vena cava diameter during lung inflation allowed discrimination between responders and non-responders to volume loading, with a positive predictive value of 93% and a negative predictive value of 92% [12]. The great merit of this work is to propose a noninvasive parameter to evaluate volume loading. Moreover, this echocardiographic measurement is very easy at the bedside, and requires only minimal experience in echocardiography (Fig. 6). The findings of Feissel et al. are confirmed in an identical study by Barbier et al. [13], which appears in the same issue. It remains to be seen whether this index is still reliable in patients with a significant increase in intra-abdominal pressure, which could limit IVC diameter variations.

Another phenomenon occasionally observed in the IVC during mechanical ventilation is backward flow, which is not caused by tricuspid regurgitation but by cyclic compression of the right atrium by lung inflation. Such a sudden compression boosts blood backward from the right atrium to the IVC and does not concern tricuspid valve competency [14]. This backward flow might explain in part the inaccuracy of the thermodilution method in

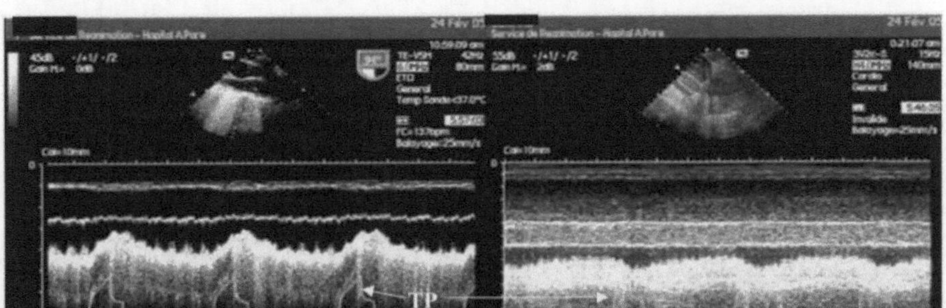

Fig. 6a,b Ultrasonographic examination of the superior (**a**) and inferior (**b**) venae cavae in the same mechanically ventilated patient, who exhibited hypotension. Transesophageal echocardiography demonstrated a partial collapse of the SVC at each inflation, whereas echocardiography by a subcostal approach demonstrated a marked increase in IVC diameter. After blood volume expansion cardiac index significantly increased, hypotension was corrected, and variations in vena cava diameter disappeared. TP: tracheal pressure

measuring cardiac output in mechanically ventilated patients [14].

In conclusion, ultrasonographic examination of the venae cavae provides new and accurate indices of fluid responsiveness in mechanically ventilated patients exhibiting circulatory failure. In our opinion, a complete evaluation of volume status in these patients should include both IVC and SVC examination.

References

1. Mellander S, Johanson B (1968) Control of resistance, exchange and capacitance functions in the peripheral circulation. Pharmacol Rev 20:117–196
2. Rushmer R (1970) Peripheral vascular control. In Rushmer R (ed) Cardiovascular dynamics. WB Saunders, Philadelphia, pp 113–147
3. Vieillard-Baron A, Augarde R, Prin S, Page B, Beauchet A, Jardin F (2001) Influence of superior vena caval zone conditions on cyclic changes in right ventricular outflow during respiratory support. Anesthesiology 95:1083–1088
4. Vieillard-Baron A, Chergui K, Rabiller A, Peyrouset O, Page B, Beauchet A, Jardin F (2004) Superior vena caval collapsibility as a gauge of volume status in ventilated septic patients. Intensive Care Med 30:1734–1739
5. Mintz G, Kotler M, Parry W, Iskandrian A, Kane S (1981) Real-time inferior vena caval ultrasonography: normal and abnormal findings and its use in assessing right heart function. Circulation 64:1018–1025
6. Moreno F, Hagan A, Holmen J, Pryor A, Strickland R, Castle H (1984) Evaluation of size and dynamics of the inferior vena cava as an index of right-sided cardiac function. Am J Cardiol 52:579–585
7. Nakao S, Come P, McKay R, Ransil B (1987) Effects of positional changes on inferior vena caval size and dynamics and correlations with right-sided cardiac pressures. Am J Cardiol 59:125–132
8. Guyton A, Lindsey A, Abernathy A, Richardson T (1957) Venous return at various right atrial pressures and the normal venous return curve. Am J Physiol 189:609–615
9. Jardin F, Farcot JC, Boisante L, Prost JF, Guéret P, Bourdarias JP (1982) Mechanism of paradoxal pulse in bronchial asthma. Circulation 66:887–894
10. Himelman R, Kircher B, Rockey D, Schiller N (1988) Inferior vena cava plethora with blunted respiratory response: a sensitive echocardiographic sign of cardiac tamponade. J Am Coll Cardiol 12:1470–1477
11. Jue J, Chung W, Schiller N (1992) Does inferior vena cava size predict right atrial pressure in patients receiving mechanical ventilation. J Am Soc Echocardiogr 5:613–619
12. Feissel M, Michard F, Faller JP, Teboul JL (2004) The respiratory variation in inferior vena cava diameter as a guide to fluid therapy. Intensive Care Med 30:1834–1837
13. Barbier C, Loubières Y, Schmit C, Hayon J, Ricôme JL, Jardin F, Vieillard-Baron A (2004) Respiratory changes in inferior vena cava diameter are helpful in predicting fluid responsiveness in ventilated septic patients. Intensive Care Med 30:1740–1746
14. Jullien T, Valtier B, Hongnat JM, Dubourg O, Bourdarias JP, Jardin F (1995) Incidence of tricuspid regurgitation and vena caval backward flow in mechanically ventilated patients. A color Doppler and contrast echocardiographic study. Chest 107:488–493

Xavier Monnet
Jean-Louis Teboul

Passive leg raising

Abstract *Objective:* To assess whether the passive leg raising test can help in predicting fluid responsiveness. *Design:* Nonsystematic review of the literature. *Results:* Passive leg raising has been used as an endogenous fluid challenge and tested for predicting the hemodynamic response to fluid in patients with acute circulatory failure. This is now easy to perform at the bedside using methods that allow a real time measurement of systolic blood flow. A passive leg raising induced increase in descending aortic blood flow of at least 10% or in echocardiographic subaortic flow of at least 12% has been shown to predict fluid responsiveness. Importantly, this prediction remains very valuable in patients with cardiac arrhythmias or spontaneous breathing activity. *Conclusions:* Passive leg raising allows reliable prediction of fluid responsiveness even in patients with spontaneous breathing activity or arrhythmias. This test may come to be used increasingly at the bedside since it is easy to perform and effective, provided that its effects are assessed by a real-time measurement of cardiac output.

Keywords Fluid responsiveness · Passive leg raising · Volume expansion · Cardiac preload

Physiological changes in hemodynamics during PLR

Lifting the legs in the event of circulatory collapse is a rescue maneuver that has been used for years by first-aid rescuers. Passive leg raising (PLR) has recently gained interest as a test for monitoring functional hemodynamic and assessing fluid responsiveness since it is a simple way to transiently increase cardiac preload. Lifting the legs passively from the horizontal plane in a lying subject obviously induces a gravitational transfer of blood from the lower part of the body toward the central circulatory compartment and especially toward the cardiac cavities. Using radiolabeled erythrocytes a physiological study in humans demonstrated that the volume of blood contained in the calves was reduced during PLR, a reduction corresponding to the transfer of approx. 150 ml blood [1]. Thus PLR recruits a part of blood contained in the venous reservoir and converts unstressed volume to stressed volume. In turn PLR increases right cardiac preload, likely through an increase in the mean circulatory pressure which is the driving pressure for venous return. If the right ventricle is preload responsive, the increase in systemic venous return results in an increase in right cardiac output and hence in the left ventricular filling. Clinical studies conducted in various hemodynamic conditions have reported an increase in pulmonary artery occlusion pressure [2–5], left ventricular end-diastolic dimension [2, 6], E wave of the mitral flow [2, 3, 7], and left ventricular ejection time [8] during PLR, supporting the evidence that the volume of

M.R. Pinsky et al. (eds.), *Applied Physiology in Intensive Care Medicine 2: Physiological Reviews and Editorials*,
DOI 10.1007/978-3-642-28233-1_6, © Springer-Verlag Berlin Heidelberg 2012

blood transferred to the heart during PLR is sufficient to increase left cardiac preload. Nonetheless, if the preload reserve of the right heart is limited, the increase in right cardiac preload should not result in an increased flow toward the left ventricle, and thus PLR should not increase left-side preload in such cases. The response to PLR of the markers of right preload (e. g., central venous pressure) and of left preload may therefore differ.

As a result of the increase in left ventricular preload PLR may ultimately result in an increase in cardiac output, depending on the degree of left ventricular preload reserve. Interestingly, Wong and colleagues [9] reported that the increase in stroke volume induced by a 45° leg lifting in healthy subjects was of larger magnitude after withdrawal of 500 ml blood, suggesting that PLR affects cardiac output differently according to the central volume status and thus the degree of cardiac preload reserve. An important point is that the PLR-induced increase in cardiac preload vanishes completely when the legs are returned to horizontal position [5, 8, 10, 11]. Therefore PLR can be considered as a brief and completely reversible "self-volume challenge". It must also be stressed that the effect of PLR on cardiac output—when it occurs—is not always sustained when the leg elevation is prolonged. In septic shock patients capillary leak may account for this attenuation. In a study including critically ill patients with circulatory failure we observed that the increase in the blood flow of the descending thoracic aorta induced by PLR in "preload-dependent" patients occurred in few seconds and was maximal approx. 1 min after starting the PLR maneuver [8]. In patients who did not have a sustained response to PLR the response to volume infusion also was not sustained. Thus the hemodynamic effects of PLR should be assessed during the time frame of 30–90 s after the onset of the test.

Postural changes during PLR are important to consider. If the trunk is in the semirecumbent position before the maneuver, PLR consists in pivoting the entire body, with the legs lifted up and the trunk ultimately in the horizontal position. With this method one would expect that PLR induces the transfer of a larger blood volume than if the trunk is initially lying horizontally since not only the venous blood of the legs but also that contained into the large splanchnic compartment is mobilized in such a case (Fig. 1; Electronic Supplementary Material, ESM). This should increase the total amount of blood that is mobilized during the postural maneuver.

The response to PLR may also depend upon the ability of the venous reservoir to be recruited. In a patient who is vasoconstricted because of hypovolemic/cardiogenic shock the venous reservoir is likely reduced, and the volume recruited by the PLR would be expected to be less. By contrast, in a patient with a vasodilatory state such as septic shock a higher unstressed volume is expected to be recruited by PLR. Based on this hypothesis, PLR should theoretically increase right ventricle preload less in patients with hypovolemic than in those with septic shock. However, in volume-depleted patients with high volume responsiveness even a moderate increase in preload can result in a significant change in cardiac output. In support of this, the increase in cardiac output in normal subjects in response to PLR has been shown to be increased after blood removal [12].

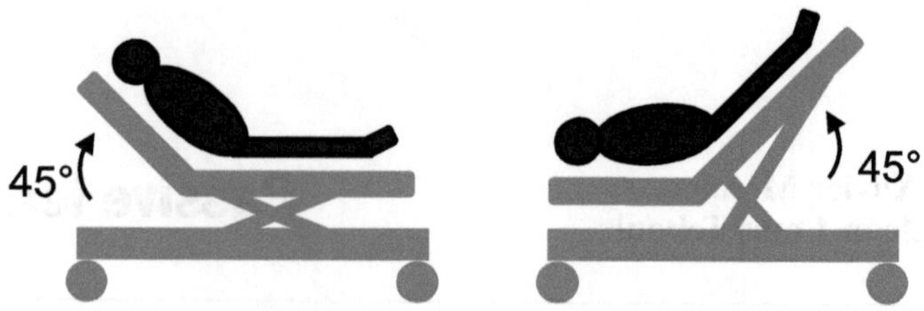

Fig. 1 Postural change during passive leg raising. If at baseline the patient is not lying horizontally but is in semirecumbent position, PLR consists of a simple pivoting of the entire bed. Compared to a case in which the trunk of the patient lies horizontally at baseline, this method is advantageous because (a) it does not change the hip angle, and (b) it may induce the transfer of a larger volume of blood

PLR for testing fluid responsiveness in the critically ill

Facing a hemodynamic failure, the clinician is often tempted to give fluid in order to increase cardiac output by fueling the reservoir in which the heart is pumping. However, fluid administration does not always result in cardiac output enhancement. This comes from the curvilinearity of the Frank–Starling relationship: if the heart is operating on the initial and steep part of the curve, it should have some preload reserve, and any increase in cardiac preload results in an increase in stroke volume. In this case the patient "responds" positively to fluid administration (Fig. 2). In contrast, if the heart is operating on the distal and flat part of the Frank–Starling curve (absence of preload reserve), no significant increase in stroke volume is expected from volume loading. In this case fluid administration may induce harmful effects (e. g., lung inflation, worsening of gas exchange in the case of pulmonary injury, worsening of tissue oxygen transfer) that would not be counterbalanced by any hemodynamic benefit. Thus the need has risen to find diagnostic tools for predicting which shocked patients will respond to fluid administration [13].

Predicting fluid responsiveness solely on the basis of measures of preload must be discouraged. Not only one but a family of Frank–Starling curves rely cardiac preload and stroke volume according to individual factors such as cardiac contractility (Fig. 2). Accordingly, a given value of preload could be associated with preload reserve in patients with normal cardiac contractility but with absence of preload reserve in the case of patients with profoundly

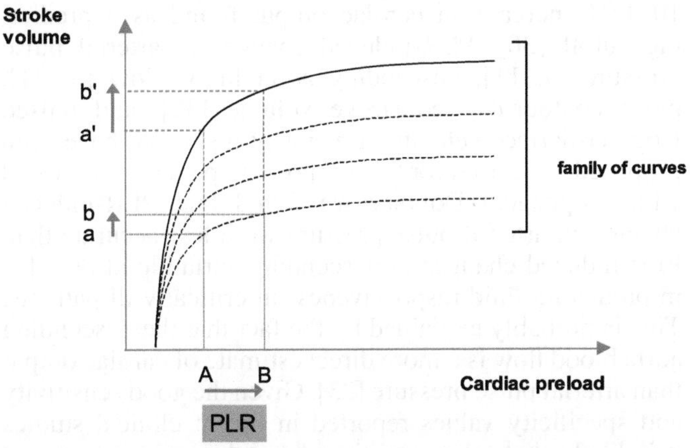

Fig. 2 Challenging the Frank–Starling curve with the passive leg raising (*PLR*). In patients with circulatory failure it is not possible to predict the response to volume administration because not just one but numerous curves rely stroke volume and cardiac preload. PLR induces a change in preload that enables to challenge the relationship. If the increase in cardiac preload occurring during the test (*from A to B*) produces a large increase in stroke volume (*from a' to b'*), preload responsiveness is likely and the patient should respond to fluid administration. If the increase in stroke volume during the test is of small amplitude (*from a to b*), preload responsiveness is unlikely and fluid administration should be avoided

impaired contractility because they are on the steep part of their cardiac function curve. Numerous studies now support the evidence that static measures of cardiac preload are not appropriate to assess preload reserve [14, 15]. In this regard cardiac filling pressures such as central venous pressure and pulmonary artery occlusion pressure cannot differentiate between patients responding and patients not responding to fluid administration [16]. Fluid responsiveness assessment must be rather based on the response to dynamic tests which induce transient changes in cardiac preload [17].

Since mechanical ventilation is able to induce cyclic changes in cardiac preload, the respiratory variation in stroke volume has been proposed to assess preload reserve [17]. Accordingly, the respiratory variations in surrogates of stroke volume such as arterial pulse pressure [18], Doppler subaortic flow [19], pulse contour derived stroke volume [20, 21], descending aortic blood flow [22], and even pulse oximetry wave [23] have been demonstrated to predict fluid responsiveness in the critically ill. Nonetheless, such heart–lung interaction indices can be used in only specific conditions, such as regular sinus cardiac rhythm and full adaptation of the patient to the ventilator as during deep sedation or coma. If not, the irregularity of the cardiac rhythm or of the respiratory cycle also account for variability in stroke volume such that fluid responsiveness can no longer be predicted by the variations in stroke volume [8, 24]. In patients with spontaneous ventilation respiratory variation in the central venous pressure has been proposed as an alternative [25]. Conflicting results have subsequently been reported [24], perhaps because the test is effective only in cases of no forced expiration [26].

PLR is an alternative means to predict the hemodynamic response to fluid administration since it can be used as a "self-volume challenge" at the bedside [27]. In mechanically ventilated patients fully adapted to their ventilator PLR-induced changes in stroke volume have been found to be closely correlated with the changes in stroke volume induced by a subsequent 300 ml colloid infusion [5]. Importantly, the hemodynamic changes induced by PLR are not affected by arrhythmias or by ventilator triggering. Therefore the PLR can be still used in circumstances where heart–lung interaction indices are misleading. In a study including 71 shocked patients monitored by esophageal Doppler we investigated whether the response of descending aortic blood flow to PLR predicts fluid responsiveness [8]. Interestingly, PLR increased the aortic flow time—a marker of left cardiac preload—to the same proportion in both responders and nonresponders, suggesting that this test actually performs as a volume challenge. The changes in the descending aortic blood observed during a PLR test were closely correlated with those induced by the subsequent volume expansion. Moreover, a PLR-induced increase in aortic blood flow by more than 10% predicted a fluid-induced increase in aortic blood flow by more than 15% (i. e., fluid responsiveness) with very good sensitivity and specificity [8] (Fig. 3). In the subgroup of patients fully adapted to their ventilator the response to PLR performed equally to pulse pressure respiratory variation in predicting volume responsiveness [8]. More importantly, in the subgroup of patients who triggered their ventilator or who experienced arrhythmias we found that the aortic blood flow response to PLR to predict fluid responsiveness retained its predictive value while pulse pressure variation was no longer reliable [8]. These findings emphasize the specific interest of PLR under conditions where heart–lung interactions

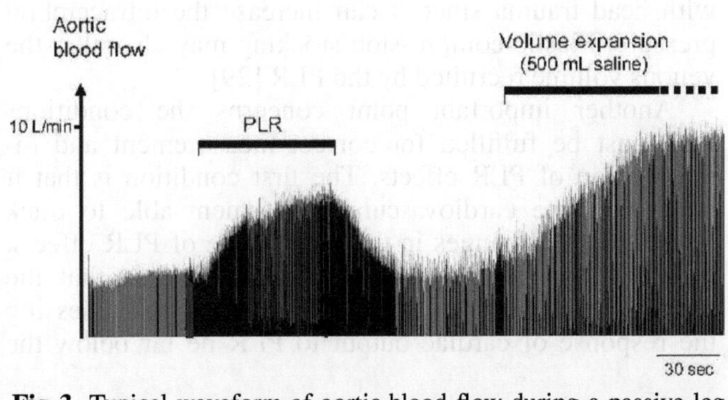

Fig. 3 Typical waveform of aortic blood flow during a passive leg raising (*PLR*) test and volume expansion in a patient with preload reserve. In this patient with an acute circulatory failure the increase in aortic blood flow observed during PLR can predict the positive response to volume expansion

indices cannot be interpretable. Recently two studies performed in patients with spontaneous breathing activity demonstrated that an increase in echocardiographic stroke volume by more than 12% in response to PLR well distinguished between responders and nonresponders to fluid administration [11, 28]. In addition, stroke volume response to PLR performed far better than static ultrasonographic indices of cardiac filling such as left ventricular end-diastolic area and Doppler estimates of left ventricular filling pressure [11].

As with any method for predicting response to fluid administration, the cutoff value found for the PLR effects should not be considered as a magic number. Furthermore, sensitivity and specificity values are not absolute. They should be interpreted differently depending upon the clinical context. For instance, the risk of giving fluid unduly may be more dangerous in patients with acute lung injury or acute respiratory distress syndrome. In these cases the physician should administer fluid if the effects of PLR on the cardiac output estimate are clearly above the proposed cutoff value.

Practical aspects of the PLR test

A simple way to perform PLR is to transfer the patient from the 45° semirecumbent to the PLR position by using the automatic pivotal motion of the patient's bed [8] (Fig. 1; see ESM). In addition to its ease of use, this method allows PLR to be performed rapidly without inducing hip flexion and femoral catheters motion. This is important since such procedures should avoid any pain-induced sympathetic stimulation that can result in erroneous interpretation of the hemodynamic effects of PLR. Accordingly, when performed in such a way, PLR did not increase heart rate, suggesting that no confusing sympathetic alteration occurred during the test [8]. Additionally, keeping the thorax in the horizontal position, and not lower, may avoid the risk of gastric inhalation. Nevertheless, it is reasonable to avoid PLR in patients with head trauma since it can increase the intracerebral pressure. Elastic compression stocking may also alter the venous volume recruited by the PLR [29].

Another important point concerns the conditions that must be fulfilled for correct measurement and interpretation of PLR effects. The first condition is that it be a real-time cardiovascular assessment able to track hemodynamic changes in the time frame of PLR effects, i. e., 30–90 s [30] (see ESM). The second is that the limits of precision in the technique used for assessing the response of cardiac output to PLR be far below the 10–15% increase in cardiac output found as a predicting cutoff [30]. PLR-induced changes in arterial pulse pressure [5, 11], descending aorta blood flow [8, 31], pulse contour-derived stroke volume [32], and pulsed Doppler-derived velocity–time integral [11, 28] have been proposed to be used for this purpose. In patients monitored with esophageal Doppler we found that PLR-induced changes in arterial pulse pressure were less accurate than PLR-induced changes in descending aorta blood flow [8] in predicting fluid responsiveness in critically ill patients. This is probably explained by the fact that the descending aorta blood flow is a more direct estimate of cardiac output than arterial pulse pressure [33]. Given the good sensitivity and specificity values reported in recent clinical studies it is likely that other real-time hemodynamic assessment methods such as transthoracic echocardiography (pulsed Doppler subaortic flow) [11, 28] and pulse contour cardiac output monitor [32] can be also appropriately used for quantifying the short-term hemodynamic response to PLR. The third requirement is to ensure that there is actually a change in preload in response to PLR before trying to determine whether there is an increase in cardiac output or preload. In the case of increase in cardiac preload with PLR the absence of increase in stroke volume should indicate that the patient is not fluid responsive. On the other hand, in the case of insufficient increase in preload with PLR (insufficient volume recruitment) the absence of PLR-induced increase in stroke volume cannot be interpreted. In such cases the PLR cannot be used to predict volume responsiveness. Thus it should be recommended to follow the changes in a marker of cardiac preload as a prerequisite to a correct interpretation of the PLR test [34]. Central venous pressure, duration of the aortic flow measured by esophageal Doppler, or end-diastolic dimensions at echocardiography can be used for this purpose. Finally, the level of the intra-abdominal pressure may be important to consider since it can impede the PLR-induced blood transfer when elevated. This point may be one of those that should be addressed by further studies concerning PLR.

In summary, the physiological effects of PLR consist of an increase in venous return and cardiac preload. The PLR thus acts as a self-volume challenge which is easy-to-perform and completely reversible. It has gained an increasing interest in the field of functional hemodynamic monitoring since it can help to detect fluid responsiveness in critically ill patients even in cases of ventilator spontaneous triggering or cardiac arrhythmias. Its optimal use requires a real-time cardiovascular assessment device able to quantify accurately the short-term hemodynamic response.

References

1. Rutlen DL, Wackers FJ, Zaret BL (1981) Radionuclide assessment of peripheral intravascular capacity: a technique to measure intravascular volume changes in the capacitance circulation in man. Circulation 64:146–152
2. Pozzoli M, Traversi E, Cioffi G, Stenner R, Sanarico M, Tavazzi L (1997) Loading manipulations improve the prognostic value of Doppler evaluation of mitral flow in patients with chronic heart failure. Circulation 95:1222–1230
3. Takagi S, Yokota M, Iwase M, Yoshida J, Hayashi H, Sotobata I, Koide M, Saito H (1989) The important role of left ventricular relaxation and left atrial pressure in the left ventricular filling velocity profile. Am Heart J 118:954–962
4. Rocha P, Lemaigre D, Leroy M, Desfonds P, De Zuttere D, Liot F (1987) Nitroglycerin-induced decrease of carbon monoxide diffusion capacity in acute myocardial infarction reversed by elevating legs. Crit Care Med 15:131–133
5. Boulain T, Achard JM, Teboul JL, Richard C, Perrotin D, Ginies G (2002) Changes in BP induced by passive leg raising predict response to fluid loading in critically ill patients. Chest 121:1245–1252
6. Kyriakides ZS, Koukoulas A, Paraskevaidis IA, Chrysos D, Tsiapras D, Galiotos C, Kremastinos DT (1994) Does passive leg raising increase cardiac performance? A study using Doppler echocardiography. Int J Cardiol 44:288–293
7. Paelinck BP, van Eck JW, De Hert SG, Gillebert TC (2003) Effects of postural changes on cardiac function in healthy subjects. Eur J Echocardiogr 4:196–201
8. Monnet X, Rienzo M, Osman D, Anguel N, Richard C, Pinsky MR, Teboul JL (2006) Passive leg raising predicts fluid responsiveness in the critically ill. Crit Care Med 34:1402–1407
9. Wong DH, O'Connor D, Tremper KK, Zaccari J, Thompson P, Hill D (1989) Changes in cardiac output after acute blood loss and position change in man. Crit Care Med 17:979–983
10. Bertolissi M, Broi UD, Soldano F, Bassi F (2003) Influence of passive leg elevation on the right ventricular function in anaesthetized coronary patients. Crit Care 7:164–170
11. Lamia B, Ochagavia A, Monnet X, Chemla D, Richard C, Teboul JL (2007) Echocardiographic prediction of volume responsiveness in critically ill patients with spontaneously breathing activity. Intensive Care Med 33:1125–1132
12. Wong DH, Tremper KK, Zaccari J, Hajduczek J, Konchigeri HN, Hufstedler SM (1988) Acute cardiovascular response to passive leg raising. Crit Care Med 16:123–125
13. Michard F, Teboul JL (2002) Predicting fluid responsiveness in ICU patients: a critical analysis of the evidence. Chest 121:2000–2008
14. Bendjelid K, Romand JA (2003) Fluid responsiveness in mechanically ventilated patients: a review of indices used in intensive care. Intensive Care Med 29:352–360
15. Monnet X, Teboul JL (2006) Invasive measures of left ventricular preload. Curr Opin Crit Care 12:235–240
16. Osman D, Ridel C, Ray P, Monnet X, Anguel N, Richard C, Teboul JL (2007) Cardiac filling pressures are not appropriate to predict hemodynamic response to volume challenge. Crit Care Med 35:64–68
17. Pinsky MR, Teboul JL (2005) Assessment of indices of preload and volume responsiveness. Curr Opin Crit Care 11:235–239
18. Michard F, Boussat S, Chemla D, Anguel N, Mercat A, Lecarpentier Y, Richard C, Pinsky MR, Teboul JL (2000) Relation between respiratory changes in arterial pulse pressure and fluid responsiveness in septic patients with acute circulatory failure. Am J Respir Crit Care Med 162:134–138
19. Feissel M, Michard F, Mangin I, Ruyer O, Faller JP, Teboul JL (2001) Respiratory changes in aortic blood velocity as an indicator of fluid responsiveness in ventilated patients with septic shock. Chest 119:867–873
20. Berkenstadt H, Margalit N, Hadani M, Friedman Z, Segal E, Villa Y, Perel A (2001) Stroke volume variation as a predictor of fluid responsiveness in patients undergoing brain surgery. Anesth Analg 92:984–989
21. Reuter DA, Felbinger TW, Schmidt C, Kilger E, Goedje O, Lamm P, Goetz AE (2002) Stroke volume variations for assessment of cardiac responsiveness to volume loading in mechanically ventilated patients after cardiac surgery. Intensive Care Med 28:392–398
22. Monnet X, Rienzo M, Osman D, Anguel N, Richard C, Pinsky MR, Teboul JL (2005) Esophageal Doppler monitoring predicts fluid responsiveness in critically ill ventilated patients. Intensive Care Med 31:1195–1201
23. Feissel M, Teboul JL, Merlani P, Badie J, Faller JP, Bendjelid K (2007) Plethysmographic dynamic indices predict fluid responsiveness in septic ventilated patients. Intensive Care Med 33:993–999
24. Heenen S, De Backer D, Vincent JL (2006) How can the response to volume expansion in patients with spontaneous respiratory movements be predicted? Crit Care 10:R102
25. Magder SA, Goeogiadis G, Tuck C (1992) Respiratory variations in right atrial pressure predict response to fluid challenge. J Crit Care 7:76–85
26. Magder S (2006) Predicting volume responsiveness in spontaneously breathing patients: still a challenging problem. Crit Care 10:165
27. Monnet X, Richard C, Teboul JL (2007) Passive leg raising. In: Vincent JL (ed) Yearbook of intensive care and emergency medicine. Springer, Berlin Heidelberg New York, pp 542–548
28. Maizel J, Airapetian N, Lorne E, Tribouilloy C, Massy Z, Slama M (2007) Diagnosis of central hypovolemia by using passive leg raising. Intensive Care Med 33:1133–1138
29. Zogheib E, Defouilloy C, Mahjoub Y, Cherradi N, Moubarak M, Beloucif S, Dupont H (2007) Modification of hemodynamic effect after passive leg raising test by the use of elastic compression stocking (abstract). Intensive Care Med 33:S72
30. De Backer D (2006) Can passive leg raising be used to guide fluid administration? Crit Care 10:170
31. Lafanechere A, Pene F, Goulenok C, Delahaye A, Mallet V, Choukroun G, Chiche J, Mira J, Cariou A (2006) Changes in aortic blood flow induced by passive leg raising predict fluid responsiveness in critically ill patients. Crit Care 10:R132
32. Ridel C, Lamia B, Monnet X, Richard C, Teboul JL (2006) Passive leg raising and fluid responsiveness during spontaneous breathing: pulse contour evaluation. Intensive Care Med 32:S81
33. De Backer D, Pinsky MR (2007) Can one predict fluid responsiveness in spontaneously breathing patients? Intensive Care Med 33:1111–1113
34. Antonelli M, Levy M, Andrews PJ, Chastre J, Hudson LD, Manthous C, Meduri GU, Moreno RP, Putensen C, Stewart T, Torres A (2007) Hemodynamic monitoring in shock and implications for management. Intensive Care Med 33:575–590

Sairam Parthasarathy
Martin J. Tobin

Sleep in the intensive care unit

Abstract Abnormalities of sleep are extremely common in critically ill patients, but the mechanisms are poorly understood. About half of total sleep time occurs during the daytime, and circadian rhythm is markedly diminished or lost. Judgments based on inspection consistently overestimate sleep time and do not detect sleep disruption. Accordingly, reliable polygraphic recordings are needed to measure sleep quantity and quality in critically ill patients. Critically ill patients exhibit more frequent arousals and awakenings than is normal, and decreases in rapid eye movement and slow wave sleep. The degree of sleep fragmentation is at least equivalent to that seen in patients with obstructive sleep apnea. About 20% of arousals and awakenings are related to noise, 10% are related to patient care activities, and the cause for the remainder is not known; severity of underlying disease is likely an important factor. Mechanical ventilation can cause sleep disruption, but the precise mechanism has not been defined. Sleep disruption can induce sympathetic activation and elevation of blood pressure, which may contribute to patient morbidity. In healthy subjects, sleep deprivation can decrease immune function and promote negative nitrogen balance. Measures to improve the quantity and quality of sleep in critically ill patients include careful attention to mode of mechanical ventilation, decreasing noise, and sedative agents (although the latter are double-edged swords).

Keywords Sleep · Critical illness · Mechanical ventilation · Artificial respiration · Arousal

Introduction

In his roman-a-clef, "Ravelstein", the Nobel Laureate Saul Bellow [1] describes being admitted to an intensive care unit and receiving mechanical ventilation:

"I was now the dying man. My lungs had failed. A machine did my breathing for me. Unconscious, I had no more idea of death than the dead have. But my head (I assume it was my head) was full of visions, delusions, and hallucinations. These were not dreams or nightmares. Nightmares have an escape hatch...."

Despite the obvious importance of sleep and its desirability in a patient with a serious illness, we know nothing of the visions, hallucinations and dreams experienced by a critically ill patient such as Bellow. Indeed, we know little of the sleep experienced by a critically ill patient. But we do know that sleep is commonly disrupted in critically ill patients [2, 3, 4, 5, 6, 7, 8, 9, 10, 11, 12, 13, 14, 15, 16], and that sleep disruption may adversely affect patient outcome [8, 17]. In this review, we discuss the nature of sleep disturbances in critically ill patients, potential causes, and possible therapies.

Normal sleep and circadian rhythm

Healthy young adults experience two distinct states of sleep: rapid eye movement (REM) sleep and non-REM (NREM) sleep. REM sleep accounts for about 25% of sleep time and is characterized by episodic bursts of rapid

DOI 10.1007/978-3-642-28233-1_7,

Table 1 Studies of sleep in critically ill patients

More than 24 h	Number of patients	Patient type	Sleep staging	Arousals and awakenings per hour	Mechanical ventilation (%)
Polysomnography performed over 24 h					
Hilton [2]	10	Medical	Yes	Not listed	Not listed
Aurell [3]	9	Postoperative	Yes	Not listed	Some patients
Gottschlich [4]	11	Burn patients	Yes	>63	100
Cooper [5]	20	Medical	Yes	39	100
Freedman [6]	22	Medical	Yes	>11	100
Valente [7]	24	Head trauma	Yes	Not listed	100
Gabor [8]	7	Medical	Yes	22	100
Polysomnography performed only at nighttime					
Johns [9]	5	Postoperative	Yes	Not listed	Not listed
Orr 10	9	Postoperative	Yes	Not listed	Not listed
Broughton [11]	12	Medical	Yes	>21	NA
Knill [12]	12	Postoperative	Yes	>21	Not listed
Edwards [13]	21	Medical	Yes	Not listed	95
Aaron [14]	6	Medical	Yes	>19	Not listed
Parthasarathy [15]	11	Medical	Yes	58	100
Richards [16]	64	Medical	Not listed	Not listed	0
Polysomnography not performed					
Woods [18]	4	Postoperative			Not listed
Helton [19]	62	Not listed			Not listed
Tweedie [20]	15	Medical and postoperative			80
Kong [21]	60	Medical			100
Hurel [22]	223	Medical and postoperative			0
Freedman [23]	203	Medical and postoperative			0
Simini [24]	162	Medical and postoperative			0
Treggiari [25]	40	Postoperative			0
Walder [26]	17	Postoperative			60
Shilo [27]	8	Medical			50
Olson [28]	843	Medical and postoperative			Not listed
Topf [29]	97	Postoperative			Not listed
Nelson [30]	100	Medical			60
Mundigler [31]	24	Medical and postoperative			100
McKinley [32]	14	Medical and postoperative			0

eye movements, irregularities in respiration and heart rate, and paralysis of major muscle groups with the exception of the diaphragm and upper airway muscles. NREM sleep is divided into four stages (1, 2, 3 and 4). The progression of sleep from stage 1 through to stage 4 is accompanied by a progressive increase in the arousal threshold (the ability to wake in response to a stimulus). Stage 1 occurs at sleep onset and is also a transitional state between sleep stages. Up to 50% of the night is spent in stage 2 sleep, which is characterized by spindles and K complexes on the electroencephalograph (EEG). Progression of stage 2 is accompanied by the gradual appearance of high-voltage slow wave activity on the EEG (greater than 75 μV and less than 2 Hz). When such slow-wave activity exceeds 20% of the time in a 30-s epoch, sleep is categorized as stage 3; when it exceeds 50%, sleep is categorized as stage 4. Slow wave sleep is considered the most restorative. NREM sleep normally cycles with REM sleep every 90 min. The cycling of sleep and wakefulness, in turn, is regulated by a biological clock that operates over a 24-h period (circadian rhythm). In addition to sleep, the biological clock regulates several physiological, behavioral, and biochemical rhythms. Hormone secretion (cortisol, growth hormone), body temperature, immune function, coronary artery muscle tone, and bronchial smooth muscle tone, to name a few, exhibit marked circadian variability.

Abnormalities of sleep in critically ill patients

Just as with ambulatory patients, sleep in critically ill patients is assessed in terms of quantity, distribution over 24 h, and lack of continuity. Also assessed is the type and depth of sleep—rapid eye movement (REM) and non-REM (stages 1, 2, 3 and 4)—and the pattern from day to day in the distribution of sleep over a 24-h period (circadian rhythm). Accurate measurement of sleep quantity and quality requires reliable polygraphic recordings. Judgments based on inspection consistently overestimate sleep time [3] and do not detect sleep disruption [3, 13]. Table 1 classifies research reports on sleep in critically ill patients into studies involving polysomnographic recordings over 24 h [2, 3, 4, 5, 6, 7, 8], polysomnographic recordings during nighttime alone [9, 10, 11, 12, 13, 14, 15, 16], and studies without polysomnographic recordings [18, 19, 20, 21, 22, 23, 24, 25, 26, 27, 28, 29, 30, 31, 32]. Also indicated is the type of patient population, whether patients were receiving mechanical ventilation, and whether sleep stages and disruption were adequately reported. Of the 28 studies listed in Table 1, 15 employed polysomnography [2, 3, 4, 5, 6, 7, 8, 9, 10, 11, 12, 13, 14, 15, 16], and 7 included continuous recordings for 24 h or longer [2, 3, 4, 5, 6, 7, 8]. These studies reveal that almost half of total sleep time in critically ill patients can occur during the daytime [5, 8].

Investigators differ in their conclusions as to whether critically ill patients are sleep deprived. Three groups of investigators found that critically ill patients have a normal or near normal total sleep time, an average of 7–10.4 h a day [4, 5, 6]. Three other groups of investigators found a decrease in total sleep time, 3.6–6.2 h a day [2, 3, 8]. The investigators in one of the studies revealing decreased sleep time had deliberately restricted sedatives and hypnotics [3], although patients received sedatives in the other two studies that revealed sleep deprivation [2, 8]. Even in the studies revealing adequate amounts of sleep, the investigators noted large variations in total sleep time among the patients. Cooper and co-workers found that some patients slept for hardly an hour and other patients for nearly 15 of 24 h [5] (Fig. 1). Total sleep time in the study of Freedman and co-workers varied from 1.7 to 19.4 h [6]. Patients falling in the lowest quartile for total sleep time in these studies are clearly suffering from major sleep deprivation. In addition to variation in sleep quality from patient to patient, sleep quality may vary from night to night within a patient as a result of changes in acuity of illness [33], pain, and sedative and analgesic infusions. As such, sleep deprivation occurs in many, if not all, critically ill patients. To achieve better clarification of the frequency and severity of sleep deprivation, longitudinal studies in a large number of patients are needed; it will be essential to control for the effects of sedation, analgesia, and acuity of illness when conducting such studies.

In 11 critically ill patients, Parthasarathy and Tobin [15] noted 19 arousals (abrupt shifts in EEG frequency lasting more than 3 s) and 35 awakenings (EEG features compatible with wakefulness) per hour. Total sleep disruption, 54 arousals and awakenings per hour, was more than twice that seen in healthy individuals similarly instrumented. Cooper and co-workers [5] also reported frequent sleep disruption, with 42 arousals and awakenings per hour, and Gabor and co-workers [8] reported somewhat less frequent disruption, 22 arousals and awakenings per hour. With the exception of the three preceding studies [5, 8, 15], the remaining investigators who obtained EEG recordings in critically ill patients did not specify the sum of arousals and awakenings [3, 7, 9, 10, 16], making it impossible to compare studies in that respect (Table 1). The degree of sleep fragmentation in studies of critically ill patients, however, is equivalent to that in patients with obstructive sleep apnea [34].

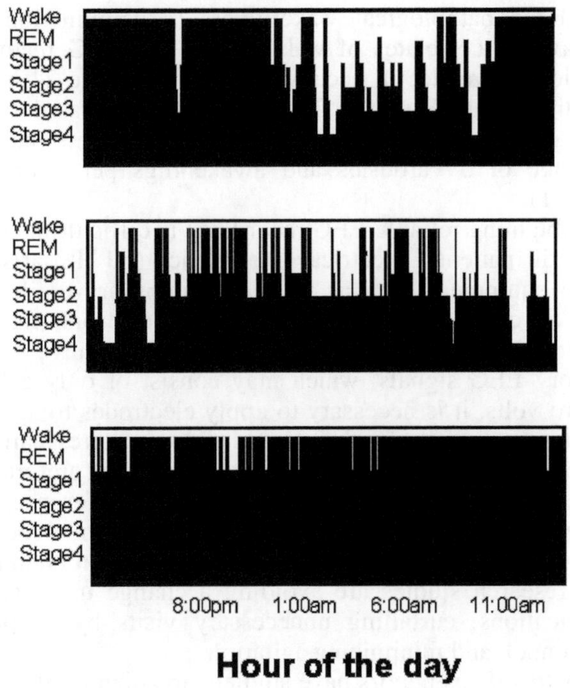

Fig. 1 Sleep stages, along the vertical axis, over a 24-h period in three critically ill patients with disrupted sleep. The hypnogram in patient 1 (*top*) reveals a normal nocturnal sleep pattern. Patients 2 (*middle*) slept for 65% of time, predominantly stages 1 and 2, and wakened repeatedly. Patient 3 (*bottom*) had isolated episodes of stage 1 sleep but was awake for most of 24 h. (Modified from [5] with permission)

Sleep is normally divided into rapid eye movement (REM) and non-REM (NREM) sleep. Critically ill patients spend 6% or less of sleep time in REM sleep as opposed to the normal of 25% [5, 6, 12]. The decrease in REM sleep has been attributed to medications (narcotics) [12], lack of sustained sleep needed to reach REM sleep [6], disturbance of circadian rhythm, underlying disease, and endotoxin release [35, 36]. The reduction in REM sleep might also be an adaptive response to critical illness because REM is a time of sympathetic-parasympathetic imbalance and increased susceptibility to breathing abnormalities. Critically ill patients also experience less of stages 3 and 4 of NREM, which are characterized by stable respiratory control and are devoid of sympathetic-parasympathetic imbalances.

Critically ill patients may not exhibit the EEG features of sleep and wakefulness conventionally seen in ambulatory patients [5]. Cooper and co-workers found that 7 of 20 mechanically ventilated patients were in coma and 5 patients did not exhibit EEG characteristics of stage 2 sleep (spindles or K complexes). Four patients exhibited pathological wakefulness (a combination of behavioral correlates of wakefulness and EEG features of slow wave sleep), occupying 26–68% of the 24-h recording. Only 8 of the 20 patients demonstrated EEG characteristics of sleep, and even these patients had an average of 39 arousals and awakenings per hour [5] (Fig. 1).

Obtaining reliable EEG recordings is difficult in critically ill patients. Electrical interference (60 Hz) arising from equipment such as infusion pumps or ventilators [37] is common; interference also arises from muscle contractions in agitated patients [38]. To achieve satisfactory EEG signals, which may consist of only a few micro volts, it is necessary to apply electrodes to appropriate areas of the scalp; the skin also requires careful preparation to ensure low contact impedance (preferably less than 5 Ohms). To further minimize interference, all wires between a patient and preamplifier must be as short as possible [37]. Additional challenges in conducting research studies are avoiding a change in sedative medications, curtailing unnecessary visits by hospital personnel, and minimizing agitation.

A few investigators have studied circadian rhythms in critically ill patients. Mundeglier and co-workers [31] measured urinary 6-sulfatoxymelatonin every 4 h over 24 h. Compared with 7 non-septic critically ill patients and 21 healthy volunteers, the amplitude of circadian fluctuation in this melatonin metabolite was markedly lower in 17 critically ill patients suffering from septic shock.

Relationship between sedation and sleep

Critically ill patients are often given sedatives to increase patient comfort, decrease anxiety and agitation, and promote amnesia and sleep [25, 39]. Continuous infusion of sedatives, however, may prolong the duration of mechanical ventilation by 2.5 days and prolong ICU stay by 3.5 days [40]. The effect of sedative agents on the depth of sedation has been rigorously studied [39, 41, 42], although little is known about its effect on sleep quality in critically ill patients [43]. Over a 5-day period, 40 non-intubated critically ill patients were randomized to nocturnal midazolam and propofol [25]. On a 10-point self-rating scale, both groups reported a tendency towards improved sleep quality: from 6.3 to 7.2. The infusions were titrated to achieve a score of 3 or greater on the Ramsay sedation scale (a score of 3 indicates that a patient is asleep but awakens with a brisk response to a glabellar tap or a loud auditory stimulus) [42]. Self-perception of sleep quality was not different for propofol and midazolam (range 0.1–9.7; mean of 7.2). Some patients continued to rate sleep quality close to zero on the fifth day. These data indicate that self-perception of sleep quality can be poor with high dosages of sedatives despite achieving adequate levels of sedation. Severe sleep fragmentation may also occur in mechanically ventilated patients despite sedatives and analgesics [4, 5].

Some of the discrepancies between bedside assessment of sedation and subjective scoring of sleep may reflect known limitations in the Ramsay sedation scale [43]. Kong and co-workers studied the efficacy of midazolam and isoflurane in reducing plasma levels of catecholamines when similar levels of sedation (on the Ramsay scale) were achieved. Although both agents achieved comparable levels of sedation, isoflurane, but not midazolam, lowered the plasma levels of catecholamines from baseline [21]. The persistently elevated catecholamines in the patients receiving midazolam may have produced sleep disruption, although the explanation is no more than a possibility because polysomnography was not performed.

Benzodiazepines, narcotic analgesics, and propofol are commonly used to sedate critically ill patients [39]. Benzodiazepines improve behavioral aspects of sleep. They decrease the time needed to fall asleep, decrease awakenings, increase sleep duration, and increase sleep efficiency (duration of sleep as a percentage of time in bed). Benzodiazepines, however, also increase the number of spindles, increase cortical EEG frequency (at low doses), decrease EEG amplitude and frequency (at high doses), *and* suppress REM and slow wave sleep [44]. Although the clinical importance of these EEG alterations is not totally clear, an ideal hypnotic should not disturb the normal sleep pattern. Narcotics can also suppress REM sleep, cause a dose-dependent slowing of EEG, and suppress slow wave sleep—the most restorative stage of sleep [12, 44, 45]. In sum, a medicated state may resemble sleep on the surface, but may not provide the physiological benefits associated with true sleep.

Factors contributing to sleep disruption

Noise and hospital staff

The level of noise in the ICU ranges from 50 to 75 dB, with peaks of up to 85 dB [8, 26, 46, 47, 48, 49, 50, 51, 52]. This level of noise is comparable to that in a factory (80 dB) or a busy office (70 dB), and is louder than noise in a bedroom (40 dB) [51]. (The decibel scale is logarithmic, and an increase of 10 dB represents a doubling of noise.) When studying the relationship between ICU noise and sleep disruption, investigators commonly attribute arousals to noise when they occur within 3 s of a measurable (greater than 15 dB) increase in noise [5, 6]. In these studies, 11–20% of arousals were attributed to noise [5, 6]. Because critically ill patients have frequent arousals and awakenings (20–68 per hour, Table 1) some arousals may mistakenly be attributed to noise. In a study of healthy volunteers subjected to audio recordings of ICU noise, a greater than normal number of awakenings and less REM and total sleep time were observed [50, 53]. Findings in healthy subjects, however, may not apply to critically ill patients, who may have a higher arousal threshold secondary to sleep deprivation, sedative agents, or coma.

Gabor and co-workers [8] recorded audio and video signals in synchrony with polysomnography in seven patients receiving mechanical ventilation. Twenty percent of the arousals and awakenings were related to noise peaks, and only 10% were related to patient care activities. The cause of 68% of arousals and awakenings could not be identified [8].

Mechanical ventilation

About 40% of patients in an ICU receive mechanical ventilation [54], but investigations into the precise mechanisms of the effect of mechanical ventilation on sleep are only commencing. Mechanically ventilated patients experience considerable sleep disruption, with as many as 20–63 arousals and awakenings per hour [4, 5, 8]. At first glance, a comparison of mechanically ventilated patients with spontaneously breathing critically ill patients should provide a reasonable method for investigating the effect of mechanical ventilation on sleep (Table 1). Such comparisons might prove misleading for a number of reasons. First, acuity of illness may be greater in ventilated patients than in spontaneously breathing patients. Second, spontaneously breathing patients are vulnerable to obstructive apneas, which will be prevented by an endotracheal tube. Third, factors associated with ventilation, such as masks, tracheal tubes, suctioning, mouth guards, nasogastric tubes, and physical restraints, may contribute to sleep fragmentation [55]. Fourth, sedatives and analgesics are more likely during mechanical ventilation. An attractive way to study the effect of mechanical ventilation on sleep might be to study tracheostomized patients while connected and disconnected from a ventilator over a short time period.

Notwithstanding methodological concerns with the studies, data suggest that the mode of ventilation can influence sleep quality [56, 57]. Meza and co-workers [56] showed that pressure support induces central apneas in healthy subjects during sleep. In a study of 11 critically ill patients during one night of sleep, Parthasarathy and Tobin observed greater sleep fragmentation during pressure support than during assist-control ventilation: 79 versus 54 arousals and awakenings per hour (Fig. 2). Six of the 11 patients developed central apneas during pressure support, but not during assist-control ventilation [15]. Heart failure was more common in the patients who developed apneas than in the patients without apneas: 83% versus 20%. The findings emphasize that research on sleep in critically ill patients needs to be controlled for the ventilator mode. In these 11 patients, the most important determinant of apneas was the difference between PCO_2 during resting breathing and the patient's apnea threshold. When a patient's resting PCO_2 was close to the apnea threshold, central apneas were more likely to develop. The addition of dead space caused a further increase in resting PCO_2 above the apnea threshold and decreased the sum of arousals and awakenings from 83 to 44 events per hour (in the patients who developed central apneas during pressure support). Sleep efficiency (time asleep as a percentage of study duration) increased from 63 to 81% with the addition of dead space (Fig. 2).

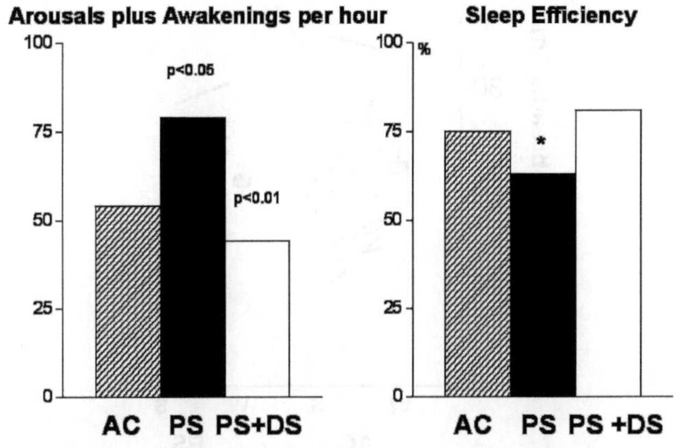

Fig. 2 Sleep fragmentation (*left panel*) and sleep efficiency (*right panel*) during assist-control ventilation and pressure support with and without dead space. Sleep fragmentation, measured as the number of arousals and awakenings, was greater during pressure support (*solid bars*) than during assist-control ventilation (*hatched bars*) or pressure support with dead space (*open bars*). Sleep efficiency (*right panel*) was also lower during pressure support (*solid bars*) than during assist-control ventilation (*hatched bars*) or pressure support with dead space (*open bars*). (Modified from [15] with permission)

Other factors

Factors that contribute to sleep abnormalities in critically ill patients include acute illness [2, 3, 11, 12], pain, light, and patient discomfort [17]. Noxious stimuli that contribute to patient discomfort and arousal include increased respiratory effort [58, 59], hypoxemia [58], and hypercapnia [58]. Swings in intrathoracic pressures are potent stimuli for inducing arousals in healthy subjects [60] and in patients with upper airway resistance syndrome [34].

Clinical implications

Clinical outcomes

Sleep fragmentation may influence morbidity and mortality in critically ill patients. Patients in coma and pa-

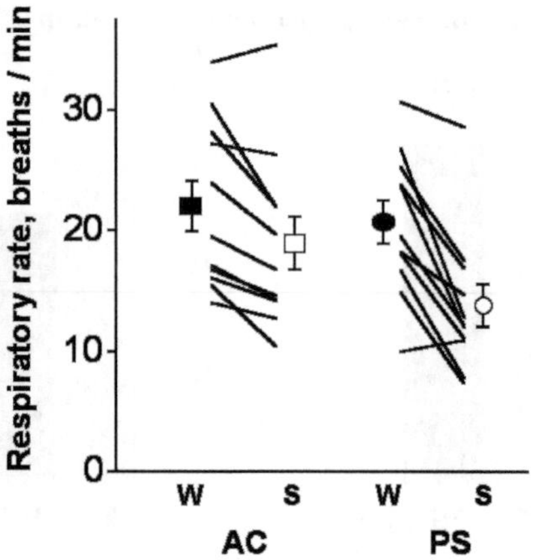

Fig. 3 Respiratory rate during assist-control ventilation (*AC*) and pressure support (*PS*) in 11 critically ill patients. For each mode, the lines connect the mean value for each patient during wakefulness (*W, left*) and sleep (*S, right*). Compared with wakefulness, group mean respiratory rate was lower during sleep (*closed symbols*) than during wakefulness (*open symbols*). The difference between sleep and wakefulness was greater for pressure support than for assist-control ventilation. (Modified from [15] with permission)

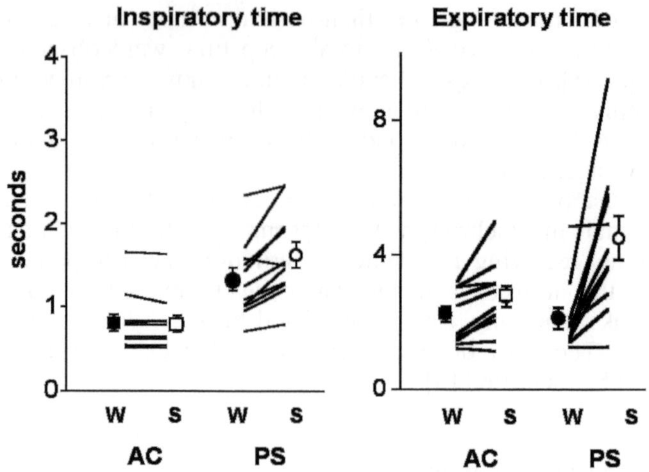

Fig. 4 Inspiratory time (*left panel*) and expiratory time (*right panel*) during assist-control ventilation (*AC*) and pressure support (*PS*) in 11 critically ill patients. The lines connect the mean value for each patient during wakefulness (*W, left*) and sleep (*S, right*). During pressure support, group mean inspiratory time and expiratory time were greater during sleep (*closed symbols*) than during wakefulness (*open symbols*). The difference between sleep and wakefulness was greater for pressure support than for assist-control ventilation. (Modified from [15] with permission)

tients who lack well-defined EEG characteristics of stage 2 sleep have higher acute physiological scores than do patients with identifiable but fragmented sleep [5]. Some investigators have reported no association between the acuity of illness and sleep disruption [6]. As such, the contribution of acuity of illness to sleep disturbances is unclear. Animal data suggest that sleep deprivation may lead to death [61]. It is thought that death is unlikely to result with sleep deprivation in human subjects [62, 63], but the consequence of sleep deprivation has been studied only in healthy subjects and not in critically ill patients.

Among 24 patients with post-traumatic coma, 5 of 6 patients who had organized sleep patterns survived as opposed to 3 of 7 patients who had low voltage theta-delta or mixed frequency activity without definable features of sleep; functional outcome was also better in the patients with organized sleep patterns [7]. Freedman and co-workers found that 5 of 22 patients exhibited EEG features of mild to moderate encephalopathy before other features of sepsis manifested [6]; none of the non-septic patients demonstrated such EEG features.

Ventilator settings

Physicians typically adjust ventilator settings during the daytime and without knowing whether a patient is asleep or awake. Compared with wakefulness, sleep caused a 33% decrease in respiratory rate during pressure support and a 15% decrease in rate during assist-control (Fig. 3) [15]. The level of pressure support is commonly titrated to respiratory rate, which provides reasonable guidance as to a patient's inspiratory effort [64, 65]. If, however, physicians titrate pressure support to respiratory rate while the patient is asleep, patient effort will increase considerably on awakening.

Changes in ventilator settings are commonly based on arterial blood gas measurements. End-tidal CO_2 was greater in 11 critically ill patients during sleep than during wakefulness: by 11% during pressure support and by 5% during assist-control ventilation. Patients who repeatedly slip in and out of sleep display marked fluctuations in end-tidal CO_2. The coefficient of variation of end-tidal CO_2 was 8.7% during pressure support and 4.7% during assist-control ventilation [15]. In some patients receiving pressure support, end-tidal CO_2 can be as much as 7 mmHg higher during sleep than during wakefulness. Differences in PCO_2 between sleep and wakefulness of this magnitude may cause physicians to change ventilator settings when a change is not necessary. Consequently, under-ventilation or over-ventilation may result [66]. Compared with wakefulness, sleep caused a 23% increase in inspiratory time and a 126% increase in expiratory time in patients receiving pressure support (Fig. 4). The increase in inspiratory time that accompanied change from wakefulness to sleep was also associated with an increase in tidal volume, and the likely accompaniment of hypocapnia may explain the development of apneas during pressure support [67, 68]. These findings indicate that the effect of sleep on breathing pattern and gas exchange has important implications for research on patient-ventilator interaction.

Cardiorespiratory consequences

In ambulatory patients, sleep fragmentation can result in elevations of arterial blood pressure, elevations of urinary and serum catecholamines, arrhythmias, progression of cardiac failure, and even death [69, 70]. Sleep-disordered breathing might cause similar abnormalities in critically ill patients, although direct evidence is lacking. Apneas and hypopneas cause hypoxemia [16], which, in turn, may produce sympathetic activation and arrhythmias in critically ill patients; evidence on this issue, however, is anecdotal [71] and inconclusive [72].

Sleep fragmentation induced by auditory stimuli can increase nocturnal blood pressure in dogs [73]. In patients who have central sleep apnea, the major cause of oscillations in blood pressure is ventilatory oscillations, with a significant contribution from arousals [73]. These investigations [73, 74] suggest that arousals may elevate nocturnal blood pressure, secondary to increases in sympathetic activity, and contribute to cardiovascular complications [75]. Preliminary data suggests that sleep fragmentation in critically ill patients may be associated with elevations in blood pressure [76], but the effect on morbidity and mortality is unknown.

The effect of sleep deprivation [77] on the ventilatory responses to hypoxia and hypercapnia is controversial [78]. Sleep deprivation has long been believed to depress chemoreceptor function [78]. Spengler and colleagues [78], however, recently found that sleep deprivation did not alter the hypercapnic ventilatory response in healthy subjects. The situation in critically ill patients has not been studied. Blunting of the chemoreceptor response can decrease the ability of the respiratory system to compensate for respiratory loads during or after the withdrawal of mechanical ventilation [68].

At least some postoperative patients experience an increase in REM sleep on the third to fourth postoperative day secondary to the earlier suppression of REM sleep by anesthetics and analgesics [12]. Because REM sleep is characterized by unstable breathing patterns and sympathetic-parasympathetic imbalances, the increase in REM sleep in the early postoperative period may aggravate the risk of postoperative atelectasis, pneumonia, hypoxemia, and cardiovascular morbidity.

Neurological consequences

Sleep deprivation may contribute to delirium and agitation [19, 79]. In a study of 62 critically ill patients, Helton and colleagues [19] noted that 24% experienced severe sleep deprivation and 16% experienced moderate deprivation. One third of the patients with severe sleep disruption suffered from delirium, 10% of patients with moderate sleep disruption suffered from delirium, but only 3% of patients with adequate sleep had delirium. The study has limitations. Sleep was assessed at the bedside by nursing staff rather than polysomnography. No intervention was performed, and a cause and effect relationship between sleep deprivation and delirium cannot be inferred. Agitation can cause elevations in plasma catecholamines [21]. Large doses of sedative agents are often used in agitated and delirious patients; when the agitation resolves, however, the sedative agent may remain in adipose tissue and interfere with weaning from mechanical ventilation.

Immunological and metabolic consequences

Sleep deprivation can unfavorably alter immune function [80, 81, 82, 83, 84, 85, 86]. In 42 healthy volunteers, Irwin and co-workers found that sleep deprivation resulted in almost a 50% decrease in natural killer cell activity and a 50% decrease in lymphokine killer cell activity. One night of sleep returned natural killer cell activity to baseline.

Sleep deprivation can promote negative nitrogen balance and increase energy expenditure [62, 63, 87]. In six healthy volunteers, 24 h of sleep deprivation produced a 7% increase in nitrogen excretion. Some subjects experienced as much as a 20% increase in nitrogen excretion. It is not known whether similar changes occur in critically ill patients.

Long-term consequences

Critical illness may have long-term consequences on sleep [22]. When 329 patients were interviewed 6 months after discharge from an ICU, 223 (67%) reported severe alterations in sleep. The lack of a control group makes it impossible to distinguish the role of critical illness from previous health status, underlying medical diagnosis, persistent disability, or other factors.

Strategies to decrease sleep disruption

Gabor and co-workers studied the effect of reducing noise in six healthy volunteers while they slept in an ICU [8]. The average level of noise was 51 dB in an open ICU and 43 dB in an isolated single room (the respective peak levels were 65 and 54 dB). Total sleep time was greater in the isolated room than in the open ICU, 9.5 versus 8.2 h, although the number of arousals and awakenings were virtually identical in the two settings (14 to 15 events per hour) [8]. In six healthy volunteers attempting to sleep in a noisy environment, Wallace and co-workers found that use of earplugs increased REM sleep (20 versus 15%) and decreased REM latency (107 versus 148 min), although the number of awakenings was not affected (25 versus 27 per hour). Because only 20% of sleep fragmentation in critically ill patients appears to be attributable to noise [8], reducing noise in the ICU may be of limited value.

Shilo and co-workers undertook a double blind, placebo-controlled study of melatonin in eight critically ill patients with chronic obstructive pulmonary disease [27]. The authors conclude that melatonin achieved greater sleep time and less fragmentation, although the conclusions are not well supported by the data.

Conclusion

Research into sleep disorders in ambulatory patients over the last 30 years has provided us with a strong set of physiological principles. The time is ripe for applying these principles to critically ill patients. A major challenge, as with most research in critically ill patients, is the difficulty in controlling for confounding influences in order to achieve high fidelity recordings.

References

1. Bellow S (2000) Ravelstein. Penguin, New York, pp 208
2. Hilton BA (1976) Quantity and quality of patients' sleep and sleep-disturbing factors in a respiratory intensive care unit. J Adv Nurs 1:453–468
3. Aurell J, Elmqvist D (1985) Sleep in the surgical intensive care unit: continuous polygraphic recording of sleep in nine patients receiving postoperative care. BMJ 290:1029–1032
4. Gottschlich MM, Jenkins ME, Mayes T, Khoury J, Kramer M, Warden GD, Kagan RJ (1994) The 1994 Clinical Research Award. A prospective clinical study of the polysomnographic stages of sleep after burn injury. J Burn Care Rehabil 15:486–492
5. Cooper AB, Thornley KS, Young GB, Slutsky AS, Stewart TE, Hanly PJ (2000) Sleep in critically ill patients requiring mechanical ventilation. Chest 117:809–818
6. Freedman NS, Gazendam J, Levan L, Pack AI, Schwab RJ (2001) Abnormal sleep/wake cycles and the effect of environmental noise on sleep disruption in the intensive care unit. Am J Respir Crit Care Med 163:451–457
7. Valente M, Placidi F, Oliveira AJ, Bigagli A, Morghen I, Proietti R, Gigli GL (2002) Sleep organization pattern as a prognostic marker at the subacute stage of post-traumatic coma. Clin Neurophysiol 113:1798–1805
8. Gabor JY, Cooper AB, Crombach SA, Lee B, Kadikar N, Bettger HE, Hanly PJ (2003) Contribution of the intensive care unit environment to sleep disruption in mechanically ventilated patients and healthy subjects. Am J Respir Crit Care Med 167:708–715
9. Johns MW, Large AA, Masterton JP, Dudley HA (1974) Sleep and delirium after open heart surgery. Br J Surg 61:377–381
10. Orr WC, Stahl ML (1977) Sleep disturbances after open heart surgery. Am J Cardiol 39:196–201
11. Broughton R, Baron R (1978) Sleep patterns in the intensive care unit and on the ward after acute myocardial infarction. Electroencephalogr Clin Neurophysiol 45:348–360
12. Knill RL, Moote CA, Skinner MI, Rose EA (1990) Anesthesia with abdominal surgery leads to intense REM sleep during the first postoperative week. Anesthesiology 73:52–61
13. Edwards GB, Schuring LM (1993) Pilot study: validating staff nurses' observations of sleep and wake states among critically ill patients, using polysomnography. Am J Crit Care 2:125–131
14. Aaron JN, Carlisle CC, Carskadon MA, Meyer TJ, Hill NS, Millman RP (1996) Environmental noise as a cause of sleep disruption in an intermediate respiratory care unit. Sleep 19:707–710
15. Parthasarathy S, Tobin MJ (2002) Effect of ventilator mode on sleep quality in critically ill patients. Am J Respir Crit Care Med 166:1423–1429
16. Richards KC, Anderson WM, Chesson AL Jr, Nagel CL (2002) Sleep-related breathing disorders in patients who are critically ill. J Cardiovasc Nurs 17:42–55
17. Krachman SL, D'Alonzo GE, Criner GJ (1995) Sleep in the intensive care unit. Chest 107:1713–1720
18. Woods NF (1972) Patterns of sleep in postcardiotomy patients. Nurs Res 21:347–352
19. Helton MC, Gordon SH, Nunnery SL (1980) The correlation between sleep deprivation and the intensive care unit syndrome. Heart Lung 9:464–468
20. Tweedie IE, Bell CF, Clegg A, Campbell IT, Minors DS, Waterhouse JM (1989) Retrospective study of temperature rhythms of intensive care patients. Crit Care Med 17:1159–1165
21. Kong KL, Willatts SM, Prys-Roberts C, Harvey JT, Gorman S (1990) Plasma catecholamine concentration during sedation in ventilated patients requiring intensive therapy. Intensive Care Med 16:171–174
22. Hurel D, Loirat P, Saulnier F, Nicolas F, Brivet F (1997) Quality of life 6 months after intensive care: results of a prospective multicenter study using a generic health status scale and a satisfaction scale. Intensive Care Med 23:331–337
23. Freedman NS, Kotzer N, Schwab RJ (1999) Patient perception of sleep quality and etiology of sleep disruption in the intensive care unit. Am J Respir Crit Care Med 159:1155–1162
24. Simini B (1999) Patients' perceptions of intensive care. Lancet 354:571–572
25. Treggiari-Venzi M, Borgeat A, Fuchs-Buder T, Gachoud JP, Suter PM (1996) Overnight sedation with midazolam or propofol in the ICU: effects on sleep quality, anxiety and depression. Intensive Care Med 22:1186–1190
26. Walder B, Francioli D, Meyer JJ, Lancon M, Romand JA (2000) Effects of guidelines implementation in a surgical intensive care unit to control nighttime light and noise levels. Crit Care Med 28:2242–2247
27. Shilo L, Dagan Y, Smorjik Y, Weinberg U, Dolev S, Komptel B, Shenkman L (2000) Effect of melatonin on sleep quality of COPD intensive care patients: a pilot study. Chronobiol Int 17:71–76
28. Olson DM, Borel CO, Laskowitz DT, Moore DT, McConnell ES (2001) Quiet time: a nursing intervention to promote sleep in neurocritical care units. Am J Crit Care 10:74–78
29. Topf M, Thompson S (2001) Interactive relationships between hospital patients' noise-induced stress and other stress with sleep. Heart Lung 30:237–243
30. Nelson JE, Meier DE, Oei EJ, Nierman DM, Senzel RS, Manfredi PL, Davis SM, Morrison RS (2001) Self-reported symptom experience of critically ill cancer patients receiving intensive care. Crit Care Med 29:277–282

31. Mundigler G, Delle-Karth G, Koreny M, Zehetgruber M, Steindl-Munda P, Marktl W, Ferti L, Siostrzonek P (2002) Impaired circadian rhythm of melatonin secretion in sedated critically ill patients with severe sepsis. Crit Care Med 30:536–540
32. McKinley S, Nagy S, Stein-Parbury J, Bramwell M, Hudson J (2002) Vulnerability and security in seriously ill patients in intensive care. Intensive Crit Care Nurs 18:27–36
33. Parthasarathy S, Tobin MJ (2003) Is sleep disruption related to severity of critical illness (abstract)? Am J Respir Crit Care Med 167:A968
34. Guilleminault C, Partinen M, Quera-Salva MA, Hayes B, Dement WC, Nino-Murcia G (1988) Determinants of daytime sleepiness in obstructive sleep apnea. Chest 94:32–37
35. Young GB, Bolton CF, Austin TW, Archibald YM, Gonder J, Wells GA (1990) The encephalopathy associated with septic illness. Clin Invest Med 13:297–304
36. Trachsel L, Schreiber W, Holsboer F, Pollmacher T (1994) Endotoxin enhances EEG alpha and beta power in human sleep. Sleep 17:132–139
37. Prior PF (1985) EEG monitoring and evoked potentials in brain ischaemia. Br J Anaesth 57:63–81
38. Riker RR, Fraser GL, Simmons LE, Wilkins ML (2001) Validating the sedation agitation scale with the bispectral index and visual analog scale in adult ICU patients after cardiac surgery. Intensive Care Med 27:853–858
39. Kress JP, Pohlman AS, Hall JB (2002) Sedation and analgesia in the intensive care unit. Am J Respir Crit Care Med 166:1024–1028
40. Kress JP, Pohlman AS, O'Connor MF, Hall JB (2000) Daily interruption of sedative infusions in critically ill patients undergoing mechanical ventilation. N Engl J Med 342:1471–1477
41. Sessler CN, Gosnell MS, Grap MJ, Brophy GM, O'Neal PV, Keane KA, Tesoro EP, Elswick RK (2002) The Richmond Agitation-Sedation Scale: validity and reliability in adult intensive care unit patients. Am J Respir Crit Care Med 166:1338–1344
42. Ramsay MA, Savege TM, Simpson BR, Goodwin R (1974) Controlled sedation with alphaxalone-alphadolone. BMJ 2:656–659
43. Jacobi J, Fraser GL, Coursin DB, Riker RR, Fontaine D, Wittbrodt ET, Chalfin DB, Masica MF, Bjerke HS, Coplin WM, Crippen DW, Fuchs BD, Kelleher RM, Marik PE, Nasraway SA Jr, Murray MJ, Peruzzi WT, Lumb PD (2002) Clinical practice guidelines for the sustained use of sedatives and analgesics in the critically ill adult. Crit Care Med 30:119-141
44. Wauquier A (1993) EEG and neuropharmacology. In: Niedermeyer E and Da Silva FL (eds) Elelctroencephalography. Basic principles, clinical applications, and related fields. Williams and Wilkins, Baltimore, pp 619–629
45. Sebel PS, Bovill JG, Wauquier A, Rog P (1981) Effects of high-dose fentanyl anesthesia on the electroencephalogram. Anesthesiology 55:203–211
46. Cropp AJ, Woods LA, Raney D, Bredle DL (1994) Name that tone. The proliferation of alarms in the intensive care unit. Chest 105:1217–1220
47. Bentley S, Murphy F, Dudley H (1977) Perceived noise in surgical wards and an intensive care area: an objective analysis. BMJ 2:1503–1506
48. Soutar RL, Wilson JA (1986) Does hospital noise disturb patients? BMJ 292:305
49. Topf M, Davis JE (1993) Critical care unit noise and rapid eye movement (REM) sleep. Heart Lung 22:252–258
50. Topf M (1992) Effects of personal control over hospital noise on sleep. Res Nurs Health 15:19–28
51. Woods NF, Falk SA (1974) Noise stimuli in the acute care area. Nurs Res 23:144–150
52. Kahn DM, Cook TE, Carlisle CC, Nelson DL, Kramer NR, Millman RP (1998) Identification and modification of environmental noise in an ICU setting. Chest 114:535–540
53. Wallace CJ, Robins J, Alvord LS, Walker JM (1999) The effect of earplugs on sleep measures during exposure to simulated intensive care unit noise. Am J Crit Care 8:210–219
54. Esteban A, Anzueto A, Alia I, Gordo F, Apezteguia C, Palizas F, Cide D, Goldwaser R, Soto L, Bugedo G, Rodrigo C, Pimentel J, Raimondi G, Tobin MJ (2000) How is mechanical ventilation employed in the intensive care unit? An international utilization review. Am J Respir Crit Care Med 161:1450–1458
55. Mehta S, Hill NS (2001) Noninvasive ventilation. Am J Respir Crit Care Med 163:540–577
56. Meza S, Mendez M, Ostrowski M, Younes M (1998) Susceptibility to periodic breathing with assisted ventilation during sleep in normal subjects. J Appl Physiol 85:1929–1940
57. Hotchkiss JR Jr, Adams AB, Stone MK, Dries DJ, Marini JJ, Crooke PS (2002) Oscillations and noise: inherent instability of pressure support ventilation? Am J Respir Crit Care Med 165:47–53
58. Gleeson K, Zwillich CW, White DP (1990) The influence of increasing ventilatory effort on arousal from sleep. Am Rev Respir Dis 142:295–300
59. Preas HL 2nd, Jubran A, Vandivier RW, Reda D, Godin PJ, Banks SM, Tobin MJ, Suffredini AF (2001) Effect of endotoxin on ventilation and breath variability: role of cyclooxygenase pathway. Am J Respir Crit Care Med 164:620–626
60. Issa FG, Sullivan CE (1983) Arousal and breathing responses to airway occlusion in healthy sleeping adults. J Appl Physiol 55:1113–1119
61. Rechtschaffen A, Gilliland MA, Bergmann BM, Winter JB (1983) Physiological correlates of prolonged sleep deprivation in rats. Science 221:182–184
62. Rechtschaffen A, Bergmann BM, Everson CA, Kushida CA, Gilliland MA (1989) Sleep deprivation in the rat: X. Integration and discussion of the findings. Sleep 12:68–87
63. Bonnet MH (2000) Sleep deprivation. In: Kryger MH, Roth T, Dement WC (eds) Principles and practice of sleep medicine. Saunders, Philadelphia, pp 53–71
64. Jubran A, Van de Graaff WB, Tobin MJ (1995) Variability of patient-ventilator interaction with pressure support ventilation in patients with chronic obstructive pulmonary disease. Am J Respir Crit Care Med 152:129–136
65. Tobin MJ, Jubran A, Laghi F (2001) Patient-ventilator interaction. Am J Respir Crit Care Med 163:1059–1063
66. Younes M (1994) Mechanisms of respiratory load compensation. In: Dempsey JA, Pack AI (eds) Regulation of breathing. Lung biology in health and disease. Vol. 79. Dekker, New York, pp 867–922
67. Dempsey JA, Skatrud JB (2001) Apnea following mechanical ventilation may be caused by nonchemical neuromechanical influences. Am J Respir Crit Care Med 163:1297–1298
68. Younes M (2001) Apnea following mechanical ventilation may not be caused by neuromechanical influences. Am J Respir Crit Care Med 163:1298–1301

69. Leung RS, Bradley TD (2001) Sleep apnea and cardiovascular disease. Am J Respir Crit Care Med 164:2147–2165
70. Sin DD, Logan AG, Fitzgerald FS, Liu PP, Bradley TD (2000) Effects of continuous positive airway pressure on cardiovascular outcomes in heart failure patients with and without Cheyne-Stokes respiration. Circulation 102:61–66
71. Wellens HJ, Vermeulen A, Durrer D (1972) Ventricular fibrillation occurring on arousal from sleep by auditory stimuli. Circulation 46:661–665
72. Marin JM, Carrizo SJ, Kogan I (1998) Obstructive sleep apnea and acute myocardial infarction: clinical implications of the association. Sleep 21:809–815
73. Brooks D, Horner RL, Kozar LF, Render-Teixeira CL, Phillipson EA (1997) Obstructive sleep apnea as a cause of systemic hypertension. Evidence from a canine model. J Clin Invest 99:106–109
74. Trinder J, Merson R, Rosenberg JI, Fitzgerald F, Kleiman J, Douglas Bradley T (2000) Pathophysiological interactions of ventilation, arousals, and blood pressure oscillations during Cheyne-Stokes respiration in patients with heart failure. Am J Respir Crit Care Med 162:808–813
75. Leuenberger U, Jacob E, Sweer L, Waravdekar N, Zwillich C, Sinoway L (1995) Surges of muscle sympathetic nerve activity during obstructive apnea are linked to hypoxemia. J Appl Physiol 79:581–588
76. Parthasarathy S, Laghi F, Jubran A, Tobin MJ (2002) Does ventilator mode influence blood pressure oscillations in critically ill patients (abstract)? Am J Respir Crit Care Med 165:A165
77. Cheshire K, Engelman H, Deary I, Shapiro C, Douglas NJ (1992) Factors impairing daytime performance in patients with sleep apnea/hypopnea syndrome. Arch Intern Med 152:538–541
78. Spengler C, Shea S (2001) Sleep deprivation per se does not decrease the hypercapnic ventilatory response in humans. Am J Respir Crit Care Med 161:1124–1128
79. McGuire BE, Basten CJ, Ryan CJ, Gallagher J (2000) Intensive care unit syndrome: a dangerous misnomer. Arch Intern Med 160:906–909
80. Irwin M, McClintick J, Costlow C, Fortner M, White J, Gillin JC (1996) Partial night sleep deprivation reduces natural killer and cellular immune responses in humans. FASEB J 10:643–653
81. Dinges DF, Douglas SD, Hamarman S, Zaugg L, Kapoor S (1995) Sleep deprivation and human immune function. Adv Neuroimmunol 5:97–110
82. Dinges DF, Douglas SD, Zaugg L, Campbell DE, McMann JM, Whitehouse WG, Orne EC, Kapoor SC, Icaza E, Orne MT (1994) Leukocytosis and natural killer cell function parallel neurobehavioral fatigue induced by 64 hours of sleep deprivation. J Clin Invest 93:1930–1939
83. Palmblad J, Petrini B, Wasserman J, Akerstedt T (1979) Lymphocyte and granulocyte reactions during sleep deprivation. Psychosom Med 41:273–278
84. Moldofsky H, Lue FA, Davidson JR, Gorczynski R (1989) Effects of sleep deprivation on human immune functions. FASEB J 3:1972–1977
85. Boyum A, Wiik P, Gustavsson E, Veiby OP, Reseland J, Haugen AH, Opstad PK (1996) The effect of strenuous exercise, calorie deficiency and sleep deprivation on white blood cells, plasma immunoglobulins and cytokines. Scand J Immunol 43:228–235
86. Brown R, Pang G, Husband AJ, King MG (1989) Suppression of immunity to influenza virus infection in the respiratory tract following sleep disturbance. Reg Immunol 2:321–325
87. Scrimshaw NS, Habicht JP, Pellet P, Piche ML, Cholakos B (1966) Effects of sleep deprivation and reversal of diurnal activity on protein metabolism of young men. Am J Clin Nutr 19:313–319

Luis J. Noronha
George M. Matuschak

Magnesium in critical illness: metabolism, assessment, and treatment

Introduction

Magnesium is the second most abundant intracellular cation and the fourth most common cation in the body [1]. Its importance as an essential nutrient has been recognized since 1932, when Kruse et al. [2] reported the effects of acute Mg deficiency in rats. Even recently Mg was considered the "forgotten cation" in clinical practice [3]; however, this is no longer the case [4]. Estimates of Mg deficiency range from 20% to 61% [5, 6, 7], while a recent study found that reductions in total serum Mg on admission are associated with increased mortality [8].

Nonetheless, the relevance of such data to intensive care is problematic. Controlled data are lacking on how circulating total Mg concentrations are related to levels of biologically active ionized Mg (Mg^{2+}). Data are likewise sparse concerning the interplay between serum total and ionized Mg levels during specific critical illnesses and their treatment. In particular, the efficacy of therapeutic Mg supplementation on Mg^{2+}, organ function, inflammatory events, and mortality are poorly understood. This lack of information on the biology of Mg contrasts with well established correlations between serum total and ionized calcium (Ca^{2+}) concentrations, manifestations of acute Ca^{2+} deficiency, and the physiological effects of correcting ionized hypocalcemia [9, 10, 11, 12].

This review summarizes key aspects of Mg metabolism in adult intensive care patients, emphasizing the interdependence of Mg homeostasis with that of other cations such as Ca^{2+} and K^{+}. Thereafter we examine the justification for the trend of increasingly frequent measurements of serum total Mg in the critically ill, and how this information is related to emerging data concerning circulating Mg^{2+}. In this context, the limitations of current treatment recommendations for hypomagnesemia in the ICU are analyzed as well as research developments likely to alter our diagnostic and therapeutic algorithms in the near future. The use of therapeutic doses of Mg independent of hypomagnesemia or titration to serum total Mg levels to treat conditions such as preeclampsia and asthma are covered since this is beyond the scope of this review.

Compartmental distribution and metabolism of Mg

The body normally contains 21–28 g Mg [13]. Approximately 53% of total Mg stores are in bone, 27% in muscle, 19% in soft tissues, 0.5% in erythrocytes, and 0.3% in serum [14]. The Mg in muscle, soft tissues, and erythrocytes is considered to be intracellular [1], and mostly bound to chelators such as adenosine triphosphate (ATP), adenosine diphosphate (ADP), proteins, RNA, DNA, and citrate [14]. Although only 5–10% of intracellular Mg is ionized, this fraction is essential for regulating intracellular Mg homeostasis [15] (Fig. 1).

Traditionally, extracellular Mg in serum was considered to be 33% protein bound, 7% complexed to citrate, PO_4^{2-}, and HCO_3^- [16], and 55% circulating in the diva-

M.R. Pinsky et al. (eds.), *Applied Physiology in Intensive Care Medicine 2: Physiological Reviews and Editorials*,
DOI 10.1007/978-3-642-28233-1_8, © Springer-Verlag Berlin Heidelberg 2012

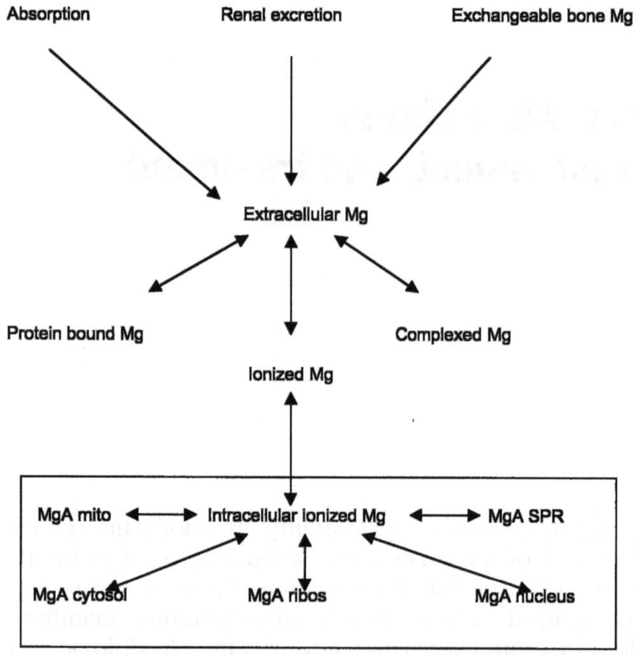

Fig. 1 Mg homeostasis. Extracellular Mg levels are maintained via absorption, renal excretion, and bone contribution. Extracellular Mg comprises protein-bound, complexed, and ionized fractions. Ionized extracellular Mg is in exchanging equilibrium with the intracellular ionized Mg fraction. *MgA cytosol, MgA ribos, MgA nucleus, MgA SPR, MgA mito* refer to Mg bound in the cytosol, ribosomes, nucleus, sarcoplasmic reticulum, and mitochondria, respectively

lent ionized form (Mg^{2+}). However, the newer methods of ion-selective Mg electrodes, atomic absorption spectroscopy, and ultrafiltration indicate that serum Mg is 67% ionized, 19% protein bound, and 14% complexed [17]. Standard clinical determinations of serum total Mg reflect all three forms. Of note, protein-bound and complexed Mg are unavailable for most biochemical processes [1]. The important issue of the dynamics of equilibration among the various states of extracellular Mg has not been extensively studied. Since serum contains only 0.3% of total body Mg stores, serum total Mg measurements poorly reflect total body status. Serum total Mg concentrations normally average 1.7–2.3 mg/dl (1.4–2.1 mEq/l) [13], depending on the laboratory and measurement technique. Mg concentrations are commonly expressed in units of milligrams, millimoles, or milliequivalents; for conversion one can use the following formula: 1 g Mg sulfate contains 98 mg= 4.06 mmol=8.12 mEq elemental Mg.

Daily Mg intake in adults normally averages 6–10 mg/kg [18]. Absorption occurs primarily in the jejunum and ileum [19]. Several lines of evidence suggest that absorption involves a transcellular, saturable process involving facilitated diffusion and a passive intercellular mechanism mediated by cationic electrochemical gradients and solvent drag [20]. Although 30–40% of dietary Mg is absorbed [19, 20], factors controlling intestinal absorption are unclear. An inverse curvilinear relationship was shown in healthy volunteers between Mg intake and its fractional absorption ranging from 65% absorption at low intake to 11% at high intake [21]. Thus, estimating the amount of oral Mg salts to correct hypomagnesemia in ICU patients who commonly have ileus and other forms of gastrointestinal dysfunction is problematic. The effects of vitamin D and parathyroid hormone (PTH) on enteral Mg absorption are minor [22].

Renal function is central to Mg homeostasis. Of the approx. 2.4 g Mg filtered per day (i.e., the 77% of total serum Mg that is not protein bound), 5% (120 mg) is normally excreted in the urine [23]. Glomerular filtration and tubular reabsorption both influence renal Mg handling [24]. Specifically, 20–30% of filtered Mg is reabsorbed in the proximal tubule and 60% in the thick ascending loop of Henlé [25]. This is where ionic regulators, hormones, and medications affect Mg excretion. Mg reabsorption in the thick ascending loop of Henlé is linked with NaCl transport and is therefore influenced by tubular flow [24, 25]. Conservation of Mg by normal kidneys during Mg deprivation may decrease fractional excretion to less than 0.5% (12 mg/day) [23]. Conversely, the kidneys increase excretion of Mg to approximate the filtered load during increased intake or excessive Mg administration [26]. During renal failure the fractional excretion of Mg progressively increases, and normal serum total Mg levels are maintained until the later stages when hypermagnesemia supervenes [27].

Mg homeostasis and compensatory mechanisms

Mg homeostasis involves interaction between three organ systems: kidneys, small bowel, and bone (Fig. 1). Acute Mg deprivation increases tubular reabsorption and intestinal absorption [28]. The mechanisms for such compensatory alterations in Mg transport are not fully understood. Several reports indicate a lack of correlation of these alterations with serum total Mg concentrations [29, 30, 31]. In Mg deficient rats a fall in urinary Mg excretion was found to occur without changes in plasma total Mg concentrations [28]. This adaptation was rapid (within 5 h) and specific (without changes in Na^+ or Ca^{2+} reabsorption). If Mg deprivation continues, exchangeable bone Mg starts contributing to extracellular Mg levels [32]. Up to 30% of bone Mg is rapidly exchangeable [33].

The threshold of negative Mg balance that triggers compensatory mechanisms is not known. Even so, ionized intracellular Mg $[Mg^{2+}]_i$ appears to be the ultimate regulatory signal [28]. $[Mg^{2+}]_i$ and intracellular bound Mg are exchangeable and are in equilibrium with extracellular Mg^{2+} [34]. Thus, ionized and bound intracellular

Mg represent buffers whose chief function appears to be maintaining constancy of the intracellular concentration of free $[Mg^{2+}]_i$. In human erythrocytes and other cells an increase in $[Mg^{2+}]_i$ by Mg loading is associated with Mg efflux via the Na^{2+}/Mg^{2+} antiport until $[Mg^{2+}]_i$ is normalized. Furthermore, reductions in $[Mg^{2+}]_i$ stimulate cationic diffusion down a concentration gradient from higher levels of extracellular Mg^{2+} [35, 36]. Consequently, Mg homeostasis is regulated chiefly by $[Mg^{2+}]_i$ which is in equilibrium with both intracellular bound Mg and extracellular Mg^{2+}. Neither the magnitude nor the efficiency of these compensatory mechanisms is known for critically ill patients, in whom counterregulatory hormone release, insulin administration, and de novo renal and gastrointestinal dysfunction are common.

Biochemical, biological, and physiological effects of Mg

Mg is important in physiological processes involving energy storage, transfer, and utilization [13, 37]. Mg complexed to ATP is a substrate for signal-transducing enzymes including phosphatases and phosphokinases on the plasma membrane and within intracellular compartments. Enzymatic reactions involving ATP require Mg^{2+}, which neutralizes the negative charge on ATP to facilitate binding to enzymes and assists hydrolysis of the terminal PO_4^{2-} bond [38]. Intracellular Mg^{2+} regulates intermediary metabolism by activating rate-limiting glycolytic and tricarboxylic acid cycle enzymes [39]. Mg^{2+}-ATPases include Mg^{2+}-(Na^+-K^+) ATPase, Mg^{2+}-(HCO_3^-) ATPase, and Ca^{2+}-Mg^{2+} ATPase, which are involved in Na^+, proton, and Ca^{2+} transport, respectively [40]. Mg indirectly affects protein synthesis by four mechanisms: (a) facilitation of nucleic acid polymerization, (b) enhanced binding of ribosomes to mRNA, (c) acceleration of the synthesis and degradation of DNA, and (d) regulation of protein:DNA interactions and thus transcriptional activity [41, 42]. Adenylate cyclase also requires Mg to generate the intracellular second messenger cAMP [40].

Intracellular Mg^{2+} significantly affects Ca^{2+} and K^+ metabolism. As a divalent cation Mg^{2+} competes with Ca^{2+} for membrane-binding sites and modulates Ca^{2+} binding and release from the sarcoplasmic reticulum [43]. Complementary effects include maintenance of low resting levels of intracellular Ca^{2+}, thereby modulating muscle contraction by noncompetitive inhibition of inositol 1,4,5-triphosphate gated Ca^{2+} channels [44]. Calcium metabolism is controlled chiefly through PTH; substantial evidence indicates that Mg modulates Ca balance by its actions on PTH itself [45]. For example, impaired PTH secretion associated with hypomagnesemia results in hypocalcemia. This is attributed to reduced Mg-dependent activation of adenylate cyclase in parathyroid tissue [46, 47]. Whether Mg deficiency also contributes to skeletal muscle resistance to PTH is controversial [48].

Mg^{2+} regulates K^+ transport via the Na^+-K^+-ATPase system as a cofactor. This action influences Na^+ and K^+ extracellular fluxes, which determine the electrical potential across cell membranes [49]. $[Mg^{2+}]_i$ blocks outward movement of K^+ through K^+ channels in cardiac cells. Decreases in $[Mg^{2+}]_i$ cause excessive outward movement of K^+ even as intracellular K^+ falls, thereby inducing depolarization [50]. This critical role of Mg^{2+} to maintain intracellular K^+ concentrations is termed "inward rectification" [51]. Mg^{2+} deficiency also impairs K^+-Na^+-Cl^- cotransport [52].

In the nervous system Mg has a depressant effect at the synapses; this is related to competition with calcium in the stimulus-secretion coupling processes in transmitter release. The best described of these is presynaptic inhibition of acetylcholine release at the neuromuscular junction [53]. The action of Mg as an anticonvulsant is related to noncompetitive blockade of *N*-methyl-D-aspartate receptors. These are a group of glutamate receptors, stimulation of which leads to excitatory postsynaptic potentials causing seizures [54].

Overall, Mg^{2+} deficiency has the potential to impair oxidative phosphorylation, protein metabolism, and transmembrane electrolyte flux in cardiac and neural tissues.

Assessment of Mg status

Assessing Mg status in the critically ill beyond serum total Mg levels is difficult. No single laboratory test tracks total body Mg stores. In all, three groups of tests are available: (a) estimates of tissue Mg using concentrations in serum, red blood cells, blood mononuclear cells, or muscle; (b) metabolic assessments of Mg balance encompassing isotopic analyses and evaluation of renal Mg excretion and retention, and (c) determination of Mg^{2+} levels which utilize fluorescent probes, nuclear magnetic resonance spectroscopy, or ion-selective electrodes (ISE).

Measuring total Mg concentrations in serum rather than plasma has been preferred because additives such as anticoagulants may be contaminated with Mg or otherwise affect the assay. For example, citrate binds Ca^{2+} as well as Mg^{2+} to affect fluorometric (8-hydroxyquinoline) and colorimetric procedures for Mg estimation [55]. As indicated above, serum total Mg levels reflect Mg^{2+}, the protein-bound Mg fraction, and Mg complexed to anions, and each component of the total value may change independently and in a nonlinear manner with respect to the other Mg fractions.

Most clinical laboratories report serum total Mg concentrations using colorimetric methods with calmagite or methylthymol blue as the chromophore [56]. As mentioned above, the chief limitation is that serum concentrations represent only 0.3% of total body Mg content [14]. Moreover, with the exception of bone, serum total Mg concentrations are not correlated with other tissue pools of Mg [57]. As for Ca, normal total Mg levels may coexist with ionized hypomagnesemia and vice versa [58]. Red blood cell Mg determinations have no advantage over serum levels and also are not correlated with other tissue fractions [57]. In normal subjects there is no correlation among Mg levels in mononuclear cells compared with serum or erythrocytes [59]. In a prospective controlled study measuring skeletal muscle Mg concentrations in 32 ICU patients with respiratory failure no correlation was found between serum total and muscle Mg concentrations [60]. Lower muscle Mg levels were associated with reduced intracellular K^+ levels, a higher incidence of ventricular extrasystoles, and a longer ICU stay.

Physiological assessments of Mg balance require steady-state conditions for accurate results, conditions that are infrequent in the critically ill. A 24-h urine collection for renal Mg excretion takes into account the circadian rhythm of cationic urinary losses [61]. However, existence of this rhythm during critical illness is unknown. Even so, a 24-h Mg excretion rate of less than 12 mg/day is acceptable evidence of Mg deficiency in the presence of serum total hypomagnesemia and normal renal function [23]. The Mg tolerance test has been used for many years as a fairly reliable means of assessing total body Mg status in patients at risk of hypomagnesemia [62]. Subjects with normal Mg balance and renal function excrete most of a parenterally administered Mg load within 24 h [28, 62]. A generally accepted protocol includes: (a) a baseline 24-h urine collection for Mg, followed immediately by (b) an infusion of 2.4 mg Mg per kilogram of lean body weight in 50 ml 5% dextrose over 4 h, and (c) a second 24-h urine collection. Differences in Mg content between the two urine collections represent the retained Mg fraction. Retention of more than 20% of administered Mg is suggestive of Mg deficiency, whereas retention of more than 50% is confirmatory [40]. This test is contraindicated when serum creatinine exceeds 200 μmol/l. Furthermore, drugs or conditions producing renal Mg wasting invalidate the results. Using the Mg loading test, serum ionized Mg levels were found to be insensitive markers of Mg deficiency in 44 ICU patients without renal insufficiency [63]. However, confounding variables, such as the use of diuretics, prevent any firm conclusions to be drawn.

A major advance in evaluating Mg deficiency is the ability to measure Mg^{2+}. In 1989 Raju et al. [64] modified the calcium fluoroprobe fura-2 to improve selectivity for Mg^{2+}. The resulting compound furaptra (mag fura-2) exhibits a shift in the peak excitation wavelength for fluorescence when bound to Mg^{2+} or Ca^{2+}. The change in fluorescence corresponds to Mg^{2+} and Ca^{2+} concentrations weighted by their respective dissociation constants. For Mg^{2+}, these probes work well within the cell. Other fluorescent probes for Mg^{2+} have been described [65]. Nuclear magnetic resonance spectroscopy estimates Mg^{2+} noninvasively. Although several isotopes ($^{19}F^-$, $^{25}Mg^{2+}$, and $^{31}P^{-2}$) have been used to estimate Mg^{2+}, the α- and β-phosphate moieties of ATP have been used most frequently [66].

Three ISEs for Mg^{2+} determination are currently available: (a) the NOVA 8 analyzer (NOVA, Waltham, Mass., USA); (b) the Microlyte 6 analyzer (Kone, Espoo, Finland); and (c) the AVL 988/4 analyzer (AVL, Schaffhausen, Switzerland). In May 1993 the United States Food and Drug Administration approved the NOVA 8 electrode for clinical use, and most studies of Mg^{2+} have used the NOVA 8 instrument. These ISEs employ ionophores and neutral carrier-based membranes designed to function in the presence of Ca^{2+} and other cations. Mg^{2+}-specific ISEs yield rapid results on whole blood, plasma, and serum using samples between 100–200 μl. Ionized Mg concentrations in healthy subjects using the NOVA 8 average 0.54–0.67 mmol/l [58, 67]. Serum reference intervals for the Kone and AVL analyzers are 0.47–0.57 mmol/l and 0.55–0.63 mmol/l, respectively [68]. No gender-related differences in Mg^{2+} have been described [67]. To date ISEs have been found to be selective for Mg^{2+}; physiological concentrations of Ca^{2+}, Na^+, K^+, H^+ and NH_4^+ have negligible effects. Therefore the precision of these analyzers is suitable for determining Mg^{2+} in intensive care [67].

The NOVA 8 and AVL analyzers correct signals from the Mg^{2+} electrode for concurrent Ca^{2+}. Calculations of Mg^{2+} and Ca^{2+} are normalized to a pH of 7.4 in the NOVA 8 instrument, which also estimates Na^+, K^+, Ca^{2+}, hematocrit, and pH [69]. The binding capacity and affinity of albumin for Mg^{2+} and Ca^{2+} varies with pH [70]; hence the Mg^{2+} and Ca^{2+} levels are pH dependent. Because of pH changes during specimen storage, measured Mg^{2+} can be reported as the Mg^{2+} at the pH of the blood sample (preferably) or as Mg^{2+} normalized to a pH of 7.4.

Mg deficiency in intensive care

Ideally, Welt and Gitelman's [71] definition of hypomagnesemia as "a reduction in total body magnesium content" defines true Mg deficiency. Unfortunately, this definition of Mg deficiency is not in keeping with commonly available laboratory technology. In spite of its imperfections serum total Mg is still used as the standard for defining hypomagnesemia in intensive care patients.

Clinical manifestations of hypomagnesemia

Most hypomagnesemia in intensive care is asymptomatic. In theory, symptoms and signs occur when the serum total Mg concentrations fall below 1.2 mg/dl (0.5 mmol/l) [72], as summarized below:

- Neuromuscular manifestations
  - Positive Chvostek's sign
  - Positive Trousseau's sign
  - Carpopedal spasm (tetany)
  - Muscle cramps
  - Muscle fasciculations and tremor
  - Muscle weakness
- Neurological manifestations
  - Convulsions
  - Nystagmus
  - Athetoid movements
  - Apathy
  - Delirium
  - Coma
- Cardiac manifestations
  - Supraventricular arrhythmias
  - Ventricular arrhythmias
  - Torsades de pointes
  - Enhanced sensitivity to digitalis intoxication
- Electrolyte disturbances
  - Hypokalemia
  - Hypocalcemia

However, manifestations of hypomagnesemia may depend more on the rate of development of the deficiency, on serum ionized rather than total hypomagnesemia, or on tissue Mg deficits rather than on circulating levels [73]. Consequently symptoms and signs ascribed to Mg deficiency may be absent even with severe hypomagnesemia (serum total Mg levels <0.8 mg/dl) [72]. Such dissociations between serum total Mg levels and clinical findings make it difficult to infer total body Mg deficiency, the need for correction of hypomagnesemia, and the physiological benefit of such correction in individual patients.

Neuromuscular manifestations of hypomagnesemia: relationship to hypocalcemia

Serum total hypomagnesemia is usually corrected because of concerns over neuromuscular irritability (e.g., positive Chvostek's and Trousseau's signs, tremors, fasciculations, and tetany) or weakness [74]. In particular, the possibility of weakness and resultant delays in ventilatory weaning attributable to hypomagnesemia have resulted in the widespread practice of frequent measurements and vigorous normalization of serum total Mg levels in ventilated patients. However, no controlled data support this practice, and its putative physiological benefit to respiratory muscle function remains obscure. Indeed, neuromuscular manifestations of serum total hypomagnesmia may be due more to concomitant hypocalcemia, even though tetany attributable solely to hypomagnesemia can occur independently of reduced serum total Ca levels [75]. Overall, neuromuscular irritability and weakness appear to be related to the combined actions of ionized hypomagnesemia and ionized hypocalcemia on the neuromuscular apparatus. Hypocalcemia does not usually develop until serum total Mg is below 1.2 mg/dl; serum total hypocalcemia occurs in one-third of hypomagnesemic medical ICU patients [76]. Hypocalcemia is usually refractory to Ca repletion unless Mg is first administered [76, 77].

Neurological manifestations of hypomagnesemia

Reported neurological manifestations of hypomagnesemia include convulsions, athetoid movements, nystagmus, apathy, delirium, and coma [40]. As mentioned above, the anticonvulsant effect of Mg appears to be via a voltage-gated antagonist action at the *N*-methyl-D-aspartate receptor [54].

Cardiac electrophysiology, hypomagnesemia, and hypokalemia

The frequency and pathogenesis of cardiac arrhythmias during hypomagnesemia [78] are hard to establish because coexisting hypokalemia is common. Whang et al. [79] reported hypokalemia in 42% of hypomagnesemic patients. Such hypokalemia is also refractory to treatment unless Mg is first repleted [74]. Although Mg per se does not participate in the production of the cardiac action potential [80], Watanabe and Dreifus [81] showed that Mg's effects on cardiac transmembrane potentials varied in perfused rat hearts according to extracellular K^+ levels. Increases or decreases in Mg levels with normal extracellular K^+ concentrations causes minor electrophysiological changes. Alterations in serum total Mg concentrations are unlikely to destabilize sinus rhythm unless accompanied by changes in other cations [80].

Serum total Mg levels below 0.7 mmol/l are associated with electrocardiographic changes indistinguishable from hypokalemia-related effects, including ST segment depression, flattened T waves, and prolongation of PR and QT/QTc intervals [38]. Arrhythmias associated with serum total hypomagnesemia include premature atrial contractions, atrial fibrillation, multifocal atrial tachycardia, premature ventricular contractions, ventricular tachycardia, and ventricular fibrillation [82, 83]. Hypomagnesemia promotes digitalis-induced arrhythmias [84]. The mechanisms are unclear but include: (a) increased myocardial uptake of digoxin, (b) augmented inhibitory action of digoxin on Na^+-K^+-ATPase causing a reduction in intracellular K^+ [82], and (c) loss of the membrane-stabilizing effect Mg^{2+} on the myocardial cell membranes [84]. Mg therapy is recommended for torsades de pointes [85]. Despite these associations of low serum total Mg levels with cardiac electrophysiological changes, purported links between low Mg and arrhythmias do not confirm a cause and effect relationship. Lack of a standard by which to define a Mg-deficient state, coexistence of other electrolyte abnormalities, varying methods of arrhythmia monitoring, and inability to distinguish between spontaneous and drug-induced arrhythmia termination are all factors [80]. Moreover, a prospective uncontrolled study of 23 heart failure patients found no correlation between serum total Mg and myocardial Mg concentrations [86].

Causes of Mg deficiency in intensive care

Singly or combined, Mg deficiency in intensive care has three main causes – (a) reduced intestinal absorption, (b) increased renal losses, and (c) compartmental redistribution, as detailed below.

Gastrointestinal causes include:

- Nutritional disturbances
  - Inadequate intake
  - Mg-free fluids and total parenteral nutrition
  - Refeeding syndrome
- Reduced absorption
  - Malabsorption syndromes
  - Short bowel syndrome
  - Chronic diarrhea
- Increased intestinal losses
  - Intestinal and biliary fistulae
  - Prolonged nasogastric suction
- Pancreatitis

Causes related to renal Mg wasting include:

- Intrinsic tubular defect
  - Interstitial nephropathy
  - Postobstructive diuresis
  - Diuretic phase of ATN
  - Postrenal transplantation
- Drug-induced renal Mg wasting
  - Loop and thiazide diuretics
  - Cisplatin
  - Cyclosporine A
  - Aminoglycosides
  - Amphotericin B
  - Pentamidine and foscarnet
  - Colony-stimulating factor therapy
- Hypophosphatemia
- Hypercalcemia/hypercalciuria

Endocrine causes include:

- Hyperaldosteronism
- Hyperparathyroidism
- Hyperthyroidism
- Syndrome of inappropriate antidiuretic hormone
- Diabetic ketoacidosis
- Alcoholic ketoacidosis

Causes related to the redistribution of Mg include:

- Acute pancreatitis
- Administration of epinephrine
- "Hungry bone" syndrome
- Massive blood transfusion
- Acute respiratory alkalosis

Other causes include:

- Cardiopulmonary bypass
- Severe burns
- Excessive sweating
- Chronic alcoholism and alcoholic withdrawal

Nearly all data concerning hypomagnesemia during critical illness comes from measurements of circulating total Mg. These do not shed light on the causes of Mg deficiency and likely underestimate ionized hypomagnesemia and total body Mg depletion.

Gastrointestinal causes

Prolonged administration of Mg-free parenteral nutrition formulae and other intravenous fluids can precipitate Mg deficiency, especially in patients with preexisting marginal stores of Mg [87]. Vomiting and nasogastric suctioning further contribute to Mg depletion [48], since the Mg content of upper intestinal fluids is about 1 mEq/l. Diarrheal fluids and fistula drainage contain up to 15 mEq/l total Mg ions [88]. Hemorrhagic pancreatitis is an additional cause of acute hypomagnesemia with hypocalcemia due to formation of Mg and Ca fatty acid soaps in sites of tissue necrosis [89].

Renal causes

Renal Mg wasting is traditionally diagnosed when the 24 h urinary Mg excretion exceeds 24 mg in the presence of hypomagnesemia as assessed by serum total Mg levels [23]. Random or "spot" urinary tests for Mg are interesting albeit unvalidated diagnostic tests. Renal Mg wasting has been reported with tubulointerstitial renal diseases, postobstructive diuresis, the diuretic phase of acute tubular necrosis, and following renal transplantation [90]. Since Mg absorption in the thick ascending loop of Henlé depends on the positive transmembrane potential created by NaCl absorption, alterations in NaCl transport by loop diuretics, 0.9% NaCl infusion, or osmotic diuresis promote Mg excretion. Loop diuretics (furosemide, bumetamide, and ethacrynic acid) are potent inhibitors of Mg reabsorption and are a common cause of hypomagnesemia in the ICU. Thiazide diuretics act on the distal tubule, where less than 5% of Mg is absorbed. Short-term administration of thiazides does not produce significant renal Mg wasting, whereas long-term administration may produce substantial Mg deficiency [40].

Several drugs cause excessive renal losses of Mg. Cisplatin causes hypomagnesemia in more than 50% of treated patients [91]; the incidence increases with the cumulative dose. Likewise, aminoglycosides induce magnesuria; 4.5% of 200 patients treated with 400 courses of aminoglycosides developed hypomagnesemia [92]. The total dose of aminoglycoside treatment in these studies varied from 1.3–40 g and recovery from hypomagnesemia varied from 2–8 weeks. A recent prospective study showed ionized hypomagnesemia secondary to renal Mg wasting in cystic fibrosis patients treated with a 2-week course of 33 mg/kg amikacin daily and 250 mg/kg ceftazidime daily [93], although no clinical correlation with ionized hypomagnesemia was performed. Amphotericin B causes mild and reversible hypomagnesemia [94]. Barton et al [94]. reported that reversal of amphotericin B-induced renal Mg wasting could take as long as 1 year following treatment. As with amphotericin B, cyclosporine A causes Mg deficiency secondary to defects in renal tubular function [95]. Parenteral pentamidine has also been implicated in hypomagnesemia secondary to renal Mg wasting [96].

Hypophosphatemia is common during intensive care, particularly in insulin-dependent diabetics and during Gram-negative bacterial sepsis [97]. Although hypophosphatemia promotes magnesuria, the mechanism is unclear [79]. Serum total Mg levels are inversely correlated with the fasting blood sugar level in diabetics in whom glycosuria, ketoaciduria, and hypophosphatemia contribute to renal Mg wasting [98]. Primary [99] and secondary [100] hyperaldosteronism are associated with renal Mg wasting secondary to volume expansion, causing increased tubular flow rates and decreased NaCl reabsorption [99]. The exact mechanism, however, remains controversial. Other hormonal conditions associated with hypomagnesemia are the syndrome of inappropriate antidiuretic hormone secretion [101] and hyperthyroidism [102].

Redistribution of Mg

"Hungry bone syndrome" after parathyroidectomy [103] or diffuse osteoblastic metastasis [104] can result in hypomagnesemic, hypocalcemic tetany from osseous deposition of Mg and Ca. Epinephrine and other β-agonists (e.g., salbutamol) cause transient hypomagnesemia in healthy subjects [105]. This is thought to occur from uptake of Mg into adipose tissue as fatty acids are released. Release of fatty acids into the blood may also lead to the formation of insoluble fatty acid–Mg^{2+} and fatty acid–Ca^{2+} complexes [40]. Massive blood transfusion (>10 U/24 h) may cause hypomagnesemia from the chelating effects of citrate [106]. Hypomagnesemia occurs during and after cardiopulmonary bypass surgery [84, 107]. Potential mechanisms include hemodilution from large-volume infusion of Mg-free fluids, removal of Mg by the bypass pump, and catecholamine-induced intracellular Mg shifts, and binding to free fatty acids [107]. A retrospective study of 30 patients undergoing elective cardiopulmonary bypass surgery demonstrated ionized hypomagnesemia in 73% [108]. Of note, the relationship between Mg^{2+} and Ca^{2+} during CPB was variable, and Ca^{2+} levels did not predict Mg^{2+} levels [108]. Significant hypomagnesemia (i.e., serum total Mg level <1.40±0.15 mEq/l) occurs in up to 30% of alcoholics. Multiple mechanisms are likely, including decreased Mg intake accompanying poor nutritional status, vomiting, chronic pancreatitis-induced steatorrhea, and Mg malabsorption [109].

Collectively, the above data indicate that hypomagnesemia (serum total Mg level <1.5 mEq/l) may have multiple causes in the ICU patient. Even so, three critical questions remain: (a) to what extent does ionized hypomagnesemia parallel reductions in serum total Mg levels and in total body Mg stores? (b) Does Mg replacement to correct levels of serum total Mg also correct ionized hypomagnesemia? (c) Is correction of serum total or ionized hypomagnesemia associated with definable clinical changes in biochemistry, electrophysiology, inflammatory responses or organ function? Until the answers to these questions are forthcoming, we may be spending considerable effort and expense merely to make serum total Mg levels "look better."

Mg, sepsis, and shock

Novel immunoregulatory effects of Mg deficiency and supplementation are increasingly reported [110, 111,

112]. Such data suggest that reductions in circulating and intracellular Mg have important, albeit clinically occult immunomodulatory consequences during severe sepsis and shock states. By enhancing generation of reactive O_2 species [111] and cytokine biosynthesis, hypomagnesemia can promote inflammatory tissue injury [112].

Altura et al. [113] proposed that circulating free Mg^{2+} ions are "natural" Ca^{2+} antagonists that modulate lethal cellular Ca^{2+} entry during shock. Lower Mg^{2+} concentrations have been found to be correlated with efflux of Ca^{2+} from the sarcoplasmic reticulum of frog myocytes over a 0.3- to 3-mmol concentration range of Mg^{2+} [114]. A direct effect of low $[Mg^{2+}]_i$ to increase the voltage-gated calcium current (I_{Ca}) was implicated. Based on this and other reports [115], Mg^{2+} deficiency may promote abnormal cellular Ca^{2+} entry during sepsis; this may in turn increase free cytosolic and mitochondrial Ca^{2+} to cause cell death. In support of this, intracellular Ca^{2+} has been reported to increase as tissue Mg^{2+} levels decline in a rat endotoxic shock model [116]. Concomitant depression of mitochondrial respiration was restored after Mg^{2+} supplementation.

Since considerable intracellular Mg^{2+} is complexed to ATP, sepsis, or ischemia/reperfusion-induced ATP hydrolysis or falls in ATP production release intracellular Mg^{2+} ions. Subsequently $[Mg^{2+}]_i$ concentrations rise, and Mg^{2+} effluxes from cells [115, 117]. Three negative consequences may result: (a) impaired Na^+-K^+ ATPase pump activity, (b) reduced inwardly rectifying K^+ ion channels, and (c) dysfunctional cell membrane and sarcolemmal Ca^{2+} ion channels [61]. These changes may partly account for the increased lethality of endotoxemia seen in rats during hypomagnesemia as well as the protective effects of Mg replacement from endotoxin challenge [118].

Mg^{2+} ions modulate key immunological functions, including macrophage activation, leukocyte adherence, and bactericidal activity [119], granulocyte oxidative burst, lymphocyte proliferation, and endotoxin binding to monocytes [118]. In Mg-deficiency models time-dependent increases are seen in circulating interleukin-1, tumor necrosis factor-α, interferon-γ, substance P, and calcitonin gene related peptide [110, 112, 120]. Such effects may result from altered DNA binding of transcription factors notable for their suppression of inflammatory cytokine gene activation, including the cyclic AMP response element binding protein [42]. Likewise, Mak et al. [121] reported overproduction of nitric oxide in an Mg-deficient rat model. In that report increased nitric oxide production was considered secondary to Mg deficiency-related stimulation of inducible nitric oxide synthase and activation of Ca-sensitive nitric oxide synthase from increased intracellular Ca^{2+}. Cytotoxic effects of NO include those resulting from its combination with superoxide to form peroxynitrite [121]. Inhibition of mitochondrial respiration, interference with the O_2 carrying ability of hemoglobin and myoglobin due to interaction with heme proteins, and inhibition of enzymes containing heme and nonheme iron-sulfur centers all contribute to toxicity [122]. Overall, emerging data showing interrelated links among biochemical, physiological, and immunoregulatory effects of Mg deficiency during sepsis and shock suggest the corollary thesis that titrated Mg supplementation can alter outcomes. Further experimental and clinical data are needed to confirm this notion.

Ionized Mg and intensive care

Serum total Mg levels are not correlated with serum Mg^{2+} in the critically ill because of accompanying variations in plasma protein concentrations, acid-base balance, metabolic derangements, and drugs that affect Mg balance [58, 123]. Külpmann et al. [123] showed that reduced serum total Mg concentrations maymight reflect "pseudohypomagnesemia" from hypoalbuminemia when concomitant Mg^{2+} concentrations are normal. Such findings have led to the suggestion that the terms hypo-, normo-, and hypermagnesemia should be restricted to Mg^{2+} levels. Of note, $[Mg^{2+}]_i$ levels are correlated well with serum Mg^{2+} by ^{31}P-nuclear magnetic resonance spectroscopy [124]. In aortic endothelium $[Mg^{2+}]_i$ levels change within 5 min of increasing extracellular Mg^{2+}, suggesting that extracellular Mg^{2+} dynamically equilibrates with $[Mg^{2+}]_i$ [125]. Additional studies are needed to confirm whether extracellular Mg^{2+} accurately tracks total body Mg balance. In spite of in vitro studies demonstrating the superiority of ionized Mg measurements over total Mg estimations; few studies have attempted to demonstrate the importance of measuring ionized Mg levels in the critical care setting and to examine the correlation of ionized hypomagnesemia with clinical manifestations and outcomes.

Salem et al. [126] measured Mg^{2+} and serum total Mg concentrations in 180 critically ill patients. Serum total Mg values were sensitive (75%) but not specific (38%) in predicting ionized hypomagnesemia. Increased supraventricular and ventricular dysrhythmias, seizures, hypotension, and death were associated with ionized hypomagnesemia (normal range 0.52–0.60 mmol/l). Recently, Huijgen and colleagues [127] evaluated the relationships between serum Mg^{2+}, total body Mg estimated by Mg content in blood mononuclear cells and erythrocytes, serum albumin, and 30-day mortality in 115 critically ill patients. A normal serum Mg^{2+} was found in 71% of patients with total serum hypomagnesemic values. Moreover, neither total nor ionized Mg measurement was correlated with cellular Mg levels or with outcome. With respect to the cardiovascular effects of hypomagnesemia, Kasaoka et al. [128] found that supraventricular and ventricular extrasystoles decreased by 50% and ventricular tachycardia was abolished by a 0.15 mmol/kg intravenous bolus of Mg sulfate ($MgSO_4$) over 10 min, which increased serum Mg^{2+} from 0.35±0.06 mmol/l to 0.54±0.09 mmol/l. $MgSO_4$ had no effect in patients with a normal serum Mg^{2+}. The ratio of Mg^{2+} to Ca^{2+} as a modulator of vascular tone also increased after intravenous $MgSO_4$ and was thought to contribute to the antiarrhythmic effect. Bertschat et al. [129] determined serum Mg^{2+} levels on days 1, 2, 3, 5, and 7 after myocardial infarction in 42 patients, in addition to concomitant serum total Mg, free fatty acids, Ca^{2+}, and total Ca. Compared with serum total Mg concentrations, Mg^{2+} levels fell on the 1st day of myocardial infarction and were inversely correlated with serum free fatty acids. The ionized hypomagnesemia was attributed to β-adrenergic induced lipolysis and binding of Mg^{2+} by fatty acids. Since the benefit of intravenous $MgSO_4$ during acute myocardial infarction is not established, the authors suggest that serum Mg^{2+} rather than total Mg be measured in coronary care patients, and that those with ionized hypomagnesemia be treated [129].

Frankel et al. [130] noted a poor correlation between serum total and Mg^{2+} values in 113 trauma patients, although injury severity or blood ethanol levels did not predict ionized hypomagnesemia. It has been hypothesized that decreased serum Mg^{2+} levels after trauma result from increases in circulating catecholamines and corticosteroids, and to Mg redistribution within injured tissues [131]. Ionized hypomagnesemia occurs after experimental head trauma [132] and in brain-injured patients [133]. In vivo animal studies have shown that pre- or posttreatment with $MgCl_2$ 15 min after cerebral injury restores brain Mg^{2+} levels, improves motor function [134], attenuates cognitive deficits [135], and reduces cerebral edema [136]. In a traumatic brain injury rat model Bareyre et al. [137] studied serum Mg^{2+} levels 24 h postinjury and neuromotor outcome after 1 and 2 weeks. Supplemental Mg treatment given to rats with ionized hypomagnesemia reduced posttraumatic impairments. No such correlation was found using blood total Mg levels, which did not change postinjury. In other in vivo animal studies Mg treatment has been shown to reduce posttraumatic edema and cortical damage, in association with concomitant changes in gene expression for c-fos, heat shock protein-70, neurotrophins, and cyclooxygenase-2 [136, 138]. In addition to Mg's multiple effects on intermediary metabolism, oxidative phosphorylation, protein synthesis, regulation of membrane permeability to Ca^{2+} and K^+ ions, and potential anti-inflammatory effects, it has also been recently shown in murine cortical cell cultures to be a potent antioxidant to iron-dependent oxidative injury [139]. By increasing the physiologically active ionized Mg fraction, $MgCl_2$ possibly restores the ability of cells to maintain homeostasis [137]. Available data therefore suggest that early measurement of blood ionized Mg levels and supplementation when indicated may be of value in reducing morbidity after head injury or cerebral infarction. The positive data correlating neuromotor outcomes after head injury and correcting ionized hypomagnesemia are currently limited to animal studies only; more investigation needs to be carry out to determine whether the same holds true in human head-injured patients in prospective randomized controlled trials.

Treatment of hypomagnesemia

Treatment recommendations for hypomagnesemia in intensive care are confounded by the lack of controlled clinical data regarding the directional changes in time-matched serum total and ionized Mg levels, particularly in relation to concomitant ionized Ca^{2+}, K^+, and PO_4 concentrations. In addition, renal insufficiency, administration of drugs which promote renal Mg wasting, and varying recommendations for Mg repletion are problematic [140, 141]. An ideal ICU study to clarify these issues would therefore have to first attempt to define the measure of true Mg deficiency (total body, extracellular ionized, etc.) that is correlated with clinical manifestations. The study would further need to control for disturbances in other cations and drugs that interfere with Mg balance and renal function and determine the clinical, biochemical, and hemodynamic effects of correcting Mg deficiency with the ultimate goal of determining patient outcomes.

Nonetheless, several generalizations are appropriate regarding the treatment of Mg deficiency:

- Emergency (intravenous route):
  - 8–12 mmol Mg over 1–2 min
  - 40 mmol Mg over next 5 h
- Severely ill (intravenous or intramuscular route)
  - 40 mmol Mg on day 1
  - 16–24 mmol Mg on days 2–5
- Oral maintenance
  - 12–24 mmol per day

Kidney function must be assessed prior to the initiation of Mg therapy. Since the major route of Mg excretion is via the kidney, significant hypermagnesemia can occur in the setting of compromised renal function. In general, when rapid Mg administration is needed, as for cardiac arrhythmias, the intravenous route is safe. It should, however, be performed with hemodynamic and electrocardiographic monitoring as there may be significant prolongation of intra-atrial and atrioventricular nodal conduction times [142] as well as hypotension. Davies et al. [143] noted hypotension in three patients during

Gram-negative bacteremic sepsis when Mg sulfate ($MgSO_4$) was given using a rapid regimen (8 mmol intravenously over 5 min). The authors did not mention the degree of hypotension that occurred, nor the baseline blood pressure and the use of vasopressors (if any) prior to Mg administration. No hypotension occurred when 48 mmol $MgSO_4$ was infused over 24 h. Such hypotensive responses may reflect the combined effects of sepsis-induced myocardial dysfunction together with Mg infusion-induced reductions in systemic vascular resistance. In the critical care setting treatment recommendations must therefore be tempered with the urgency of replacing Mg deficits. Slower infusions (mentioned below) are appropriate unless cardiac arrhythmias or seizures are present. Slow replacement can be achieved by giving 8–12 g $MgSO_4$ intravenously over 24 h, followed by 4–6 g daily for another 3–4 days [40]. Since up to 50% of administered Mg may be lost in the urine, continuous infusions of Mg or repeated doses may be preferable. However, there are no controlled data with regard to the efficacy of this approach in critically ill patients. Oral Mg salts can be used as maintenance therapy in conditions associated with chronic Mg loss, for example, short or long-term use of diuretics. An initial daily dose of 300–600 mg elemental Mg may be used. The Mg is given in divided doses to decrease its cathartic effect. Significant hypermagnesemia can complicate Mg replacement when the glomerular filtration rate is less than 30 ml/min [13]. Elevation in serum total Mg to levels higher than 2 mmol/l are usually accompanied by symptoms. The effects of increasing rise in serum total Mg levels include hypotension (1.5–2.5 mmol/l), electrocardiographic changes (2.5–5 mmol/l), areflexia (5 mmol/l), respiratory paralysis (7.5 mmol/l), and cardiac arrest (>12.5 mmol/l) [38]. Physiological antagonism of hypermagnesemia with intravenous calcium gluconate can be used until dialysis can be initiated.

With respect to cardiac arrhythmias and ventricular arrhythmias in particular, recommended protocols for Mg treatment are unclear as no large-scale controlled studies comparing replacement regimens, their effects on total vs. ionized Mg levels, and clearcut physiological endpoints have been performed. In general, 2 g $MgSO_4$ constituting 8 mmol intravenously over 1–2 min, followed by an additional 40 mmol over the next 5 h is considered safe and probably effective [141]. As discussed above, an antiarrhythmic dose of 0.15 mmol/kg $MgSO_4$ given as an intravenous bolus over 10 min was used by Kasaoka et al. [128] to correct ionized hypomagnesemia (<0.40 mmol/l). Simultaneous administration of K^+ and Ca may be necessary because concomitant losses of these cations are common in Mg deficiency. Emerging data underscore the lack of a predictable relationship between serum total and ionized Mg levels, either before or after intravenous Mg supplementation. Barrera et al. [144] were unable to predict serum Mg^{2+} levels from serum total Mg values in 33 ICU patients, in whom intravenous treatment with 4.1 mmol (1 g) had no effect on ionized Ca^{2+} or K^+ concentrations, although both serum ionized and total Mg levels were increased.

Summary

Mg metabolism and the important physiological roles of Mg as they relate to the critically ill have been reviewed. However, fundamental aspects of Mg metabolism, assessment of Mg deficiency, and efficacy of treatment of hypomagnesemia, whether total or ionized, remain poorly understood. Although serum total Mg continues to be the most frequently used tool for diagnosing and treating hypomagnesemia, randomized clinical studies are needed to determine whether newer methods of Mg assessment, including the measurement of Mg^{2+}, are superior. Newer insights into the immunomodulatory roles of Mg in vivo, improvements in estimating whole-body and compartmental Mg concentrations, and clearer documentation of the biochemical and physiological effects of correcting hypomagnesemia will undoubtedly assist the intensivist in determining the the rationale and the mode for correcting a low Mg value.

References

1. Elin RJ (1994) Magnesium: the fifth but forgotten electrolyte. Clin Chem 102:616–622
2. Kruse HD, Orent ER, McCollum EV (1932) Studies on magnesium deficiency in animals. I. Symptomatology resulting from Mg deprivation. J Biol Chem 96:519–539
3. Whang R (1987) Routine serum magnesium determination: a continuing unrecognized need. Magnesium 6:1–4
4. Toffaletti J (1995) Physiology and regulation: ionized calcium, magnesium and lactate measurements in critical care settings. Am J Clin Pathol 104 [Suppl 1]:S88–S94
5. Reinhart RA, Desbiens NA (1985) Hypomagnesemia in patients entering the ICU. Crit Care Med 13:506–507
6. Ryzen E, Wagers PW, Singer FR, Rude RK (1985) Magnesium deficiency in a medical ICU population. Crit Care Med 13:19–21
7. Chernow B, Bamberger S, Stoiko M, Vadnais M, Mills S, Hoellrich V, Warshaw AL (1989) Hypomagnesemia in patients in postoperative intensive care. Chest 95:391–397
8. Rubeiz GJ, Thill-Baharozian M, Hardie D, Carlson RW (1993) Association of hypomagnesemia and mortality in acutely ill medical patients. Crit Care Med 21:203–209

9. Drop LJ (1985) Ionized calcium, the heart, and hemodynamic function. Anesth Analg 64:432–451
10. Kost GJ (1993) The significance of ionized calcium in cardiac critical care. Arch Pathol Lab Med 117:890–896
11. Desai TK, Carlson RW, Thill-Baharozian M, Geheb MA (1988) A direct relationship between ionized calcium and arterial pressure among patients in an intensive care unit. Crit Care Med 16:578–582
12. Broner CW, Stidham GL, Westenkirchner DF, Tolley EA (1990) Hypermagnesemia and hypocalcemia as predictors of high mortality in critically ill pediatric patients. Crit Care Med 18:921–928
13. Wacker WEC, Parisi AF (1968) Magnesium metabolism. N Engl J Med 278:658–663
14. Elin RJ (1987) Assessment of magnesium status. Clin Chem 33:1965–1970
15. Günther T (1993) Mechanisms of regulation of Mg efflux and Mg influx. Miner Electrolyte Metab 19:259–265
16. Speich M, Bousquet B, Nicolas G (1981) Reference values for ionized, complexed and protein-bound plasma magnesium in men and women. Clin Chem 27:246–248
17. Altura BT, Altura BM (1994) A method for distinguishing ionized, complexed and protein-bound Mg in normal and diseased subjects. Scand J Clin Lab Invest 54, Suppl 217:83–87
18. Seelig MS (1981) Magnesium requirements in human nutrition. Magnesium Bull 3 [Suppl 1A]:26–47
19. Graham LA, Caessar JJ, Burgen ASV (1960) Gastrointestinal absorption of Mg28 in man. Metabolism 9:646–659
20. Kayne LH, Lee DBN (1993) Intestinal magnesium absorption. Miner Electrolyte Metab 19:210–217
21. Fine KD, Santa Ana CA, Porter JL, Fordtran JS (1991) Intestinal absorption of magnesium from food and supplements. J Clin Invest 88:396–402
22. Hodgkinson A, Marshall DH, Nordin BEC (1979) Vitamin D and magnesium absorption in man. Clin Sci (Colch) 57:121–123
23. Sutton RAL, Domrongkitchaiborn S (1993) Abnormal renal magnesium handling. Miner Electrolyte Metab 19:232–240
24. Quamme GA, Dirks JH (1986) The physiology of renal magnesium handling. Renal Physiol 9:257–269
25. Quamme GA (1989) Control of magnesium transport in the thick ascending limb. Am J Physiol 256:F197–F210
26. Wong NLM, Dirks JH, Quamme GA (1983) Tubular reabsorptive capacity for magnesium in the dog kidney. Am J Physiol 244:F78–F83
27. Coburn JW, Popovtzer MM, Massry SG, Kleeman CR (1969) The physicochemical state and renal handling of divalent ions in chronic renal failure. Arch Intern Med 124:302–311
28. Quamme GA (1993) Laboratory evaluation of magnesium status. Renal function and free intercellular magnesium concentration. Clin Lab Med 13:209–223
29. Dunn MJ, Walser MR (1964) Magnesium depletion in normal man. Metabolism 15:884–895
30. Fitzgerald MG, Fourman P (1956) An experimental study of magnesium deficiency in man. Clin Sci (Colch) 15:635
31. Rude RK, Bethune JR, Singer FR (1980) Renal tubular maximum for magnesium in normal, hypoparathyroid and hyperparathyroid man. J Clin Endocrinol Metab 51:1425
32. Alfrey AC, Miller NL, Trow R (1974) Effect of age and magnesium depletion on bone magnesium pools in rats. J Clin Invest 54:1074–1081
33. Alfrey AC, Miller NL (1973) Bone magnesium pools in uremia. J Clin Invest 52:3019–3027
34. Günther T (1990) Functional compartmentation of intracellular magnesium. In: Sigel H, Sigel A (eds) Metal ions in biological systems, vol 26. Dekker, New York, pp 193–213
35. Quamme GA (1997) Renal magnesium handling: new insights in understanding old problems. Kidney Int 52:1180–1195
36. Beyenbach KW (1990) Transport of magnesium across biological membranes. Magnes Trace Elem 9:223–254
37. Aikawa JK (1981) Magnesium: its biological significance. CRC, Boca Raton
38. Reinhart RA (1988) Magnesium metabolism: a review with special reference to the relationship between intracellular content and serum levels. Arch Intern Med 148:2415–2420
39. Garfinkel L, Garfinkel D (1985) Magnesium regulation of the glycolytic pathway and the enzymes involved. Magnesium 4:60–72
40. Al-Gamadi SMG, Cameron EC, Sutton RAL (1994) Magnesium deficiency: pathophysiologic and clinical overview. Am J Kidney Dis 24:737–752
41. Vernon WB (1988) The role of magnesium in nucleic acid and protein metabolism. Magnesium 7:234–248
42. Schumacher MA, Goodman RH, Brennan RG (2001) The structure of a CREB bZIP.somatostatin CRE complex reveals the basis for selective dimerization and divalent cation-enhanced DNA binding. J Biol Chem 10:35242–35247
43. Ryan MF (1991) The role of magnesium in clinical biochemistry: an overview. Ann Clin Biochem 28:19–26
44. Volpe P, Vezu L (1993) Intracellular magnesium and inositol 1:4,5 triphosphate receptor: molecular mechanisms of interaction, physiology and pharmacology. Magnes Res 6:267–274
45. Rude RK, Oldham SB, Sharpe CF, Singer FR (1978) Parathyroid hormone secretion in magnesium deficiency. J Clin Endocrinol Metab 47:800–806
46. Rude RK, Singer FR (1981) Magnesium deficiency and excess. Annu Rev Med 32:245–259
47. Targovnik JH, Rodman JS, Sherwood LM (1971) Regulation of parathyroid hormone secretion in vitro: quantitative aspects of calcium and magnesium ion control. Endocrinology 88:1477–1482
48. Nadler JL, Rude RK (1995) Disorders of magnesium metabolism. Endocrinol Metab Clin North Am 24:623–641
49. Dyckner T, Wester PO (1984) Intra-/extracellular shifts of potassium after administration of Mg in patients with cardiovascular diseases. Magnesium 3:339–345
50. White RE, Hartzell HC (1989) Magnesium ions in cardiac function. Regulator of ion channels and second messengers. Biochem Pharmacol 38:859–867
51. Vandenberg CA (1987) Inward rectification of a potassium channel in cardiac ventricular cells depends on internal magnesium ions. Proc Natl Acad Sci USA 84:2560–2564
52. Whang R, Whang DD, Ryan MR (1992) Refractory potassium repletion. Arch Intern Med 152:40–45
53. Borzeix MG, Akimjak JP, Charles P, Lenfant M, Cahn R (1994) Effect of magnesium on GABA inhibition-induced convulsions in mice. Effect of three salts. In: Golf S, Dralle D, Vecchiet L (eds) Magnesium 1993. Libbey, London, pp 177–180
54. Mason BA, Standley CA, Irtenkauf SM, Bardicef M, Cotton DB (1994) Magnesium is more efficacious than phenytoin in reducing N-methyl-D-aspartate seizures in rats. Am J Obstet Gynecol 171:999–1002
55. Caddell JL, Erickson M, Byrne PA (1974) Interference from citrate using the titan yellow method and two fluorometric methods for magnesium determination in plasma. Clin Chim Acta 41:435–438
56. Elin RJ (1991) Determination of serum magnesium concentration by clinical laboratories. Magnes Trace Elem 10:60–66
57. Alfrey AC, Miller NL, Butkus D (1974) Evaluation of body magnesium stores. J Lab Clin Med 84:153–162
58. Altura BT, Altura BM (1992) Measurement of ionized magnesium in whole blood, plasma and serum with a new ion-selective electrode in healthy and diseased human subjects. Magnes Trace Elem 10:90–98

59. Elin RJ (1988) Status of the determination of magnesium in mononuclear blood cells in humans. Magnesium 7:300–305
60. Fiaccadori E, Del Canale S, Coffrini E, Melej R, Vitali P, Guariglia A, Borghetti A (1988) Muscle and serum magnesium in pulmonary intensive care unit patients. Crit Care Med 16:751–760
61. Luce GG (1970) Biological rhythms in psychiatry and medicine. Publication no 2088. Public Health Service, Washington
62. Ryzen E, Elbaum N, Singer FR, Rude RK (1985) Parenteral magnesium tolerance testing in the evaluation of magnesium deficiency. Magnesium 4:137–147
63. Hébert P, Mehta N, Wang J, Hindmarsh T, Jones G, Cardinal P (1997) Functional magnesium deficiency in critically ill patients identified using a magnesium-loading test. Crit Care Med 25:749–755
64. Raju B, Murphy E, Levy LA, Hall RD, London RE (1989) A fluorescent indicator for measuring cytosolic free magnesium. Am J Physiol 256:C540–C548
65. Illner H, McGuigan JAS, Lüthi D (1992) Evaluation of Mag-fura-5, the new fluorescent indicator for free magnesium measurements. Pflugers Arch 422:179–184
66. London RE (1991) Methods for measurement of intracellular magnesium: NMR and fluorescence. Annu Rev Physiol 53:241–258
67. Altura BT, Shirey TL, Young CC, Hiti J, Orfano KD, Handwerker M, Altura BM (1992) A new method for the rapid determination of ionized Mg in whole blood, serum and plasma. Methods Find Exp Clin Pharmacol 14:297–304
68. Huijgen HJ, Sanders R, Cecco SA, Rehak NN, Sanders GT, Elin RJ (1999) Serum ionized magnesium: comparison of results obtained with three ion-selective analyzers. Clin Chem Lab Med 37:465–470
69. Anonymous (1997) NOVA 8 reference manual. Nova Biomedical, Waltham
70. Fogh-Andersen N, Bjerrum PJ, Siggaard-Andersen O (1993) Ionic binding, net charge, and Donnan effect of human serum albumin as a function of pH. Clin Chem 39:48–52
71. Welt LG, Gitelman H (1965) Disorders of magnesium metabolism. DM 11:1–32
72. Kingston ME, Al-Siba'i MB, Skooge WC (1986) Clinical manifestations of hypomagnesemia. Crit Care Med 14:950–954
73. Sutton RL, Dirks JH (1991) Disturbances of calcium and magnesium metabolism. In: Brenner BM, Rector FR (ed) The kidney, vol 1, 4th edn. Saunders, Philadelphia, pp 841–887
74. Shills ME (1969) Experimental human magnesium depletion. Medicine (Baltimore) 48:61–85
75. Wacker WEC, Moore FD, Ulmer DD, Vallee BL (1962) Normocalcemic magnesium deficiency tetany. JAMA 180:161–163
76. Ryzen E, Wagers PW, Singer FR, Rude RK (1985) Magnesium deficiency in a medical ICU population. Crit Care Med 13:19–21
77. Abdulrazzaq YM, Smigura FC, Wettrell G (1989) Primary infantile hypomagnesemia; report of two cases and review of literature. Eur J Pediatr 148:459–461
78. Iseri LT, Allen BJ, Brodsky MA (1989) Magnesium therapy of cardiac arrhythmias in critical care medicine. Magnesium 8:299–306
79. Whang R, Oei TO, Aikawa JK, Vannatta J, Fryer A, Markanich M (1984) Predictors of clinical hypomagnesemia. Arch Intern Med 144:1794–1796
80. Keller P, Aronson R (1990) The role of magnesium in cardiac arrhythmias. Prog Cardiovasc Dis 32:433–448
81. Watanabe Y, Dreifus LS (1972) Electrophysiological effects of magnesium and its interaction with potassium. Cardiovasc Res 6:79–88
82. Iseri LT, Freed J, Bures AR (1975) Magnesium deficiency and cardiac disorders. Am J Med 58:837–844
83. Burch GE, Giles TD (1977) The importance of magnesium deficiency in cardiovascular disease. Am Heart J 94:649–657
84. Fawcett WJ, Haxby EJ, Male DA (1999) Magnesium: physiology and pharmacology. Br J Anaesth 83:302–320
85. Tzivoni D, Banai S, Schuger C, Benhorin J, Keren A, Gottlieb S, Stern S (1988) Treatment of torsade de pointes with magnesium sulfate. Circulation 77:392–397
86. Ralston MA, Murnane MR, Kelley RE, Altschuld R, Unverferth DV, Leier CV (1989) Magnesium content of serum, circulating mononuclear cells, skeletal muscle, and myocardium in congestive heart failure. Circulation 80:573–580
87. Hall RCW, Joffre JR (1973) Hypomagnesemia: physical and psychiatric symptoms. JAMA 224:1749–1751
88. Booth CC, Babouris N, Hanna S, MacIntyre I (1963) Incidence of hypomagnesemia in intestinal malabsorption. BMJ 2:141–144
89. Edmondson HA, Berne CJ, Homann RE, Wertman M (1952) Calcium, potassium, magnesium and amylase disturbances in acute pancreatitis. Am J Med 12:34–42
90. Davis BB, Preuss HG, Murdaugh HV Jr (1975) Hypomagnesemia following the diuresis of post-renal obstruction and renal transplant. Nephron 14:275–280
91. Schilsky RL, Anderson T (1979) Hypomagnesemia and renal magnesium wasting in patients receiving cisplatin. Ann Intern Med 90:929–931
92. Shah GM, Kirschenbaum MA (1991) Renal magnesium wasting associated with therapeutic agents. Miner Electrolyte Metab 17:58–64
93. Von Vigier RO, Truttmann AC, Zindler-Schmocker K, Bettinelli A, Aebischer CC, Wermuth B, Bianchetti MG (2000) Aminoglycosides and renal magnesium homeostasis in humans. Nephrol Dial Transplant 15:822–826
94. Barton CH, Pahl M, Vaziri ND, Cesario T (1984) Renal magnesium wasting associated with amphotericin B therapy. Am J Med 77:471–474
95. Barton CH, Vaziri ND, Martin DC, Choi S, Alikhani S (1987) Hypomagnesemia and renal magnesium wasting in renal transplant recipients receiving cyclosporine. Am J Med 83:693–699
96. Shah GM, Alvarado P, Kirschenbaum MA (1990) Symptomatic hypocalcemia and hypomagnesemia with renal magnesium wasting associated with pentamidine therapy in a patients with AIDS. Am J Med 89:380–382
97. Knochel JP (1977) The pathophysiology and clinical characteristics of severe hypophosphatemia. Arch Intern Med 137:203–220
98. Martin HE, Smith K, Wilson ML (1958) The fluid and electrolyte therapy of severe diabetic acidosis and ketosis. Am J Med 24:376–389
99. Delva P, Pastori C, Degan M, Montesi G, Brazzarola P, Lechi A (2000) Intralymphocyte free magnesium with primary aldosteronism. Hypertension 35:113–117
100. Lim P, Jacob E (1972) Magnesium deficiency in liver cirrhosis. Q J Med 41:291–300
101. Hellman ES, Tschudy DP, Bartter FC (1962) Abnormal electrolyte and water metabolism in acute intermittent porphyria. The transient inappropriate secretion of antidiuretic hormone. Am J Med 32:734–746
102. Jones JE, Desper PC, Shane SR, Flink EB (1966) Magnesium metabolism in hyperthyroidism and hypothyroidism. J Clin Invest 45:891–900
103. Davies DR, Friedman M (1966) Complications after parathyroidectomy. Fractures from low calcium and magnesium convulsions. J Bone Joint Surg Br]48:117–126
104. Navarro J, Oster JR, Gkonos PJ, Ruiz JP, Rhamy RK, Perez GO (1991) Tetany induced on separate occasions by administration of potassium and magnesium in a patient with hungry-bone syndrome. Miner Electrolyte Metab 17:340–344

105. Whyte KF, Addis GJ, Whitesmith R, Reid JL (1987) Adrenergic control of plasma magnesium in man. Clin Sci (Colch) 72:135–138
106. McLellan BA, Reid SR, Lane PL (1984) Massive blood transfusion causing hypomagnesemia. Crit Care Med 12:146–147
107. England MR, Gordon G, Salem M, Chernow B (1992) Magnesium administration and dysrhythmia after cardiac surgery. JAMA 268:2395–2402
108. Aziz S, Haigh WG, Van Norman GA, Kenny RJ, Kenny MA (1996) Blood ionized magnesium concentrations during cardiopulmonary bypass and their correlation with other circulating cations. J Card Surg 11:341–347
109. Shane SR, Flink EB (1992) Magnesium deficiency in alcohol addiction and withdrawal. Magnes Trace Elem 10:263–268
110. Weglicki WB, Phillips TM (1992) Pathobiology of magnesium deficiency: a cytokine/neurogenic inflammation hypothesis. Am J Physiol 32:R734–737
111. Weglicki WB, Freedman AM, Bloom S, Atrakchi AH, Cassidy MM, Dickens BF (1992) Antioxidants and the cardiomyopathy of Mg-deficiency. Am J Cardiovasc Pathol 4:210–215
112. Weglicki WB, Phillips TM, Freedman AM, Cassidy MM, Dickens BF (1992) Magnesium-deficiency elevates circulating levels of inflammatory cytokines and endothelin. Mol Cell Biochem 110:169–173
113. Altura BM, Altura BT (1990) Role of magnesium in the pathogenesis of hypertension: relationship to its actions on cardiac and vascular smooth muscle. In: Laragh JH, Brenner BM (ed) Hypertension: pathophysiology, diagnosis and management. Raven, New York, pp 1003–1025
114. White RE, Hartzell HC (1988) Effects of intracellular free magnesium on calcium current in isolated cardiac myocytes. Science 239:778–780
115. Murphy E, Steenbergen C, Levy LS, Raju B, London RE (1989) Cytosolic free magnesium levels in ischemic rat heart. J Biol Chem 264:5622–5627
116. Sayeed MM, Zhu M, Maitra SR (1989) Alterations in cellular calcium and magnesium during circulatory/septic shock. Magnesium 8:179–189
117. Günther T, Ebel H (1990) Membrane transport of magnesium. Metal Ions Biol Syst 26:216–225
118. Salem M, Kasinski N, Munoz R, Chernow B (1995) Progressive magnesium deficiency increases mortality from endotoxin challenge: protective effects of acute magnesium replacement. Crit Care Med 23:108–118
119. Johnson JS, Hand WL, King-Thompson NL (1980) The role of divalent cations in interactions between lymphokines and macrophages. Cell Immunol 53:236–245
120. Weglicki WB, Mak IT, Stafford RE, Dickens BF, Cassidy MM, Philliips TM (1994) Neurogenic peptides and the cardiomyopathy of Mg-deficiency: effects of substance P receptor inhibition. Mol Cell Biochem 130:103–109
121. Mak IT, Komarov AM, Wagner TL, Stafford RE, Dickens BF, Weglicki WB (1996) Enhanced NO production during Mg deficiency and its role in mediating red blood cell glutathione loss. Am J Physiol 271:C385–C390
122. Schmidt HH, Walter U (1994) NO at work. Cell 78:919–925
123. Külpmann WR, Gerlach M (1996) Relationship between ionized and total magnesium in serum. Scand J Clin Lab Invest 56 [Suppl 224]:251–258
124. Altura BM, Altura BT (1996) Role of magnesium in patho-physiological processes and the clinical utility of magnesium ion selective electrodes. Scand J Clin Lab Invest 56 [Suppl 224]:211–234
125. Zhang A, Cheng TPO, Altura BT, Altura BM (1992) Extracellular magnesium regulates intracellular free Mg in vascular smooth muscle cells. Pflugers Arch 421:391–393
126. Salem M, Stacey J, Chernow B (1993) Ionized magnesium values in critically ill patients – a novel ion selective electrode for determining free extracellular magnesium concentrations. Crit Care Med:S256
127. Huijgen HJ, Soesan M, Sanders R, Mairuhu WM, Kesecioglu J, Sander GT (2000) Magnesium levels in critically ill patients: what should we measure? Am J Clin Pathol 114:688–695
128. Kasaoka S, Tsuruta R, Nakashima K, Soejima Y, Miura T, Sadamitsu D, Tateishi A, Maekawa T (1996) Effect of intravenous magnesium sulfate on cardiac arrhythmias in critically ill patients with low serum ionized magnesium. Jpn Circ J 60:871–875
129. Bertschat F, Ising H, Günther T, Jeremias A, Jeremias E (1995) Changes of ionized magnesium and free fatty acids in serum after myocardial infarction. Eur J Clin Chem Clin Biochem 33:553–558
130. Frankel H, Haskell R, Lee SY, Miller D, Rotondo M, Schwab CW (1999) Hypomagnesemia in trauma patients. World J Surg 23:966–969
131. Sawyer RB, Drew MA, Gesink MH, Sawyer KC Jr, Sawyer DC (1970) Post-operative magnesium metabolism. Arch Surg 100:343–348
132. Heath DL, Vink R (1998) Blood-free magnesium concentration declines following graded experimental traumatic brain injury. Scand J Clin Invest 58:161–166
133. Altura BM, Memon ZS, Altura BT, Cracco RQ (1995) Alcohol-associated acute head trauma in human subjects is associated with early deficits in serum ionized Mg and Ca. Alcohol 12:433–437
134. Heath DL, Vink R (1998) Neuroprotective effects of $MgSO_4$ and $MgCl_2$ in closed head injury: a comparative phosphorous NMR study. J Neurotrauma 15:183–189
135. Smith DH, Okiyama K, Gennarelli TA, McIntosh TK (1993) Magnesium and ketamine attenuate cognitive dysfunction following experimental brain injury. Neurosci Lett 157:211–214
136. Kinoshita Y, Ueyuama T, Senba E, Terada T, Nakai K, Itakura T (2001) Expression of c-fos, heat shock protein 70, neurotrophins, and cyclooxygenase-2 mRNA in response to focal cerebral ischemia/reperfusion in rats and their modification by magnesium sulfate. J Neurotrauma 18:435–445
137. Bareyre FM, Saatman KE, Helfaer MA, Sinson G, Weisser JD, Brown AL, McIntosh TK (1999) Alterations in ionized and total blood magnesium after experimental traumatic brain injury: relationship to neurobehavioral outcome and neuroprotective efficacy of magnesium chloride. J Neurochem 73:271–280
138. Feldman Z, Gurevitch B, Artru A, Oppenheim A, Shohami E, Reichenthal E, Shapira Y (1996) Effect of magnesium given 1 hour after head trauma on brain edema and neurological outcome. J Neurosurg 85:131–137
139. Regan RF, Jasper E, Guo Y, Panter SS (1998) The effect of magnesium on oxidative neuronal injury in vitro. J Neurochem 70:77–85
140. James MFM (1991) Magnesium in critical care medicine. Care Crit Ill 7:233–237
141. Iseri LT, Freed J, Bures AR (1975) Magnesium deficiency and cardiac disorders. Am J Med 58:837–846
142. Rasmussen HS, Thomsen PEB (1989) The electrophysiological effects of intravenous magnesium sulfate on human sinus node, atrioventricular node, atrium, and ventricle. Clin Cardiol 12:85–90
143. Davies GE, Cudworth P, Lawler PG (1992) Intravenous magnesium in critically ill patients. Anaesthesia 47:1104
144. Barrera R, Fleischer M, Miletic J, Groeger J (2000) Ionized magnesium supplementation in critically ill patients: comparing ionized and total magnesium. J Crit Care 15:36–40

S. E. Orfanos
I. Mavrommati
I. Korovesi
C. Roussos

Pulmonary endothelium in acute lung injury: from basic science to the critically ill

Abstract *Background:* Pulmonary endothelium is an active organ possessing numerous physiological, immunological, and metabolic functions. These functions may be altered early in acute lung injury (ALI) and further contribute to the development of acute respiratory distress syndrome (ARDS). Pulmonary endothelium is strategically located to filter the entire blood before it enters the systemic circulation; consequently its integrity is essential for the maintenance of adequate homeostasis in both the pulmonary and systemic circulations. Noxious agents that affect pulmonary endothelium induce alterations in hemodynamics and hemofluidity, promote interactions with circulating blood cells, and lead to increased vascular permeability and pulmonary edema formation. *Objective:* We highlight pathogenic mechanisms of pulmonary endothelial injury and their clinical implications in ALI/ARDS patients.

Keywords Endothelium · Lungs · Acute lung injury · Acute respiratory distress syndrome

Introduction

The intimal lining of all blood vessels is composed of a single continuous layer of simple squamous epithelial cells of mesenchymal origin which are called endothelial cells (ECs). In the human lung ECs occupy a surface area of approximately 130 m^2 [1]. Vascular endothelium was considered for many years to be nothing more than a nucleated layer, functioning as a semipermeable barrier that separates blood from the surrounding tissues and, in the lungs, blood from air. However, extensive research over the past 25 years has confirmed that vascular endothelium is a highly specialized metabolically active organ possessing numerous physiological, immunological, and synthetic functions (Table1). The strategic location of the lungs and the tremendous surface area of the pulmonary capillary endothelium allow the latter to filter the entire circulating blood volume before it enters the systemic circulation. Thus pulmonary endothelial functional and structural integrity are essential for adequate pulmonary and systemic cardiovascular homeostasis.

Pulmonary endothelium is a major component of the alveolar-capillary unit; it is therefore vulnerable to injury from noxious agents (mechanical, chemical, or cellular) that are either inhaled or delivered to the lung through the pulmonary circulation and may cause acute lung injury (ALI) in animals and humans (Table 2).

ALI represents a pathological continuum characterized by acute respiratory distress and severe oxygenation impairment, occurring as a consequence of the host response after exposure to noxious external or endogenous agents. The most severe extreme of ALI is the acute respiratory distress syndrome (ARDS), an overt noncardiogenic pulmonary edema that carries high morbidity and mortality

DOI 10.1007/978-3-642-28233-1_9, © Springer-Verlag Berlin Heidelberg 2012

Table 1 Major pulmonary endothelial functions

Synthesis and release of several vasoactive compounds such as angiotensin II, prostacyclin, thromboxane A_2, nitric oxide (NO), and endothelins; regulation of vascular tone
Expression of enzymes such as angiotensin converting enzyme, endothelin converting enzyme, nucleotidases, NO synthase and lipoprotein lipase
Expression of receptors and signal transduction molecules
Cell surface redox activity (transplasma membrane electron transport systems)
Removal and biotransformation of drugs
Regulation of coagulation and thrombolysis; promotion of hemofluidity
Participation in immune reactions
Binding of immune complexes
Interaction with bacteria (phagocytosis) and blood components such as leukocytes and platelets
Expression of adhesion molecules
Production of growth factors
Production of cytokines and chemokines
Production of reactive oxygen species
Barrier function

Table 2 Major agents that cause pulmonary endothelial injury

Endotoxin
Cytokines, chemokines
Activated leukocytes
Proteolytic enzymes
Partially reduced O_2 species
Immune complexes
Microbes (e.g., rickettsial infection)
Hyperoxia
Radiation
Drugs
Ischemia/reperfusion
Hyperlipidemia
Fibrin split products
Actin and actin complexes
Toxins
Mechanical stretch

[2]. ALI/ARDS is caused by an autodestructive inflammatory process characterized by the activation of intrapulmonary and circulating cells and by a tremendous influx of neutrophils (although ARDS occurs in neutropenia) and cytokine production, resulting in a breakdown of the lung barrier and gas exchange functions. ALI pathogenesis is still only partly understood; however, pulmonary endothelium plays a major role by: (a) altering its metabolic activity, thus affecting pulmonary and systemic homeostasis; (b) mediating cell-cell adhesions, especially with neutrophils; and (c) changing its barrier permeability, thus promoting pulmonary edema formation [3].

Pulmonary endothelial functions

The various pulmonary endothelial metabolic properties were identified using isolated perfused lung preparations, in vivo animal studies, and EC culture techniques. It is well recognized now that the pulmonary endothelium possesses numerous enzymes, receptors, and transduction molecules, and that it interacts with other vessel wall constituents and circulating blood cells. Major physiological properties of the pulmonary endothelium include: (a) the promotion of antiaggregation and hemofluidity, (b) an enforced barrier function, and (c) the synthesis, metabolism, or uptake of vasoactive compounds that modulate the systemic (endocrinelike action) and/or pulmonary vascular tone (paracrinelike action) [4, 5]. The latter appears to contribute in the induction of hypoxic pulmonary vasoconstriction (HPV), a unique physiological feature of the pulmonary circulation that maintains proper ventilation/perfusion match and optimizes systemic oxygenation. Although the exact role of EC in HPV is still under investigation, EC-derived vasoactive compounds such as nitric oxide, endothelin (ET) 1, and a yet unidentified agent that may cause Ca^{2+} sensitization in the smooth muscle have been implicated [6]. Consequently, pulmonary endothelial injury is expected to compromise adequate HPV and contribute to the ventilation/perfusion abnormalities seen in ALI/ARDS.

The most important endothelial functions are presented in Table 1. Most of these functions are constitutive while others are induced upon endothelial activation after exposure to proinflammatory stimuli such as endotoxin and/or cytokines. In this respect the activated pulmonary endothelium (a) expresses leukocyte adhesion molecules, (b) produces cytokines, (c) induces changes in vascular integrity and tone, (d) becomes procoagulant, and (e) upregulates HLA molecules [7]. ALI is associated with an intense pulmonary inflammatory response with accumulation of both pro- and anti-inflammatory mediators [8]. If the proinflammatory process dominates, endothelial activation is followed by functional and, at a second stage, structural endothelial injury, leading to alterations in all the above critical metabolic functions that contribute to ARDS pathogenesis. ARDS-related structural endothelial injury has been identified in humans: Postmortem studies of patients who died of sepsis-related ARDS revealed patchy EC swelling and injury [9], while a recent study found circulating ECs to be increased (i.e., increased EC shedding) in sepsis and septic shock, suggesting a widespread endothelial damage that should also include the pulmonary endothelium [10].

Cytokines and pulmonary endothelium

Cytokines are soluble polypeptides serving as chemical messengers between cells; they are involved in processes such as cell growth and differentiation, tissue repair and remodeling, and regulation of the immune response [11]. ECs are both targets and cytokine producers. Among the more than 250 known cytokines, tumor necrosis factor

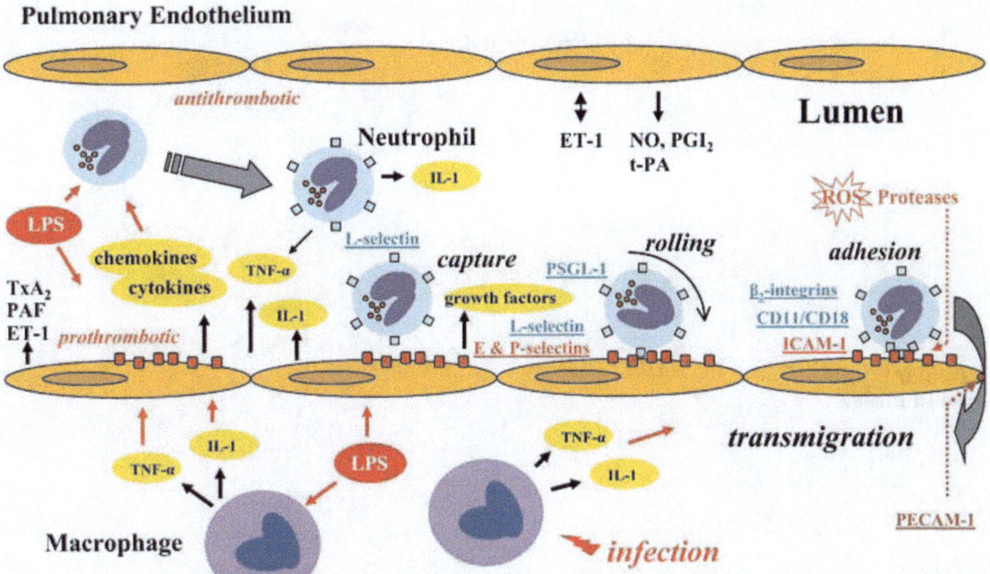

Fig. 1 Schematic illustration demonstrating major endothelial functional properties in the normal lung (upper endothelial cell layer), and mechanisms of pulmonary endothelial injury induced by infection, encompassing many of the major inflammatory interactions among cytokines, macrophages, neutrophils, and pulmonary endothelium. *LPS* Lipopolysaccharide; *TNF-α* tumor necrosis factor-α; *IL-1* interleukin-1; *NO* nitric oxide; *ET-1* endothelin-1; *PGI₂* prostacyclin; *TxA₂* thromboxane A₂; *PAF* platelet-activating factor; *t-PA* tissue plasminogen activator; *ROS* reactive oxygen species; *PSGL-1* P-selectin glycoprotein-1; *ICAM-1* intercellular adhesion molecule-1; *PECAM-1* platelet-endothelial cell adhesion molecule-1. *Underlined* Adhesion molecules; *red arrows* action; *black arrows* synthesis (and uptake for ET-1); *dotted arrows* location

(TNF) α and interleukin (IL) 1 are produced mostly by mononuclear phagocytes, and natural killer cells. In the lung they are mainly produced by activated interstitial and alveolar cells (primarily macrophages), as well as ECs, and have a major role in the early ALI stage. TNF-α and IL-1 share a number of biological properties and markedly amplify each other's biological actions. They act on EC mainly by inducing a functional program that promotes thrombosis and inflammation [12]. Among other things they induce (a) a prothrombotic EC phenotype, (b) the production of several cytokines including chemokines, colony-stimulating factors, IL-6 which has both pro- and anti-inflammatory properties, and IL-1 itself, (c) the production of several autacoids such as prostanoids including prostacyclin (PGI_2) and thromboxane A_2, platelet-activating factor (PAF) and nitric oxide (NO), and (d) the upregulation of adhesion molecules (Fig. 1). All these functions, with the latter being the most important, contribute to ALI/ARDS development [11, 12].

Several animal studies have revealed the pro- or anti-inflammatory contribution of cytokine–EC interaction in the pathogenesis of ALI occurring from different insults. In this respect acid aspiration induced lung injury in rabbits is mediated mainly by neutrophils recruited in the lung by IL-8 and the subsequent endothelial injury [13], while IL-8 also mediates injury from smoke inhalation to both pulmonary endothelium and epithelium in the same animal model [14]. In contrast to this, cardiotrophin-1, a member of the gp130 cytokine family that carries anti-inflammatory properties, appears to attenuate the endotoxin-induced impairment of endothelium-dependent pulmonary vasorelaxation in an ALI ex vivo rat model [15]. Partial liquid ventilation with perflubron decreases serum TNF-α concentrations in a rat acid aspiration model, thus reducing the systemic sequelae of ALI [16]. The above anti-inflammatory phenomenon might be related in part to attenuated leukocyte activation, which would consequently attenuate leukocyte–EC interaction. Interestingly, it has recently been shown that TNF-α installation into the alveolar space sends inflammatory signals to the adjoining capillary endothelium, which in minutes upregulates the expression of the adhesion molecule P-selectin enhancing leukocyte–EC interaction [17].

The cytokine-EC interaction in ALI pathogenesis has also been shown in humans or human tissues. Pulmonary microvascular EC (PMEC) from ARDS patients present an upregulation of TNF-R2 receptors and a higher constitutive production of IL-6 and IL-8 than control PMEC, suggesting either a stronger EC activation occurring during the ALI/ARDS process or that PMEC are constitutively more reactive in subjects who subsequently develop ARDS [18]. Additionally, TNF-α induces IL-8 production by pulmonary EC via the p38 mitogen-activated protein kinase pathway; the underlying mechanism is regulated by the EC redox status, suggesting that anti-oxidant therapy might be of value in the ALI treatment [19].

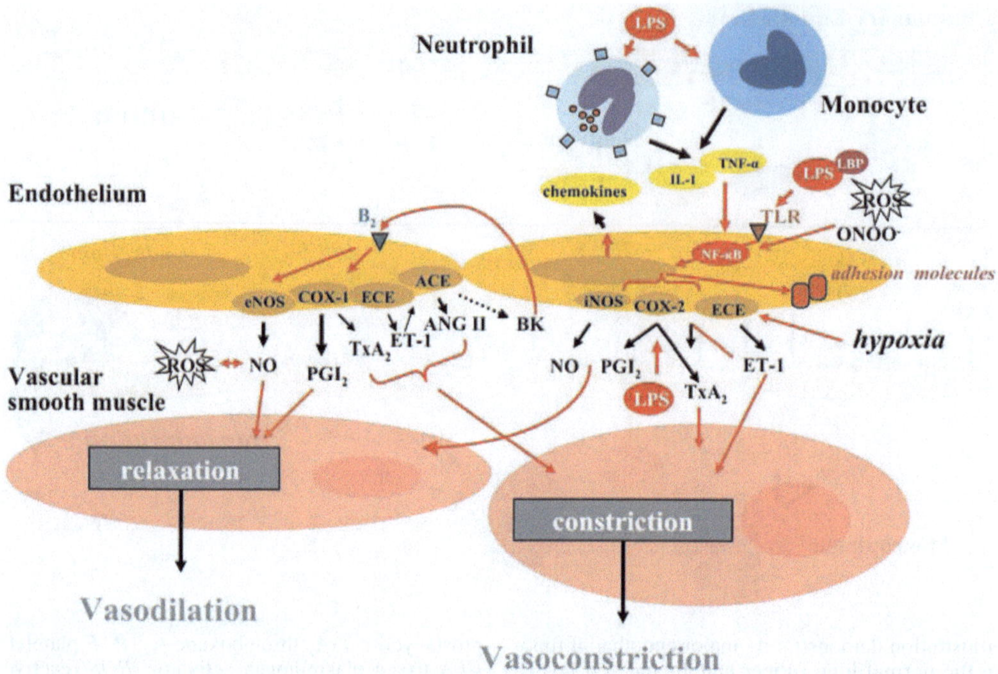

Fig. 2 Schematic illustration of major endothelial–smooth muscle interactions under normal conditions and after endothelial exposure to inflammatory stimuli. Inflammatory stimuli induce vasoactive mediator synthesis via the activation of nuclear factor-κB (*NF-κB*) or other transcription factors. Lipopolysaccharide (*LPS*) activates signaling pathways, leading to NF-κB through binding to Toll-like receptors (*TLR*) on the endothelial surface. TLR responsiveness depends on LPS-binding protein (*LBP*) and other factors. *TNF-α* Tumor necrosis factor-α; *IL-1* interleukin-1; *NO* nitric oxide; *ONOO⁻* peroxynitrite; *ET-1* endothelin-1; *PGI_2* prostacyclin; *TxA_2* thromboxane A_2; *ANG II* angiotensin II; *BK* bradykinin; *ROS* reactive oxygen species; *eNOS* endothelial NO synthase; *iNOS* inducible NO synthase; *COX-1* constitutive cyclooxygenase; *COX-2* inducible cyclooxygenase; *ACE* angiotensin-converting enzyme; *ECE* endothelin-converting enzyme; *B_2* B_2 kinin receptor. *Red arrows* Action; *black arrows* synthesis (and uptake for ET-1); *dotted arrow* breakdown

A particular pro-inflammatory process of high clinical importance is the ventilator-induced lung injury (VILI). This highly morbid clinical entity is believed to be caused by excessive mechanical stress that alters epithelial and endothelial barrier properties and stimulates pro-inflammatory responses of several cell types including macrophages and neutrophils [20]. Conventional mechanical ventilation in ARDS patients can induce ventilator-associated lung injury (VALI) that leads to pro-inflammatory cytokine production, attenuated by a protective ventilatory strategy [21]. In this respect "protective" low tidal volumes appear to attenuate epithelial and endothelial injury [estimated by plasma von Willebrand factor (vWF) and permeability to albumin] in a rat model of acid-induced ALI, demonstrating the role of endothelial injury in this pathology [22].

Transcriptional mechanisms in ALI

Transcription factors (i.e., DNA-binding proteins that regulate gene expression) are major components of the molecular mechanism underlying the cytokine-induced EC activation. Among these, nuclear factor-κB (NF-κB) is a crucial factor for the maximal expression of many cytokines involved in ALI pathogenesis. NF-κB enhances the transcription of several genes including cytokines, growth factors, vasoactive mediators, adhesion molecules, immunoreceptors, and acute-phase proteins (Fig. 2) [23]. NF-κB regulates the cytokine-mediated inducibility of adhesion molecules and cytokines in EC [24]. NF-κB activation is the final target of a signal transduction pathway that leads from the cell surface to the nucleous. Numerous inducers have been implicated in NF-κB stimulation including proinflammatory cytokines (mainly TNF-α and IL-1), bacterial and viral products [such as lipopolysaccharide (LPS)], and reactive oxygen species (ROS) [23].

ROS at low (subcytotoxic) concentrations function as important signaling molecules, while at higher concentrations they induce cell injury and death (see below) [25]. NF-κB activation is a major redox-sensitive transcription factor: Thiol antioxidants such as *N*-acetylcysteine abolish LPS-induced activation of NF-κB and improve lung function in ARDS patients [23]. Similarly, high intracellular glutathione concentrations inhibit NF-κB activation, an inhibition also induced by high levels of glutathione disulfide, the oxidized form of glutathione [25]. Redox regulation of NF-κB appears to be complex and mediated by both oxidant and antioxidant mechanisms; it is cell-type specific and in several cases is more facilitatory than causal [23, 25]. Cathecholamines that are often administered in ALI/ARDS subjects also affect NF-κB activation via several mechanisms, including ROS generation [26].

Activation of NF-κB is a critical step in the initiation of neutrophilic inflammation in animals and has been linked to ALI/ARDS pathogenesis. NF-κB activation is inhibited in vivo by treatment with antioxidants, corticosteroids, and the induction of endotoxin tolerance [24]. In a similar respect NF-κB dependent expression of EC adhesion molecules were downregulated by antioxidant treatment [23]. Dexamethasone administration in isolated rat lungs inhibited the TNF-α and IL-1 induced upregulation of pulmonary vascular ET, possibly via NF-κB dependent mechanisms [27]. These findings suggest that a specific NF-κB inhibition would contribute to ALI/ARDS treatment.

Reactive oxygen and nitrogen species

Patients with ARDS are subjected to an oxidant burden that results in molecular/cellular damage and arises from an increased generation of ROS and reactive nitrogen species (RNS) and/or a deficiency of antioxidant defenses. ROS include superoxide anion (O_2^-), hydrogen peroxide (H_2O_2) and hydroxyl radical (OH). Various ROS sources such as the mitochondrial respiratory chain, the protease-mediated enzyme xanthine oxidase, the metabolic cascade of arachidonic acid, and the oxidative burst of activated neutrophils are present in ARDS [28]. RNS consist of species such as NO, nitrogen dioxide (NO_2), and peroxynitrite ($ONOO^-$). NO is highly reactive with free radicals; the reaction between NO and O_2^- produces the very powerful and cell toxic $ONOO^-$ [28].

Following the exposure to various inflammatory stimuli, pulmonary endothelial, epithelial, and alveolar macrophages are among the lung cell types that contribute to the production of ROS and RNS, with deleterious effects on pulmonary endothelium [29]. Among other features, oxidant stress alters endothelial barrier function and increases endothelial permeability through activations of protein kinace C, myosin light chain kinase and other signaling pathways [25, 29]. ARDS nonsurvivors reveal higher levels of oxidative stress and damage than survivors as well as histochemical evidence of RNS-modified proteins in the lungs, while the antioxidant protective system in ARDS is severely compromised [28, 29].

Leukocytes and pulmonary endothelium

Pulmonary endothelial-leukocyte interaction is a key step in ALI/ARDS development since alterations in cell-cell adhesion is the initial step in leukocyte migration from the capillaries into the lung parenchyma, and the subsequent inflammatory response. Neutrophils appear to be the key cell type related to pulmonary injury in ALI/ARDS, while eosinophils [30, 31] and macrophages have also been implicated [30, 31, 32]. The latter might be responsible for ALI occurring in neutropenic patients [32].

Neutrophil adhesion to EC is a multistage process and a sine qua non for successful neutrophil migration and extravasation (Fig. 1). The initial phase, neutrophil capture and rolling, is mediated by cell adhesion molecules of the selectin family: L-selectin is constitutively expressed on neutrophils, P-selectin is found on platelets and EC, while E-selectin is expressed solely on EC [32, 33]. P-selectin is expressed within minutes on EC surface after EC activation by stimuli such as histamine, thrombin, bradykinin, leukotriene C_4 or free radicals; P-selectin interacts with neutrophil counterreceptors such as the P-selectin glycoprotein-1. E-selectin is rapidly synthesized by EC after cell activation by cytokines such as TNF-α and IL-1, or endotoxin [33].

The second phase is firm neutrophil adhesion (Fig. 1). It requires the interaction of the β_2 (CD18) integrin family (more specifically the CD11/CD18 integrins) expressed on neutrophils, mainly with the intercellular adhesion molecule (ICAM) 1, a member of the immunoglobulin superfamily expressed on EC [33]. ICAM-1 expression on EC is augmented by inflammatory mediators such as TNF-α, IL-1, γ-interferon, and endotoxin. Although ICAM-1 is constitutively expressed by EC in relatively high levels, it appears that the additional expression induced by cytokines is important for the neutrophil–EC interaction [33]. Oxidant stress promotes neutrophil adhesion [25]. Once neutrophils firmly adhere on the pulmonary endothelial layer, they create a microenviroment for injury, mainly via the production of proteases and ROS (i.e., oxidant burst) that induce cell injury and death. Neutrophil adherence to EC or matrix proteins appears to prime the former for a massive burst lasting 1–3 h in response to stimuli such as TNF-α. Activated EC also generate ROS, contributing in maintaining an oxidant-rich environment at injury site [25].

Neutrophil transmigration through the endothelium is the third phase of the adhesion cascade. It does not necessarily accompany firm adherence and depends on the presence of a chemeotactic gradient and the platelet–EC adhesion molecule 1 (PECAM-1) expressed on EC junctions [33]. ROS appear to increase endothelial permeability, facilitating leukocyte transmigration [25].

A large body of evidence has demonstrated the critical role of the neutrophil interaction with pulmonary endothelium in ALI in animals and humans and has examined potential therapeutic interventions. In this respect the dysfunction of endothelium-dependent and endothelium-independent pulmonary vasorelaxation in an endotoxin-induced ALI rat model is attenuated by neutrophil depletion [34], while neutralization of CD18 attenuates ALI caused by acid installation in the rabbit [35]. Activated neutrophils, as revealed by elastase and superoxide production, are involved in an oleic acid induced ALI guinea pig model [36], while E-selectin and ICAM-1 play important roles in the bleomycin-induced ALI and the subsequent lung fibrosis, through the induction of neutrophil recruitment in the pulmonary circulation [37, 38]. Pulmonary endothelial P-selectin upregulation appears to play a crucial role in the leukocyte recruitment occurring in the pulmonary microcirculation in a pancreatitis-induced ALI rat model, a process that is possibly related to free radicals generated by xanthine-oxidase released by the injured pancreas. Constitutive pulmonary endothelial ICAM-1 contributes to the pathogenic process [39].

Numerous human studies have been performed focusing on EC–neutrophil interaction indices in ALI in an effort to both investigate the underlying pathogenic mechanisms and possibly provide endothelial markers that could predict ALI/ARDS development or outcome [3]. In this respect granulocyte aggregation occurring in the pulmonary microcirculation after activation by transfusion-derived antibodies or biologically active lipids appears to be involved in transfusion-related ALI in man [40]. Soluble plasma P-selectin was found elevated in ALI patients, especially in those who subsequently died [41], while plasma vWF antigen, soluble ICAM-1, and soluble E-selectin measured in patients at risk for ARDS were elevated in septic but not in trauma subjects [42].

In a different study, plasma soluble (s)L-selectin measured in ARDS at-risk patients were significantly lower in those who subsequently progressed to ARDS than in those who did not or in normal controls. Significant correlations were found between the above low sL-selectin levels and the requirement for ventilation, the degree of respiratory failure, and patient mortality, elucidating the interactions between neutrophils and ECs at the early ARDS stage [43]. Additionally, PMEC purified from ARDS patients who died revealed a significantly higher constitutive expression of ICAM-1 than in control human PMEC. When treated with TNF-α, both cell lines showed a dose-dependent increase in ICAM-1 expression that was significantly higher in the ARDS-derived EC [18]. The question remains, however, of whether the observed stronger EC activation occurred during the ALI/ARDS process, or, more importantly, whether PMEC are constitutively more reactive in subjects who will subsequently develop the syndrome.

A more recent study used the endothelial specific E-selectin promoter to express a selective β_2 CD11/CD18 integrin antagonist in a cell- and inflammation-specific manner. This treatment prevented neutrophil adhesion to human pulmonary artery ECs that had been activated by LPS; it additionally prevented neutrophil sequestration in the lungs and ALI development in mice that had received *Escherichia coli* intraperitoneally. These data suggest that conditionally blocking of β_2 integrin function at sites where the endothelium is activated is feasible and might offer in the future a means of locally preventing neutrophil activation that leads to ALI/ARDS [44].

Pulmonary endothelium and pulmonary vascular permeability

Increased pulmonary vascular permeability is a hallmark of ALI/ARDS pathogenesis since it is a sine qua non for noncardiogenic pulmonary edema formation. ARDS patients exhibit persistent pulmonary endothelial permeability that was revealed in vivo by means of a dual-isotope technique; the severity of vascular permeability appeared related to lung injury score as proposed by Murray et al. [45] and the number of neutrophils in bronchoalveolar lavage [46].

Increased pulmonary endothelial permeability may be induced by ALI-related cytokines, other agents, and via EC cytoskeletal-related mechanisms in response to stimuli such as thrombin or mechanical stretch. For a detailed analysis the reader is referred to [47]. Vascular endothelial growth factor (VEGF) is a potent vascular permeability inducer. VEGF was higher in the plasma of ARDS patients, especially in subsequent nonsurvivors as compared to that from patients at risk of ARDS or controls; VEGF may be another important factor in the pathogenesis of noncardiogenic pulmonary edema in ARDS [48].

Pulmonary endothelium and hemofluidity

ECs possess a sophisticated metabolic machinery of interactive factors that modulates all three components of the hemostatic system: platelet aggregation, blood coagulation, and fibrinolysis [49]. In the healthy lung the combined effect of these factors promotes hemofluidity, while under pathological conditions the injured pulmonary endothelium becomes thrombogenic.

Platelets and pulmonary endothelium

Pulmonary endothelium affects platelet function mainly through the production of the platelet aggregation inhibitors PGI_2 and NO; the production of vWF; the conversion of adenosine diphosphate (which can induce platelet aggregation) to adenosine monophosphate, mediated by the endothelial ectoenzyme adenosine diphoshatase; and the removal of serotonin from the pulmonary circulation [49]. In ALI all the above features may be altered leading to enhanced platelet aggregation. In this respect several agents that could cause ALI, such as oxidative injury generated from reactive oxygen species and hyperoxia, alter the synthesis and release of PGI_2 [49], while the pulmonary endothelium-mediated extraction of serotonin is decreased in ARDS patients [50].

Numerous studies have shown that vWF is altered in ALI/ARDS, and that vWF is a sensitive marker denoting the existence of EC injury or activation [3]. vWF is synthesized predominantly by vascular ECs. Markedly elevated levels of plasma vWF were reported in patients with acute respiratory failure 22 years ago [51]; this phenomenon appears to occur in early ALI, prior to significant endothelial damage [52]. Since then investigators have focused on the validity of vWF as a predictor of ARDS development. Elevated plasma vWF in patients with nonpulmonary sepsis had a predictive value for ALI development, especially in patients who had concomitant dysfunction of at least one organ [53]. However, more recent studies confirmed that vWF is increased in ARDS at risk patients, but it does not predict ALI development in a heterogeneous patient population [54, 55].

Pulmonary endothelium and coagulation

Pulmonary endothelium possesses both anticoagulant and procoagulant properties. Antithrombin III (AT III) is a major inhibitor of blood coagulation that inhibits thrombin. EC possess heparinlike glycosaminoglycans and sulfated proteoglycans on their surface that sequester AT III and thrombin from the circulation, facilitating their reaction [49]. Additionally, AT III binding to glycosaminoglycans promotes PGI_2 release [56], a feature that among other things prevents LPS-induced pulmonary vascular injury in rats, possibly by inhibiting lung leukocyte accumulation [57].

Thrombomodulin (TM) is an anticoagulant proteoglycan located on the EC surface. TM reacts with thrombin producing a marked increase in the thrombin-catalyzed activation of protein C, which in turn inactivates coagulation factors VA and VIIIA [49]. Plasma TM is increased in ARDS patients, possibly through proteolytic release from the injured pulmonary endothelium, an event mediated by activated neutrophils [58]. Similarly, plasma TM is increased in preterm infants with respiratory distress syndrome, especially in those treated with mechanical ventilation [59]. The critical role of TM dysfunction on ALI/ARDS development was recently demonstrated by blocking pulmonary endothelial TM in mice by means of glucose oxidase (the H_2O_2 generating enzyme) immunotargeting. This treatment caused lung injury that combined oxidative, prothrombotic, and inflammatory components, characteristic of the ALI/ARDS pathology in humans [60].

Endothelial procoagulant properties under normal conditions are covered by its predominant anticoagulant activity. In this respect the activity of thromboplastin, an EC-associated procoagulant factor, is normally low but can be induced by various ALI-related stimuli such as endotoxin, IL-1, and thrombin [49].

Pulmonary endothelium and fibrinolysis

Pulmonary endothelium is actively involved in the fibrinolytic process, expressing tissue-type (t-PA) and urokinase-type (u-PA) plasminogen activators as well as plasminogen activator inhibitors [49]. The EC fibrinolytic activity appears to be affected by several ALI-related mediators including endotoxin, IL-1, TNF-α, and thrombin [49, 61]. In a more recent study human PMECs isolated from ARDS patients expressed higher procoagulant activity and plasminogen activator inhibitor (PAI) 1 as well as lower fibrinolytic potential (i.e., t-PA/PAI-1) than the controls, confirming the procoagulant pulmonary endothelial profile in ARDS [61].

Pulmonary endothelium-derived vasoactive mediators

Nitric oxide

NO is a free radical (RNS) with a very short half-life and is very unstable in biological systems. NO is formed from L-arginine by NO synthase (NOS). There are three known NOS isoenzymes: (a) neuronal (n) NOS, also expressed in pulmonary arterial smooth muscle cells (SMC), (b) inducible (i) NOS, induced by several pro-inflammatory mediators, which upon expression produces NO at very high rates with profound effects on cardiovascular homeostasis, and (c) endothelial (e) NOS, a constitutive isoenzyme expressed principally in EC (Fig. 2) [62]. The latter is the main isoenzyme involved in vascular tone regulation. Deficiency of L-arginine or the NOS cofactor tetrahydrobiopterin may result in eNOS-generated $O_2^{\bullet-}$ instead of or along with NO, promoting the formation of highly reactive RNS such as $ONOO^-$. NO activates soluble guanylate cyclase, thus producing 3,5-cyclic monophosphate (cGMP) and eliciting cGMP-mediated SMC relaxation and other cell-specific functions [62].

In addition to vascular SMC relaxation, NO inhibits (a) platelet aggregation, (b) leukocyte adhesion, and (c) cellular proliferation [7]. In the pulmonary circulation NO synthesis is reduced under hypoxia, and as such it may modulate HPV [63], a feature that is lost in ARDS. Several studies have reported that NO can in addition exert either pro- or anti-oxidative effects, depending on the type and the quantity of oxygen radicals present; NO can additionally attenuate ARDS-associated lung leak [64]. Therapeutic NO inhalation improves oxygenation in several ALI animal models and in responder ARDS patients, while in addition it inhibits neutrophil activation, platelet adhesion, and the production of inflammatory mediators in the injured lungs [64].

Endothelins

Endothelins (ETs) are the most potent naturally occurring vasoconstrictors. Three isoforms have been identified, ET-1, ET-2, and ET-3 all formed from "big endothelin" by ET-converting enzyme [7]. ET-1 is produced mainly by EC, and its production is induced by several factors including hypoxia, endotoxin, TNF-α, interferon, and epinephrine (Fig. 2) [7]. ET-1 release occurs mainly in the abluminal direction towards SMC, and its signaling is mediated by two distinct receptors, ET_A and ET_B. ET_A is expressed on SMC, signaling vasoconstriction; ET_B is expressed primarily on EC and elicits transient vasodilation by signaling NO and prostaglandin release, revealing a cross-talk between the ET-1 and NO pathways [62]. Similarly, EC activation is characterized by a reciprocal ET-1 and eNOS regulation, with most pro-inflammatory stimuli increasing ET-1 and decreasing eNOS expression [62].

The human lung is an important site for both ET-1 clearance and production: approximately 50% of circulating ET-1 is cleared in a single transpulmonary passage via the ET_B receptor, with a simultaneous equal production [65]. This balance between pulmonary ET-1 clearance and release was found decreased early in ALI, reversing in patients who subsequently recovered [66]. Additionally, plasma ET-1 values are increased in septic patients with and without ARDS [67], possibly contributing to the ALI-associated pulmonary hypertension.

Prostaglandins

Among the several cyclo-oxygenase (COX) products PGI_2 and thromboxane A_2 are probably the most important in ALI. PGI_2 is a potent vasodilator and an important inhibitor of platelet aggregation. Thromboxane A_2 is a potent pulmonary vasoconstrictor secondary to endotoxin infusion; Thromboxane A_2 also increases capillary permeability and platelet aggregation [7]. Prostaglandin E_1 (PGE_1) is another COX product with EC protective properties. As with PGI_2, PGE_1 is a vasodilator and platelet aggregation inhibitor, also impairing neutrophil chemotaxis and macrophage activation [68]. COX products contribute to HPV; however, their vasoactive action varies with the size of the artery and the species involved. A particular role of eicosanoids in several ALI models is their contribution to the regulation of perfusion redistribution that diverts blood flow to healthier lung regions. Pretreatment of rabbits with indomethacin, under partial lung microvascular recruitment, protects against PMA-induced pulmonary endothelial enzyme dysfunction, probably by diverting flow to previously unperfused (i.e., unexposed to PMA) capillaries. Under nearly full microvascular recruitment, the above protective effect of indomethacin is abolished [69]. In a similar respect selective inhibition of the inducible COX isoform protects against the endotoxin-related loss of perfusion redistribution in an oleic acid induced dog ALI model, an effect mediated by PGI_2 [70].

Platelet activating factor

Pulmonary ECs release the phospholipid PAF, a highly reactive mediator that has been reported to cause both vasodilation and vasoconstriction in vivo, depending on its concentration [49]. PAF has been additionally reported to increase lung permeability, to activate platelets, neutrophils, and macrophages and to cause EC release of t-PA and PGI_2. PAF synthesis by EC may be induced by H_2O_2 and other reactive oxygen species [49]. *E. coli* injection in rats induced pulmonary hypertension stimulated by PAF and partly mediated by ET-1; it additionally induced PAF-mediated microvascular injury and leak as well as neutrophil activation-sequestration in the lungs. Pretreatment with a PAF receptor antagonist completely blocked all the above events, suggesting a potential future therapeutic application for this compound [71].

Pulmonary endothelial angiotensin-converting enzyme

Angiotensin-converting enzyme (ACE) hydrolyzes angiotensin I to angiotensin II and breaks down bradykinin [72, 73]. Pulmonary endothelium-bound (PE) ACE has a central role in maintaining adequate local and systemic homeostasis, revealing the dynamic interaction between EC and other cell types schematically shown in Fig. 2. In this respect angiotensin II induces SMC constriction, proliferation, and growth. In contrast to this, bradykinin that escapes ACE inactivation exerts vasodilatory, anti-inflammatory and antithrombotic actions through stimulation of endothelial B_2 kinin receptors, causing the synthesis and release of substances such as NO and PGI_2, generated by eNOS and constitutive COX (COX-1), respectively [73]. PE-ACE pro-inflammatory action is further revealed by the fact that angiotensin II can generate $O_2^{\cdot -}$ via the activation of NADH/NADPH oxidases in EC and SMC [73]. Superoxide anions interact with NO to generate $ONOO^-$, while free radicals from several sources cause molecular and cellular damage and decrease ACE activity [74]. It has recently been proposed that the PE-ACE activity reduction seen in ALI is related to enzyme downregulation, mediated by overproduction of $ONOO^-$ and other ROS/RNS, aimed at reducing oxidant stress in the microenvironment [74]. The role of PE-ACE in lung injury and repair may be more complex since recent investigation provided evidence that ACE possesses characteristics of a signal transduction molecule, involved in EC outside-in signaling [75].

Pulmonary endothelial ACE is an ectoenzyme uniformly distributed throughout the luminal EC surface, with its catalytic site exposed to the blood stream; it is directly accessible to blood-borne substrates, and its activity may be measured in vivo by means of indicator-dilution type techniques [5, 72, 76]. Due to the very high enzyme concentrations in the capillaries, monitoring pulmonary endothelial ACE activity in this type of studies, is in practical terms equal to monitoring pulmonary capillary endothelium-bound (PCEB) ACE activity [72]. This method offers quantifiable indices that may distinguish between abnormalities secondary to endothelial dysfunction per se and decreased pulmonary vascular surface area. PCEB-ACE activity estimations have been recently validated in humans [77].

Plasma soluble ACE (sACE) activity is decreased in ARDS patients [78]. However, in contrast to PCEB-ACE, sACE activity is a surrogate index of pulmonary endothelial function. PCEB-ACE activity reduction is among the earliest signs in various ALI animal models, preceding changes in parameters such as acid-base balance, gas exchange, hemodynamic parameters, increased permeability, and morphological changes at the light and electron-microscopic level. This is the case following administration of bleomycin to rabbits [79], exposure of rabbits to hyperoxia [80], PMA administration to rabbits and dogs [69, 81], and chest irradiation to rabbits [82, 83]. Similarly, pulmonary endothelial ACE activity depression, determined by the decreased pulmonary uptake of an anti-ACE monoclonal antibody, occurs in rats secondary to normoxic lung ischemia/reperfusion [84].

PCEB-ACE activity was estimated in mechanically ventilated patients belonging to high-risk groups for ARDS development and suffering from various degrees of ALI/ARDS [85]. Enzyme activity was expressed as transpulmonary substrate hydrolysis (reflecting enzyme activity per capillary) and as the functional capillary surface area (FCSA) index A_{max}/K_m (reflecting enzyme activity per vascular bed) related to both enzyme quantity and functional integrity [72, 77]. Both indices decreased early during the ALI/ARDS continuum and were inversely related to the lung injury score [45], suggesting that the clinical severity of the syndrome is related to the degree of PCEB-ACE activity depression (i.e., the underlying pulmonary endothelial dysfunction). Further analysis of the FCSA data revealed two different profiles in the A_{max}/K_m vs. cardiac output relationships, probably distinguishing patients with reserves of healthy or mildly injured capillaries from those without; the former had better survival, raising the possibility that FCSA could be of value as an outcome predictor in ARDS [85].

Marshall et al. [86] have recently shown that ACE insertion/deletion polymorphism is associated with the susceptibility and outcome in ARDS, with the DD genotype frequency being increased and associated with mortality in these patients. This first description of a specific allele association with ARDS development suggests a major role for the renin-angiotensin system in the pathophysiology of the syndrome. Although the D allele has been associated with higher ACE activity, this does not necessarily contradict the reported PCEB-ACE activity reduction in ALI/ARDS [85]. The former could affect mostly other lung compartments or, alternatively, the latter might be related to either damaged ECs or to PCEB-ACE downregulation as a host response aimed at reducing local inflammation.

Endothelium-related therapies in ALI/ARDS

Pulmonary endothelial functional and structural alterations are key components of ALI pathogenesis. Consequently EC-related therapies may have beneficial effects in ALI/ARDS. Such therapies should restore adequate endocrine and paracrine EC functions, and protect ECs against harmful insults as well as against pro-inflammatory cell-cell interactions [68, 87]. Several therapeutic interventions, most of them related to endothelium-derived vasoactive (and anti-inflammatory) mediators are already in place, in an effort to improve arterial oxygenation and treat ARDS-related pulmonary hypertension [68]. In this respect inhaled or intravenous PGI_2, inhaled or intravenous (in either native or liposomal form) PGE_1, and, mainly, inhaled NO have been used, with mixed results [68, 87]. Additional agents include antioxidants such as *N*-acetylcysteine and hyperoncotic albumin, and the thromboxane synthetase inhibitor ketoconazole [87]. Several agents already in clinical use for treating pathologies other than ALI, such as ET-1 receptor antagonists, phosphodiesterase inhibitors, and ACE inhibitors might have beneficial effects. For a comprehensive analysis of this topic the reader is referred to [68] and [87]. Throughout this review several experimental studies with future therapeutic potential have been reported. More recent experimental work focus on unmasking EC diversity in an effort to develop means that will target the injured pulmonary endothelium and allow specific drug and/or gene delivery.

Conclusion and future directions

In addition to gas exchange, pulmonary vasculature filters the entire circulating blood before the latter enters the systemic circulation, affecting both local and systemic vascular tones, inflammatory processes, and whole-body homeostasis. Pulmonary circulation possesses two major distinct features: in health it responds to hypoxia with HPV to maintain adequate ventilation/perfusion match; in critical illness pulmonary hypertension may develop, as opposed to the often occurring systemic hypotension. As these responses strongly depend on pulmonary endothelial functional and structural integrity, further understanding of the pulmonary endothelial properties will provide insights into ALI pathophysiology and how the latter affects systemic cardiovascular homeostasis. In this respect recent investigations revealed the existence of pulmonary EC heterogeneity that might contribute to ALI pathogenesis: neutrophil adhesion through ICAM-1 induces cytosceletal changes in pulmonary microvascular ECs (where the site of neutrophil emigration) and not in pulmonary arterial ECs [88]. Additionally, Ca^{2+} communication from pulmonary septal capillaries appears to establish a pro-inflammatory state in downstream venular capillaries, probably amplifying lung inflammation [89]. Specific pulmonary ECs that locally enhance or amplify lung injury might be the targets of future genetic or other therapies.

A National Heart, Lung and Blood Institute workshop has recently proposed future research directions in ALI/ARDS [90]. Pulmonary ECs appear to be the first lung cells altered in ALI/ARDS generated by sepsis, trauma, and other systemic conditions. Among other things, EC heterogeneity should be further investigated along with the EC functional changes involving new gene expression or constitutive pathways, the molecular mechanisms that govern pulmonary EC responses, their interaction with alveolar epithelium, and the responses of systemic endothelium in ALI/ARDS. New EC-related therapies targeting pulmonary microvascular inflammation and thrombosis, and the value of newly implanted pulmonary ECs derived by intravenous infusion of bone marrow stem cells should be investigated [90]. In relation to the former, studies of activated protein C administration in ARDS patients are already under way.

In conclusion, pulmonary EC dysfunction is a key component of ALI pathogenesis. Future investigations of pulmonary endothelial dysfunction may provide additional information on ALI pathophysiology, markers that could predict ARDS development or outcome, and new therapeutic approaches.

References

1. Simionescu M (1991) Lung endothelium: structure-function correlates. In: Crystal RG, West JB (eds) The Lung: scientific foundations. Raven, New York, pp 301–331
2. Bernard GR, Artigas A, Brigham KL, Carlet J, Falke A, Hudson L, Lamy M, LeGall JR, Morris A, Spragg R, the Consensus Committee (1994) The American-European Consensus Conference on ARDS: definitions, mechanisms, relevant outcomes, and clinical trial coordination. Am J Respir Crit Care Med 49:818–824
3. Pittet JF, Mackersie RC, Martin TR, Matthay MA (1997) Biological markers of acute lung injury: prognostic and pathogenic significance. Am J Respir Crit Care Med 155:1187–1205
4. Hassoun PM, Fanburg BL, Junod AF (1991) Metabolic functions. In: Crystal RG, West JB (eds) The lung: scientific foundations. Raven, New York, pp 313–327
5. Orfanos SE, Catravas JD (1993) Metabolic functions of the pulmonary endothelium. In: Yacoub M, Pepper J (eds) Annual review of cardiac surgery, 6th edn. Current Science, London, pp 52–59
6. Aaronson PI, Robertson TP, Ward JPT (2002) Endothelium-derived mediators and hypoxic pulmonary vasoconstriction. Respir Physiol Neurobiol 132:107–120
7. Wort SJ, Evans TW (1999) The role of endothelium in modulating vascular control in sepsis and related conditions. Br Med Bull 55:30–48
8. Park WY, Goodman RB, Steinberg KP, Ruzinski JT, Radella F 2nd, Park DR, Pugin J, Skerrett SJ, Hudson LD, Martin TR (2001) Cytokine balance in the lungs of patients with acute respiratory distress syndrome. Am J Respir Crit Care Med 164:1896–1903
9. Meyrick B (1986) Pathology of the adult respiratory distress syndrome. Crit Care Clin 2:405–428
10. Mutunga M, Fulton B, Bullock R, Batchelor A, Gascoigne A, Gillespie JI, Baudouin SV (2001) Circulating endothelial cells in patients with septic shock. Am J Respir Crit Care Med 163:195–200
11. Oberholzer A, Oberholzer C, Moldawer LL (2000) Cytokine signalling-regulation of the immune response in normal and critically ill states. Crit Care Med 28 [Suppl 4]:N3–N12
12. Mantovani A, Bussolini F, Introna M (1997) Cytokine regulation of endothelial cell function: from molecular level to the bedside. Immunol Today 18:231–239
13. Folkesson HG, Matthay MA, Hebert CA, Broaddus VC (1995) Acid aspiration induced lung injury in rabbits is mediated by interleukin-8 dependent mechanisms. J Clin Invest 96:107–116
14. Laffon M, Pittet JF, Modelska K, Matthay MA, Young DM (1999) Interleukin-8 mediates injury from smoke inhalation to both the lung endothelial and the alveolar epithelial barriers in rabbits. Am J Respir Crit Care Med 160:1443–1449
15. Pulido EJ, Shames BD, Pennica D, O'Leary RM, Bensard DD, Cain BS, McIntyre RC Jr (1999) Cardiotrophin-1 attenuates endotoxin-induced acute lung injury. J Surg Res 84:240–246
16. Kawamae KK, Pristine G, Chiumello D, Tremblay LN, Slutsky AS (2000) Partial liquid ventilation decreases serum tumor necrosis factor-α concentrations in a rat acid aspiration lung injury model. Crit Care Med 28:479–483
17. Kuebler WM, Parthasarathi K, Wang PM, Bhattacharya J (2000) A novel signalling mechanism between gas and blood compartments of the lung. J Clin Invest 105:905–913
18. Grau GE, Mili N, Lou JN, Morel DR, Ricou B, Lucas R, Suter PM (1996) Phenotypic and functional analysis of pulmonary microvascular endothelial cells from patients with acute respiratory distress syndrome. Lab Invest 74:761–770

19. Hashimoto S, Gon Y, Matsumoto K, Takeshita I, Takashi H (2001) N-acetylcysteine attenuates TNF-α induced p38 MAP kinase activation and p38 MAP kinase-mediated IL-8 production by human pulmonary vascular endothelial cells. Br J Pharmacol 132:270–276
20. Matthay MA, Bhattacharya S, Gaver D, Ware LB, Lim LHK, Syrkina O, Eyal F, Hubmayr R (2002) Ventilator-induced lung injury: in vivo and in vitro mechanisms. Am J Physiol Lung Cell Mol Physiol 283:L678–L682
21. Ranieri VM, Suter PM, Tortorella C, De Tullio R, Dayer JM, Brienza A, Bruno F, Slutsky AS (1999) Effect of mechanical ventilation on inflammatory mediators in patients with acute respiratory distress syndrome. JAMA 282:54–61
22. Frank JA, Gutierrez JA, Jones KD, Allen L, Dobbs L, Matthay MA (2002) Low tidal volume reduces epithelial and endothelial injury in acid-injured rat lungs. Am J Respir Crit Care Med 165:242–249
23. Fan J, Ye RD, Malik AB (2001) Transcriptional mechanisms of acute lung injury. Am J Physiol Lung Cell Mol Physiol 281:L1037–L1050
24. Blackwell TS, Christman JW (1997) The role of nuclear factor-kappa B in cytokine gene regulation. Am J Respir Cell Mol Biol 17:3–9
25. Lum H, Roebuck KA (2001) Oxidant stress and endothelial cell dysfunction. Am J Physiol Cell Physiol 280:C719–C741
26. Abraham E (2000) NF-κB activation Crit Care Med 28 [Suppl 4]:N100–N104
27. Dschietzig T, Richter C, Pfannenschmidt G, Bartsch C, Laule M, Baumann G, Stangl K (2001) Dexamethasone inhibits stimulation of pulmonary endothelins by pro-inflammatory cytokines: possible involvement of a nuclear factor κB dependent mechanism. Intensive Care Med 27:751–756
28. Quinlan GJ, Upton RL (2002) Oxidant/antioxidant balance in acute respiratory distress syndrome. In: Evans TW, Griffiths MJD, Keogh BF (eds) European respiratory monograph: ARDS, vol 7, monograph 20. European Respiratory Society Journals, Sheffield, pp 33–46
29. Bhatia M, Moochhala S (2004) Role of inflammatory mediators in the pathophysiology of acute respiratory distress syndrome. J Pathol 202:145–156
30. Haligren R, Samuelson T, Veng P, Modig I (1987) Eosinophil activation in the lung is related to lung damage in adult respiratory distress syndrome. Am Rev Respir Dis 135:639–642
31. Rowen JL, Hyde DM, McDonald RJ (1990) Eosinophils cause acute edematous injury in isolated perfused rat lungs. Am Rev Respir Dis 142:215–220
32. Hasleton PS, Roberts TE (1999) Adult respiratory distress syndrome-an update. Histopathology 34:285–294
33. Albelda SM, Smith CW, Ward PA (1994) Adhesion molecules and inflammatory injury. FASEB J 8:504–512
34. Sheridan BC, McIntyre RC Jr, Moore EE, Meldrum DR, Agrafojo J, Fullerton DA (1997) Neutrophils mediate pulmonary vasomotor dysfunction in endotoxin-induced acute lung injury. J Trauma 42:391–397
35. Folkesson HG, Matthay MA (1997) Inhibition of CD18 or CD11b attenuates acute lung injury after acid instillation in rabbits. J Appl Physiol 82:1743–1750
36. Moriuchi H, Zaha M, Fukumoto T, Yuizono T (1998) Activation of polymorphonuclear leukocytes in oleic acid-induced lung injury. Intensive Care Med 24:709–715
37. Azuma A, Takahashi S, Nose M, Araki K, Araki M, Takahashi T, Hirose M, Kawashima H, Miyasaka M, Kudoh S (2000) Role of E-selectin in bleomycin induced lung fibrosis in mice. Thorax 55:147–152
38. Sato N, Suzuki Y, Nishio K, Suzuki K, Naoki K, Takeshita K, Kudo H, Miyao N, Tsumura H, Serizawa H, Suematsu M, Yamaguchi K (2000) Roles of ICAM-1 for abnormal leukocyte recruitment in the microcirculation of bleomycin-induced fibrotic lung injury. Am J Respir Crit Care Med 161:1681–1688
39. Folch E, Salas A, Panes J, Gelpi E, Roselo-Catafau J, Anderson DC, Navarro S, Pique JM, Fernandez-Cruz L, Closa D (1999) Role of P-selectin and ICAM-1 in pancreatitis-induced lung inflammation in rats. Ann Surg 230:792–799
40. Dry SM, Bechard KM, Milford EL, Churchill WH, Benjamin RJ (1999) The pathology of transfusion-related acute lung injury. Am J Clin Pathol 112:216–221
41. Sakamaki F, Ishizaka A, Handa M, Fujishima S, Urano T, Sayama K, Nakamura H, Kanazawa M, Kawashiro T, Katayama M, Ikeda Y (1995) Soluble form of P-selectin in plasma is elevated in acute lung injury. Am J Respir Crit Care Med 151:1821–1826
42. Moss M, Gillespie MK, Ackerson L, Moore FA, Moore EE, Parsons PE (1996) Endothelial cell activity varies in patients at risk for the adult respiratory distress syndrome. Crit Care Med 24:1782–1786
43. Donelly SC, Haslett C, Dransfield I, Robertson CE, Carter DC, Ross JA, Grant IS, Tedder TF (1994) Role of selectins in development of adult respiratory distress syndrome. Lancet 344:215–219
44. Xu N, Rahman A, Minshall RD, Tiruppathi C, Malik AB (2000) β_2-integrin blockade driven by E-selectin promoter prevents neutrophil sequestration and lung injury in mice. Circ Res 87:254–260
45. Murray JF, Matthay MA, Luce JM, Flick MR (1988) An expanded definition of the adult respiratory distress syndrome. Am Rev Respir Dis 138:720–723
46. Sinclair DG, Braude S, Haslam PL, Evans TW (1994) Pulmonary endothelial permeability in patients with severe lung injury. Clinical correlates and natural history. Chest 106:535–539
47. Dudek SM, Garcia JGN (2001) Cytoskeletal regulation of pulmonary vascular permeability. J Appl Physiol 91:1487–1500
48. Thickett DR, Armstrong L, Christie SJ, Millar AB (2001) Vascular endothelial growth factor may contribute to increased vascular permeability in acute respiratory distress syndrome. Am J Respir Crit Care Med 164:1601–1605
49. Block ER (1992) Pulmonary endothelial cell pathobiology: implications for acute lung injury. Am J Med Sci 304:136–144
50. Morel Dr, Dargent F, Bachmann M, Suter PM, Junod AF (1985) Pulmonary extraction of serotonin and propranolol in patients with adult respiratory distress syndrome. Am Rev Respir Dis 132:479–484
51. Carvalho AC, Bellman SM, Saullo VJ, Quinn D, Zapol WM (1982) Altered factor VIII in acute respiratory failure. N Engl J Med 307:1113–1119
52. Sabharwal AK, Bajaj SP, Ameri A, Tricomi SM, Hyers TM, Dahms TE, Taylor FB, Bajaj MS (1995) Tissue factor pathway inhibitor and von Willebrand factor antigen levels in adult respiratory distress syndrome and in a primate model of sepsis. Am J Respir Crit Care Med 151:758–767
53. Rubin DB, Wiener-Kronish JP, Murray JF, Green DR, Turner J, Luce JM, Montgomery AB, Marks JD, Matthay MA (1990) Elevated von Willebrand factor antigen is an early plasma predictor of acute lung injury in nonpulmonary sepsis syndrome. J Clin Invest 86:474–480
54. Moss M, Ackerson L, Gillespie MK, Moore FA, Moore EE, Parsons PE (1995) Von Willebrand factor antigen levels are not predictive for the adult respiratory distress syndrome. Am J Respir Crit Care Med 151:15–20

55. Bajaj MS, Tricomi SM (1999) Plasma levels of the three endothelial-specific proteins von Willebrand factor, tissue factor pathway inhibitor, and thrombomodulin do not predict the development of acute respiratory distress syndrome. Intensive Care Med 25:1259–1266
56. Fisele B, Lamy M, Thijs LG, Keinecke H-O, Schuster H-P, Matthias FR, Fourrier F, Heinrichs H, Delvos U (1998) Antithrombin III in patients with severe sepsis. A randomized, placebo-controlled, double-blind multicenter trial plus a meta-analysis on all randomized, placebo-controlled, double-blind trials with antithrombin III in severe sepsis. Intensive Care Med 24:663–672
57. Uchiba M, Okajima K (1997) Antithrombin III (AT III) prevents LPS-induced pulmonary vascular injury: a novel biological activity of AT III. Semin Thromb Hemost 23:583–590
58. McGregor IR, Perrie AM, Donnelly SC, Haslett C (1997) Modulation of human endothelial thrombomodulin by neutrophils and their release products. Am J Respir Crit Care Med 155:47–52
59. Distefano G, Romeo MG, Betta P, Rodono A, Amato M (1998) Thrombomodulin serum levels in ventilated preterm babies with respiratory distress syndrome. Eur J Pediatr 157:327–330
60. Christoforidou-Solomidou M, Kennel S, Scherpereel A, Wiewrodt R, Solomides CC, Pietra GG, Murciano JC, Shah SA, Ischiropoulos H, Albelda SM, Muzykantov VR (2002) Vascular immunotargeting of glucose oxidase to the endothelial antigens induces distinct forms of oxidant acute lung injury: targeting to thrombomodulin, but not to PECAM-1, causes pulmonary thrombosis and neutrophil transmigration. Am J Pathol 160:1155–1169
61. Grau GE, de Moerloose P, Bulla O, Lou J, Lei Z, Reber G, Mili N, Morel DR, Suter PM (1997) Haemostatic properties of human pulmonary and cerebral microvascular endothelial cells. Thromb Haemost 77:585–590
62. Mawji IA, Mardsen PA (2003) Perturbations in paracrine control of the circulation: role of the endothelial-derived vasomediators, endothelin-1 and nitric oxide. Microsc Res Tech 60:46–58
63. Liu S, Crawley DE, Barnes PJ, Evans TW (1991) Endothelium derived relaxing factor inhibits hypoxic pulmonary vasoconstriction in rats. Am Rev Respir Dis 143:32–37
64. Hart CM (1999) Nitric oxide in adult lung disease. Chest 115:1407–1417
65. Dupuis J, Stewart DJ, Cernacek P, Gosselin G (1996) Human pulmonary circulation is an important site for both clearance and production of endothelin-1. Circulation 94:1578–1584
66. Langleben D, Demarchie M, Laporta D, Spanier AH, Schlesinger D, Stewart DJ (1993) Endothelin-1 in acute lung injury and the adult respiratory distress syndrome. Am Rev Respir Dis 148: 1646–1650
67. Sanai L, Haynes WG, MacKenzie A, Grant IS, Webb DJ (1996) Endothelin in sepsis and the adult respiratory distress syndrome. Intensive Care Med 22:52–56
68. Moloney ED, Evans TW (2003) Pathophysiology and pharmacological treatment of pulmonary hypertension in acute respiratory distress syndrome. Eur Respir J 21:720–727
69. Chen XL, Orfanos SE, Catravas JD (1992) Effects of indomethacin on PMA-induced pulmonary endothelial enzyme dysfunction in vivo. Am J Physiol 262:L153–L162
70. Gust R, Kozlowski K, Stephenson AH, Schuster DP (1999) Role of cyclooxygenase-2 in oleic acid-induced acute lung injury. Am J Respir Crit Care Med 160:1165–1170
71. Clavijo LC, Carter MB, Matheson PJ, Wills-Frank LA, Wilson MA, Wead WB, Garrison RN (2000) Platelet activating factor and bacteremia-induced pulmonary hypertension. J Surg Res 88:173–180
72. Orfanos SE, Kotanidou K, Roussos C (2002) Pulmonary endothelial angiotensin converting enzyme in lung injury. In: Vincent JL (ed) 2002 Yearbook of intensive care and emergency medicine. Springer, Berlin Heidelberg New York; pp 100–110
73. Linz W, Wohlfart P, Scholkens BA, Malinski T, Wiemer G (1999) Interactions among ACE, kinins and NO. Cardiovasc Res 43:549–561
74. McCloud L, Parkerson JB, Freant L, Hoffman WH, Catravas JD (2004) β-hydroxybutyrate induces acute pulmonary endothelial dysfunction in rabbits. Exp Lung Res 30:193-206
75. Kohlstedt K, Brandes RP, Muller-Esterl W, Busse R, Fleming I (2004) Angiotensin converting enzyme is involved in outside-in signalling in endothelial cells. Circ Res 94:60–67
76. Ryan US, Ryan JW, Whitaker C, Chiu A. (1976) Localization of angiotensin-converting enzyme (kinase II). Immunocytochemistry and immunofluorescence. Tissue Cell 8:125–146
77. Orfanos SE, Langleben D, Khoury J, Schlesinger RD, Dragatakis L, Roussos C, Ryan JW, Catravas JD (1999) Pulmonary capillary endothelium-bound angiotensin converting enzyme activity in humans. Circulation 99:1593–1599
78. Casey L, Krieger B, Kohler J, Rice C, Oparil S, Szidon P (1982) Decreased serum angiotensin converting enzyme in adult respiratory distress syndrome associated with sepsis: a preliminary report. Crit Care Med 9:651–654
79. Lazo JS, Catravas JD, Gillis CN (1981) Reduction in rabbit serum and pulmonary angiotensin converting enzyme after subacute bleomycin treatment. Biochem Pharmacol 30:2577–2584
80. Dobuler KJ, Catravas JD, Gillis CN (1982) Early detection of oxygen-induced lung injury in conscious rabbits: reduced in vivo activity of angiotensin converting enzyme and removal of 5-hydroxytryptamine. Am Rev Respir Dis 126:534–539
81. Ehrhart IC, Orfanos SE, McCloud LL, Sickles DW, Hoffman WF, Catravas JD (1999) Vascular recruitment increases evidence of lung injury. Crit Care Med 27:120–129
82. Orfanos SE, Chen XL, Burch SE, Ryan JW, Chunk AYK, Catravas JD (1994) Radiation-induced early pulmonary endothelial ectoenzyme dysfunction in vivo: effect of indomethacin. Toxicol Appl Pharmacol 124:112–122
83. Catravas JD, Burch SE, Sprulock BO, Mills LR (1988) Early effects of ionising radiation on pulmonary endothelial angiotensin converting enzyme and 5'-nucleotidase, in vivo. Toxicol Appl Pharmacol 94:342–355
84. Atochina EN, Muzykantov VR, Al-Medhi AB, Danilov SM, Fisher AB (1997) Normotoxic lung ischemia/reperfusion accelerates shedding of angiotesin converting enzyme from the pulmonary endothelium. Am J Respir Crit Care Med 156:1114–1119
85. Orfanos SE, Armaganidis A, Glynos C, Psevdi E, Kaltsas P, Sarafidou P, Catravas JD, Dafni UG, Langleben D, Roussos C (2000) Pulmonary capillary endothelium-bound angiotensin converting enzyme activity in acute lung injury. Circulation 102:2011–2018
86. Marshall RP, Webb S, Bellingan GJ, Montgomery HE, Chaudhari B, McAnulty RJ, Humphries SE, Hill MR, Laurent GJ (2002) Angiotensin converting enzyme insertion/deletion polymorphism is associated with susceptibility and outcome in acute respiratory distress syndrome. Am J Respir Crit Care Med 166:646–650
87. Groeneveld ABJ (2003) Vascular pharmacology of acute lung injury and acute respiratory distress syndrome. Vascul Pharmacol 39:247–256

88. Wang Q, Pfeiffer GR, Stevens T, Doerschuck CM (2002) Lung microvascular and arterial endothelial cells differ in their responses to intercellular adhesion molecule-1 ligation. Am J Respir Crit Care Med 166:872–877

89. Parthasarathi K, Ichimura H, Bhattacharya J (2003) Septal capillaries communicate pro-inflammatory signals to downstream vascular segments in lung (abstract). Am J Respir Crit Care Med 167:A121

90. Matthay MA, Zimmerman GA, Esmon C, Bhattacharya J, Coller B, Doerschuck CM, Floros J, Gimbrone MA Jr, Hoffman E, Hubmayr RD, Leppert M, Matalon S, Munford R, Parsons P, Slutsky AS, Tracey KJ, Ward P, Gail DB, Harabin AL (2003) Future research directions in acute lung injury. Summary of a National Heart, Lung and Blood Institute working group Am J Respir Crit Care Med 167:1027–1035

C. S. A. Macmillan
I. S. Grant
P. J. D. Andrews

Pulmonary and cardiac sequelae of subarachnoid haemorrhage: time for active management?

Abstract Cardiac injury and pulmonary oedema occurring after acute neurological injury have been recognised for more than a century. Catecholamines, released in massive quantities due to hypothalamic stress from subarachnoid haemorrhage (SAH), result in specific myocardial lesions and hydrostatic pressure injury to the pulmonary capillaries causing neurogenic pulmonary oedema (NPO). The acute, reversible cardiac injury ranges from hypokinesis with a normal cardiac index, to low output cardiac failure. Some patients exhibit both catastrophic cardiac failure and NPO, while others exhibit signs of either one or other, or have subclinical evidence of the same.Hypoxia and hypotension are two of the most important insults which influence outcome after acute brain injury. However, despite this, little attention has hitherto been devoted to prevention and reversal of these potentially catastrophic medical complications which occur in patients with SAH. It is not clear which patients with SAH will develop important cardiac and respiratory complications. An active approach to investigation and organ support could provide a window of opportunity to intervene before significant hypoxia and hypotension develop, potentially reducing adverse consequences for the long-term neurological status of the patient. Indeed, there is an argument for all SAH patients to have echocardiography and continuous monitoring of respiratory rate, pulse oximetry, blood pressure and electrocardiogram. In the event of cardio-respiratory compromise developing i.e. cardiogenic shock and/or NPO, full investigation, attentive monitoring and appropriate intervention are required immediately to optimise cardiorespiratory function and allow subsequent definitive management of the SAH.

Keywords Subarachnoid · haemorrhage · Neurogenic pulmonary oedema · Cardiac injury · Critical care Electrocardiogram

Abbreviations *ALI* acute lung injury · *CI* cardiac index · *CK-MB* creatine phosphokinase-myocardial fraction · *CVP* central venous pressure · *ECHO* echocardiogram · *ARDS* acute respiratory distress syndrome · *CPP* cerebral perfusion pressure · *EVLW* extravascular lung water · *HDU* high dependency unit · *ICP* intracranial pressure · *ICU* intensive care unit · *MAP* mean arterial pressure · *MPAP* mean pulmonary artery pressure · *Neuro obs* neuroligical observation/assessment · *NPO* neurogenic pulmonary oedema · *ODM* oesophageal Doppler monitor · *PAC* pulmonary artery catheter · *PAOP* pulmonary artery occlusion pressure · *PAP* pulmonary artery pressure · *PEEP* positive end expiratory pressure · *SAH* subarachnoid haemorrhage · *SBP* systolic blood pressure · *WFNS* World Federation of Neurosurgeons grading for SAH

DOI 10.1007/978-3-642-28233-1_10,

Introduction

Subarachnoid haemorrhage (SAH), which affects predominantly women of working age, has devastating consequences with a mortality exceeding 40% and a morbidity so high that less than 25% make a complete recovery [1]. Improved management over recent years has included optimal timing of surgery [2], endovascular coiling [3]and nimodipine therapy [4, 5, 6]. Recently published recommendations support active intensive care for patients with complications of SAH [7], yet research and clinical resources have focused on other major causes of mortality following SAH – direct pressure effects, rebleed and vasospasm, each of which accounts for a quarter of the deaths. However, in a recent study involving more than 450 SAH patients, medical complications accounted for a similar proportion of deaths [8]. Clearly, there is room for improvement.

Medical complications after SAH have been neglected both in terms of research and their importance to outcome in clinical practice. This review will focus on cardiorespiratory compromise – cardiac dysfunction and pulmonary oedema – associated with acute SAH, where the experience of intensivists may have a crucial influence. Evidence will be assessed to clarify the pathophysiological processes that result in life-threatening clinical deterioration. Treatment options will be reviewed and a evidence-based practical approach to patient management will be discussed.

Medical complications of SAH

The most comprehensive study of medical complications after SAH to date followed 457 adult patients for 3 months after ictus [8]. Patients were recruited between 1987 and 1989, none received a calcium antagonist but corticosteroids were given to 70%, anticonvulsant therapy to 80%, and nearly two-thirds had surgery within 3 days. Complying with current recommendations [7] and practice [9] for 'triple H' therapy, 80% had *H*ypervolaemia (average daily fluid intake during the first 2 weeks was 4.1 l) and over 30% had induced *H*ypertension. In terms of *H*aemodilution, the third '*H*', 30% had 'anaemia'. Medical complications accounted for 23% of deaths. Other deaths were caused by the primary bleed (19%), re-bleed (22%) and vasospasm (23%). While little can be done for the primary bleed, much effort has been directed towards reducing the impact of re-bleed and vasospasm, but relatively little has been aimed at identifying the causes, reducing the incidence or improving the management of medical complications. Indeed, not only is a significant proportion of mortality directly attributable to medical complications, but also a significant degree of morbidity as 83% of those who died had a life-threatening medical complication compared to 30% of survivors [8].

The scope of medical complications in these SAH patients was representative of many intensive care patient groups and included renal, hepatic, haematological, metabolic and endocrine dysfunction. However, the most frequent were pulmonary and cardiovascular complications [8]. Cardiac dysfunction is a well-known and frequently reported complication of SAH, most often recognised on the electrocardiogram (ECG) by arrhythmias, including ventricular fibrillation and conduction abnormalities. Cardiac failure is less commonly reported in the literature, but was found in 4% of patients reported by Solenski et.al. This has also been the subject of several studies of cardiac function after SAH [10, 11, 12, 13, 14, 15]. Pulmonary oedema, sometimes severe enough to be life-threatening, was identified in a quarter of patients. As will be discussed later, pulmonary oedema associated with SAH has a different aetiology from the inflammatory response that produces acute lung injury (ALI) and the acute respiratory distress syndrome (ARDS), although SAH can also trigger a systemic inflammatory response leading to this lung pathology.

Cardiac dysfunction and pulmonary oedema may occur together or independently after SAH. Secondary brain injury caused by hypoxia and hypotension – the two most influential factors on poor outcome after acute traumatic brain injury [16] – are situations where intensive care clinicians have arguably the greatest experience and therefore potentially have the most to offer patients. Logical treatment of cardiac and respiratory deterioration requires an understanding of the underlying pathophysiology.

Cardiac injury

Electrical cardiac disturbances

Rhythm and conduction disturbances are almost universal after SAH [17] and have been regularly reported in the last 50 years [18]. Anything from fatal ventricular fibrillation to bradycardia is possible [20]; common findings include QRS, ST segment and T-wave abnormalities, and prolongation of the QT interval [21, 22, 23]. These changes may mimic myocardial infarction or ischaemia on a 12-lead ECG [21], but clinical diagnoses of myocardial infarction have been refuted at post-mortem examination due to lack of coronary artery disease [22, 23, 24]. In survivors of SAH the ECG changes are usually reversible, although they may persist for several weeks [11, 22, 25] and can recur in patients with re-bleed. Experimental evidence may explain these ECG abnormalities. Stimulation of the posterior hypothalamus in cats caused a marked pressor response, multifocal ectopic beats, T wave inversion and S-T segment changes [27]. Hypothalamic stress (from ischaemia and/or pressure) is the common link between SAH and its cardiac sequelae.

Clinical relevance of ECG abnormalities

SAH is almost universally associated with cardiac electrical disturbance [17], but its clinical relevance is questionable. There is no consistent association between ECG abnormalities and the mechanical hypokinesis found on echocardiography, histological cardiac lesions or serum markers of cardiac injury [10, 11, 12, 13, 14, 17]. In relation to brain secondary insults, a low cardiac output with reduced cerebral perfusion could be important to outcome; markers of impending clinical deterioration would thus be helpful.

Arrhythmias make a significant contribution to mortality and most occur within the first week [20, 28]. In monitored patients, rhythm disturbances occurred in 35%, most commonly sinus tachy or bradycardia, and were considered a moderate threat to life. In addition, ventricular arrhythmias such as asystole and fibrillation were recorded [8], with 5% suffering a life-threatening arrhythmia. These ECG abnormalities were not associated with cardiac failure. Arrhythmias causing haemodynamic changes have been detected in more than 40% of patients, and were life-threatening in 10% [8, 20, 29]. ECGs repeated regularly during hospital admission of 37 SAH patients did not reveal any association between abnormalities and outcome [23]. There were conflicting opinions when neurological state was compared with arrhythmias, some finding no association [12, 20, 29] while others concluded the opposite. However, in a recent study of 61 SAH patients with continuous ECG monitoring, poor outcome was associated with tachyarrhythmias and/or cardiac ischaemia, although this did not hold true for individual ECG abnormalities such as T wave changes [17]. Continuous ECG monitoring in an area with immediate cardiac resuscitation facilities could save lives. In terms of neurological outcome, patients with the most to benefit are those with good neurological grades who may suffer a life-threatening arrhythmia.

Virtually every possible static ECG abnormality has been described after SAH, but clinical relevance is uncertain. Electrolyte disturbance of sodium, calcium and potassium do not seem to be relevant to morphology [12, 22, 30], although, not surprisingly, serious arrhythmias occurred in SAH patients with low serum potassium [29]. Increased urinary catecholamine metabolite and plasma cortisol concentrations were significantly associated with tachycardia, large P waves, short PR interval (<0.13 s), peaked or inverted T waves, and prolonged QTc interval [30]. However, this was refuted in a more recent study [25]. Perhaps ECG abnormalities known to be associated with serious arrhythmias, such as an increased QTc interval, should be measured and thus encourage clinicians to increase their vigilance.

Prolongation of the QT interval after SAH is well documented [10, 11, 13, 17, 19, 20, 21, 22, 25, 30]. A more recent measure, QT dispersion (the difference between the longest and shortest QT interval on a standard 12-lead ECG) – which is associated with fatal arrhythmogenic potential [31] – is increased in SAH patients [32, 33]. The exact mechanism for these changes is unclear, but may be related to imbalance of autonomic tone [22, 25], catecholamines [30, 34, 35] or electrolyte disturbance.

Whatever the truth is in relation to ECG changes, clinical course and outcome, the practical relevance may be a delay in surgery to clip or coil aneurysms as a consequence of additional investigations deemed necessary because of such ECG abnormalities. It could be argued that the standard 12-lead ECG should be discounted in relation to risk assessment for anaesthesia for SAH.

Ventricular dysfunction

Mechanical pump failure causing a reduction in cardiac output occurs less frequently than conduction problems, but can be fatal. The aetiology is controversial. Myocardial 'stunning' is a term that has been applied to sudden and sometimes unexpected ventricular hypokinesis. Sudden onset of ventricular failure (often hypotensive) with or without pulmonary oedema has been reported in SAH case series [8, 11, 36, 37, 38]. In fact, any acute intracranial pathology may result in a stunned myocardium [39]; endogenous catecholamines are the most likely cause.

Surrogate markers for impaired myocardial function include a reduction in blood pressure and cardiac output, or an increase in pulmonary artery occlusion pressure. Direct evidence of ventricular systolic dysfunction can be obtained using echocardiography or nucleotide ventriculography. There are few studies in the literature because these are relatively new investigative tools, but animal experiments provide some insight. SAH induced in nine dogs resulted in motion abnormalities in each, particularly hypokinesis of the left ventricle, detected by transoesophageal echocardiography [34]. SAH causes similar ventricular dysfunction in patients. Case studies after SAH demonstrate general hypokinesia [11, 40, [41]and reduced ejection fraction [37, 41]. Of 19 SAH patients who had thallium scintigraphy, 6 had areas of reversible reduced uptake, indicating perfusion abnormality [10]. Of 12 patients with SAH, more than half had abnormal ventriculography and echocardiography [13]In a larger series of 45 patients, 4 had ventricular hypokinesis 12, as did 4 of 13 SAH patients in another report [14]. A case series of five SAH patients, all with severe neurogenic pulmonary oedema (NPO), demonstrated low ejection fractions requiring inotropic support. Such cases illustrate that NPO and myocardial wall motion abnormalities can occur concurrently [11], i.e. left ventricular failure, but one does not necessarily follow the other [14]. Wall-motion abnormalities are temporary and normal cardiac function usually returns [10, 11, 13, 14, 41]. Interestingly, ventricular dysfunction and ECG changes can occur independently or together [14], but large vessel coronary artery disease has been excluded by angiography as a contributing factor in wall-motion abnormality [13]. This is supported by autopsy [42]; transmural myocardial infarction typically caused by coronary atheroma thrombus was not seen at post-mortem in SAH victims; instead discrete focal lesions occurred [10, 12, 13, 43].

Markers of myocardial cell injury

The myocardium is injured in many patients with SAH; an abnormal increase in plasma creatine phosphokinase-myocardial fraction (CK-MB) concentration is a common finding. The CK-MB was increased in all patients after SAH, but more so in those with echocardiographic evidence of wall-motion abnormalities [14]. More recently, a case series of five SAH patients suffering acute hypotension and NPO was reported [11]. All patients had significantly increased serum CK-MB and wall-motion abnormalities on echocardiography. This pattern has also been described in case reports [40], but there is no association between the increase in CK-MB after SAH and ECG changes [44]. However, there may be an association between cerebral vasospasm after SAH and increased CK-MB [37, 45]. Another marker of cardiac injury, troponin I, was increased in approximately one-fifth of SAH patients, but only a fraction of these had clinically detectable cardiac abnormalities [46]. The reasons for myocardial injury are not clear, but are probably related to hypothalamic stimulation and catecholamine secretion. In animal experiments, stimulation of the midbrain caused myocyte degeneration throughout the heart [27], but most dense in the subendocardium, and surrounded by normal tissue, as is found in SAH patients [47]. Hypothalamic stimulation in cats resulted in cardiac dysfunction and ECG changes similar to those found after SAH. After several hours of stimulation, the hearts had evidence of small haemorrhages and infarcted myocardial fibres with homogeneous cytoplasm, loss of cross striation and loss of nuclei.

Haemodynamic changes

After SAH clinical manifestations of cardiac injury and NPO may occur simultaneously [11, 24, 37, 38, 40, 48, 49] or in isolation [10, 12, 13, 14, 38, 47, 50, 51, 52, 53, 54, 55, 56], depending on the individual's response to the pathophysiological insult [42]. A recent retrospective case series included 16 SAH patients with NPO [48]. All were mechanically ventilated and 4 received vasoactive agents (3 epinephrine and 1 dobutamine) prior to baseline haemodynamic recordings. Their initial mean derivatives included a mean arterial pressure (MAP) of 84 mmHg (range 74–104), mean pulmonary artery pressure (MPAP) 29 mmHg (14–44), CVP 10 mmHg (1–29), PAOP 16 mmHg (5–29), cardiac index (CI) 2.5 $l.min^{-1}m^{-2}$ (1.6–4.5) and a PaO_2:FiO_2 ratio (kPa) of 22 (13–34). The clinical picture was thus one of normal blood pressure, reduced cardiac output and pulmonary oedema diagnosed by chest X-ray findings and hypoxaemia (PaO_2:FiO_2 <40), but with a wide range of PAOP. Most patients had a very low left ventricular stroke work index indicating LVF, but markedly elevated pulmonary vascular resistance implying a pulmonary component in addition to the cardiac aetiology of the NPO. Thus there was a marked variation amongst patients, measured and derived variables being heterogeneous in relation to cardiac and pulmonary lesions.

As the above report shows, NPO occurs in the presence of reduced, normal or increased haemodynamic measures, including PAOP, which ranged from 5 to 29 mmHg at pulmonary artery catheter insertion. It should be noted that insertion of pulmonary catheters in that intensive care unit was not routine, but required the patient to be unstable, for example with hypoxaemia, frank pulmonary oedema or hypotension; five patients had had prior therapy with ephedrine, methoxamine or dobutamine. Another case series of five SAH patients with severe NPO demonstrated a variable cardiac index (1.9–3.0 $l.min^{-1}$. m^{-2}), increased PAOP (17–36 mmHg) and reduced ejection fraction (20–35%) on echocardiography with global impairment of the left ventricle [41]. Examining extravascular lung water (EVLW), initial recordings in 21 patients with intracerebral haemorrhage and 4 with SAH showed no difference in PAOP between those with the greatest EVLW and those without increased EVLW (7.8 vs 7.9 mmHg) [54]. Another case report of SAH demonstrated pulmonary oedema, after which a low systemic blood pressure (90/60 mmHg) and high PAOP (22 mmHg) developed, indicating cardiac dysfunction [37]. This was confirmed on cardiac echocardiography and radionuclide ventriculography where a hypokinetic septum and basal segments were associated with a low ejection fraction of approximately 35%. These case series describes small numbers of patients; therefore, caution should be applied when interpreting the results. However, they do illustrate the variable clinical picture at any one point in time.

Other papers demonstrate temporal haemodynamic changes. Although these, too, are drawn from case reports, it is important to acknowledge the cardiovascular changes described, which do not conform to a single clinical picture. A patient with NPO had PAOP values that ranged from 0 to 15 mmHg over a 3-day period with a maximum recorded PAP of 50/17 mmHg [53]. The recordings were infrequent (every 4 h or less), so it is possible that more extreme pressures were missed. Similarly, in a series of four SAH patients who developed NPO

[12], initially normal PAOP values increased to above 16 mmHg. Another patient with SAH developed NPO [55] where the initial right ventricular pressure was 40/2 mmHg and PAOP 0–4 mmHg, although he had several episodes of severe systemic hypertension (up to 410/200 mmHg) with corresponding PAP 110/60 mmHg and PAOP 48 mmHg. Each episode lasted for approximately 5 min before returning to baseline. Other reports confirm rapidly changing PAOP and systemic blood pressure after SAH [57]. These cases underline the rapid and volatile change in pressures that may occur and could easily be missed.

The closest approximation to pulmonary capillary pressure is an estimate somewhere between PAP and PAOP [58]. Indeed, in experimental animals the left ventricular end diastolic pressure exceeded PAP when epinephrine was used to induce pulmonary oedema [59]. The pulmonary veins were the first vessels to develop increased pressure [60]. In response to experimentally induced SAH, the systemic pressure increased, followed by pulmonary venous then pulmonary arterial pressure, with little change in CVP [61]. Resistance in pulmonary veins of rats increases as constrictions or valves within the vessels increase their tone immediately after a blow to the head [62]. Thus pressure increases in the pulmonary veins precede those in the pulmonary capillaries and may not be reflected by PAOP, PAP or CVP [61]. In addition, if the left ventricle fails, it may contribute to the increase in pulmonary venous pressure.

Neurogenic pulmonary oedema

Any factor reducing diffusion across the alveolar-capillary barrier, including interstitial and frank alveolar oedema, will increase the likelihood of hypoxaemia. Post-mortem studies of intracranial pathology recorded an incidence of pulmonary oedema of 46 [63] and 52% [64]. A Minnesota study of sudden deaths found that over 90% of patients with intracranial bleeds had pulmonary oedema [65]. Furthermore, NPO can develop within seconds of a neurological insult. In a series of 56 Vietnam casualties (aged 17–37 years) killed from head wounds, it was found that most had oedema, congestion and haemorrhage of the lungs [66]. Indeed, even 17 of 20 soldiers killed almost instantaneously had these findings at autopsy. Interestingly, casualties with cervical cord transection or massive haemorrhage had normal lungs. The development of NPO requires an adequate systemic circulating volume. Rabbits given epinephrine infusions to induce pulmonary oedema [67] had increased lung-to-body weight ratios and reduced static compliance, but animals rendered hypovolaemic by bleeding prior to epinephrine administration had no evidence of oedema. Similarly, autopsy findings in soldiers with serious head trauma showed no evidence of pulmonary oedema if significant hypovolaemia had occurred [66].

NPO, defined as bilateral pulmonary infiltrates on chest X-ray and reduced PaO_2 not attributable to another cause, was identified in 23% of all SAH patients surviving to reach hospital and was considered to be a threat to life in 6% [8]. This is probably an underestimate because to meet the definitions of severe (life-threatening) pulmonary oedema for the purposes of the study, a pulmonary artery catheter was required to confirm a PAOP>22 mmHg associated with severe impairment of gas exchange (PaO_2 <6.7 kPa with FiO_2 ≥0.4). Pulmonary oedema occurred on days 0–14 but most frequently on day 3, and was associated with increasing age (>30 years), poorer grades (WFNS grading [68]) and day of surgery, but not with 'triple H' therapy, cerebral angiography, past history of cardiac disease, ECG changes or lung disease. The time scale noted also coincides with catecholamine hypersecretion that may last for 10 days or more after SAH [69]. Curiously, hepatic dysfunction was associated with pulmonary oedema [8], perhaps owing to hypoxia or to liver congestion, which has been noted at autopsy [47]. NPO is a serious and common complication after SAH that threatens both survival and good neurological outcome.

Pulmonary oedema fluid

Several investigations into the nature of SAH-induced pulmonary oedema fluid have been conducted to determine if its evolution is hydrostatic (low protein content) or permeable (high protein content) in nature. The ratio of oedema fluid to plasma colloid oncotic pressure separates transudates from exudates. In a study examining pulmonary oedema fluid from multiple causes, left ventricular failure oedema fluid usually had a ratio of <0.6 [49, 70], i.e. a low protein content and therefore hydrostatic in origin. However, in SAH-induced pulmonary oedema, a spectrum of ratios occur. One of the earliest case reports to document this found a high protein content [53], while more recently a study in 12 SAH patients found an increased ratio (>0.7, permeability lesion) in 5 patients and a low ratio (<0.6) in 7 [38]. SAH-induced NPO with a range of protein concentrations requires further explanation because the findings by Smith et al. [38]suggest that some patients have permeability oedema and others hydrostatic oedema. However, there may be only one pathological process at work. Pulmonary oedema developing after SAH is caused by increasing capillary pressures that damage the endothelium and, as the pressure increases further, disrupts the basement membrane causing fluid and protein extravasation [58]. This is supported by animal work where intense pulmonary vascular constriction induced using endothelin produced an increase in pulmonary pressure and EVLW causing oedema [71]. Microscopic changes have been found in animal experiments using rabbits [72]. When transmural pressures exceeded 40 mmHg, the pulmonary capillary endothelium became disrupted. As the transmural pressure increased further, the basement membranes of the capillaries and alveoli and the alveolar endothelium were also injured to the point where red blood cells, protein and fluid escaped into the alveolar lumen. Thus, oedema fluid is initially low in protein (low permeability, hydrostatic) but, as barriers are disrupted with increasing capillary pressure, the oedema fluid becomes proteinaceous (high permeability). The time course for this is very variable. Patient data are limited and have not examined cardiovascular markers such as PAOP, PAP and central venous pressure (CVP), in relation to hydrostatic and permeability oedema.

Catecholamines as the common link

There is a remarkable similarity between the cardiorespiratory compromise found after SAH and that of phaeochromocytoma crises. Sudden onset of ventricular failure (often hypotensive) with or without pulmonary oedema has been reported in case series of SAH [8, 11, 36, 37, 38] and phaeochromocytoma [73, 74]. Pulmonary oedema [75], cardiogenic shock and arrhythmias are common to both, as is the high concentration of catecholamines [25, 30, 32, 35, 47, 69, 76, 77]. Conclusions from many reports on catecholamines in relation to SAH describe a catecholamine 'storm'. In addition, a recent report has found evidence in SAH patients of prolonged and massive sympathetic nervous activation [69]. A three-fold increase in norepinephrine spill-over into the plasma was detected, which was sustained for at least 10 days, but was normal at the 6-month follow-up.

Catecholamine induced cardiac injury

Experimental evidence linking catecholamines to cardiac injury exists in animals and man. Specific myocardial lesions in animals subjected to infusions of l-norepinephrine [78]are the same as those found in shocked patients treated with epinephrine and l-norepinephrine. In mongrel dogs an increase in plasma catecholamines as a consequence of induced SAH caused specific cardiac lesions on electron microscopy within 4 h of induced SAH [79]. Others have found histological contraction band lesions within 5 min of beginning a catecholamine infusion [80]. Such contraction-band necrosis is unevenly distributed, being most dense at the apex and subendocardial areas of the ventricles [81], i.e. in the regions of heart muscle most responsible for cardiac output.

Focal myocytolysis [82] or myofibrillar degeneration [where dense eosinophilic bands replace the normal striated appearance of the cytoplasm, and the muscle fibres appear as 'empty' sarcolemic sheaths (Fig. 1)] have been described in patients dying from SAH [47] and phaeochromocytoma [73]. Further human post-mortem evidence of myocytolysis and contraction-band necrosis of the heart in neurosurgical patients, including those dying after SAH, has been described by Connor [50], who considered these lesions to be the same as those caused by catecholamines. Furthermore, in a case series of 54 consecutive SAH deaths [42], 42 cadavers (including a 12-year-old boy) had myocardial lesions described as foci of necrotic muscle fibres, haemorrhage and inflammatory cells that were not found in the control group. An interesting finding was that the SAH victims with more variable pulse and blood pressure recorded prior to death (presumably from autonomic fluctuation) were more likely to have myocardial lesions. In addition, hypertensive heart disease was associated with significantly fewer myocardial lesions than SAH victims without hypertensive heart disease. Perhaps patients with hypertensive heart disease are less sensitive to catecholamines and are thus protected from their acute effects. It is not clear if

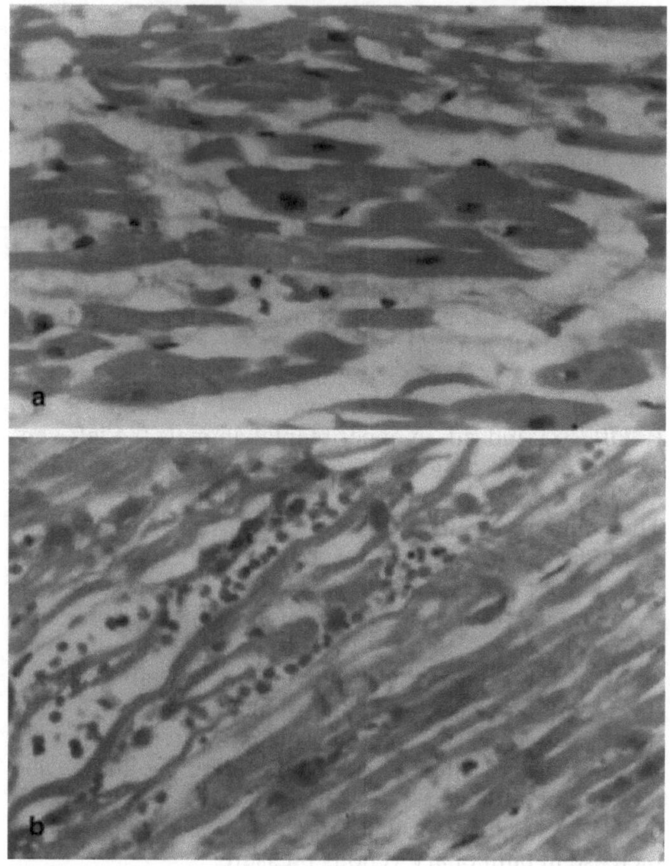

Fig. 1 Histological section (100) of the myocardium demonstrating **a** normal ventricle and **b** myofibrillar degeneration, myocytolysis and inflammatory cell infiltration

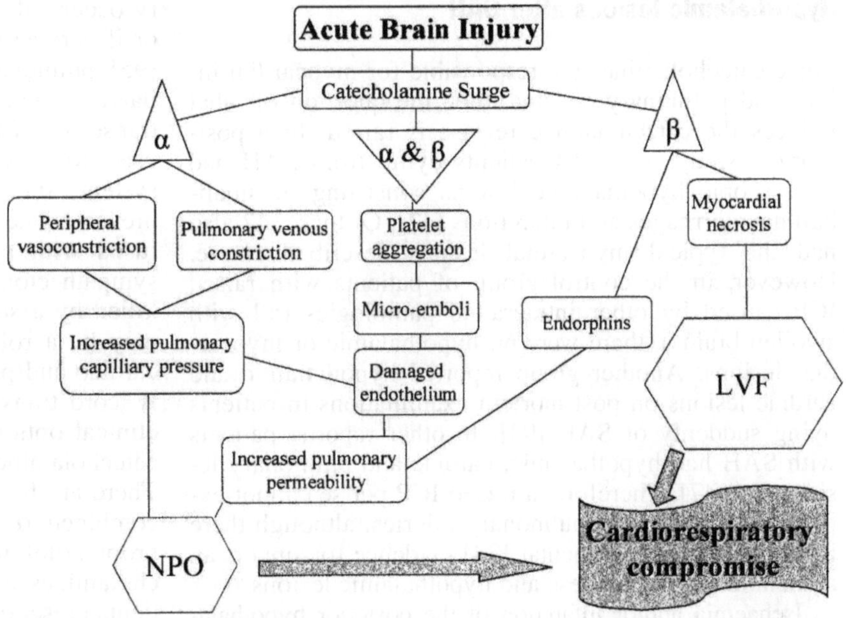

Fig. 2 Subarachnoid haemorrhage can result in sympathetic activation that causes pulmonary oedema and cardiac failure (α alpha-adrenoceptor, β beta-adrenoceptor, *LVF* left ventricular pressure)

anti-hypertensive medication such as beta-blockers or some intrinsic property of the hypertensive myocardium to resist a catecholamine 'storm' play a part. In another SAH post-mortem study, those who died suddenly were compared to those with WFNS grade 5 who subsequently died. NPO was much more common in the 68 sudden-death patients; histological examination of the myocardium was performed in 6 patients which showed contraction band necrosis in every case [28]. Multifocal transmural myocardial injury was the post-mortem finding in most SAH patients, but not in the control group [43]. Catecholamine induced myocardial injury poses challenges for prophylaxis and therapy.

Catecholamine-induced pulmonary oedema

Catecholamines can cause pulmonary oedema. They increase transmural pulmonary vascular pressures [83] by a combination of α- and β-adrenoceptor activation, and cardiac injury (Fig. 2). Frank pulmonary oedema can be induced experimentally by epinephrine infusion [59, 61], or seen clinically in phaeochromocytoma crisis [75, 84, 85, 86]. The largest initial effect is increased pulmonary venous pressure [61]. Pulmonary arterial pressure may then increase and this is *sometimes* reflected in the central venous pressure. A rise in pulmonary capillary pressure was demonstrated in 11 baboons where brain death was induced by acute intracranial hypertension. Between brain injury and death, significant increases in circulating catecholamines occurred, causing an increase in systemic vascular resistance and acute left ventricular failure. In this study mean PAOP increased above the mean PAP in most animals, and more than 70% of blood volume pooled in the lungs. The high pressures within the pulmonary circulation caused pulmonary oedema and alveolar haemorrhage in 4 of the animals [87].

An increase in EVLW, whether extensive enough to result in frank pulmonary oedema or not, reduces compliance [83]. Using the double-indicator dilution method to calculate EVLW in 25 patients with SAH, Tuoho et.al. [54] found a significant positive correlation between increased alveolar-arterial oxygen difference ($AaDO_2$) and increasing EVLW. An increase in EVLW occurs in animal models of raised ICP and massive sympathetic discharge [88, 89]and was proportional to pressures in the pulmonary circulation. The essential physiological phenomenon was the requirement for a massive, but not necessarily prolonged, rise in PAP [88, 90]. Studies in humans during maximum exercise have shown PAP and PAOP to reach maximal mean values of 37 and 21 mmHg, respectively [91]; capillary pressure should fall between the two pressures at approximately 30 mmHg. Pathological states may exceed such pressures. After SAH the increase in catecholamine concentration can occur in seconds and be 1200, 145 and 35 times the normal limit for epinephrine, norepinephrine and dopamine, respectively [92]. Furthermore, epinephrine can remain increased in the circulation for at least 10 days [69]. This could explain why NPO can be seen anytime from ictus up to 14 days [8, 41, 66].

Hypothalamic lesions after SAH

Since catecholamines are responsible for myocardial injury and pulmonary oedema, then the question of what induces the catecholamine release is raised. In a post-mortem study, 49 of 54 patients dying from SAH had microscopic hypothalamic lesions consisting of small-ball haemorrhages and infarctions [42]. Of these, 42 also had the typical myocardial lesions described above. However, in the control group of patients with raised ICP caused by other intracranial pathologies (all with swollen brains), there were no hypothalamic or myocardial lesions. Another group reported hypothalamic and cardiac lesions on post-mortem examinations in patients dying suddenly of SAH [93]. In other reports, patients with SAH had hypothalamic, cardiac and pulmonary lesions [24, 47]. Therefore, a raised ICP per se cannot explain the cardiac and pulmonary injuries, although there is clinical and experimental [34] evidence to support an association between these and hypothalamic lesions.

Ischaemia and/or infarction of the posterior hypothalamus is the most likely initiating event that causes sympathetic activation. In a series of 106 patients dying from SAH, 65 had hypothalamic lesions which had histological evidence of ischaemia, microhaemorrhages, massive haemorrhage or a combination of ischaemia and haemorrhage [94]. Perhaps the close proximity of subarachnoid blood from the ruptured aneurysm influences the fine perforating arteries to the hypothalamus, causing microvascular spasm.

Management

There are two important reasons for being proactive in the treatment of patients with cardiac and/or respiratory complications of SAH. Firstly, secondary brain injury caused by hypoxia and hypotension should be prevented [2]. Secondly, mechanical cardiac dysfunction and NPO are very treatable with potentially good outcomes, despite affected patients appearing moribund [41]

Identifying patients at risk

It is not clear which SAH patients will develop cardiac and respiratory complications, but risk factors include poor neurological grade, age over 30 years, hypertension, ventricular repolarisation abnormalities, and the timing of surgery [8, 33]. These patients may benefit from early intensive monitoring.

Prophylaxis

Regardless of where the trigger zone is within the brain, experimental evidence shows that when acute brain injury occurs, if the cervical cord is transected [47, 61, 66] or if cardiac sympathetic nerves are severed or blocked [95], pulmonary oedema does not develop [27, 93]. Similarly, cardiac lesions do not occur if the cervical cord is transected [27]. Prophylactic pharmacological drugs used to block the effects of the autonomic nervous system, such as α-blockade with phenoxybenzamine, prevented death and pulmonary oedema in rabbits infused with epinephrine [59]. Pharmacological cardiac sympathectomy prevented myocardial injury in baboons killed by a sudden massive increase in ICP [95]. There may be a role for prophylactic intervention to prevent cardiac and pulmonary complications after SAH. Clearly, cord transection is not a therapeutic or prophylactic clinical option, but pharmacological shielding from the catecholamine storm deserves further evaluation.

There are few data from clinical trials, but prophylactic combined α- and β-blockade using phentolamine and propranolol may reduce myocardial injury from catecholamines after SAH [93]. In this study 90 SAH patients presenting within 48 h of ictus and without a history of cardiac disease were randomised to receive both propranolol 80 mg 8 hourly and phentolamine 20 mg 3 hourly, or placebo. There was no difference in the mortality (perhaps because of small numbers) but, at autopsy, focal necrosis of the myocardium was only present in the placebo group, implying a protective cardiac effect. Another report by the same group showed benefit in terms of survival and neurological state in SAH patients given prophylactic phentolamine and propranolol [96]. They surmised this was due to a reduction in complications such as NPO and cardiac lesions. An interesting suggestion that deserves further consideration is stellate ganglion block [66]. A more contemporary therapy that may have benefit is infusion of magnesium, which inhibits catecholamine release and may reduce cerebral vasospasm [97]. These therapies require caution, however, as a reduction in MAP and CPP could result.

Impaired cardiac function

It may be difficult to identify patients with ventricular dysfunction, as the ECG is non-specific [10, 11, 12, 17], while isoenzyme markers of myocardial injury take time to become apparent and may be inconclusive [11, 44]. Once pulmonary oedema and/or cardiac compromise is evident, echocardiography to assess LV function would be useful to guide therapy. In addition, invasive monitoring may produce helpful information, despite the risks [98], as almost any combination of normal and abnormal pulmonary pressures is possible [48], and these may change with time [55]. A new alternative is the oesophageal Doppler monitor, which gives objective and subjective information about left ventricular function and the systemic circulation [99, 100], although not the pulmonary circulation. This method is now used in preference to the pulmonary artery catheter in some intensive care units.

Surprisingly, inotropic support may improve matters, despite catecholamines causing ventricular injury and NPO. In patients with reduced left ventricular work, dobutamine has proved effective [37, 41, 56, 96]. A recent series of SAH patients with pulmonary oedema, increased PAOP and variable cardiac index (but all with low ejection fractions on echocardiography) were treated successfully with dobutamine and a combination of epinephrine and/or norepinephrine (although one patient did also received intra-aortic balloon pump assistance) [41]. This report is not unique. Patients with SAH (or other intracranial pathology) and myocardial impairment treated with dobutamine rapidly normalised their cardiac index, and improved PAOP and ventricular work with consequent benefit to oxygenation [48]. It is difficult to reconcile the fact that endogenous catecholamines cause cardiac and pulmonary complications and that patients may then be treated using similar agents. Perhaps it is the magnitude of the endogenous catecholamine surge that causes the pathology, and thereafter the levels quickly decline, perhaps to the point where catecholamine depletion at the receptor level exists so that low-to-moderate exogenous administration has a beneficial therapeutic effect.

Pulmonary oedema

Traditional management strategies for cardiac failure induced pulmonary oedema, such as positive pressure ventilation and diuretics are often used for SAH patients [48, 101]. Systemic circulating volume overload is, however, not the cause of SAH-associated NPO. The pulmonary circulation may be severely over-loaded [87] as a result of catecholamines shunting blood, so that the systemic circulation is rendered acutely hypovolaemic. Therefore, volume resuscitation may be more appropriate than diuretic therapy to restore circulating volume acutely and optimise right ventricular preload [41].

These clinical reports confirm the potential of functional reversibility of cardiac and pulmonary pathophysiology. Cardiac involvement may be overt or subclinical in a substantial number of SAH patients, and a proactive approach to identify them, for example using echocardiography, with a subsequent increase in the level of monitoring and care would seem appropriate for this relatively young patient group. At the very least, patients exhibiting any clinical evidence of NPO and/or cardiac impairment should have a pulmonary artery catheter or oesophageal Doppler assessment of cardiac function to guide therapy. A guide to management is shown in Fig. 3.

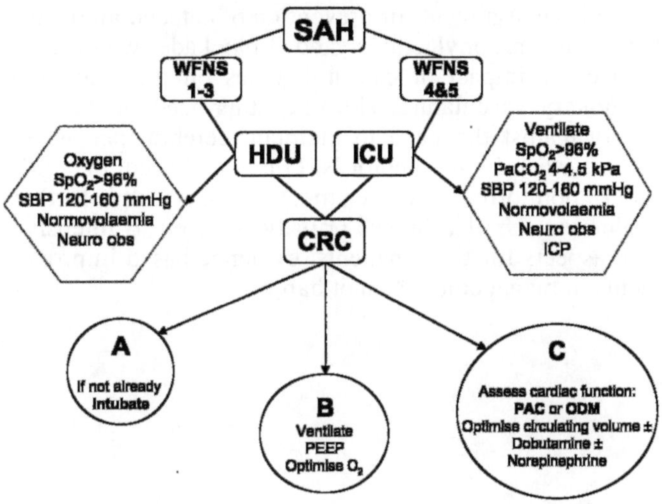

Fig. 3 Management of cardiorespiratory compromise after subarachnoid haemorrhage. Neurogenic pulmonary oedema and cardiac dysfunction can manifest clinically as separate entities or together. They should be considered together as part of a clinical syndrome – 'CRC'- which requires assessment of cardiac function for optimal treatment

Implications for management of brain-stem dead organ donors

Most cadaver organs for transplant in the UK come from patients dying of intracranial catastrophes, i.e. trauma and haemorrhage. Catecholamine-induced myocardial injury (although reversible with time) and pulmonary endothelial injury, with or without gross pulmonary oedema, is not ideal preparation for these organs. In essence, recipients may not be getting the healthy organs that would be predicted from the donor's pre-morbid health. Perhaps management aimed at reducing cardiac and respiratory pathology after SAH should be more aggressive when it becomes clear that the neurological prognosis is hopeless. It may even be appropriate under these circumstances to institute therapies that are organ preserving, such as α- and β-blockade, particularly when cerebral perfusion is no longer a consideration. Some authorities have cautioned against the use of organs from SAH donors because of organ dysfunction, as they do less well than organs from trauma victims [102]. Yet there is such a demand for organs [102] that optimisation of the cadaver until harvest is complete should be a continuing aim [103, 104, 105].

Need for clinical trials

There is a compelling argument for well-conducted trials to be undertaken in order to identify patients who will develop cardiac failure, pulmonary oedema or both.

There is an argument for prevention of catecholamine effects using prophylactic α- and β-blockade, which may reduce the impact of catecholamines on the heart and pulmonary vasculature. However, this needs to be balanced against the need to maintain cerebral perfusion. Once cardiac failure and/or NPO is established, the optimum monitoring and treatment choices need further evaluation. Until a higher priority is given to intensive care aspects for these patients, evidence-based improvements in management cannot happen.

Conclusions

There is substantial clinical and experimental evidence to support the conclusion that catecholamines cause cardiac failure and pulmonary oedema after an acute neurological event such as SAH. The range of symptoms caused by catecholamines should be considered part of a syndrome of cardiorespiratory compromise, so monitoring and therapy can be rationalised (Fig. 3). The subsequent development of hypoxaemia and hypotension, which adds to the neurological insult and may have long-term physical, cognitive and financial consequences for patients and society, could thus be minimised. The intensivist has a major role to play in pre-empting and treating such complications and must aim to improve management for these patients.

References

1. Ingall TJ, Whisnant JP, Wiebers DO O'Fallon WM (1989) Has there been a decline in subarachnoid hemorrhage mortality? Stroke 20:718–724
2. Haley EC, Jr. Kassell NF Torner JC (1992) The International Cooperative Study on the Timing of Aneurysm Surgery. The North American experience. Stroke 23:205–214
3. National CEPOD (2000) Interventional vascular radiology and interventional neurovascular radiology. Callum KG, Whimster F (eds). NCEPOD, London 2000
4. Allen GS, Ahn HS, Preziosi TJ, Battye R, Boone SC, Boone SC, Chou SN, Kelly DL, Weir BK, Crabbe RA, Lavik PJ, Rosenbloom SB, Dorsey FC, Ingram CR, Mellits DE, Bertsch LA, Boisvert DP, Hundley MB, Johnson RK, Strom JA, Transou CR (1983) Cerebral arterial spasm – a controlled trial of nimodipine in patients with subarachnoid hemorrhage. N Engl J Med 308:619–624
5. Pickard JD, Murray GD, Illingworth R, ShawMD, Teasdale GM, Foy PM, Humphrey PR, Lang DA Nelson R, Richards P (1989) Effect of oral nimodipine on cerebral infarction and outcome after subarachnoid haemorrhage: British aneurysm nimodipine trial. BMJ 298:636–642
6. Petruk KC, West M, Mohr G, Weir BK, Benoit BG, Gentili F, Disney L, Khan M, Grace M, Holness R (1988) Nimodipine treatment in poor-grade aneurysm patients. Results of a multicenter double-blind placebo-controlled trial. J Neurosurg 68:505–517
7. Mayberg MR, Batjer HH, Dacey R, Diringer M, Haley EC, Heros RC, Sternau LL, Torner J, Adams HPJr, Feinberg W (1994) Guidelines for the management of aneurysmal subarachnoid hemorrhage. A statement for healthcare professionals from a special writing group of the Stroke Council, American Heart Association. Stroke 25:2315–2328
8. Solenski NJ, Haley ECJ, Kassell NF, Kongable G, Germanson T, Truskowski L Torner JC (1995) Medical complications of aneurysmal subarachnoid hemorrhage: a report of the multicenter, cooperative aneurysm study. Participants of the Multicenter Cooperative Aneurysm Study. Crit Care Med 23:1007–1017
9. Miller JA, Dacey RGJ, Diringer MN (1995) Safety of hypertensive hypervolemic therapy with phenylephrine in the treatment of delayed ischemic deficits after subarachnoid hemorrhage. Stroke 26:2260–2266
10. Szabo MD, Crosby G, Hurford WE Strauss HW (1993) Myocardial perfusion following acute subarachnoid hemorrhage in patients with an abnormal electrocardiogram. Anesth Analg 76:253–258
11. Mayer SA, Fink ME, Homma S, Sherman D, LiMandri G, Lennihan L, Solomon RA, Klebanoff LM, Beckford A, Raps EC (1994) Cardiac injury associated with neurogenic pulmonary edema following subarachnoid hemorrhage. Neurology 44:815–820
12. Davies KR, Gelb AW, Manninen PH, Boughner DR Bisnaire D (1991) Cardiac function in aneurysmal subarachnoid haemorrhage: a study of electrocardiographic and echocardiographic abnormalities. BJA 67:58–63
13. Kono T, Morita H, Kuroiwa T, Onaka H, Takatsuka H Fujiwara A (1994) Left ventricular wall motion abnormalities in patients with subarachnoid hemorrhage: neurogenic stunned myocardium. J Am Coll Cardiol 24:636–640
14. Pollick C, Cujec B, Parker S Tator C (1988) Left ventricular wall motion abnormalities in subarachnoid hemorrhage: an echocardiographic study. J Am Coll Cardiol 12:600–605
15. Mayer SA, LiMandri G, Sherman D, Lennihan L, Fink ME, Solomon RA, DiTullio M, Klebanoff LM, Beckford AR, Homma S (1995) Electrocardiographic markers of abnormal left ventricular wall motion in acute subarachnoid hemorrhage. J Neurosurg 83:889–896
16. Gentleman D, Jennett B (1990) Audit of transfer of unconscious head-injured patients to a neurosurgical unit. Lancet 335:330–334
17. Brouwers PJ, Wijdicks EF, Hasan D, Vermeulen M, Wever, EF, Frericks H van Gijn J (1989) Serial electrocardiographic recording in aneurysmal subarachnoid hemorrhage. Stroke 20:1162–1167
18. Burch GE, Meyers R Abildskov JA (1954) A new electrocardiographic pattern observed in cerebrovascular accidents. Circulation 9:719–723
19. Marion DW, Segal R Thompson ME (1986) Subarachnoid hemorrhage and the heart. Neurosurgery 18:101–106
20. Andreoli A, di PG, Pinelli G, Grazi P, Tognetti F Testa C (1987) Subarachnoid hemorrhage: frequency and severity of cardiac arrhythmias. A survey of 70 cases studied in the acute phase. Stroke 18:558–564

21. Cropp GJ, Manning GW (1960) Electrocardiographic changes simulating myocardial ischaemia and infarction associated with spontaneous intracranial haemorrhage. Circulation 22:25–38
22. Shuster S (1960) The electrocardiogram in subarachnoid haemorrhage. Br Heart J 22:316–320
23. Galloon S, Rees GA, Briscoe CE, Davies S Kilpatrick GS (1972) Prospective study of electrocardiographic changes associated with subarachnoid haemorrhage. BJA 44:511–516
24. Hammermeister KE, Reichenbach DD (1969) QRS changes, pulmonary edema, and myocardial necrosis associated with subarachnoid hemorrhage. Am Heart J 78:94–100
25. Svigelj V, Grad A Kiauta T (1996) Heart rate variability, norepinephrine and ECG changes in subarachnoid hemorrhage patients. Acta Neur Scand 94:120–126
26. Lanzino G, Kongable GL Kassell NF (1994) Electrocardiographic abnormalities after nontraumatic subarachnoid hemorrhage. J Neurosurg Anesthesiol 6:156–162
27. Melville KI, Blum B, Shister HE, Silver MD (1963) Cardiac ischaemic changes and arrhythmias induced by hypothalamic stimulation. Am J Cardiol 12:781–4
28. Kitahara T, Masuda T Soma K (1993) The etiology of sudden cardiopulmonary arrest in subarachnoid hemorrhage. No Shinkei Geka (Neurological Surgery) 21:781–786
29. di Pasquale G. Pinelli G, Andreoli A, Manini G, Grazi P Tognetti F (1987) Holter detection of cardiac arrhythmias in intracranial subarachnoid hemorrhage. Am J Cardiol 59:596–600
30. Cruickshank JM, Neil-Dwyer G Stott AW (1974) Possible role of catecholamines, corticosteroids, and potassium in production of electrocardiographic abnormalities associated with subarachnoid haemorrhage. Br Heart J 36:697–706
31. Barr CS, Naas A, Freeman M, Lang CC Struthers AD (1994) QT dispersion and sudden unexpected death in chronic heart failure. Lancet 343:327–329
32. Randell T, Tanskanen P, Scheinin M, Kytta J, Ohman J Lindgren L (1999) QT dispersion after subarachnoid hemorrhage. J Neurosurg Anesthesiol 11:163–166
33. Andrews PJD (2000) Medical management of complications following aneurysmal sub-arachnoid haemorrhage. In: Galley HF (ed) Neurological injury. BMJ Books, London, pp 28–38
34. Elrifai AM, Bailes JE, Shih SR, Dianzumba S Brillman J (1996) Characterization of the cardiac effects of acute subarachnoid hemorrhage in dogs. Stroke 27:737–741
35. Grad A, Kiauta T Osredkar J (1991) Effect of elevated plasma norepinephrine on electrocardiographic changes in subarachnoid hemorrhage. Stroke 22:746–749
36. Knudsen K, Abrahamsson J (1995) Antiarrhythmic effects of magnesium sulphate. Report of three cases. Acta Anaesthesiol Scand 39:850–854
37. Schell AR, Shenoy MM, Friedman SA Patel AR (1987) Pulmonary edema associated with subarachnoid hemorrhage. Evidence for a cardiogenic origin. Arch Intern Med 147:591–592
38. Smith WS, Matthay MA (1997) Evidence for a hydrostatic mechanism in human neurogenic pulmonary edema. Chest 111:1326–1333
39. Harari A, Rapin M, Regnier B, Comoy J Caron JP (1976): Normal pulmonary-capillary pressures in the late phase of neurogenic pulmonary oedema. Lancet i:494
40. Raymer K, Choi P (1997) Concurrent subarachnoid haemorrhage and myocardial injury. Can J Anaesth 44:515–519
41. Parr MJ, Finfer SR Morgan MK (1996) Reversible cardiogenic shock complicating subarachnoid haemorrhage. BMJ 313:681–683
42. Doshi R, Neil-Dwyer G (1980) A clinicopathological study of patients following a subarachnoid hemorrhage. J Neurosurg 52:295–301
43. Kolin A, Norris JW (1984) Myocardial damage from acute cerebral lesions. Stroke 15:990–993
44. Rudehill A, Gordon E, Sundqvist K, Sylven C, Wahlgren NG. (1982) A study of ECG abnormalities and myocardial specific enzymes in patients with subarachnoid haemorrhage. Acta Anaesthesiol Scand 26:344–350
45. Fabinyi G, Hunt D McKinley L (1977) Myocardial creatine kinase isoenzyme in serum after subarachnoid haemorrhage. J Neurol Neurosurg Psych 40:818–820
46. Horowitz MB, Willet D Keffer J (1998) The use of cardiac troponin-I (cTnI) to determine the incidence of myocardial ischemia and injury in patients with aneurysmal and presumed aneurysmal subarachnoid hemorrhage. Acta Neurochirurgica 140:87–93
47. Greenhoot JH, Reichenbach DD (1969) Cardiac injury and subarachnoid hemorrhage. A clinical, pathological, and physiological correlation. J Neurosurg 30:521–531
48. Deehan SC, Grant IS (1996) Haemodynamic changes in neurogenic pulmonary oedema: Effect of dobutamine. Intensive Care Med 22:672–676
49. Carlson RW, Schaeffer RC, Jr. Carpio M Weil MH (1981) Edema fluid and coagulation changes during fulminant pulmonary edema. Chest 79:43–49
50. Connor RC (1969) Myocardial damage secondary to brain lesions. Am Heart J 78:145–148
51. Connor RC (1970) Fuchsinophilic degeneration of myocardium in patients with intracranial lesions. Br Heart J 32:81–84
52. Ducker TB (1968) Increased intracranial pressure and pulmonary edema. 1. Clinical study of 11 patients. J Neurosurg 28:112–117
53. Fein IA, Rackow EC (1982) Neurogenic pulmonary edema. Chest 81:318–320
54. Touho H, Karasawa J, Shishido H, Yamada K Yamazaki Y (1989) Neurogenic pulmonary edema in the acute stage of hemorrhagic cerebrovascular disease. Neurosurgery 25: 762–768
55. Wray NP, Nicotra MB (1978) Pathogenesis of neurogenic pulmonary edema. Am Rev Respir Dis 118:783–786
56. Melon E, Bonnet F Lepresle E (1985) Altered capillary permeability in neurogenic pulmonary oedema. Intensive Care Med 11:323–325
57. Wiener F, Carlson RW, Puri VK Weil MH (1983) Mathematical model to study fluid and protein transfer in pulmonary edema in man. Crit Care Med 11:132–141
58. West JB, Mathieu-Costello O (1992) Stress failure of pulmonary capillaries in the intensive care setting. Schweiz Med Wochenschr 122:751–757
59. Siwadlowski W, Aravanis C, Worthen M Luisada AA (1970) Mechanism of adrenalin pulmonary edema and its prevention by narcotics and autonomic blockers. Chest 57:554–557
60. Maron MB (1990) Pulmonary vasoconstriction in a canine model of neurogenic pulmonary edema. J Appl Physiol 68:912–918
61. Ducker TB, Simmons RL (1968) Increased intracranial pressure and pulmonary edema. 2. The hemodynamic response of dogs and monkeys to increased intracranial pressure. J Neurosurg 28:118–123
62. Schraufnagel DE, Patel KR (1990) Sphincters in pulmonary veins. An anatomic study in rats. Am Rev Respir Dis 141:721–726
63. Richards.P (1963) Pulmonary oedema and intracranial lesions. BMJ ii:83
64. Paine R, Smith JR, Howard FA (1952) Pulmonary oedema in patients dying with disease of the central nervous system. JAMA 149: 643–646

65. Schievink WI, Wijdicks EF, Parisi JE, Piepgras DG Whisnant JP (1995) Sudden death from aneurysmal subarachnoid hemorrhage. Neurology 45:871–874
66. Simmons RL, Martin AM, Jr. Heisterkamp CA, III Ducker TB (1969) Respiratory insufficiency in combat casualties. II. Pulmonary edema following head injury. Ann Surg 170:39–44
67. Estanol BV, Marin OS (1975) Cardiac arrhythmias and sudden death in subarachnoid hemorrhage. Stroke 6:382–386
68. Drewes LR (1988) Report of World Federation of Neurological Surgeons Committee on a universal subarachnoid haemorrhage grading scale. J Neurosurg 68:985–986
69. Naredi S, Lambert G, Eden E, Zall S, Runnerstam M, Rydenhag B Friberg P (2000) Increased sympathetic nervous activity in patients with nontraumatic subarachnoid hemorrhage. Stroke 31:901–906
70. Carlson RW, Schaeffer RC, Jr. Michaels SG Weil MH (1979) Pulmonary edema fluid. Spectrum of features in 37 patients. Circulation 60:1161–1169
71. Poulat P, Couture R (1998) Increased pulmonary vascular permeability and oedema induced by intrathecally injected endothelins in rat. Eur J Pharmacol 344:251–259
72. West JB, Mathieu-Costello O (1992) Stress failure of pulmonary capillaries: Role in lung and heart disease. Lancet 340:762–767
73. Kline IK (1961) Myocardial alterations associated with phaeochromocytomas. Am J Pathol 38:539–551
74. Northfield TC (1967) Cardiac complications of phaeochromocytoma. Br Heart J 29:588–593
75. Blom HJ, Karsdorp V, Birnie R Davies G (1987) Phaeochromocytoma as a cause of pulmonary oedema. Anaesthesia 42:646–650
76. Sato K, Masuda T, Kikuno T, Kobayashi A, Ikeda Y, Ohwada T Kikawada R (1990) Left ventricular asynergy and myocardial necrosis accompanied by subarachnoid hemorrhage: contribution of neurogenic pulmonary edema. Jpn J Cardiol 20:359–367
77. Hanley DF, Ulatowski JA (1995) Medical management of aneurysmal subarachnoid hemorrhage. Crit Care Med 23:992–993
78. Szakacs JE, Mehlman B (1960) Pathological changes induced by l-norepinephrine: quantitative aspects. Am J Cardiol 5:619–627
79. Elrifai AM, Bailes JE, Shih SR, Dianzumba S Brillman J (1996) Characterization of the cardiac effects of acute subarachnoid hemorrhage in dogs. Stroke 27:737–741
80. Todd GL, Baroldi G, Pieper GM, Clayton FC Eliot RS (1985) Experimental catecholamine-induced myocardial necrosis. II. Temporal development of isoproterenol-induced contraction band lesions correlated with ECG, hemodynamic and biochemical changes. J Mol Cell Cardiol 17:647–656
81. Todd GL, Baroldi G, Pieper GM, Clayton FC Eliot RS (1985) Experimental catecholamine-induced myocardial necrosis. I. Morphology, quantification and regional distribution of acute contraction band lesions. J Mol Cell Cardiol 17:317–338
82. Schlesinger MJ, Reiner L (1955) Focal myocytolysis of the heart. Am J Pathology 31:443
83. Davidson JT, Charuzi I (1973) Epinephrine-induced changes in the pulmonary pressure-volume curve of the intact and hypovolemic rabbit. Chest 63:250–253
84. Greaves DJ, Barrow PM (1989) Emergency resection of phaeochromocytoma presenting with hyperamylasaemia and pulmonary oedema after abdominal trauma. Anaesthesia 44:841–842
85. Platts JK, Drew PJ Harvey JN (1995) Death from phaeochromocytoma: lessons from a post-mortem survey. JRCPL. 29:299–306
86. Ross EJ, Griffith DN (1989) The clinical presentation of phaeochromocytoma. Q J Med 71:485–496
87. Novitzky D, Wicomb WN, Rose AG, Cooper DK Reichart B (1987) Pathophysiology of pulmonary edema following experimental brain death in the chacma baboon. Ann Thorac Surg 43:288–294
88. Maron MB, Holcomb PH, Dawson CA, Rickaby DA, Clough AV Linehan JH (1994) Edema development and recovery in neurogenic pulmonary edema. J Appl Physiol 77:1155–1163
89. Gupta YK, Chugh A, Kacker V, Mehta VS Tandon PN (1998) Development of neurogenic pulmonary edema at different grades of intracranial pressure in cats. Indian J Physiol Pharmacol 42:71–80
90. Maron MB (1985) A canine model of neurogenic pulmonary edema. J Appl Physiol 59:1019–1025
91. Wagner PD, Gale GE, Moon RE, Torre-Bueno JR, Stolp BW Saltzman HA (1986) Pulmonary gas exchange in humans exercising at sea level and simulated altitude. J Appl Physiol 61:260–270
92. Graf CJ, Rossi NP (1978) Catecholamine response to intracranial hypertension. J Neurosurg 49:862–868
93. Neil-Dwyer G, Walter P, Cruickshank JM, Doshi B O'Gorman P (1978) Effect of propranolol and phentolamine on myocardial necrosis after subarachnoid haemorrhage. BMJ ii:990–992
94. Crompton MR (1963) Hypothalamic lesions following the rupture of cerebral berry aneurysms. Brain 86: 301–318
95. Novitzky D, Wicomb WN, Cooper DK, Rose AG Reichart B (1986) Prevention of myocardial injury during brain death by total cardiac sympathectomy in the Chacma baboon. Ann Thorac Surg 41:520–524
96. Walter P, Neil-Dwyer G Cruickshank JM (1982) Beneficial effects of adrenergic blockade in patients with subarachnoid haemorrhage. BMJ 284:1661–1664
97. Watson VF, Vaughan RS (2001) Magnesium and the anaesthetist. Br J Anaesth CEPD Reviews 1:16–20
98. Rosenwasser RH, Jallo JI, Getch CC Liebman KE (1995) Complications of Swan-Ganz catheterization for hemodynamic monitoring in patients with subarachnoid hemorrhage. Neurosurgery 37:872–875
99. Singer M, Bennett ED (1991) Noninvasive optimization of left ventricular filling using esophageal Doppler. Crit Care Med 19:1132–1137
100. Singer M, Clarke J Bennett ED (1989) Continuous hemodynamic monitoring by esophageal Doppler. Crit Care Med 17: 447–452
101. Lagerkranser M, Pehrsson K Sylven C (1982) Neurogenic pulmonary oedema. A review of the pathophysiology with clinical and therapeutic implications. Acta Medica Scand 212:267–271
102. Cohen B, D'Amaro J, De Meester J Persijn GG (1997) Changing patterns in organ donation in Eurotransplant, 1990–1994. Transplant Int 10:1–6
103. Power BM, Van Heerden PV (1995) The physiological changes associated with brain death–current concepts and implications for treatment of the brain dead organ donor. Anaesth Intensive Care 23:26–36
104. MacLean A, Dunning J (1997) The retrieval of thoracic organs: donor assessment and management. Br Med Bull 53:829–843
105. Bodenham A, Park GR (1989) Care of the multiple organ donor. Intensive Care Med 15:340–348

John G. Laffey
Donall O'Croinin
Paul McLoughlin
Brian P. Kavanagh

Permissive hypercapnia — role in protective lung ventilatory strategies

Abstract 'Permissive hypercapnia' is an inherent element of accepted protective lung ventilation. However, there are no clinical data evaluating the efficacy of hypercapnia per se, independent of ventilator strategy. In the absence of such data, it is necessary to determine whether the potential exists for an active role for hypercapnia, distinct from the demonstrated benefits of reduced lung stretch. In this review, we consider four key issues. *First*, we consider the evidence that protective lung ventilatory strategies improve survival and we explore current paradigms regarding the mechanisms underlying these effects. *Second*, we examine whether hypercapnic acidosis may have effects that are additive to the effects of protective ventilation. *Third*, we consider whether direct elevation of CO_2, in the absence of protective ventilation, is beneficial or deleterious. *Fourth*, we address the current evidence regarding the buffering of hypercapnic acidosis in ARDS. These perspectives reveal that the potential exists for hypercapnia to exert beneficial effects in the clinical context. Direct administration of CO_2 is protective in multiple models of acute lung and systemic injury. Nevertheless, several specific concerns remain regarding the safety of hypercapnia. At present, protective ventilatory strategies that involve hypercapnia are clinically acceptable, provided the clinician is primarily targeting reduced tidal stretch. There are insufficient clinical data to suggest that hypercapnia per se should be independently induced, nor do outcome data exist to support the practice of buffering hypercapnic acidosis. Rapidly advancing basic scientific investigations should better delineate the advantages, disadvantages, and optimal use of hypercapnia in ARDS.

Keywords Hypercapnic acidosis · Mechanical ventilation · Acute lung injury · ARDS · Ventilation-induced lung injury · Buffering

Introduction

'Permissive hypercapnia' is an inherent element of accepted protective lung ventilatory strategies. However, the precise role of hypercapnia remains unclear, with no clinical data comparing the efficacy of protective lung ventilatory strategies in the presence and absence of hypercapnia. Furthermore, it is unlikely that such a trial will be carried out, at least in the medium term. In the absence of such data, it is appropriate to investigate whether the potential exists for an active role for hypercapnia per se, distinct from the demonstrated benefits of reduced lung stretch. This review first considers the evidence that protective lung ventilatory strategies reduce lung injury and improve survival. We examine current paradigms regarding the mechanisms underlying this protective effect, and the passive role presently attributed to hypercapnia. We focus on whether

M.R. Pinsky et al. (eds.), *Applied Physiology in Intensive Care Medicine 2: Physiological Reviews and Editorials*,
DOI 10.1007/978-3-642-28233-1_11,

hypercapnia and/or acidosis may have effects that are distinct from the effects of protective ventilator parameters. In addition, the current status of buffering hypercapnic acidosis is reviewed.

Protective lung ventilatory strategies — current paradigms

It is increasingly clear that mechanical ventilation can potentiate or even cause lung injury and worsen outcome in ARDS patients [1, 2]. The likely mechanisms underlying this 'ventilator associated lung injury' (VALI) are increasingly well characterized [3], and several plausible theories have been proposed. Mechanotrauma, which results from repetitive over-stretching and damage of lung tissue and cyclic recruitment-derecruitment of collapsed areas of lung [4–9], plays a pivotal role (Fig. 1). These effects may be particularly important, because increased mechanical stress may directly activate the cellular and humoral immune response in the lung [8–11], although this is controversial, with conflicting results reported [12]. The potential for intrapulmonary mediators and pathogens to access the systemic circulation is clear from experiments demonstrating translocation of prostaglandins [13], cytokines [14] endotoxin [15], and bacteria [16], across an impaired alveolar-capillary barrier, following high stretch mechanical ventilation. The potential for mechanical ventilation to induce a systemic cytokine response in the clinical context, and for a protective lung ventilation strategy to attenuate this response, has been demonstrated [17]. However, the contribution of cytokine release to the pathogenesis of ventilator induced ALI in the clinical context remains unclear [10, 18].

VALI may be limited by permitting hypoventilation in order to reduce mechanotrauma and the resulting inflammatory effects. This invariably involves a reduction in the tidal volume, and generally leads to an elevation in $PaCO_2$, an approach that has been termed "permissive hypercapnia". These protective lung ventilation strategies

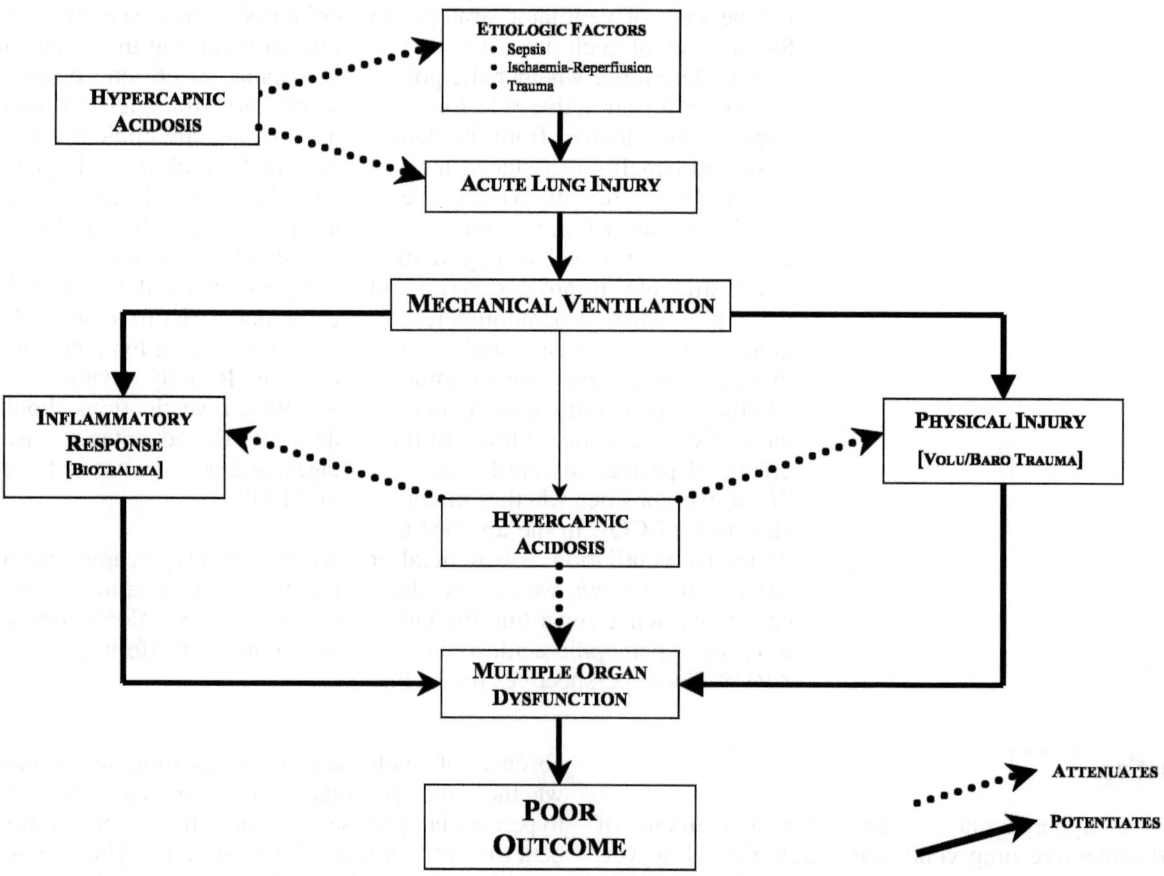

Fig. 1 Mechanical ventilation may contribute to ALI by causing direct physical injury (baro- and/or volutrauma) to the lung and by activating the inflammatory response, which in turn may lead to multiple organ dysfunction and adverse outcome. Hypercapnic acidosis may protect the lung and systemic organs via several mechanisms. These include attenuation of key etiologic factors that lead to ALI, reduction of physical lung damage, inhibition of key aspects of the inflammatory response, and direct protection of systemic organs. *Solid arrows* indicate potentiation of effect; *broken arrows* indicate inhibitory effect

improve survival in acute respiratory distress syndrome (ARDS) patients [1, 19, 20]. The reported levels of $PaCO_2$ and pH (mean maximum $PaCO_2$ 67 torr, mean pH 7.2) in the study of Hickling et al. [19] reflect typical levels observed with institution of this technique. Accordingly, there has been a shift towards greater clinical acceptability of hypercapnia in acute lung injury (ALI) and ARDS. However, current paradigms attribute the protective effect of these ventilatory strategies solely to reductions in lung stretch, with hypercapnia permitted in order to achieve this goal. Accordingly, the potential for hypercapnia to exert clinically important effects in this context has received little attention to date.

Permissive hypercapnia — potential for beneficial effects

Protective ventilatory strategies that involve hypoventilation result in both limitation of tidal volume and elevation of systemic PCO_2. Of course, lung stretch is distinct from elevated PCO_2, and by manipulation of respiratory parameters (frequency, tidal volume, dead-space, inspired CO_2) can to some extent be separately controlled in humans. The ARDSnet study [2] demonstrated that mechanical ventilation of patients with ARDS with a tidal volume of 6 ml kg^{-1} (actually, a complex protocol involving limitation of tidal volume and plateau pressure [21]) resulted in a 25% reduction in mortality when compared with a more traditional tidal volume of 12 ml kg^{-1} and a lower frequency. This study minimized the potential for hypercapnia and instead permitted increased respiratory rates (respiratory frequency of 29 min^{-1}); as a result $PaCO_2$ levels were only modestly elevated, and pH modestly decreased, in the low stretch group. In fact, the need to substantially reduce tidal volumes in order to improve outcome in ARDS patients has recently been questioned [22, 23], and it is increasingly clear that most clinicians (*including expert investigators* [24]) seldom use very low tidal volumes in practice. An acceptance of more moderate tidal volumes, whether by analysis [22], or by observation of actual current practice [25, 26] may reduce the need for — and acceptability of — permissive hypercapnia. Therefore, the context in which elevated CO_2 will be encountered in the future is less likely to be as a passive/permissive accompaniment of 'protective' ventilation.

These issues underscore the necessity for (and difficulty in) consideration of the effects of hypercapnia in isolation. If hypercapnia was proven to have independent benefit, then deliberately elevating $PaCO_2$ could provide an additional advantage over reducing lung stretch. Conversely, in patients managed with conventional permissive hypercapnia, adverse effects of elevated $PaCO_2$ might be concealed by the generally accepted benefits of lessened lung stretch. Because outcome in ICU might be related to systemic injury — as opposed to simply lung injury — it is necessary to examine the effects of hypercapnia on pathophysiologic function in the heart and brain as well as the lung. These issues are further underlined by the fact that hypercapnia has potentially severe adverse effects in some clinical settings, such as critically elevated intracranial pressure.

Clearly, the presence of an acidosis — whether hypercapnic or metabolic — indicates loss of physiologic homeostasis and the presence of disease and/or organ dysfunction. In fact, the extent and severity of acidosis is predictive of adverse outcome in diverse clinical contexts, including cardiac arrest [27, 28] sepsis [29–31] and in the immediate postpartum neonate [32]. However these data indicate an *association* rather than a cause and effect relationship, and do not indicate that acidosis is directly harmful. The systemic haemodynamic effects of hypercapnic acidosis are relatively benign, even as the pH falls to 7.15, with the typical patient experiencing no change or small increases in cardiac output and blood pressure [33, 34]. There is a body of evidence in the critical care literature attesting to the safety of hypercapnic acidosis. In many studies of patients undergoing permissive hypercapnia, a pH of well below 7.2 appeared to have been well tolerated [19, 20, 33, 35–39]. The safety of hypercapnic acidosis is further supported by reports that individuals, both adults [40] and children [41], have survived exposure to extreme levels. Therefore, although acidosis is common in the setting of critical illness, and may herald an adverse prognosis, it is likely that the aetiology of the underlying condition resulting in the acidosis, rather than the acidosis per se, is the key factor [34, 42]. Indeed acidosis may constitute a protective adaptation in the context of cellular stress, and may in fact constitute beneficial effects in the setting of acute organ injury (Table 1) [42].

The potential for hypercapnia to attenuate to the deleterious effects of high stretch mechanical ventilation in the clinical context has recently received strong support in a preliminary communication [43], where Kregenow and co-workers examined mortality as a function of permissive hypercapnia in patients enrolled in the ARDSnet study [2]. Using multivariate logistic regression analysis, and controlling for other co-morbidities and severity of lung injury, they demonstrated that permissive hypercapnia reduced mortality in patients randomized to the higher tidal volume (12 ml kg^{-1}) [43]. However, there was no additional protective effect of permissive hypercapnia in patients randomized to receive the lower tidal volume (6 ml kg^{-1}) [43]. Nevertheless, the potential for hypercapnia to protect against the deleterious effects of mechanical ventilation, is clear (Fig. 1).

Table 1 Published studies of induced hypercapnic acidosis in models of acute organ dysfunction. *ALI* acute lung injury, *IR* ischaemia-reperfusion, K_{fc} capillary filtration coefficient, P_{aw} peak airway pressure, P_{cap} pulmonary capillary pressure, P_{iso} pulmonary capillary isographic pressure, *A-a O_2 gradient* alveolar-arterial oxygen gradient, *BALF* bronchoalveolar lavage fluid, *TNFα* tumour necrosis factor alpha, *NO* nitric oxide, *NMDA* N-methyl-D-aspartate

	Animal model	Injury process	Key findings
Acute lung injury			
Shibata et al. 1998 [44]	Ex vivo isolated perfused (rabbit) lung	1. Lung free radical induced ALI 2. Lung ischemia — reperfusion-induced ALI	1. HCA attenuated indices of ALI (K_{fc}, P_{aw}, P_{cap}, P_{iso}) 2. HCA attenuated indices of ALI (K_{fc}, P_{aw}, P_{cap}, P_{iso})
Laffey et al. 2000 [45]	Ex vivo isolated perfused (rabbit) lung	Lung ischemia — reperfusion	Acidosis attenuated indices of ALI (K_{fc}, P_{aw}, P_{cap}, P_{iso}). Hypercapnic acidosis more protective than metabolic acidosis. Buffering of hypercapnic acidosis abolished protective effect.
Laffey et al. 2000 [46]	In vivo whole animal (rabbit) model	Lung ischemia — reperfusion	HCA attenuated indices of ALI (lung permeability, A-a O_2 gradient, compliance, P_{aw}) and inflammation (BALF TNFα, free radical injury) following unilateral lung IR. Potential mechanisms included attenuation of nitrotyrosine formation, and attenuation of lung apoptosis.
Broccard et al. 2001 [49]	Ex vivo isolated perfused (rabbit) lung	Ventilator-induced high lung stretch	HCA attenuated indices of ALI (lung permeability, BALF protein, K_{fc}). Potential mechanism attenuation of lung NO formation.
Sinclair et al. 2002 [50]	In vivo whole animal (rabbit) model	Ventilator-induced high lung stretch	HCA attenuated indices of ALI (lung permeability, A-a O_2 gradient, compliance, histologic injury) and inflammation (BALF neutrophils).
Laffey et al, 2003 [47]	In vivo whole animal (rat) model	Mesenteric Ischemia-Reperfusion	HCA attenuated indices of ALI (lung permeability, A-a O_2 gradient, compliance, P_{AW}) following Mesenteric IR. HCA was protective if applied following initiation of mesenteric reperfucion, indicating therapeutic potential.
Laffey et al, 2003 [51]	In vivo whole animal (rabbit) model	Ventilator-induced high lung stretch	HCA attenuated (A-a O_2 gradient) while hypocapnic alkalsois worsened (P_{AW}) indices of ALI.
Myocardial Injury			
Nomura et al. 1994 [52]	Ex vivo isolated perfused (neonatal lamb) heart	Myocardial ischemia — reperfusion	HCA improved postischemic myocardial function Metabolic acidosis to an equivalent pH did not improve postischemic function
Kitakaze et al. 1997 [53]	In vivo whole animal (rabbit) model	Myocardial ischemia — reperfusion	Acidosis (hypercapnic and metabolic) during reperfusion decreased myocardial infarct size
Neurologic Injury			
Vannucci et al. 1995 [54]	In vivo whole animal (rat) model	Unilateral common carotid artery occlusion, followed by hypoxia	HCA decreased histologic brain damage Dose response seen with 6% CO_2 more neuroprotective than 9% CO_2
Vannucci et al. 1997 [55]	In vivo whole animal (rat) model	Unilateral common carotid artery occlusion, followed by hypoxia	HCA decreased histologic brain damage Mechanisms may include improved cerebral blood flow and attenuation of NMDA receptor activation.
Vannucci et al. 2001 [73]	In vivo whole animal (rat) model	Unilateral common carotid artery occlusion, followed by hypoxia	Severe HCA (15%CO_2) *worsened* histologic brain damage

Hypercapnia and acidosis — insights from laboratory models

It is not currently feasible to examine the direct effects of hypercapnic acidosis, independent of ventilator strategy, in humans. However, important insights may be gained from evaluation of the direct effects of hypercapnia and acidosis in experimental models of organ injury (Table 1).

Protective effects of hypercapnic acidosis

There is an evolving body of evidence suggesting that hypercapnic acidosis exerts biologically important beneficial effects in experimental models (Table 1). Hypercapnic acidosis directly attenuates both primary [44–46] and secondary [47] ischaemia-reperfusion-induced ALI, without reductions in lung stretch. Hypercapnic acidosis also directly protects against free-radical-induced ALI [44] and endotoxin-induced lung injury independent of ventilation strategy [48]. In addition, hypercapnic acidosis attenuates lung injury induced by excessive lung stretch in both ex vivo [49] and in vivo [50, 51] models, by a surfactant independent mechanism [51].

Hypercapnic acidosis may also protect other vital organs from injury (Table 1). In the heart, reperfusion with a hypercapnic acidotic perfusate potentiates recovery of myocardial function following prolonged ischaemia ex vivo [52] and limits myocardial infarct size for in vivo [53] models. In the brain, hypercapnic acidosis attenuates hypoxic-ischaemic brain injury in the immature rat [54, 55]. Hypercapnic acidosis protects the porcine brain from hypoxia/reoxygenation-induced injury [56]. Hypercapnic acidosis is more effective than comparable degrees of metabolic acidosis in prevention of lipid peroxidation in cortical homogenates [57].

Beneficial effects — acidosis or hypercapnia?

While it is widely accepted that reduction in pH has profound effects on normal tissue function, it is also clear that hypercapnia per se, in the absence of alterations in pH, may exert biologically important physiologic effects distinct from those produced by acidosis. Of potential importance in the context of acute lung injury, hypercapnia per se exerts effects on systemic [58] and pulmonary vascular tone [58, 59] and pulmonary vascular remodeling [60] that are increasingly well characterized. Thus, the protective effects of hypercapnic acidosis may be a function of the acidosis or the hypercapnia per se. This issue is of particular relevance when considering the appropriateness of buffering in the clinical context. If any protective effects of hypercapnic acidosis were found to result from the acidosis, then efforts to buffer a hypercapnic acidosis would lessen such protection and should be discouraged. Conversely, if hypercapnia per se (*and not the acidemia*) were found to be protective, then further research efforts should be directed to finding better buffering strategies in order to maximise the benefits of hypercapnia.

There is increasing evidence that the protective effects of hypercapnic acidosis in ALI appear to be a function of the acidosis, rather than elevated CO_2 per se [45, 61]. Hypercapnia at normal pH caused injury to alveolar epithelial cell monolayers [61] and decreased surfactant protein A function in vitro [62]. In the isolated lung, the protective effect of hypercapnic acidosis in ischaemia reperfusion induced ALI was greatly attenuated if the pH was buffered towards normal [45]. In fact there appeared to be no significant protective effect detectable with buffered hypercapnia (Table 1). Conversely, normocapnic (i.e. metabolic) acidosis attenuates primary ischaemia-reperfusion induced ALI in an ex vivo model, although it is less effective than hypercapnic acidosis in this model [45].

The protective effects of hypercapnic acidosis in models of systemic organ injury also appear to be a function of the acidosis. The myocardial protective effects of hypercapnic acidosis are also seen with metabolic acidosis both in ex vivo [63] and in vivo [53, 64] models. In cortical brain homogenates, the protective effects of hypercapnic acidosis are also seen with metabolic acidosis, albeit to a lesser extent [57]. Metabolic acidosis appears to exert protective effects in other models of organ injury. In the liver, metabolic acidosis delays the onset of cell death in isolated hepatocytes exposed to anoxia[65] and to chemical hypoxia [66, 67]. Correcting the pH to 7.4 abolished the protective effect and in fact accelerated hepatocyte cell death [67]. Finally, isolated renal cortical tubules exposed to anoxia have improved ATP levels on reoxygenation at acidotic — compared with alkalotic — environmental pH levels [65].

Hypercapnic acidosis — underlying mechanisms

The models of ALI and ARDS are not precise representations of the clinical context; indeed most clinical scenarios differ from each other. Therefore, it is important to understand the cellular and biochemical mechanisms underlying the protective effects of hypercapnic acidosis if we are to be able to apply the findings to the bedside, and particularly, to extrapolate the principles to a variety of disease states. Hypercapnic acidosis attenuates key components of the host inflammatory response, including: lung neutrophil recruitment [48], pulmonary and systemic cytokine concentrations [46], cell apoptosis [46, 68], and both free-radical production [44, 45] and free-radical tissue injury [46, 57]. In the brain, hypercapnic acidosis attenuates glutathione depletion and lipid peroxidation [56]. One promising potential mechanism underlying these protective actions of hypercapnic acidosis is attenuation of the activation of the transcription regulator nuclear factor kappa beta (NF-κB) [69]. NF-kB regulates the expression of several genes involved in inflammatory response and its activation represents a pivotal early step in the activation of the inflammatory response.

Concerns regarding hypercapnia

There are concerns regarding the potential for hypercapnia and/or acidosis to exert deleterious effects that suggest the need for caution when considering its use in the clinical context. The potential for hypercapnic acidosis to exert adverse haemodynamic effects in patients with ARDS is clear [70]. However, the potential for detrimental effects on cardiac output [71] and on the peripheral circulation [72] may be overstated. In addition, beneficial effects of moderate hypercapnia may be counterbalanced by a potential for adverse effects at higher levels. This is supported by the experimental evidence demonstrating that protection from the adverse effects of brain ischaemia was better when the inspired CO_2 was set at 6% rather than at 9% [54]. Of concern, severe hypercapnia produced by 15% CO_2 has been more recently demonstrated to worsen neurologic injury in this context (Table 1) [73]. In isolated hepatocytes, the degree of protection from anoxic injury conferred by a metabolic acidosis was greater at pH 6.9 than at pH 6.6 [65]. Furthermore, acidosis attenuates the neutrophil respiratory burst and superoxide production, which are necessary for neutrophil bactericidal activity [74]. This may impair bacterial killing, resulting in unopposed bacterial proliferation, with deleterious consequences, in patients with sepsis induced ARDS.

There are reports of lung [75] and intestinal [76] injury following induction of metabolic acidosis by hydrochloric acid infusion in whole animal models. However, it is important to recognise that infusion of hyperosmolar solutions of strong acids into whole animal preparations may produce toxic effects close to the infusion site and adverse systemic effects, at least some of which are unrelated to any change in pH [77]. Thus, the effects of infusion of strong acid in any given experiment in vivo is likely to represent the sum of potentially beneficial and adverse actions. This contrasts with the situation with hypercapnic acidosis, which is easy to produce, is well tolerated, and does not produce toxic local effects. In ex vivo experiments, where a changes in pH and/or PCO_2 can be produced independently, and without the need for acid infusion close to the tissue, metabolic acidosis is directly protective against ischaemia-reperfusion induced ALI [45].

Of perhaps more concern is the potential for hypercapnia to increase tissue nitration. Peroxynitrite is a potent free radical produced in vivo largely by the reaction of nitric oxide with superoxide radicals, which are greatly increased in acute inflammatory states [78–80]. Peroxynitrite oxidizes a variety of biomolecules including sulfides, thiols, lipids, nucleic acids, transition metals and selenoproteins [78–80]. These oxidation reactions result in altered cellular function and tissue damage. Peroxynitrite also causes nitration of phenolic amino acid residues in proteins, including tyrosine residues, which leads to alteration of protein function [78, 79, 81, 82]. Two recent in vitro studies demonstrate that increased CO_2 and a reduction in pH below the normal physiological value inhibit oxidation by peroxynitrite while promoting nitration reactions [83, 84]. The potential for hypercapnia to promote the formation of nitration products from peroxynitrite has been clearly demonstrated in recent in vitro experiments [61, 62]. Peroxynitrite-mediated tissue nitration has been suggested to be a key mechanism of tissue damage in inflammatory conditions, including ALI [78, 79, 81, 82].

Finally, an important limitation when extrapolating to the clinical context is the relatively short duration of the ALI models in which hypercapnic acidosis has been studied to date. The common clinical scenario in ARDS patients is that of a more prolonged hypercapnia, during which time the acidosis may be partially, or even completely, compensated. As we have seen, there is reason to believe that the acidosis generated by acute hypercapnia may be the protective factor in acute models of ALI. The need to study the effects of hypercapnia in ALI models of considerably longer duration is therefore clear.

In summary, these findings demonstrate that hypercapnic acidosis, induced by direct administration of CO_2, is protective in multiple models of acute lung and systemic organ injury. These protective effects appear to be a function of the acidosis rather than the hypercapnia per se. While significant concerns remain regarding hypercapnia, in particular, its potential to increase tissue nitration, the potential for hypercapnia to attenuate acute lung and systemic organ injury is clear (Fig. 1).

Hypercapnia — with or without buffering?

Buffering of the acidosis induced by hypercapnia in ARDS patients remains a common, albeit controversial, clinical practice [85, 86]. Buffering with sodium bicarbonate was permitted in the ARDSnet study [2]. The need to examine the effects of buffering a hypercapnic acidosis is emphasised by the fact that both hypercapnia and acidosis per se may exert distinct biologic effects. However, as already discussed, there is evidence that the protective effects of hypercapnic acidosis in ALI are a function of the acidosis, rather than elevated CO_2 per se [45, 61]. In addition, there are specific concerns regarding the use of bicarbonate to correct an acidosis. These concerns have resulted in the removal of bicarbonate therapy from routine use in cardiac arrest algorithms [87, 88]. The effectiveness of bicarbonate infusion as a buffer is dependent on the ability to excrete CO_2, rendering it less effective in buffering a hypercapnic acidosis. In fact, bicarbonate may further raise systemic CO_2 levels under conditions of reduced alveolar ventilation, such as ARDS [89]. While bicarbonate may correct arterial pH, it may worsen an intracellular acidosis because the CO_2 produced when bicarbonate reacts with metabolic acids diffuses readily across cell membranes, whereas bicarbonate cannot [90]. Bicarbonate may exert detrimental effects when used to buffer a lactic acidosis. The potential for bicarbonate infusion to augment the production of lactic acid has been demonstrated in the experimental and clinical setting [91–97]. Bicarbonate infusion exerted deleterious cardiovascular effects in a model of hypoxia-induced lactic acidosis [93, 94]. The safety of bicarbonate in diabetic patients has also been questioned. Bicarbonate administration slowed the rate of decrease of ketoacids in patients with diabetic ketoacidosis [98]. Of even more concern, bicarbonate administration is associated with a four-fold increase in risk of cerebral oedema in children with diabetic ketoacidosis [99].

The administration of sodium bicarbonate constitutes a significant osmolar load, which may exert independent beneficial effects independent of any associated changes in pH. Osmolar loads, such as hypertonic saline, may improve the haemodynamic profile in hemorrhagic shock [100], attenuate key aspects of the immune response [100–102] and prevent organ injury in experimental models [101–103]. In fact, when compared with an equimolar dose of sodium chloride, bicarbonate administration does not improve the hemodynamic status of critically ill patients who have lactic acidosis [104]. A follow-up study in an in vivo model of lactic acidemia found that bicarbonate exerted haemodynamic effects (mean arterial pressure, cardiac output, left ventricular contractility), which were indistinguishable from those seen in response to an equimolar dose of sodium chloride [105]. These data give cause for concern about the practice of buffering metabolic acidosis, and comparable questions may exist in the setting of hypercapnic acidosis.

There may be a role for the use of buffers, such as the amino alcohol tromethamine (tris-hydroxymethyl aminomethane, THAM), in specific situations where the physiologic effects of hypercapnic acidosis are of concern. THAM penetrates cells easily and can buffer pH changes and simultaneously reduce PCO_2 [106]. Unlike bicarbonate, which requires an open system for CO_2 elimination in order to exert its buffering effect, THAM is effective in a closed or semi-closed system [106]. THAM rapidly restores pH and acid-base regulation in acidaemia caused by CO_2 retention [106]. A common rationale for buffering is to ameliorate the haemodynamic consequences of acidosis. In a small, but carefully performed clinical study in ARDS patients, rapid induction of a hypercapnic acidosis for a two-hour period resulted in significant hemodynamic alterations, including decreased systemic vascular resistance, increased cardiac output, decreased myocardial contractility, decreased mean arterial pressure and increased mean pulmonary arterial pressure [70]. Buffering of the hypercapnic acidosis with THAM rapidly attenuated the haemodynamic alterations and restored myocardial contractility in these patients [70].

In summary, although it is a widely accepted clinical practice, there are no long-term clinical outcome data (e.g., survival, duration of hospital stay) to support the practice of buffering a hypercapnic acidosis. Taken together, the above literature suggests that, in the absence of correcting the primary problem, buffering a hypercapnic acidosis with bicarbonate is not likely to be of benefit. If the clinician elects to buffer a hypercapnic acidosis, the rationale for this practice should be clear (e.g. to ameliorate potentially deleterious haemodynamic consequences of acidosis). THAM may have a role in these clinical situations.

Conclusions

The optimal ventilatory strategy, and the role of 'permissive hypercapnia' in that strategy, is not yet clear. The protective effect of reducing lung stretch in improving outcome in ARDS patients are beyond doubt. There is growing evidence to support the contention that hypercapnic acidosis may contribute to the benefits seen with protective lung ventilation. While direct induction of a hypercapnic acidosis is protective in multiple models of acute lung and systemic organ injury, the potential for hypercapnia to increase peroxynitrite-mediated tissue nitration is of concern and requires further investigation.

At present, ventilatory strategies that involve hypercapnia are clinically acceptable only provided the clinician is primarily targeting reduced tidal stretch. There are insufficient clinical data to suggest that hypercapnia per se should be independently induced, outside the context of a protective ventilatory strategy. Furthermore, the recent questioning of the real benefit of low — versus moderate — tidal volume ventilation for adults with ARDS may result in hypercapnia becoming less acceptable in the ventilatory management of ARDS. If that becomes the case, then the clinical study of hypercapnia will become less feasible in the setting of permissive hypercapnia, and will require the deliberate induction of hypercapnia (i.e., 'therapeutic' hypercapnia). Pre-clinical studies are urgently needed to clarify the advantages, disadvantages, and optimal use of hypercapnia in ARDS.

References

1. Amato MB, Barbas CS, Medeiros DM, Magaldi RB, Schettino GP, Lorenzi-Fihlo G, Kairalla RA, Deheinzelin D, Munoz C, Oliveira R, Takagaki TY, Carvalho CR (1998) Effect of a protective-ventilation strategy on mortality in the acute respiratory distress syndrome. N Engl J Med 338:347–354
2. The Acute Respiratory Distress Syndrome Network (2000) Ventilation with lower tidal volumes as compared with traditional tidal volumes for acute lung injury and the acute respiratory distress syndrome. N Engl J Med 342:1301–1308
3. Pinhu L, Whitehead T, Evans T, Griffiths M (2003) Ventilator-associated lung injury. Lancet 361:332–340
4. Boussarsar M, Thierry G, Jaber S, Roudot-Thoraval F, Lemaire F, Brochard L (2002) Relationship between ventilatory settings and barotrauma in the acute respiratory distress syndrome. Intensive Care Med 28:406–413
5. Maggiore SM, Jonson B, Richard JC, Jaber S, Lemaire F, Brochard L (2001) Alveolar derecruitment at decremental positive end-expiratory pressure levels in acute lung injury: comparison with the lower inflection point, oxygenation, and compliance. Am J Respir Crit Care Med 164:795–801
6. Dreyfuss D, Saumon G (1992) Barotrauma is volutrauma, but which volume is the one responsible? Intensive Care Med 18:139–141
7. Dreyfuss D, Saumon G (1998) Ventilator-induced lung injury: lessons from experimental studies. Am J Respir Crit Care Med 157:294–323
8. Dreyfuss D, Saumon G (1998) From ventilator-induced lung injury to multiple organ dysfunction? Intensive Care Med 24:102–104
9. Ricard JD, Dreyfuss D, Saumon G (2002) Ventilator-induced lung injury. Curr Opin Crit Care 8:12–20
10. Slutsky AS, Tremblay LN (1998) Multiple system organ failure. Is mechanical ventilation a contributing factor? Am J Respir Crit Care Med 157:1721–1725
11. Tremblay LN, Slutsky AS (1998) Ventilator-induced injury: from barotrauma to biotrauma. Proc Assoc Am Physicians 110:482–488
12. Ricard JD, Dreyfuss D (2001) Cytokines during ventilator-induced lung injury: a word of caution. Anesth Analg 93:251–252
13. Edmonds JF, Berry E, Wyllie JH (1969) Release of prostaglandins caused by distension of the lungs. Br J Surg 56:622–623
14. Tremblay L, Valenza F, Ribeiro SP, Li J, Slutsky AS (1997) Injurious ventilatory strategies increase cytokines and c-fos mRNA expression in an isolated rat lung model. J Clin Invest 99:944–952
15. Murphy D, Cregg N, Tremblay L, Engelberts D, Laffey JG, Slutsky AS, Romaschin A, Kavanagh BP (2000) Adverse ventilator strategy causes pulmonary to systemic translocation of endotoxin. Am J Resp Crit Care Med 162:27–33
16. Nahum A, Hoyt J, Schmitz L, Moody J, Shapiro R, Marini JJ (1997) Effect of mechanical ventilation strategy on dissemination of intratracheally instilled Escherichia coli in dogs. Crit Care Med 25:1733–1743
17. Ranieri VM, Suter PM, Tortorella C, De Tullio R, Dayer JM, Brienza A, Bruno F, Slutsky AS (1999) Effect of mechanical ventilation on inflammatory mediators in patients with acute respiratory distress syndrome: a randomized controlled trial. JAMA 282:54–61
18. Dreyfuss D, Ricard JD, Saumon G (2003) On the physiologic and clinical relevance of lung-borne cytokines during ventilator-induced lung injury. Am J Respir Crit Care Med 167:1467–1471
19. Hickling KG, Walsh J, Henderson S, Jackson R (1994) Low mortality rate in adult respiratory distress syndrome using low-volume, pressure-limited ventilation with permissive hypercapnia: a prospective study. Crit Care Med 22:1568–1578
20. Bidani A, Tzouanakis AE, Cardenas VJ Jr, Zwischenberger JB (1994) Permissive hypercapnia in acute respiratory failure. JAMA 272:957–962
21. Laffey JG, Kavanagh BP (2000) Ventilation with lower tidal volumes as compared with traditional tidal volumes for acute lung injury (Letter). N Engl J Med 343:812
22. Eichacker PQ, Gerstenberger EP, Banks SM, Cui X, Natanson C (2002) Meta-analysis of acute lung injury and acute respiratory distress syndrome trials testing low tidal volumes. Am J Respir Crit Care Med 166:1510–1514
23. Ricard JD (2003) Are we really reducing tidal volume — and should we? Am J Resp Crit Care Med 167:1297–1298
24. Rubenfeld G, Caldwell E, Hudson L (2001) Publication of study results does not increase use of lung protective ventilation in patients with acute lung injury. Am J Resp Crit Care Med 163:A295
25. Weinert CR, Gross CR, Marinelli WA (2003) Impact of randomized trial results on acute lung injury ventilator therapy in teaching hospitals. Am J Respir Crit Care Med 167:1304–1309
26. Thompson BT, Hayden D, Matthay MA, Brower R, Parsons PE (2001) Clinicians' approaches to mechanical ventilation in acute lung injury and ARDS. Chest 120:1622–1627
27. Jorgensen EO, Holm S (1999) The course of circulatory and cerebral recovery after circulatory arrest: influence of pre-arrest, arrest and post-arrest factors. Resuscitation 42:173–182
28. Suljaga-Pechtel K, Goldberg E, Strickon P, Berger M, Skovron ML (1984) Cardiopulmonary resuscitation in a hospitalized population: prospective study of factors associated with outcome. Resuscitation 12:77–95
29. Balakrishnan I, Crook P, Morris R, Gillespie SH (2000) Early predictors of mortality in pneumococcal bacteraemia. J Infect 40:256–261
30. Mathur NB, Singh A, Sharma VK, Satyanarayana L (1996) Evaluation of risk factors for fatal neonatal sepsis. Indian Pediatr 33:817–822
31. Friedman G, Berlot G, Kahn RJ, Vincent JL (1995) Combined measurements of blood lactate concentrations and gastric intramucosal pH in patients with severe sepsis. Crit Care Med 23:1184–1193
32. Anyaegbunam A, Fleischer A, Whitty J, Brustman L, Randolph G, Langer O (1991) Association between umbilical artery cord pH, five-minute Apgar scores and neonatal outcome. Gynecol Obstet Invest 32:220–223
33. Thorens JB, Jolliet P, Ritz M, Chevrolet JC (1996) Effects of rapid permissive hypercapnia on hemodynamics, gas exchange, and oxygen transport and consumption during mechanical ventilation for the acute respiratory distress syndrome. Intensive Care Med 22:182–191
34. Forsythe SM, Schmidt GA (2000) Sodium bicarbonate for the treatment of lactic acidosis. Chest 117:260–267
35. Potkin RT, Swenson ER (1992) Resuscitation from severe acute hypercapnia. Determinants of tolerance and survival. Chest 102:1742–1745
36. Tuxen DV, Williams TJ, Scheinkestel CD, Czarny D, Bowes G (1992) Use of a measurement of pulmonary hyperinflation to control the level of mechanical ventilation in patients with acute severe asthma. Am Rev Respir Dis 146:1136–1142

37. Feihl F, Perret C (1994) Permissive hypercapnia. How permissive should we be? Am J Respir Crit Care Med 150:1722–1737
38. Roupie E, Dambrosio M, Servillo G, Mentec H, el Atrous S, Beydon L, Brun-Buisson C, Lemaire F, Brochard L (1995) Titration of tidal volume and induced hypercapnia in acute respiratory distress syndrome. Am J Respir Crit Care Med 152:121–128
39. Kiely DG, Cargill RI, Lipworth BJ (1996) Effects of hypercapnia on hemodynamic, inotropic, lusitropic, and electrophysiologic indices in humans. Chest 109:1215–1221
40. Slinger P, Blundell PE, Metcalf IR (1997) Management of massive grain aspiration. Anesthesiology 87:993–995
41. Goldstein B, Shannon DC, Todres ID (1990) Supercarbia in children: clinical course and outcome. Crit Care Med 18:166–168
42. Laffey JG, Kavanagh BP (1999) Carbon dioxide and the critically ill — too little of a good thing? (Hypothesis paper). Lancet 354:1283–1286
43. Kregenow DA, Rubenfeld G, Hudson L, Swenson ER (2003) Permissive hypercapnia reduces mortality with 12 ml/kg tidal volumes in acute lung injury. Am J Resp Crit Care Med 167:A616
44. Shibata K, Cregg N, Engelberts D, Takeuchi A, Fedorko L, Kavanagh BP (1998) Hypercapnic acidosis may attenuate acute lung injury by inhibition of endogenous xanthine oxidase. Am J Resp Crit Care Med 158:1578–1584
45. Laffey JG, Engelberts D, Kavanagh BP (2000) Buffering hypercapnic acidosis worsens acute lung injury. Am J Resp Crit Care Med 161:141–146
46. Laffey JG, Tanaka M, Engelberts D, Luo X, Yiang S, Tanswell TK, Post M, Lindsay T, Kavanagh BP (2000) Therapeutic hypercapnia reduces pulmonary and systemic injury following in vivo lung reperfusion. Am J Respir Crit Care Med 162:2287–2294
47. Laffey JG, Jankov R, Engelberts D, Tanswell AK, Post M, Lindsay T, Mullen JB, Romaschin A, Stephens D, McKerlie C, Kavanagh BP (2003) Effects of therapeutic hypercapnia on mesenteric ischemia — reperfusion injury. Am J Respir Crit Care Med: 168:1383–1390
48. Honan D, Laffey JG, Hopkins N, Boylan JF, Mcloughlin P (2002) Therapeutic hypercapnia attenuates endotoxin induced acute lung injury (Abstract). Am J Resp Crit Care Med 165:A383
49. Broccard AF, Hotchkiss JR, Vannay C, Markert M, Sauty A, Feihl F, Schaller M (2001) Protective effects of hypercapnic acidosis on ventilator-induced lung injury. Am J Respir Crit Care Med 164:802–806
50. Sinclair SE, Kregenow DA, Lamm WJ, Starr IR, Chi EY, Hlastala MP (2002) Hypercapnic acidosis is protective in an in vivo model of ventilator-induced lung injury. Am J Respir Crit Care Med 166:403–408
51. Laffey JG, Engelberts D, Duggan M, Veldheuizen R, Lewis J, Kavanagh BP (2003) Carbon dioxide attenuates pulmonary impairment resulting from hyperventilation. Crit Care Med 31:2634–2640
52. Nomura F, Aoki M, Forbess JM, Mayer JE (1994) Effects of hypercarbic acidotic reperfusion on recovery of myocardial function after cardioplegic ischemia in neonatal lambs. Circulation 90:321–327
53. Kitakaze M, Takashima S, Funaya H, Minamino T, Node K, Shinozaki Y, Mori H, Hori M (1997) Temporary acidosis during reperfusion limits myocardial infarct size in dogs. Am J Physiol 272:H2071–H2078
54. Vannucci RC, Towfighi J, Heitjan DF, Brucklacher RM (1995) Carbon dioxide protects the perinatal brain from hypoxic-ischemic damage: an experimental study in the immature rat. Pediatrics 95:868–874
55. Vannucci RC, Brucklacher RM, Vannucci SJ (1997) Effect of carbon dioxide on cerebral metabolism during hypoxia-ischemia in the immature rat. Pediatr Res 42:24–29
56. Barth A, Bauer R, Gedrange T, Walter B, Klinger W, Zwiener U (1998) Influence of hypoxia and hypoxia/hypercapnia upon brain and blood peroxidative and glutathione status in normal weight and growth- restricted newborn piglets. Exp Toxicol Pathol 50:402–410
57. Rehncrona S, Hauge HN, Siesjö BK (1989) Enhancement of iron-catalyzed free radical formation by acidosis in brain homogenates: difference in effect by lactic acid and CO_2. J Cereb Blood Flow Metab 9:65–70
58. Sweeney M, Beddy D, Honner V, Sinnott B, O'Regan RG, McLoughlin P (1998) Effects of changes in pH and CO_2 on pulmonary arterial wall tension are not endothelium dependent. J Appl Physiol 85:2040–2046
59. Sweeney M, O'Regan RG, McLoughlin P (1999) Effects of changes in pH and PCO_2 on wall tension in isolated rat intrapulmonary arteries. Exp Physiol 84:529–539
60. Ooi H, Cadogan E, Sweeney M, Howell K, O'Regan RG, McLoughlin P (2000) Chronic hypercapnia inhibits hypoxic pulmonary vascular remodeling. Am J Physiol Heart Circ Physiol 278:H331–H338
61. Lang JD Jr, Chumley P, Eiserich JP, Estevez A, Bamberg T, Adhami A, Crow J, Freeman BA (2000) Hypercapnia induces injury to alveolar epithelial cells via a nitric oxide-dependent pathway. Am J Physiol Lung Cell Mol Physiol 279:L994–L1002
62. Zhu S, Basiouny KF, Crow JP, Matalon S (2000) Carbon dioxide enhances nitration of surfactant protein A by activated alveolar macrophages. Am J Physiol Lung Cell Mol Physiol 278:L1025–L1031
63. Kitakaze M, Weisfeldt ML, Marban E (1988) Acidosis during early reperfusion prevents myocardial stunning in perfused ferret hearts. J Clin Invest 82:920–927
64. Preckel B, Schlack W, Obal D, Barthel H, Ebel D, Grunert S, Thamer V (1998) Effect of acidotic blood reperfusion on reperfusion injury after coronary artery occlusion in the dog heart. J Cardiovasc Pharmacol 31:179–186
65. Bonventre JV, Cheung JY (1985) Effects of metabolic acidosis on viability of cells exposed to anoxia. Am J Physiol 249:C149–C159
66. Gores GJ, Nieminen AL, Wray BE, Herman B, Lemasters JJ (1989) Intracellular pH during "chemical hypoxia" in cultured rat hepatocytes. Protection by intracellular acidosis against the onset of cell death. J Clin Invest 83:386–396
67. Gores GJ, Nieminen AL, Fleishman KE, Dawson TL, Herman B, Lemasters JJ (1988) Extracellular acidosis delays onset of cell death in ATP-depleted hepatocytes. Am J Physiol 255:C315–C322
68. Xu L, Glassford AJ, Giaccia AJ, Giffard RG (1998) Acidosis reduces neuronal apoptosis. Neuroreport 9:875–879
69. Takeshita K, Suzuki Y, Nishio K, Takeuchi O, Toda K, Kudo H, Miyao N, Ishii M, Sato N, Naoki K, Aoki T, Suzuki K, Hiraoka R, Yamaguchi K (2003) Hypercapnic acidosis attenuates endotoxin-induced nuclear factor-κB activation. Am J Respir Cell Mol Biol 29:124–132

70. Weber T, Tschernich H, Sitzwohl C, Ullrich R, Germann P, Zimpfer M, Sladen RN, Huemer G (2000) Tromethamine buffer modifies the depressant effect of permissive hypercapnia on myocardial contractility in patients with acute respiratory distress syndrome. Am J Respir Crit Care Med 162:1361–1365
71. Prys-Roberts C, Kelman GR, Greenbaum R, Robinson RH (1967) Circulatory influences of artificial ventilation during nitrous oxide anaesthesia in man. II. Results: the relative influence of mean intrathoracic pressure and arterial carbon dioxide tension. Br J Anaesth 39:533–548
72. Ebata T, Watanabe Y, Amaha K, Hosaka Y, Takagi S (1991) Haemodynamic changes during the apnoea test for diagnosis of brain death. Can J Anaesth 38:436–440
73. Vannucci RC, Towfighi J, Brucklacher RM, Vannucci SJ (2001) Effect of extreme hypercapnia on hypoxic-ischemic brain damage in the immature rat. Pediatr Res 49:799–803
74. Allen DB, Maguire JJ, Mahdavian M, Wicke C, Marcocci L, Scheuenstuhl H, Chang M, Le AX, Hopf HW, Hunt TK (1997) Wound hypoxia and acidosis limit neutrophil bacterial killing mechanisms. Arch Surg. 132:991–996
75. Pedoto A, Caruso JE, Nandi J, Oler A, Hoffmann SP, Tassiopoulos AK, McGraw DJ, Camporesi EM, Hakim TS (1999) Acidosis stimulates nitric oxide production and lung damage in rats. Am J Respir Crit Care Med 159:397–402
76. Pedoto A, Nandi J, Oler A, Camporesi EM, Hakim TS, Levine RA (2001) Role of nitric oxide in acidosis-induced intestinal injury in anesthetized rats. J Lab Clin Med 138:270–276
77. Shams H, Peskar BA, Scheid P (1988) Acid infusion elicits thromboxane A2-mediated effects on respiration and pulmonary hemodynamics in the cat. Respir Physiol 71:169–183
78. Beckman JS, Koppenol WH (1996) Nitric oxide, superoxide, and peroxynitrite: the good, the bad, and ugly. Am J Physiol 271:C1424–C1437
79. Pryor WA, Squadrito GL (1995) The chemistry of peroxynitrite: a product from the reaction of nitric oxide with superoxide (see comments). Am J Physiol 268:L699–L722
80. Stamler JS (1994) Redox signaling: nitrosylation and related target interactions of nitric oxide. Cell 78:931–936
81. Squadrito GL, Pryor WA (1998) Oxidative chemistry of nitric oxide: the roles of superoxide, peroxynitrite, and carbon dioxide. Free Radic Biol Med 25:392–403
82. van der Vliet A, Eiserich JP, Shigenaga MK, Cross CE (1999) Reactive nitrogen species and tyrosine nitration in the respiratory tract: epiphenomena or a pathobiologic mechanism of disease? Am J Respir Crit Care Med 160:1–9
83. Denicola A, Freeman BA, Trujillo M, Radi R (1996) Peroxynitrite reaction with carbon dioxide/bicarbonate: kinetics and influence on peroxynitrite-mediated oxidations. Arch Biochem Biophys 333:49–58
84. Alvarez B, Ferrer-Sueta G, Freeman BA, Radi R (1999) Kinetics of peroxynitrite reaction with amino acids and human serum albumin. J Biol Chem 274:842–848
85. Tobin MJ (1994) Mechanical ventilation (review). N Engl J Med 330:1056–1061
86. Kollef MH, Schuster DP (1995) The acute respiratory distress syndrome (review). N Engl J Med 332:27–37
87. Levy MM (1998) An evidence-based evaluation of the use of sodium bicarbonate during cardiopulmonary resuscitation. Crit Care Clin 14:457–483
88. Grillo JA, Gonzalez ER (1993) Changes in the pharmacotherapy of CPR. Heart Lung 22:548–553
89. Sun JH, Filley GF, Hord K, Kindig NB, Bartle EJ (1987) Carbicarb: an effective substitute for $NaHCO_3$ for the treatment of acidosis. Surgery 102:835–839
90. Goldsmith DJ, Forni LG, Hilton PJ (1997) Bicarbonate therapy and intracellular acidosis. Clin Sci 93:593–598
91. Abu Romeh S, Tannen RL (1986) Amelioration of hypoxia-induced lactic acidosis by superimposed hypercapnea or hydrochloride acid infusion. Am J Physiol 250:F702–F709
92. Arieff AI, Leach W, Park R, Lazarowitz VC (1982) Systemic effects of $NaHCO_3$ in experimental lactic acidosis in dogs. Am J Physiol 242:F586–F591
93. Graf H, Leach W, Arieff AI (1985) Evidence for a detrimental effect of bicarbonate therapy in hypoxic lactic acidosis. Science 227:754–756
94. Graf H, Leach W, Arieff AI (1985) Metabolic effects of sodium bicarbonate in hypoxic lactic acidosis in dogs. Am J Physiol 249:F630–F635
95. Benjamin E, Oropello JM, Abalos AM, Hannon EM, Wang JK, Fischer E, Iberti TJ (1994) Effects of acid-base correction on hemodynamics, oxygen dynamics, and resuscitability in severe canine hemorrhagic shock. Crit Care Med 22:1616–1623
96. Rhee KH, Toro LO, McDonald GG, Nunnally RL, Levin DL (1993) Carbicarb, sodium bicarbonate, and sodium chloride in hypoxic lactic acidosis. Effect on arterial blood gases, lactate concentrations, hemodynamic variables, and myocardial intracellular pH. Chest 104:913–918
97. Fraley DS, Adler S, Bruns FJ, Zett B (1980) Stimulation of lactate production by administration of bicarbonate in a patient with a solid neoplasm and lactic acidosis. N Engl J Med 303:1100–1102
98. Okuda Y, Adrogue HJ, Field JB, Nohara H, Yamashita K (1996) Counterproductive effects of sodium bicarbonate in diabetic ketoacidosis. J Clin Endocrinol Metab 81:314–320
99. Glaser N, Barnett P, McCaslin I, Nelson D, Trainor J, Louie J, Kaufman F, Quayle K, Roback M, Malley R, Kuppermann N (2001) Risk factors for cerebral edema in children with diabetic ketoacidosis. The Pediatric Emergency Medicine Collaborative Research Committee of the American Academy of Pediatrics. N Engl J Med 344:264–269
100. Rotstein OD (2000) Novel strategies for immunomodulation after trauma: revisiting hypertonic saline as a resuscitation strategy for hemorrhagic shock. J Trauma 49:580–583
101. Shields CJ, Sookhai S, Winter DC, Dowdall JF, Kingston G, Parfrey N, Wang JH, Kirwan WO, Redmond HP (2001) Attenuation of pancreatitis-induced pulmonary injury by aerosolized hypertonic saline. Surg Infect (Larchmt) 2:215–224
102. Pascual JL, Khwaja KA, Ferri LE, Giannias B, Evans DC, Razek T, Michel RP, Christou NV (2003) Hypertonic saline resuscitation attenuates neutrophil lung sequestration and transmigration by diminishing leukocyte-endothelial interactions in a two-hit model of hemorrhagic shock and infection. J Trauma 54:121–130; discussion 130–132
103. Rizoli SB, Kapus A, Parodo J, Fan J, Rotstein OD (1999) Hypertonic immunomodulation is reversible and accompanied by changes in CD11b expression. J Surg Res 83:130–135
104. Cooper DJ, Walley KR, Wiggs BR, Russell JA (1990) Bicarbonate does not improve hemodynamics in critically ill patients who have lactic acidosis. A prospective, controlled clinical study. Ann Intern Med 112:492–498
105. Cooper DJ, Herbertson MJ, Werner HA, Walley KR (1993) Bicarbonate does not increase left ventricular contractility duringL-lactic acidemia in pigs. Am Rev Respir Dis 148:317–322
106. Nahas GG, Sutin KM, Fermon C, Streat S, Wiklund L, Wahlander S, Yellin P, Brasch H, Kanchuger M, Capan L, Manne J, Helwig H, Gaab M, Pfenninger E, Wetterberg T, Holmdahl M, Turndorf H (1998) Guidelines for the treatment of acidaemia with THAM. Drugs 55:191–224

François Jardin
Antoine Vieillard-Baron

Right ventricular function and positive pressure ventilation in clinical practice: from hemodynamic subsets to respirator settings

Introduction

When used in patients free of previous cardiorespiratory disease, mechanical ventilation with a normal tidal volume does not have any discernible hemodynamic consequences. Conversely, the presence of a pulmonary disease affecting the bronchial tree, lung parenchyma, or both, may induce extreme conditions for mechanical ventilation. In this setting, an adverse hemodynamic effect may seriously complicate respiratory support.

The drop in cardiac output occurring in extreme conditions of mechanical ventilation is usually attributed to a reduced venous return. But the terms "cardiac output"on the one hand and "venous return" on the other refer to the same phenomenon. From a physiological point of view, such an explanation is insufficient, because reduced venous return may, in the same way, be explained by the drop in cardiac output.

We have been interested for about 30 years in the hemodynamic consequences of mechanical ventilation in ARDS patients, and here we try to summarize our experience in this clinical commentary to enable a logical approach to ventilator settings. The major goal of this approach will be to avoid imposing an excessive load on the rignt ventricle. Our experience was first acquired with right heart catheterization, and later by bedside echocardiography. Recent physiological notes published in the present journal have underscored some of the drawbacks of the invasive method [1, 2] and illustrated the advantage of echocardiography [3]. The clinical results of our respiratory strategy in ARDS has been published recently [4].

The hemodynamic consequences of mechanical ventilation are easy to understand by examining the impact upon the right ventricle of applying a positive airway pressure. On the one hand, cyclic (tidal ventilation) or continuous (PEEP application) changes in transpulmonary pressure produced by respiratory support directly affect RV outflow impedance. On the other hand, cyclic (tidal ventilation) or continuous (PEEP application) increase in pleural pressure produced by respiratory support increases RV effective elastance, a factor limiting diastolic filling.

The "venous return" concept

As established by Guyton, the venous return is promoted by a forward pressure, the mean systemic pressure, and impaired by a backward pressure, the right atrial pressure [5]. For several decades it was believed that positive pressure ventilation, by increasing pleural pressure, decreased the pressure gradient for venous return. In 1991, Fessler et al., working in S. Permutt's group, demonstrated in an experimental study in dogs that positive airway

M.R. Pinsky et al. (eds.), *Applied Physiology in Intensive Care Medicine 2: Physiological Reviews and Editorials*,
DOI 10.1007/978-3-642-28233-1_12, © Springer-Verlag Berlin Heidelberg 2012

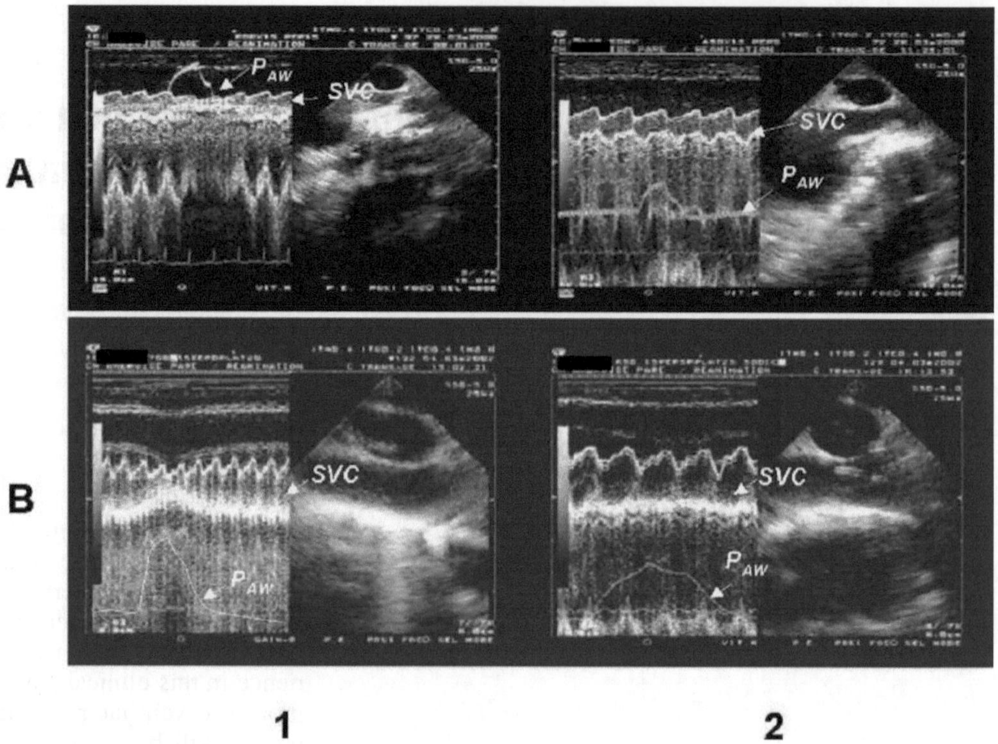

Fig. 1 Transesophageal echocardiographic examination of the superior vena cava (*SVC*) in the *long axis* (with the M-mode study on the *left* and the two-dimensional imaging on the *right* of each record) in two different patients (**A** and **B**). On the left panel (*1*), SVC collapse was observed in these patients during tidal ventilation (airway pressure, P_{AW}, was monitored on the M-mode recording). This collapse was prevented in both patients by blood volume expansion, as illustrated on the right panel (*2*)

pressure did not affect the gradient for venous return, because pleural pressure was transmitted to the same extent to both the mean systemic and right atrial pressures [6]. Van den Berg et al. [7] demonstrated in a recent clinical study that a sustained increase in airway pressure did not decrease venous return because of a concomitant increase in abdominal pressure, an operative mechanism in volume loaded patients, with the inferior vena cava in a zone 3 condition [8]. Also, Fessler et al. observed in another experimental study that venous return was actually reduced by positive pressure ventilation, despite a maintained pressure gradient [9]. They concluded that venous conductance was reduced (or venous resistance was increased) when airway pressure was increased, probably because a collapsible vascular zone was interposed between mean systemic pressure and right atrial pressure [9]. Recently, Jellinek et al. confirmed the validity of this concept in humans, and suggested that liver circulation might constitute this collapsible vascular zone sensitive to pleural pressure transmission throughout the diaphragm [10].

We have also observed another collapsible vascular zone at the level of the thoracic part of the superior vena cava [11]. Placed in a zone 2 condition in a hypovolemic patient, the superior vena cava may partially collapse during tidal ventilation, thus transiently limiting RV filling (Fig. 1, Electronic Supplementary Material Film 1A, B and C). The same phenomenon is not observed at the level of the inferior vena cava, because the thoracic part of this vessel is virtual in humans [11].

Changes in transpulmonary pressure and the impact on right ventricular outflow impedance

Applying the concept of the Starling resistor to the pulmonary circulation, S. Permutt and his co-workers described the relation between the pressures promoting blood flow through the pulmonary circulation [12]. A forward pressure, the pulmonary artery pressure, boosts blood through the pulmonary vascular bed, and a backward pressure, the pulmonary venous pressure, impedes this flow (zone 3 condition). However, alveolar pressure, which directly acts externally on the pulmonary capillary bed, may behave as backward pressure if it rises above venous pressure (zone 2 condition). During tidal volume ventilation, the increase in airway pressure produces an increased zone 2 at the expense of zone 3 (Fig. 2). Thus, during tidal ventilation, alveolar pressure, acting as the backward pressure, impedes pulmonary blood flow. This phenomenon may be important in a mechanically ventilated supine patient. If we assume an average pulmonary venous pressure at the level of the mid-axillary line of 16.5 cmH_2O (12 mmHg), and a 12 cm height between the mid-axillary line and the anterior chest wall, the pulmonary venous pressure in the anterior area of the lungs should be close to 4.5 cmH_2O (i.e., 16.5–12). Thus, in this area, a transpulmonary pressure of 5 cmH_2O would produce a permanent zone 2 condition. Conversely, because of an equal height of 12 cm between the posterior chest wall and the mid-ax-

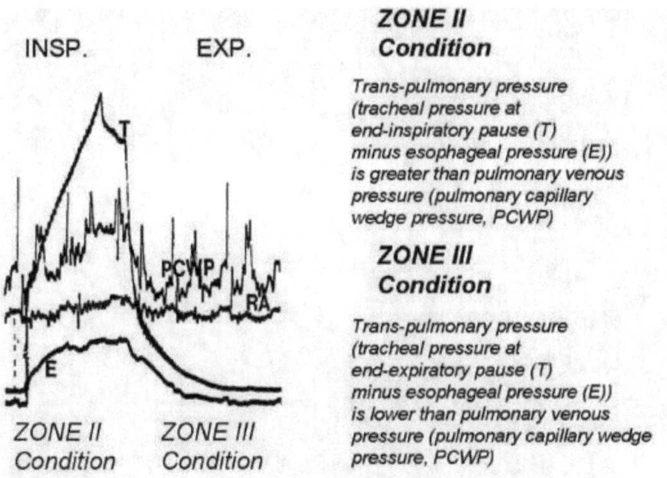

Fig. 2 An example of simultaneous recording of esophageal pressure (*E*), reflecting pleural pressure, right atrial pressure (*RA*), pulmonary capillary wedge pressure (*PCWP*), reflecting pulmonary venous pressure, and tracheal pressure (*T*). During the period of no-flow (end-inspiratory pause and end-expiration), *T* reflects alveolar pressure. Whereas a zone 3 condition is observed at end-expiration (PCWP>T), a zone 2 condition is realized at end-inspiration (T>PCWP). Also note that the increase in *E* during mechanical inspiration is accompanied by a similar increase in PCWP

illary level, dependent areas of the lung are protected against a zone 2 condition.

In fact, it is not alveolar pressure in the strict sense of the term that constitutes backward pressure during tidal ventilation, but alveolar distending pressure (i.e., transpulmonary pressure) as we have recently demonstrated in a clinical study, using chest strapping, a procedure that increases alveolar pressure without a concomitant increase in transpulmonary pressure [13].

By recording simultaneously pulmonary artery and right ventricular pressures in mechanically ventilated patients, we have observed in the past the relation between transpulmonary pressure and right ventricular outflow impedance: when tidal volume is progressively increased, the right ventricle has to develop a more and more elevated pressure to open the pulmonary artery valve (Fig. 3) [14]. We have recently confirmed these results by Doppler analysis of changes in pulmonary artery velocity (Fig. 4, Electronic Supplementary Material Film 2A, B) [13]. Increased transpulmonary pressure during tidal ventilation sharply reduces mean acceleration of blood in the pulmonary artery (Fig. 4), whereas an isolated increase in airway pressure without change in transpulmonary pressure does not affect blood velocity in the pulmonary artery [13].

Indirect evidence of RV afterloading is also provided by the frequency of tricuspid regurgitation during mechanical ventilation [15], which can also be induced by PEEP [16]. An example is given in Fig. 5.

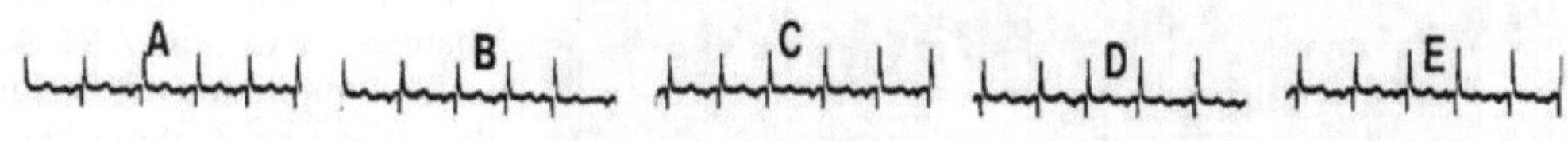

Fig. 3 Simultaneous recordings of expiratory volume (*EV*, ml), pulmonary artery pressure (*PA*, mmHg), right ventricular pressure (*RV*, mmHg), tracheal pressure (*T*, mmHg) and esophageal pressure (*E*, mmHg), during a progressive increase in tidal volume from 300 to 950 ml. This progressive increase in tidal ventilation required a progressive increase in the pressure developed by the RV during its isovolumetric contraction to open the pulmonic valve (i.e., the difference between pulmonary artery diastolic pressure, *small closed arrow*, and right ventricular end-diastolic pressure, *small closed arrow*). Note also that, with the highest tidal volume (*right panel, E*), pulmonary artery pulse became negligible (*small open arrow*)

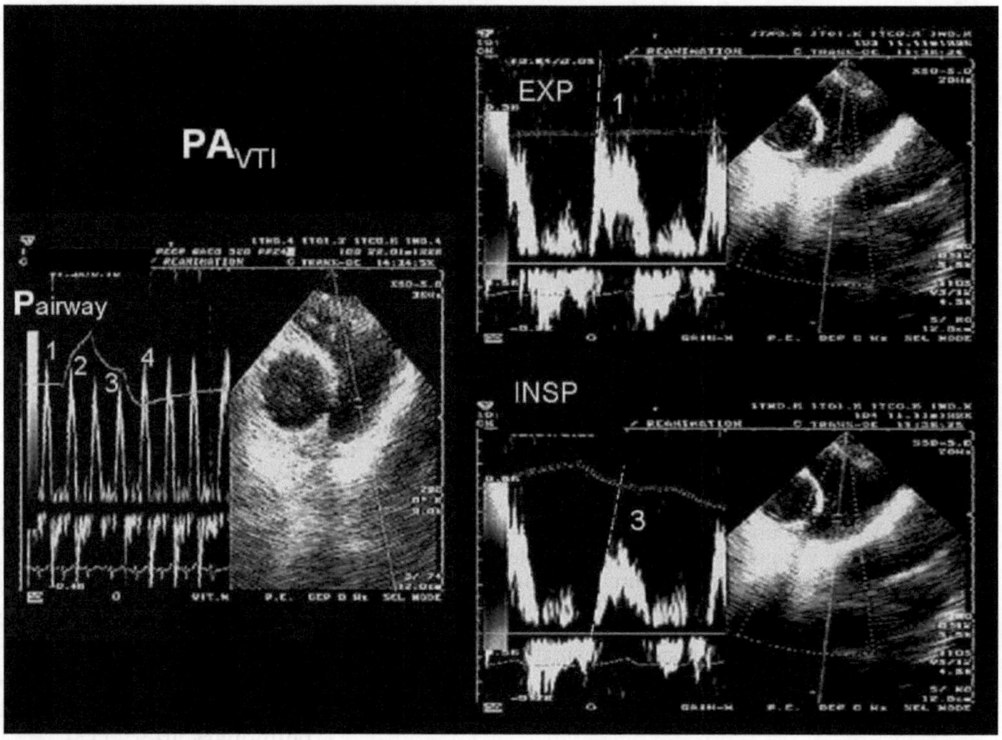

Fig. 4 Cyclic changes in pulmonary artery Doppler flow velocity during tidal ventilation. On the *left panel* these changes are recorded at low speed, illustrating the drop in peak velocity between beat 1 (end-expiratory beat) and beat 2 occurring during the dynamic phase of lung inflation. This drop was accentuated during beat 3, occurring at the end-inspiratory pause, and peak velocity start to return to its baseline value during beat 4, occurring at the onset of expiration. On the *right panel*, recording at high speed demonstrated the associated drop in mean acceleration (i.e., peak velocity divided by acceleration time), which is depicted by the slope of the *broken line* drawn on the initial part of the Doppler profile on beat 1 and beat 3

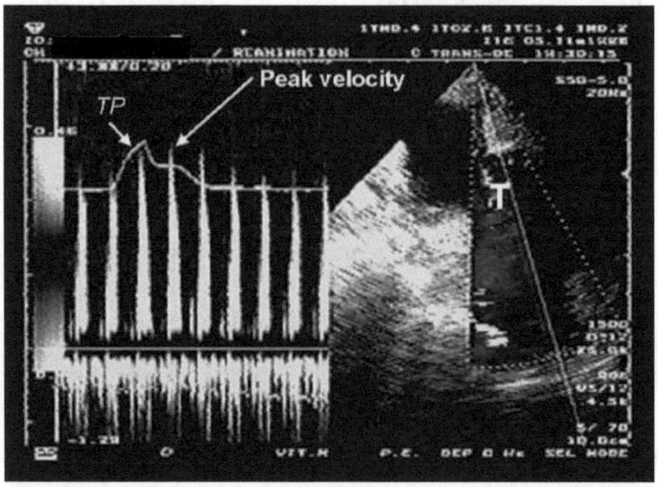

Fig. 5 Examined with a simultaneous recording of tracheal pressure (*TP*), recording of continuous Doppler backward flow velocity at the level of tricuspid valve (*T*) illustrates the increase in peak velocity produced by tidal ventilation

PEEP-related changes in transpulmonary pressure and their hemodynamic impact

In 1975, P. Suter described "best PEEP" as a PEEP resulting in "optimum" oxygen transport in ARDS patients [17]. This PEEP was easy to determine, because it was also associated with the best value of a two-point (quasi-static) compliance of the respiratory system (C_{RS}) [17].

This "best PEEP" was relatively low (8±4 cmH_2O, personal communication from P. Suter). If we assume that changes in C_{RS} in ARDS essentially reflect changes in static compliance of the lung (C_L), we can conclude that the "best PEEP" described by Suter reduced, for a given tidal volume, the required transpulmonary pressure. Thus, a lesser impact of tidal ventilation on right ventricular function should be expected when this PEEP is applied.

This hemodynamic improvement was actually present in Suter's work, where application of the "best PEEP" did not decrease cardiac output despite increased pleural pressure [17]. In accord with Suter's findings, we observed in 1981 that cardiac output was maintained at a low PEEP (<10 cmH_2O), despite pleural pressure increase (–0.6+0.4 mmHg at ZEEP, versus 0.9+1.9 mmHg with PEEP=10 cmH_2O, end-expiratory values) [18]. Conversely, above this PEEP cardiac output fell significantly [18]. Recently, we have corroborated this beneficial hemodynamic effect of a low PEEP by Doppler examination of pulmonary artery flow velocity [19] (Electronic Supplementary Material Film 3A,B).

In Suter's study, C_{RS} was a two-point compliance, calculated as tidal volume divided by plateau pressure minus end-expiratory pressure. The latter was assumed to be external PEEP, because the phenomenon of intrinsic PEEP was unknown at this time. If corrected for intrinsic PEEP [20], which was likely present in ARDS pa-

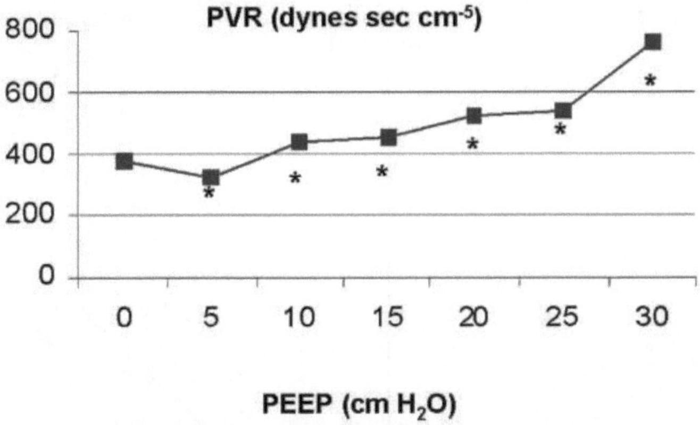

Fig. 6 Average change in pulmonary vascular resistance (*PVR*) during a progressive increase in PEEP in ten ARDS patients studied in 1981 [10]. Error bars are omitted for clarity. PVR was calculated using left ventricular end diastolic pressure measured at end-expiration by the Seldinger method, as reflecting pulmonary venous pressure. Note that PVR was significantly improved at a low PEEP, and was worsened on increasing PEEP above this level (**P*<0.05)

tients receiving a high tidal volume (13–15 ml/kg), the C_{RS} in Suter's patients would have probably been unchanged by "best PEEP" application, and the reason for the beneficial hemodynamic effect of this PEEP would probably not be an actual mechanical improvement, permitting reduction in transpulmonary pressure. In the study referred to above [18], we also observed a significant reduction in pulmonary vascular resistance with a low PEEP (between 3 and 8 cmH_2O, Fig. 6). As we have recently emphasized, a "slow compartment" is usually present at a relatively low supportive respiratory rate in ARDS patients, and produces gas trapping [21]. This gas trapping may be responsible for a permanent zone 2 condition in a limited area, and an increased vascular resistance in this specific area. Relieving gas trapping by a low PEEP [21] thus improves blood flow and reduces vascular resistance (Fig. 7).

Effect of an increase in pleural pressure on RV effective diastolic elastance

Pleural pressure is transmitted integrally to the pericardial space [22]. Thus, any increase in pleural pressure induces an increase in pericardial pressure, which limits the distending capacity of the cardiac cavities. During diastole, when pleural pressure is increased, a higher filling pressure is necessary to obtain an adequate end-diastolic volume. We have illustrated in the past the changes in left [18] and right [23] ventricular effective elastance occurring in clinical settings when pleural pressure is progressively increased by raising PEEP, and a schematic representation of theses change is shown in Fig. 8.

As a clinical consequence, a high central venous pressure (>10 mmHg) is required in a mechanically ventilated patient to put the right ventricle on the flat part of its function curve, thus rendering it somewhat insensitive to cyclic change in elastance produced by tidal ventilation

Fig. 7 A schematic representation of the adverse hemodynamic effect of the slow compartment in ARDS. On the *top left panel*, tidal ventilation with ZEEP produces a plateau pressure of 25 cmH_2O, which creates a zone 2 condition. On the *top right panel*, airway pressure in the fast compartment returns to zero at end-expiration with ZEEP, restoring a zone 3 condition, whereas the slow compartment, which cannot empty, is responsible for a permanent zone 2 condition in the corresponding vascular area. On the *bottom panel*, tidal ventilation with PEEP also creates a zone 2 condition (*left*), but the low PEEP of 7 cmH_2O suppresses the slow compartment, so that no zone 2 condition persists at expiration (*right*)

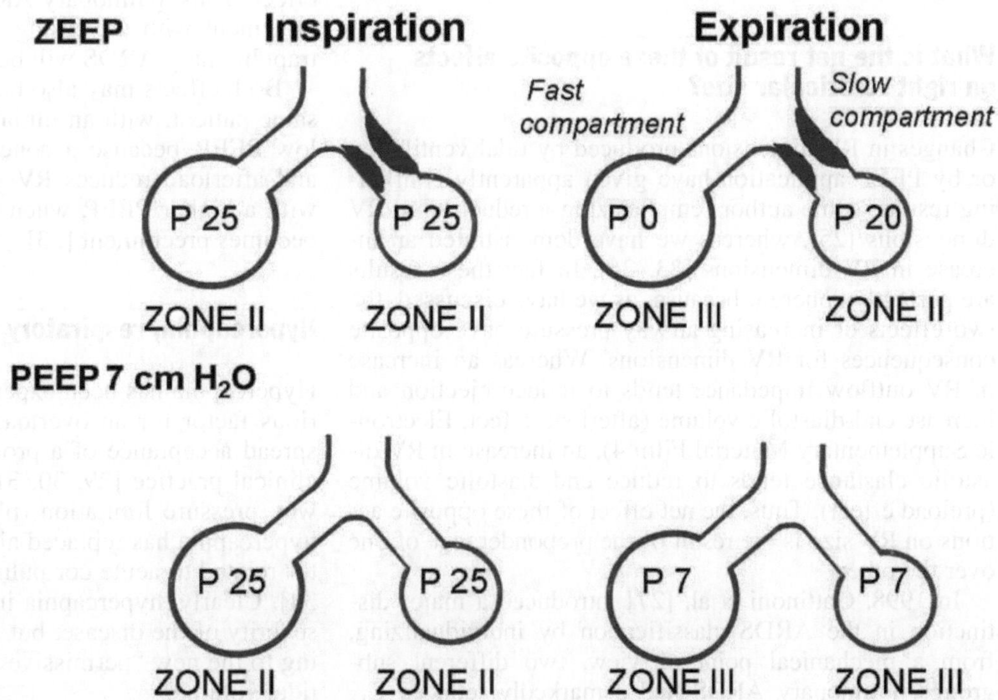

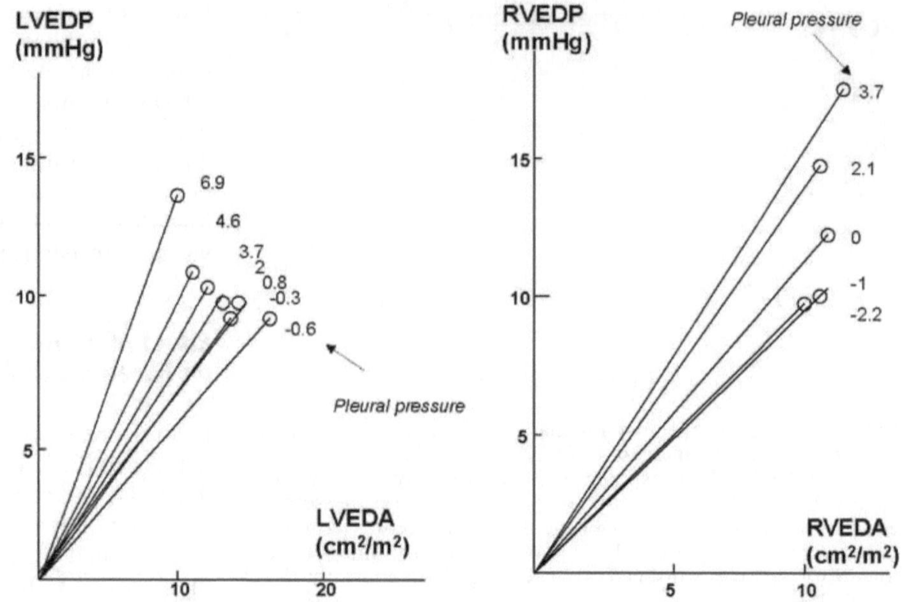

Fig. 8 Simultaneous recording of left ventricular end-diastolic pressure by left ventricular catheterization (*LVEDP*) and right ventricular end-diastolic pressure by right heart catheterization (*RVEDP*) simultaneously with left (*L*) and (*R*) ventricular end-diastolic areas (*EDA*) by two-dimensional echocardiography illustrated the changes in left (*left panel*) and right (*right panel*) ventricular elastance (the slope of the relation) occurring with a progressive increase in pleural pressure produced by a step-by-step application of PEEP. These diagrams were constructed with the data of [18, 23]

[24]. But central venous pressure may be misleading as a monitoring parameter because it is sensitive to venous elastance, which may differ from patient to patient. In our experience, observation of superior vena caval diameter by TEE is fundamental in ensuring that the right ventricle will be on the flat part of its function curve: this is likely the case when cyclic changes in pleural pressure only slightly affect vena caval diameter [11] (Electronic Supplementary Material Films 1A,B,C).

What is the net result of these opposite effects on right ventricular size?

Changes in RV dimensions produced by tidal ventilation or by PEEP application have given apparently conflicting results, some authors emphasizing a reduction in RV dimensions [25], whereas we have demonstrated an increase in RV dimensions [23, 26]. In fact these results are perfectly coherent because, as we have discussed, the two effects of increasing airway pressure have opposite consequences for RV dimensions. Whereas an increase in RV outflow impedance tends to reduce ejection and increase end-diastolic volume (afterload effect, Electronic Supplementary Material Film 4), an increase in RV diastolic elastance tends to reduce end-diastolic volume (preload effect). Thus, the net effect of these opposite actions on RV size is the result of the preponderance of one over the other.

In 1998, Gattinoni et al. [27] introduced a major distinction in the ARDS classification by individualizing, from a mechanical point of view, two different subgroups. Pulmonary ARDS had a markedly reduced C_L, whereas C_W was slightly affected in this subgroup. Extrapulmonary ARDS, on the other hand, had a markedly reduced C_W associated with a relatively preserved C_L. Thus, in pulmonary ARDS, a higher transpulmonary pressure would be required to deliver a given tidal volume. In this setting, one can expect a preeminent afterload effect. Conversely, in extrapulmonary ARDS, a given tidal volume would markedly increase pleural pressure. In this setting, one can expect a preeminent preload effect. Thus, pulmonary ARDS will be subject to RV enlargement with increasing airway pressure, whereas extrapulmonary ARDS will be subject to RV size reduction.

Both effects may also be successively observed in the same patient, with an initial reduction of RV size with a low PEEP, because a concomitant reduction in preload and afterload reduces RV size, and a final enlargement with a higher PEEP, when the increased afterload effect becomes preeminent [23].

Hypercapnia, respiratory rate and RV function

Hypercapnia has been experimentally proved as a deleterious factor for an overloaded RV [28]. With the widespread acceptance of a protective ventilation strategy in clinical practice [29, 30, 31, 32], which requires an airway pressure limitation (plateau pressure <30 cmH_2O), hypercapnia has replaced airway pressure as a direct factor related to acute cor pulmonale in ARDS patients [33, 34]. Clearly, hypercapnia in this setting results from the severity of the disease, but it may only be expressed owing to the new "permissive" respiratory strategy, limiting tidal volume.

Computed tomographic studies in ARDS have illustrated the major reduction in functional alveolar areas observed in this syndrome [35] and have led to the "baby lung" concept. In this concept, ARDS lung is compared to the lung of a baby, admitting only a small tidal volume. Because the respiratory rate of a baby is markedly greater than that of an adult, it has been proposed to limit the level of "permissive" hypecapnia by increasing the respiratory rate [36]. But adult ARDS patients actually exhibited an adult dead space [37], and increasing respiratory rate may produce an adverse intrinsic PEEP [37]. Gas trapping generated by this strategy increased right ventricular outflow impedance [37].

From a hemodynamic point of view, what are the best ventilation strategies in ARDS patients?

First of all, it should be recalled that the differences between cyclic positive airway pressure obtained by tidal ventilation and permanent airway pressure produced by PEEP are profound. Whereas transient increase in inspiratory pressure cannot be adapted because of the fleeting nature of the stress, PEEP induces a steady-state change in cardiovascular conditions, such that altering blood volume by fluid expansion and/or autonomic tone by a vasoactive support usually results in a return to baseline hemodynamic status. However, both interventions may have their own deleterious effects.

In our opinion, a first requirement for a safe mechanical ventilation is to limit transpulmonary pressure. A normal right ventricle may develop a maximal systolic pressure of 30 mmHg. During tidal ventilation, this forward pressure should work against a backward pressure, the transpulmonary pressure. In the past, excessive airway pressure was associated with a high frequency and a marked severity of acute cor pulmonale in ARDS [33]. Airway pressure limitation, which was safely obtained with a medium tidal volume (8 ml/kg of measured body weight) combined with a low PEEP (<10 cmH_2O), has reduced the incidence and clearly improved the prognosis of acute cor pulmonale in ARDS [34]. Additionally, interposing regular periods of ventilation in the prone position, by reversing hydrostatic pressure and its protective effect against a zone 2 situation, might regularly unload the most exposed upper areas of pulmonary vascular bed.

A second requirement for a safe mechanical ventilation is use of a low respiratory rate. The majority of ARDS patients have a localized expiratory flow limitation constituting a "slow compartment" [21], which requires a prolonged expiratory time of 4 s to empty [21]. Additionally, a high respiratory rate produces diffuse expiratory flow limitation and enhances gas trapping [37]. Gas trapping increases both pleural pressure and resistance to flow in the pulmonary vascular bed. However, this requirement is probably not absolute and some increase in respiratory rate may be safe, if it is not associated with intrinsic PEEP [36]. This is the case in a small number of ARDS patients, who exhibit a markedly increased elastic recoil of the lung, associated with a negligible slow compartment. Also instrumental dead space reduction may help to correct excessive hypercapnia [36, 38].

A third requirement for a safe mechanical ventilation is to use at least a low PEEP, thus improving blood flow throughout the pulmonary circulation [19]. As previously stated, the "slow compartment" can not empty with ZEEP when the respiratory rate is greater than 10 breaths/min, because its requires an expiration duration of 4 s [21]. As a result, the airway pressure remains high during the expiratory phase in this area, producing a localized and permanent zone 2. Because a low PEEP is able to reintegrate the "slow compartment" [21], it also permits the return of this area to a zone 3 condition during expiration, and a maximal efficacy of a moderate respiratory rate (15 breaths/min) [2]. This PEEP is actually close to that proposed 25 years ago by P. Suter [17].

Conclusion

The introduction of protective ventilation in 1990 by Hickling has greatly improved ARDS outcome [29]. Unknowingly, this author has also provided better working conditions for the RV, and both are probably in part related [39].

Now, the majority of authors interested in respiratory strategy in ARDS focus on complex mechanical studies to evaluate recruitment. Computed tomography (CT) scanning has been proposed for this purpose [40]. Conversely, few authors are concerned by the impact of the respiratory strategy on pulmonary circulation, and this lack of interest parallels the relative fall from grace of the Swan-Ganz catheter, an inaccurate procedure in mechanically ventilated patients [41]. While lung recruitment appears a justified goal in ARDS treatment, the procedure used for this purpose should remain compatible with the integrity of the pulmonary circulation, also required to obtain recovery [42].

References

1. Pinsky M (2003) Pulmonary artery occlusion pressure. Intensive Care Med 29:19–22
2. Pinsky M (2003) Clinical significance of pulmonary artery occlusion pressure. Intensive Care Med 29:175–178
3. Jardin F (2003) Ventricular interdependence: how does it impact on hemodynamic evaluation in clinical practice? Intensive Care Med 29:361–363

4. Page B, Vieillard-Baron A, Beauchet A, Aegerter Ph, Prin S, Jardin F (2003) Low stretch ventilation strategy in acute respiratory distress syndrome/ 8 years of clinical experience in a single center. Crit Care Med 31:765–769
5. Guyton A, Linsdsey A, Abernathy B, Richardson T (1957) Venous return at various right atrial pressures and the normal venous return curve. Am J Physiol 189:609–615
6. Fessler H, Brower R, Wise R, Premutt S (1991) Effects of positive end-expiratory pressure on the gradient for venous return. Am Rev Respir Dis 145:19–24
7. Van den Berg P, Jansen J, Pinsky M (2002) Effect of positive pressure on venous return in volume-loaded cardiac surgical patients. J Appl Physiol 92:1223–12231
8. Takata M, Wise R, Robotham J (1990) Effects of abdominal pressure on venous return: abdominal vascular zone conditions. J Appl Physiol 69:1961–1972
9. Fessler H, Brower R, Wise R, Permutt S (1992) Effects of positive end-expiratory pressure on the canine venous return curve. Am Rev Respir Dis 146:4–10
10. Jellinek H, Krenn H, Oczenski W, Veit F, Schwartz S, Fitzgerald D (2000) Influence of positive airway pressure on the pressure gradient for venous return in humans. J Appl Physiol 88:926–932
11. Vieillard-Baron A, Augarde R, Prin S, Page B, MD, Beauchet A, Jardin F (2001) Influence of superior vena caval zone conditions on cyclic changes in right ventricular outflow during respiratory support. Anethesiology 95:1083–1088
12. Permutt S, Bromberger-Barnea B, Bane H (1962) Alveolar pressure, pulmonary venous pressure, and the vascular waterfall. Med Thorac 19:239–260
13. Vieillard-Baron A, Loubières Y, Schmitt JM, Page B, Dubourg O, Jardin F (1999) Cyclic changes in right ventricular output impedance during mechanical ventilation. J Appl Physiol 87:1644–1650
14. Jardin F, Brun-Ney D, Cazaux P, Dubourg O, Hardy A, Bourdarias JP (1989) Relation between transpulmonary pressure and right ventricular isovolumetric pressure change during respiratory support. Catheter Cardiovasc Diag 16:215–220
15. Jullien T, Valtier B, Hongnat JM, Dubourg O, Bourdarias JP, Jardin F (1995) Incidence of tricuspid regurgitation and vena caval backward flow in mechanically ventilated patients. A color Doppler and contrast echocardiographic study. Chest 107:488–493
16. Artucio H, Hurtado J, Zimet L, de Paula J, Beron M (1997) PEEP-induced tricuspid regurgitation. Intensive Care Med 23:806–807
17. Suter P, Fairley H, Isenberg M (1975) Optimum end-expiratory airway pressure in patients with acute lung disease. N Engl J Med 292:284–289
18. Jardin F, Farcot JC, Boisante L, Curien N, Margairaz A, Bourdarias JP (1981) Influence of positive end-expiratory pressure on left ventricular performance. N Engl J Med 304:387–392
19. Schmitt JM, Vieillard-Baron A, Augarde R, Prin S, Page B, Jardin F (2001) PEEP titration in ARDS patients: impact on right ventricular outflow impedance evaluated by pulmonary artery Doppler flow velocity. Critical Care Med 29:1154–1158
20. Rossi A, Gottfried B, Zocchi L, Higgs B, Lennox S, Calverley M, Begin P, Grassino A, Milic-Emili J (1985) Measurements of static compliance of the total respiratory system in patients with acute respiratory failure during mechanical ventilation. The effect of intrinsic positive end-expiratory pressure. Am Rev Respir Dis 131:672–677
21. Vieillard-Baron A, Prin S, Schmitt JM, Augarde R, Page B, Beauchet A, Jardin F (2002) Pressure/volume curves in acute respiratory distress syndrome: clinical demonstration of the influence of expiratory flow limitation on the initial slope. Am J Respir Crit Care Med 165:1107–1112
22. Morgan B, Guntheroth W, Dillard D (1965) Relationship of pericardial pressure to pleural pressure during quiet respiration and cardiac tamponade. Circ Res 26:493–498
23. Jardin F, Brun-Ney D, Hardy A, Aegerter Ph, Beauchet A, Bourdarias JP (1991) Combined thermodilution and two-dimensional echocardiographic evaluation of right ventricular function during respiratory support with PEEP. Chest 99:162–168
24. Jellinek H, Krafft P, Fitzgerald R, Schwartz S, Pinsky M (2000) Right atrial pressure predicts hemodynamic response to apneic positive airway pressure. Crit Care Med 28:672–678
25. Dhainaut JF, Devaux J, Monsallier J, Brunet F, Villemant D, Huyghebaert MF (1986) Mechanism of decreased left ventricular preload during continuous positive pressure ventilation. Chest 90:74–80
26. Jardin F, Delorme G, Hardy A, Auvert B, Beauchet A, Bourdarias JP (1990) Reevaluation of hemodynamic consequences of positive pressure ventilation: emphasis on cyclic right ventricular afterloading by mechanical lung inflation. Anesthesiology 72:966–970
27. Gattinoni L, Pelosi P, Suter P, Pedoto A, Vercesi P, Lissoni A (1998) Acute respiratory distress syndrome caused by pulmonary and extrapulmonary disease. Different syndromes? Am J Respir Crit Care Med 158:3–11
28. Rose E, Van Benthuysen K, Jackson T, Tucker C, Kaiser D, Grover R, Weil J (1983) Right ventricular performance during increased afterload impaired by hypercapnic acidosis in conscious dogs. Circ Res 52:76–84
29. Hickling K, Henderson S, Jackson R (1990) Low mortality associated with low volume/pressure-limited ventilation with permissive hypercapnia in severe acute respiratory distress syndrome. Intensive Care Med 16:372–377
30. Amato M, Barbas C, Medeiraos D, Schetino G, Filho L, Kairalla R, Deheinzelin D, Morais C, Fernandes E, Tagaky T, De Carvalho C (1995) Beneficial effect of the "open lung approach" with low distending pressures in acute respiratory distress syndrome. Am J Respir Crit Care Med 152:1835–1846
31. Jardin F, Fellahi JL, Beauchet A, Vieillard-Baron A, Loubières Y, Page B (1999) Improved prognosis of acute respiratory distress syndrome 15 years on. Intensive Care Med 25:936–941
32. Ventilation with lower tidal volumes as compared with traditional tidal volumes for acute lung injury and the acute respiratory distress syndrome. The Acute Respiratory Distress Syndrome Network (2000) N Engl J Med 342:1301–1308
33. Jardin F, Gueret P, Dubourg O, Farcot JC, Margairaz A, Bourdarias JP (1985) Two-dimensional echocardiographic evaluation of right ventricular size and contractility in acute respiratory failure. Crit Care Med 13:952–956
34. Vieillard-Baron A, Schmitt JM, Beauchet A, Augarde R, Prin S, Page B, Jardin F (2001) Acute cor pulmonale in acute respiratory distress syndrome submitted to protective ventilation: incidence, clinical implications and prognosis. Crit Care Med 29:1551–1555
35. Gattinoni L, Presenti A, Torresin A, Baglioni S, Rivolta M, Rossi F, Scarani F, Marcolin R, Cappelletti G (1986) Adult respiratory distress syndrome profiles by computed tomography. J Thoracic Imaging 1:25–30

36. Richecoeur J, Q Lu Q, S Vieira, Puybasset L, Kalfon P, Coriat P, Rouby JJ (1998) Expiratory washout versus optimization of mechanical ventilation during permissive hypercapnia in patients with severe acute respiratory distress syndrome. Am J Respir Crit Care Med 160:77–85
37. Vieillard-Baron A, Prin S, Augarde R, Desfonds P, Page B, Beauchet A, MD, Jardin F (2002) Increasing respiratory rate to improve CO_2 clearance during mechanical ventilation is not a panacea in acute respiratory failure. Crit Care Med 30:1407–1412
38. Prin S, Chergui K, Augarde R, Page B, Jardin F, Vieillard-Baron A (2002) Ability and safety of a heated humidifier to control hypercapnic acidosis in severe ARDS. Intensive Care Med 28:1756–1760
39. Scherrer-Crosbie M, Streckenbach S, Zapol W (2001) Acute cor pulmonale in acute respiratory distress syndrome: a dreaded complication of the past? Crit Care Med 29:1641–1642
40. Rouby JJ, Lu Q, Goldstein I (2002) Selecting the right level of positive end-expiratory pressure in patients with acute respiratory distress syndrome. Am J Respir Crit Care Med 165:1182–1186
41. Jardin F, Bourdarias JP (1995) Right heart catheterization at bedside: a critical view. Intensive Care Med 21:291–295
42. Vieillard-Baron A, Prin S, Chergui K, Dubourg O, Jardin F (2002) Echo-doppler demonstration of acute cor pulmonale at the bedside in the medical intensive care unit. Am J Respir Crit Care Med 166:1310–1319

Alexandre Mebazaa
Peter Karpati
Estelle Renaud
Lars Algotsson

Acute right ventricular failure—from pathophysiology to new treatments

Abstract The right ventricle (RV) provides sustained low-pressure perfusion of the pulmonary vasculature, but is sensitive to changes in loading conditions and intrinsic contractility. Factors that affect right ventricular preload, afterload or left ventricular function can adversely influence the functioning of the RV, causing ischaemia and right ventricular failure (RVF). As RVF progresses, a pronounced tricuspid regurgitation further decreases cardiac output and worsens organ congestion. This can degenerate into an irreversible vicious cycle.

The effective diagnosis of RVF is optimally performed by a combination of techniques including echocardiography and catheterisation, which can also be used to monitor treatment efficacy. Treatment of RVF focuses on alleviating congestion, improving right ventricular contractility and right coronary artery perfusion and reducing right ventricular afterload. As part of the treatment, inhaled nitric oxide or prostacyclin effectively reduces afterload by vasodilating the pulmonary vasculature. Traditional positive inotropic drugs enhance contractility by increasing the intracellular calcium concentration and oxygen consumption of cardiac myocytes, while vasopressors such as norepinephrine increase arterial blood pressure, which improves cardiac perfusion but increases afterload. A new treatment, the calcium sensitiser, levosimendan, increases cardiac contractility without increasing myocardial oxygen demand, while preserving myocardial relaxation. Furthermore, it increases coronary perfusion and decreases afterload. Conversely, traditional treatments of circulatory failure, such as mechanical ventilation and volume loading, could be harmful in the case of RVF. This review outlines the pathophysiology, diagnosis and treatment of RVF, illustrated with clinical case studies.

Keywords Heart failure · Levosimendan · Vasodilator agents · Inotropic agents · Pathophysiology · Pharmacology

Introduction

Until fairly recently, right ventricular failure (RVF) was a relatively neglected medical condition. The right ventricle (RV) was considered as a moderately passive conduit between the systemic and pulmonary circulations. This belief was supported by studies showing that complete destruction of the right ventricular free wall in dogs had no detectable impairment on overall cardiac performance [1]. However, investigations in the 1970s demonstrated that RVF has significant haemodynamic and cardiac performance effects, as illustrated by Cohen et al.in six patients following a myocardial infarction involving the RV [2]. The patients had severe hypotension, diminished peripheral perfusion and severely impaired pressure generation in the RV, with almost no

M.R. Pinsky et al. (eds.), *Applied Physiology in Intensive Care Medicine 2: Physiological Reviews and Editorials*,
DOI 10.1007/978-3-642-28233-1_13, © Springer-Verlag Berlin Heidelberg 2012

pressure gradient from the right atrium to the pulmonary artery [2].

Precipitating factors for RVF are common in surgical and medical intensive care units (ICUs). These include increased pulmonary vascular resistance, such as after cardiac transplantation; acute respiratory distress syndrome; the presence of a left ventricular assist device; positive pressure mechanical ventilation and sepsis. There is also a higher incidence of RVF occurring in ICUs than is generally recognised.

Right ventricular failure has a similar incidence to left-sided heart failure, with each affecting about 1 in 20 of the population [3]. Left-sided heart failure is often a chronic, progressive disease with mortality four to eight times greater than that of the age-matched general population [4]. In contrast, the outcome of RVF is largely dependent on the underlying cause, resulting in either an acute or chronic condition. Patients in cardiogenic shock due to an infarction predominantly affecting either the left or right ventricle experience a similar rate of mortality, despite patients with RVF being younger and having a higher prevalence of single vessel disease [5]. Furthermore, ischaemia following a myocardial infarction involving both the right ventricle (RV) and the left, results in a greater risk of mortality than isolated left ventricular ischaemia [6, 7].

The pathophysiology, diagnosis and treatment of RVF in the ICU is associated with some controversy. This review provides an informed opinion on a number of these issues, the effects of some newer treatment options for RVF involving pulmonary vasodilation and enhancing cardiac contraction are described, and their therapeutic benefits are demonstrated in three case studies that are summarised here and described in full in the electronic supplementary material (ESM).

Physiology of the right ventricle and pathophysiology of right ventricular failure

The primary function of the RV is to maintain a low right atrial pressure, optimising venous return and to provide sustained low-pressure perfusion through the lungs. To achieve this, the RV ejects blood quasi-continuously from the right atria to the lungs, continuously emptying the right atria. This 'continuous' ejection is possible because of the favourable characteristics of the pulmonary vascular bed, which is a low pressure, low resistance and high compliance circuit with a pressure gradient of 5 mmHg. Conversely, the left ventricle generates high-pressure pulsatile flow through arterial vessels with low compliance. The right cardiac and pulmonary pressures observed in a healthy spontaneously breathing adult are summarised in Table 1.

The RV is anatomically adapted for the generation of a sustained low-pressure perfusion. It comprises two anatomically and functionally different cavities, termed the sinus and the cone. The sinus generates pressure during systole and the cone regulates this pressure [8]. Right ventricular contraction occurs in three phases; contraction of the papillary muscles, then movement of the right ventricular free wall towards the inter-ventricular septum and, finally, contraction of the left ventricle causes a 'wringing' which further empties the RV. The net effect is pressure generation in the sinus with a peristaltic motion starting at the apex moving towards the cone and, due to the compliance of the upper cone region of the thin-walled RV, the peak pressure is reduced and prolonged. Therefore, ejection into the pulmonary circulation is sustained until the RV has completed its emptying, end-diastolic pressure is minimal and venous return is optimal. Notably, right ventricular preload is determined by both the compliance of the RV and the venous return. The latter depends on the pressure gradient from the periphery to the right atria and the venous resistance. Despite the thin muscular walls of the RV, it adapts to small changes in venous return, such as those occurring during respiration, without altering cavity pressures or volumes. However, larger changes in venous return affect the right ventricular end-diastolic volume.

Table 1 'Normal' right atrial, right ventricular and pulmonary artery pressures for a spontaneously breathing patient

Variable	Value
Right atrial pressure	
Mean	0–7 mmHg
Right ventricular pressure	
Systolic	15–25 mmHg
Diastolic	0–8 mmHg
Pulmonary artery pressure	
Systolic	15–25 mmHg
Diastolic	8–15 mmHg
Mean	10–20 mmHg
Wedge	6–12 mmHg[a]
Pulmonary vascular resistance	100–250 dynes/s per cm^5

[a] Should be less than the pulmonary artery diastolic pressure

Effect of an increase in right ventricular afterload: chronic pulmonary hypertension or acute cor pulmonale

The pressure-volume characteristics for the RV differ markedly from those of the left ventricle (Fig. 1) [9]. The right ventricular pressure-volume loop has a more triangular shape compared with that of the left ventricle, with only brief periods of isovolaemic contraction and relaxation. There is sustained ejection during pressure development that, more importantly, continues during pressure decline. This prolonged low-pressure emptying

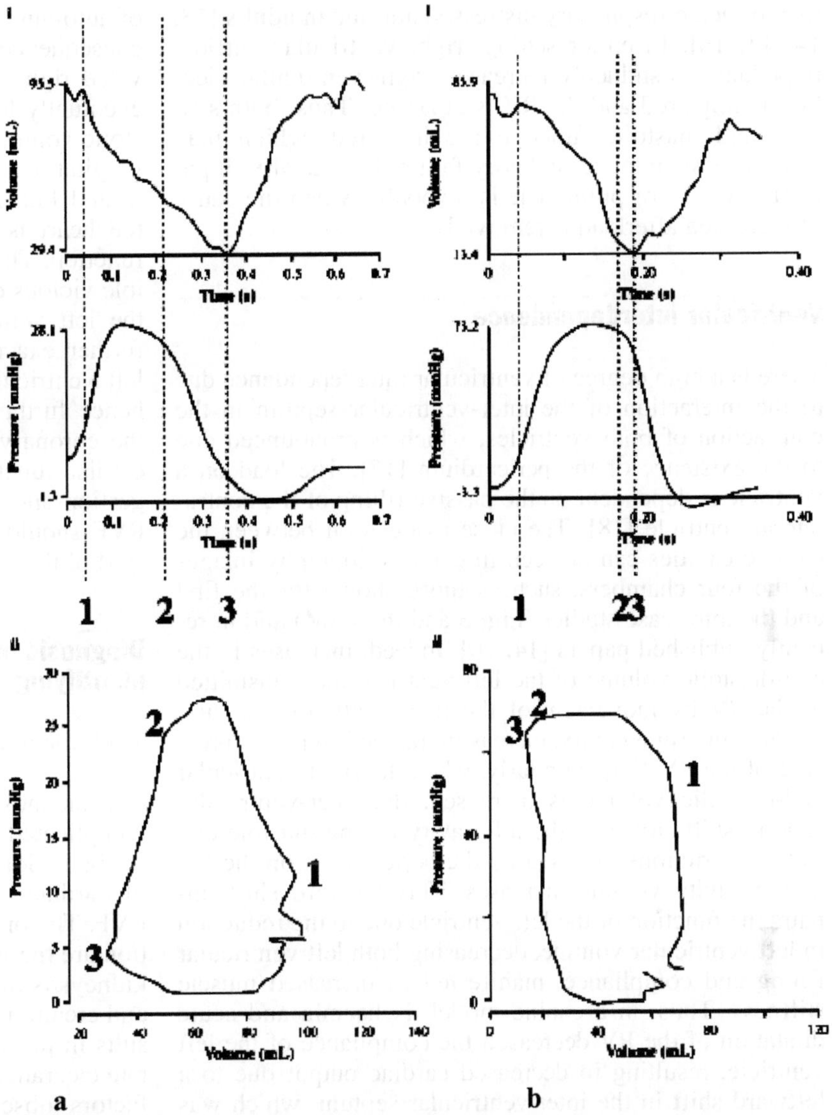

Fig. 1 Pressure and volume changes against time during a contraction cycle (i) and the pressure-volume loop derived from these measurements (ii) are shown for a normal patient (**a**) and for a patient with pulmonary stenosis (**b**). The numbers indicate: 1, the opening of the pulmonary valve marking the start of the ejection phase; 2, the onset of relaxation; 3, the closing of the pulmonary valve marking the end of the ejection phase. In (**a**), the pressure-volume loop is more triangular than that of the left ventricle. Ejection from the right ventricle starts early during the pressure increase and the isovolaemic contraction phase is consequently not well defined. It is interesting to note that ejection continued after the peak pressure during pressure decline (between points 2 and 3). In (**b**), the pressure-volume loop resembles that of the left ventricle. There is a well defined end systolic shoulder and there is no ejection during the pressure decline ([**a**] reproduced from *British Heart Journal* 1988; volume 59, pages 23–30 with permission from BMJ Publishing Group [9]; [**b**] reproduced from *British Heart Journal* 1990; volume 63, pages 45–49, with permission from BMJ Publishing Group [10])

implies that right ventricular emptying is very sensitive to changes in afterload. Thus, in a patient with pulmonary hypertension, the right ventricular pressure-volume loop is not triangular and resembles that of the left ventricle (Fig. 1b) [10]. To compensate, the RV dilates to maintain the stroke volume, though the ejection fraction is reduced [11], and the peristaltic contraction is lost, causing an accelerated increase in pulmonary artery pressure and flow.

The increased afterload also prolongs the isovolaemic contraction phase and ejection time and, therefore, increases myocardial oxygen consumption. Under physiological conditions, there may be increased perfusion of the right coronary artery. However, partial occlusion of the right coronary artery may prevent this compensatory mechanism, resulting in ischaemia [12]. Therefore, in a patient with decreased right coronary artery perfusion, it is important to reduce right ventricular afterload to improve the oxygen supply/demand ratio in the RV to maintain right ventricular function. (This is demonstrated in the first illustrative case study.)

The RV is predominantly perfused by the right coronary artery with supply of some regions by the left anterior descending branch of the left coronary artery. Physiologically, right coronary artery perfusion occurs during both diastole and systole, in contrast to the left coronary artery, that supplies the left ventricular muscle mostly during diastole. However, when pulmonary artery hypertension is present, right coronary artery perfusion occurs quasi-exclusively during diastole, potentially reducing the oxygen supply to the RV during increased oxygen demand.

Acute cor pulmonale relates to a sudden increase in afterload, most often due to a massive pulmonary embolism or acute respiratory distress syndrome in adults [13, 14, 15, 16]. In either setting, right ventricular outflow impedance is suddenly increased, right ventricular ejection is impaired and the RV is enlarged. Thus, both systolic and diastolic function are impaired, which may cause or precipitate circulatory failure in critically ill patients. Acute cor pulmonale is reversible when the cause of increased afterload is removed.

Ventricular interdependence

There is a high degree of ventricular interdependence due to the interaction of the inter-ventricular septum in the contraction of both ventricles, which is pronounced due to the existence of the pericardium [17]. The load on a ventricle is dependent on the passive filling of the contralateral ventricle [18]. The close association between the cardiac cavities can be seen in echocardiography images of the four chambers, such as those shown for the first and the third case studies (Fig. 3 and the ESM) and in recently published papers [14, 16]. Indeed, increases in the end-diastolic volume of the left ventricle are transmitted to the RV by movement of the inter-ventricular septum towards the right cavity, increasing the end-diastolic pressure of the RV [20]. Similarly, when the right ventricular end-diastolic volume is increased, the inter-ventricular septum shifts towards the left cavity during diastole due to the restrictions imposed by the pericardium on the RV as the cavity volume increases. This leftward shift impairs the function of the left ventricle due to the reduction in left ventricular volume, decreasing both left ventricular filling and compliance, manifested as increased muscle stiffness. Thus, in a canine model, ischaemia and acute dilatation of the RV decreased the compliance of the left ventricle, resulting in decreased cardiac output due to a leftward shift in the inter-ventricular septum, which was attenuated by the opening of the pericardium [21].

Ventricular interdependence can also cause RVF during left ventricular assist device support. As the left ventricular assist device unloads the left ventricle, the inter-ventricular septum is shifted left. This alters the right ventricular compliance decreasing force and rate of contraction together with a decreased afterload and increased preload. In a healthy heart, cardiac output may be maintained but, with pre-existing pathology, the decrease in contractility may result in RVF [22]. It is therefore crucial to support right ventricular function during the first days following insertion of a left ventricular assist device.

Vicious cycle of auto-aggravation

Compared to the left ventricle, RVF progresses quickly from compensated to end-stage because of a vicious cycle of auto-aggravation. This is unique to the RV and is not a consequence of isolated left ventricular failure. The elevated right atrial and ventricular end-diastolic pressures eventually lead to an increased right ventricular end-diastolic volume, insufficiency of the tricuspid valve and regurgitation. The tricuspid insufficiency aggravates hepatic and kidney congestion and decreases cardiac output; the heart is, therefore, unable to maintain an adequate function. Thus, the auto-aggravation becomes an irreversible vicious cycle. In addition, decreased venous return to the left ventricle reduces left ventricular preload. This further exacerbates the situation as it causes decreased left ventricular output and systemic blood pressure and hence further impairment of organ perfusion, including the coronary arteries. This ischaemia further diminishes cardiac function and the cycle of worsening output, congestion and ischaemia continues. Therefore, any sign of RVF should result in immediate treatment to avoid the start of the vicious cycle of auto-aggravation.

Diagnosis of right ventricular failure—identifying organ dysfunction

Traditional non-specific approach

The diagnosis of acute RVF in patients in the ICU is complicated by the lack of clinical and biological specific signs. Some biological signs which may be indicative of cardiac dysfunction appear very early during acute RVF. The organs most affected by RVF-induced congestion are the liver and kidneys. Decreased perfusion of the kidneys is manifested as a reduction in both urine output and creatinine clearance. Decreased hepatic perfusion results in increased plasma lactate due to an impaired lactate clearance, a reduction in the synthesis of coagulation factors (observed as a decrease in prothrombin time) and hepatic cytolysis. Interestingly, Fig. 2 and Fig. S1 in the ESM show two examples of the effects of very severe liver and kidney congestion related to RVF.

The sensitivity of conventional chest X-ray techniques to identify changes in right ventricular form is limited by the unusual shape of the RV and the unpredictable manner in which it dilates. Inferential diagnosis may be possible by identification of other radiographic changes, such as the state of the pulmonary circulation and the position of the heart in the chest. Changes in the left ventricle may be apparent on chest X-ray, resulting from the decreased left ventricular preload that is a consequence of RVF.

Echocardiography

Echocardiography is an alternative, more accessible technique for the diagnosis of RVF and for the intermittent repetitive follow-up of the dynamics of therapeutic responses. Its advantage is that a qualitative conclusion can be reached instantaneously. When RVF is secondary to an increase in afterload, the isovolaemic contraction phase and ejection time are prolonged, and increases in pulmonary artery pressure and flow are accelerated. Echocardiography also provides information about the mechanisms of RVF, such as pericardial effusion with or without tamponade, tricuspid insufficiency, pulmonary emboli or right ventricular ischaemia and the resulting acute cor pulmonale [14].

Additionally, echocardiography enables the simultaneous evaluation of left ventricular function, a possible component of the RVF. Due to the geometry and location of the RV, the accuracy and necessity of determining exact right ventricular dimensions remains questionable and an experienced intensivist familiar with performing and evaluating echocardiography is essential. Although echocardiography can be repeated infinitely, the continuous flow of information provided by right heart catheterisation is difficult to reproduce and when technical or human limitations render echocardiography impossible, right heart catheterisation becomes the diagnostic tool of choice.

Pulmonary artery catheterisation

Catheterisation of the pulmonary artery is more invasive but useful to evaluate right ventricular function and confirm the presence of RVF in patients in the ICU. The Swan–Ganz catheter measures both mixed venous oxygen saturation and intravascular pressures or pressure changes in the RV as well as pulmonary artery pressure and pulmonary capillary wedge pressure. Despite difficulties in the interpretation of mean intravascular pressure values, the tracings showing changes in pressure and flow enable the assessment of the impact of treatment on right ventricular function. This cautious interpretation accounts for the almost constant reflux due to the tricuspid insufficiency, which can be observed by central venous and right atrial pressure changes (see Fig. 3 and the illustrative example described in the ESM). Such regurgitation could be used as a hallmark for RVF and as a marker for treatment efficacy.

A more advanced pulmonary catheter, equipped with a fast-response thermistor, is another valuable diagnostic tool enabling clinical assessment of right ventricular volume and haemodynamic parameters by thermodilution. It may also measure cardiac output more precisely even in the presence of tricuspid insufficiency, a particular problem during mechanical ventilation. Indeed, the more widespread introduction of thermodilution techniques to assess pump function has contributed to the recognition of the inherent pathology of RVF. Values for cardiac performance obtained from this technique compare favourably with those using radionucleotides or two-dimensional echocardiography [24, 25].

If a central venous pressure or pulmonary artery catheter is in place, haemodynamic parameters that can aid in the diagnosis of RVF include an increase in right atrial pressure and a decrease in arterial blood pressure, cardiac output and mixed venous oxygen saturation, despite a usually preserved pulmonary artery pressure and pulmonary capillary wedge pressure. For difficult cases, a technique often cited in the literature for the diagnosis of RVF involves the administration of 250 ml of crystalloids or colloids over 10 min [26]. If the patient is suffering from RVF, all the above haemodynamic parameters worsen, including a dramatic increase in right atrial pressure with no change in cardiac output. This test should not be performed in patients who are in acute RVF, as there is a risk of severe aggravation of tricuspid insufficiency and organ congestion after volume loading (see below).

Management of right ventricular failure

The principal therapeutic goals of RVF depend on its underlying aetiology, but generally involve breaking the vicious cycle of reduced cardiac output by restoring adequate oxygen delivery to the myocardium and reducing right ventricular overload. Treatment usually focuses on alleviating congestion, improving right ventricular contractility and/or reducing right ventricular afterload.

When RVF is related to occlusion of the right coronary artery, reperfusion by coronary angioplasty may help restore contractile function to the ischaemic myocardium and improve the clinical outcome [27]. Revascularisation of the right coronary artery may also be prudent when inserting a left ventricular assist device in patients with right coronary artery-associated ischaemia, to avoid subsequent RVF [28]. Patients who have RVF related to atrial fibrillation may benefit from aggressive anti-arrhythmic treatment to improve cardiac output, and temporary pericardiotomy may benefit patients following sternotomy for cardiac surgery.

Volume management

Volume management is a difficult but important task in the treatment of RVF. In very few cases of RVF with normal pulmonary vascular resistance, volume loading may be useful in increasing preload, which increases right ventricular end-diastolic volume and cardiac output [29]. However in the large majority of RVF patients, this compensatory mechanism is potentially limited beyond a mean pulmonary artery pressure of 30 mmHg [30] and therefore caution is warranted when considering volume loading. Volume overload is common during RVF and volume loading may further dilate the RV, increase tricuspid regurgitation and, consequently, worsen hepatic and renal congestion and RVF. A sharp rise in left- or right-sided filling pressures without a concomitant increase in cardiac output may indicate when further volume loading is detrimental.

In this scenario, fluid withdrawal should be started with diuretics and haemofiltration. If the RV is dilated and the inter-ventricular septum shifted, one should first try diuretics. If this is unsuccessful, haemofiltration is urgently recommended, often under inotropic support.

Pulmonary vasodilators

Systemic therapy

In the presence of elevated pulmonary vascular resistances, vasodilator therapy may reduce right ventricular afterload. This will improve right ventricular function by decreasing right ventricular myocardial oxygen consumption and improving left ventricular filling, which will eventually increase systemic blood pressure and right coronary artery perfusion pressure. This will, in turn, decrease right atrial pressure and organ congestion. Thus, intravenous vasodilators such as nitroglycerin, nitroprusside or prostaglandin E1 may be beneficial in patients with isolated RVF [31, 32]. However, systemic pulmonary vasodilators reverse hypoxic pulmonary vasoconstriction, worsening ventilation-perfusion matching within the lung and decreasing arterial oxygen saturation. Also, they decrease diastolic pressure, resulting in decreased right coronary artery perfusion, which worsens ischaemia [33, 34].

Inhaled therapies

Inhalational vasodilatory agents, such as prostacyclin or its analogues and nitric oxide (NO), have a direct, selective effect on the pulmonary vasculature [23, 35, 36, 37]. NO diffuses into the pulmonary vascular smooth muscle cells, causing vasodilation, and its effects are localised as it rapidly binds to plasma proteins and haemoglobin. Following prolonged administration, rebound pulmonary hypertension has been frequently reported when NO inhalation is suddenly withdrawn [38]. Despite its haemodynamic benefits, a survival advantage for patients with RVF who respond to NO therapy has not been proven [39]. Inhaled sodium nitroprusside, a NO donor drug, is a possible alternative for the future [40].

Beneficial effects of inhaled NO have also been described in the management of RVF associated with a patent foramen ovale. As a patent foramen ovale, together with right-left shunt, is frequently found in patients who have RVF with elevated right atrial pressures, its role in maintaining (or restoring) left ventricular preload, albeit by simultaneously compromising arterial oxygenation, cannot be ignored [41, 42].

An alternative to inhaled NO is inhaled prostacyclin (= prostaglandin I_2). Besides its vasodilator properties, inhaled prostacyclin is the most potent platelet aggregation inhibitor known. Prostacyclin also stimulates endothelial release of NO, and vice versa. A potentially substantial advantage of inhaled, versus intravenous, prostacyclin is that rebound pulmonary hypertension after abrupt discontinuation has so far not been reported. This suggests that, in comparison with inhaled NO, inhaled prostacyclin may treat pulmonary hypertension more effectively. Prostacyclinhas no known toxic effects or active metabolites and it is cheaper than NO, both in terms of the equipment necessary for its administration and the substance itself [43, 44].

Iloprost is the stable carbacyclin derivative of prostacyclin. It has several advantageous properties compared to prostacyclin, including saline solubility, lower viscosity and a significantly longer duration of action with a half-life of 20–30 min and haemodynamic effects that last for 1 h [45].

Contractility enhancing agents

The right ventricular ejection can be directly increased by the insertion of a right ventricular assist device, which may be beneficial for the short-term prophylaxis in patients following cardiac surgery or transplantation, enabling the stunned heart to recover [46].

Positive inotropic agents are also commonly used to improve right ventricular function. Left ventricular contraction assists the ejection from the RV; therefore, inotropic drugs that increase the contraction of the whole heart will improve right ventricular function both by directly enhancing right-sided contractility and by their effects on the entire myocardium. Positive inotropic agents— -adrenoceptor agonists and phosphodiesterase inhibitors—enhance myocardial contractility by increasing the intracellular calcium concentration in both ventricles due to their actions on cAMP [47]. In the treatment of chronic heart failure patients, vasoactive -agonists produce a net increase in cardiac output providing a short-term benefit, but the increased contractility, working against a greater afterload, increases the workload of the heart, resulting in an increase in energy utilisation. Therefore, the oxygen consumption of the myocardium is increased without increasing oxygen supply, which may cause or worsen ischaemia and arrhythmias. Thus, the use of some of these agents has been associated with an increase in long-term mortality [48, 49, 50] and, in the case of dobutamine, tolerance develops after a short time [51]. The treatment of RVF is comparatively short and repeated dosing less common than for chronic heart failure, therefore tolerance may not be relevant in this setting. However, the effects of sympathomimetics on long-term outcome should perhaps be considered when selecting appropriate treatment for RVF.

A newer class of drugs, the calcium sensitisers, also improve cardiac function by increasing the contraction of the myocardium, but without significantly increasing intracellular calcium levels. Levosimendan, the first calcium sensitiser in clinical use, increases the sensitivity of the cardiac myofilaments to calcium during systole without affecting diastole. The increased calcium sensitivity increases the force and rate of contraction of the myocardium. Moreover, as it only increases systolic calcium sensitivity, it does not affect the relaxation kinetics, in contrast to the traditional inotropic drugs. Hence, levosimendan has no adverse effects on diastolic function [52] and is not associated with a significant increase in myocardial oxygen consumption in patients with chronic heart failure [53], though this result remains to be confirmed.

Levosimendan also induces dilatation of the pulmonary, systemic and coronary vasculature by activation of ATP-sensitive potassium channels resulting in a decreased systemic and pulmonary vascular resistance [54, 55]. This may cause under-perfusion of the myocardium, but the dilation of the coronary arteries results in improved myocardial blood flow [53]. Levosimendan improved haemodynamic performance and decreased the risk of worsening heart failure and mortality in different heart failure populations, compared with dobutamine or placebo [56, 57]. Indeed, all the evidence described comes from studies in patients with chronic heart failure, and the direct effects of levosimendan on RVF are currently unproven. However, from its known effects, including a demonstrated improvement in right ventricular contractile efficiency [53], beneficial effects in RVF may also be expected. The haemodynamic effects of levosimendan may be sustained for days, or even weeks, due to an active metabolite with a half-life of over 3 days [58].

Vasopressors

Vasopressors directly increase arterial blood pressure and improve coronary artery perfusion, though also increasing afterload. Their benefits in RVF were pioneered by Prewitt and co-workers and they may be critical in the treatment of RVF, preventing the vicious cycle by improving right coronary artery perfusion and right ventricular contraction [59, 60]. Norepinephrine, a potent -adrenergic-agonist is recommended to improve right coronary artery perfusion pressure and right ventricular function, and it is more effective than phenylephrine, another selective -adrenergic agonist [61]. In patients with septic shock, norepinephrine increased mean arterial pressure, with a moderate increase in mean pulmonary artery pressure, improving right coronary artery perfusion pressure and right ventricular contraction [60]. However, in the case report of sepsis-induced RVF (see below), norepinephrine increased organ perfusion pressure but not cardiac output, and combination with inhaled NO was therefore needed.

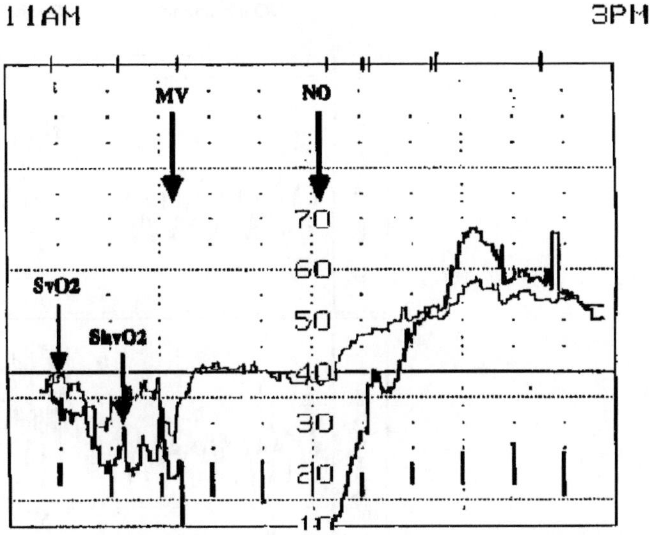

Fig. 2 Mixed venous oxygen saturation (SvO_2) increases and hepatic venous oxygen saturation ($ShvO_2$) decreases in response to the start of mechanical ventilation in a patient with predominantly right-sided congestive heart failure due to increased preload that worsens right ventricular function and hence organ congestion. Following nitric oxide inhalation, $ShvO_2$ increases indicating improved right ventricular function due to decreased preload and relieved liver congestion. *MV* start of mechanical ventilation, *NO* start of nitric oxide inhalation (18 ppm) (reproduced from Gatecel et al., 1995, with permission [23])

Mechanical ventilation

Mechanical ventilation is the usual treatment for shock, however it may worsen RVF as elevated transpulmonary pressures increase right ventricular output impedance and, hence, decrease stroke output. An example of severe hepatic and renal congestion due to subacute RVF markedly aggravated by mechanical ventilation is shown in Fig. 2 [23]. The patient had a low hepatic venous oxygen saturation caused by a high hepatic venous back-pressure that was reducing liver blood flow despite a maintained cardiac output. Due to respiratory fatigue, the patient was mechanically ventilated, which resulted in an improved mixed venous oxygen saturation, from 28 to 40%, related to the decreased respiratory work and, thus, systemic oxygen consumption. However, mechanical ventilation caused an abrupt decrease in hepatic venous oxygen saturation to an undetectable

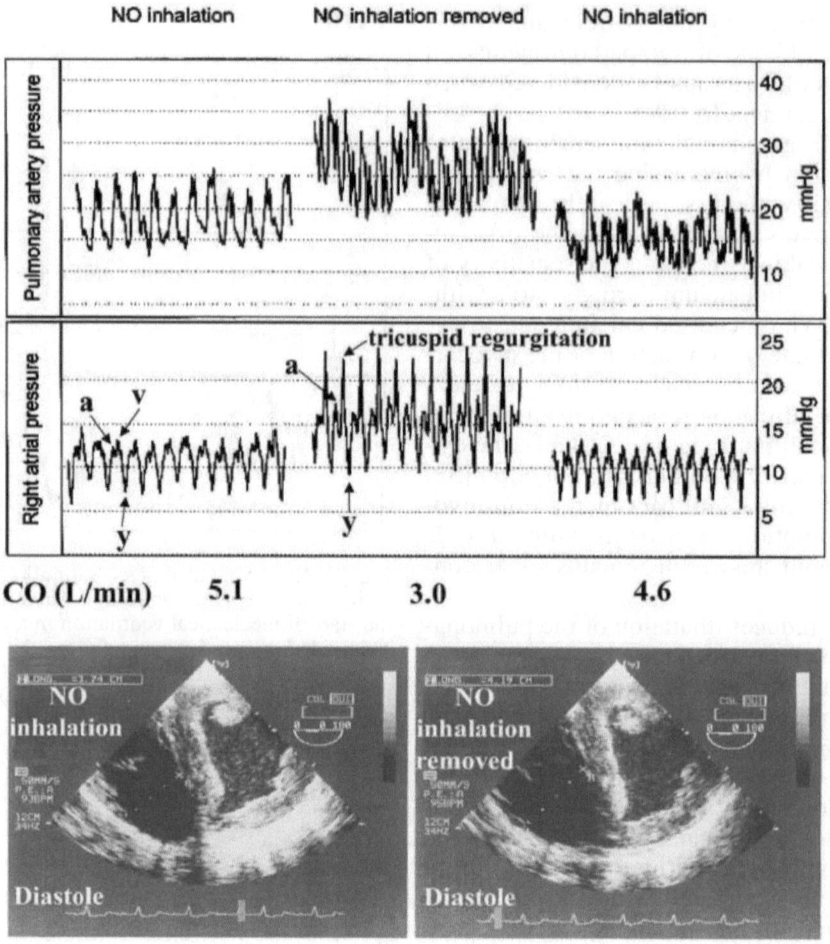

Fig. 3 Patient haemodynamics with and without inhaled nitric oxide (NO). Inhaled NO withdrawal in this patient with ischaemia-induced right ventricular failure increased mean pulmonary artery pressure from 18 to 25 mmHg. During NO inhalation and preserved right ventricular function, right atrial pressure showed 'a' waves (auricular contraction) followed by 'v' waves (passive atrial filling due to venous return) and 'y' waves (beginning of diastole: rapid ventricular filling and passive atrial emptying). When inhaled NO was removed, although pulmonary artery pressure remained in the normal range, the slight increase resulted in a deterioration of right ventricular function and dilation of the right ventricle. Right atrial pressure showed that a tricuspid insufficiency emerged (positive waves) that worsened cardiac output (CO) despite the increase in auricular contraction (increase in 'a' waves). Echocardiography shows the close association between the left and right ventricles separated by the inter-ventricular septum. An enlargement of the right ventricle can be seen, with the end-diastolic diameter increasing from 37 mm to 42 mm when NO inhalation was removed (Reproduced from 2002 Yearbook of Intensive Care and Emergency Medicine, Acute right ventricular failure: physiology and therapy by Renaud E, Karpati P, Mebazaa A, page 211, Fig. 1, and page 212, Fig. 2, 2002, Springer-Verlag, with permission [19])

level, which resulted from worsening RVF related to an increased right ventricular afterload due to positive pressure breathing. Consequently, right atrial pressure was raised, worsening the hepatic congestion. The subsequent use of NO inhalation decreased right ventricular afterload, improved right ventricular function and relieved liver congestion, demonstrated by the rapid increase in hepatic venous oxygen saturation as RVF was successfully controlled.

In summary, although several tools could be used to improve RVF, volume loading and mechanical ventilation should be used with caution because they may precipitate or aggravate RVF.

Illustrative case studies

The treatment of RVF often requires a multi-modal approach with continuous haemodynamic monitoring to observe the patient's progress. Three case studies are summarised below (and described in detail in the ESM) that highlight the diagnosis and treatment of acute RVF with therapy tailored specifically to the patient's diagnosis and haemodynamic status. These cases demonstrate that there are a number of treatment approaches that may result in a successful outcome. The new myocardial contractility-enhancing agents may obviate the use of some agents with a questionable long-term benefit.

Table 2 The treatment of sepsis-induced right ventricular failure with 'traditional' positive inotropic agents: the value of each parameter before and after the corresponding treatment (*DO* dobutamine, *NE* norepinephrine, *NO* inhaled nitric oxide, *VL* volume loading: 250 ml of colloids) had been given

Time	14:00 VL	15:30 VL	16:30 NE	20:30 DO/NO	23:30
HR (bpm)	90	90	90	94	92
BP (mmHg)	96/56	95/49	110/55	130/70	115/68
PAP (mmHg)	35/24	42/28	43/30	46/32	31/21
RAP (mmHg)	12	13	20	16	8
PCWP (mmHg)	12	12	14	15	10
SvO_2 (%)	70	71	65	63	74
CI (l/min per m^2)	2.3	2.3	2.0	1.9	2.8
Lactate (mmol/l)	3.3	3.6	3.8	4.0	4.1

HR heart rate, *BP* arterial blood pressure, *PAP* pulmonary artery pressure, *RAP* right atrial pressure, *PCWP* pulmonary capillary wedge pressure, SvO_2 mixed venous oxygen saturation, *CI* cardiac index

Effects of inhaled nitric oxide on ischaemia-related right ventricular failure following cardiac surgery

A 30-year-old male with acute RVF was treated with inhaled NO, 8 ppm, to reduce the afterload, which rapidly restored haemodynamics. When NO was withdrawn, right atrial pressure increased, cardiac output and arterial blood pressure dropped, there was tricuspid regurgitation and echocardiography showed a severe dilation of the RV (Fig. 3). NO was restored and the patient was weaned from treatment on the 7th postoperative day.

Sepsis-induced right ventricular failure treated with the combination of traditional positive inotropic agents and inhaled nitric oxide

A 55-year-old male had sepsis-induced myocardial dysfunction with a predominant RVF confirmed by echocardiography. Norepinephrine increased blood pressure but could not improve right ventricular function. The patient was subsequently treated with dobutamine, 5 g/kg per min, and inhaled NO, 5 ppm (Table 2). The combination induced a large, rapid and sustained decrease in right atrial pressure, pulmonary capillary wedge pressure was restored, mixed venous oxygen saturation and cardiac index were approaching normal values. A volume loading of 250 ml was given to improve organ perfusion pressure and subsequently the patient was haemodynamically stable and all parameters returned to values towards or within the normal range.

Ischaemia-induced right ventricular failure treated with calcium sensitiser monotherapy

Following coronary artery bypass graft surgery, a 71-year-old male was diagnosed with RVF and treated with levosimendan, 6 g/kg loading dose given over 10 min followed by a 0.1 g/kg per min infusion for 24 h. Four hours after the start of the levosimendan infusion, echocardiograhy showed an improvement in cardiac performance. At 24 h, echocardiography and haemodynamic values were almost restored to normal and the patient reported symptomatic improvement (echocardiography video available in the ESM). This improvement in right ventricular function was related to an improvement in right ventricular contractility and vasodilatory effects on the pulmonary circulation (decrease in pulmonary artery pressure).

Conclusion

It is now evident that the RV plays a pivotal role in haemodynamic homeostasis, and changes in right ventricular function can have profound effects on the pulmonary and systemic circulation. Therefore, it is important that RVF is diagnosed quickly and accurately before it degenerates into the vicious cycle of auto-aggravation with tricuspid deficiency, worsening cardiac ischaemia and multiple organ congestion. Diagnosis should include an assessment of the patient and the use of diagnostic tools that also enable the clinician to follow the progress of treatment.

The management of RVF should focus on restoring right ventricular function with the treatment dictated by the underlying aetiology. The primary cause of RVF should be corrected wherever possible. The right ventricular afterload should be reduced, if necessary, by decreasing the pulmonary artery pressure (e.g. by administering pulmonary vasodilators such as inhaled NO or prostacyclin) and limiting plateau pressure in mechanically ventilated patients, the preload should be increased cautiously with volume loading and an adequate right coronary artery perfusion maintained. Positive inotropic agents have an important role in the treatment of RVF by improving cardiac output and coronary perfusion. However, traditional inotropic drugs increase myocardial contractility by their sympathomimetic action at the expense of increasing myocardial intracellular calcium concentration and oxygen consumption. Calcium sensitisers, specifically levosimendan, enhance contractility without increasing myocardial oxygen consumption. If the beneficial effects that have been observed in chronic heart failure patients are validated in RVF in clinical studies, this class of agents may represent a valuable addition to the clinician's armamentarium for the management of this condition.

Acknowledgements We would like to acknowledge Professor Didier Payen for his critical review of the paper, Drs. Jan Eskilsson and Ulf Thilèn who performed the echocardiography shown in the ESM at the University Hospital in Lund, Sweden, and Professor Rymer and Dr Boudiaf, who performed the CT scan in Fig. S1 in the ESM.

References

1. Starr I, Jeffers WA, Meade RH (1943) The absence of conspicuous increments of venous pressure after severe damage to the RV of the dog, with discussion of the relation between clinical congestive heart failure and heart disease. Am Heart J 26:291–301
2. Cohen JN, Guiha NH, Broder MJ, Limas CJ (1974) Right ventricular infarction, clinical and hemodynamic features. Am J Cardiol 33:209–214
3. Health Central – General Encyclopaedia – right-sided heart failure http://www.healthcentral.com/mhc/top/000154.cfm. Accessed June 2002
4. Kannel WB, Belanger AJ (1991) Epidemiology of heart failure. Am Heart J 121:951–957
5. Jacobs AK, Leopold JA, Bates E, Mendes LA, Sleeper LA, White H, Davidoff R, Boland J, Modur S, Forman R, Hochman JS (2003) Cardiogenic shock caused by right ventricular infarction: a report from the SHOCK registry. J Am Coll Cardiol 41:1273–1279
6. Mehta SR, Eikelboom JW, Natarajan MK, Diaz R, Yi C, Gibbons RJ, Yusuf S (2001) Impact of right ventricular involvement on mortality and morbidity in patients with inferior myocardial infarction. J Am Coll Cardiol 37:37–43
7. Lupi-Herrera E, Lasses LA, Cosio-Aranda J, Chuquirue-Valenzuela E, Martinez-Sanchez C, Ortiz P, Gonzalez-Pacheco H, Juarez-Herrera U, Rodriguez Mdel C, Vargas-Barron J, Martinez-Rios MA (2002) Acute right ventricular infarction: clinical spectrum, results of reperfusion therapy and short-term prognosis. Coron Artery Dis 13:57–64
8. Stephanazzi J, Guidon-Attali C, Escarment J (1997) Right ventricular function: physiological and pathophysiological features. Ann Fr Anesth Reanim 16:165–186
9. Redington AN, Gray JJ, Hodson ME, Rigby ML, Oldershaw PJ (1988) Characterisation of the normal right ventricular pressure-volume relation by biplane angiography and simultaneous micromanometer pressure measurements. Br Heart J 59:23–30
10. Redington AN, Rigby ML, Shinebourne EA, Oldershaw PJ (1990) Changes in the pressure-volume relation of the right ventricle when its loading conditions are modified. Br Heart J 63:45–49
11. Matthay RA, Arroliga AC, Wiedemann HP, Schulman DS, Mahler DA (1992) Right ventricular function at rest and during exercise in chronic obstructive pulmonary disease. Chest 101:255S–262S
12. Brooks H, Kirk ES, Vokonas PS, Urschel CW, Sonnenblick EH (1971) Performance of the right ventricle under stress: relation to right coronary flow. J Clin Invest 50:2176–2183
13. Vieillard-Baron A, Page B, Augarde R, Prin S, Qandli S, Beauchet A, Dubourg O, Jardin F (2001) Acute cor pulmonale in massive pulmonary embolism: incidence, echocardiographic pattern, clinical implications and recovery rate. Intensive Care Med 27:1481–1486
14. Vieillard-Baron A, Prin S, Chergui K, Dubourg O, Jardin F (2002) Echo-Doppler demonstration of acute cor pulmonale at the bedside in the medical intensive care unit. Am J Respir Crit Care Med 166:1310–1319
15. Vieillard-Baron A, Schmitt JM, Augarde R, Fellahi JL, Prin S, Page B, Beauchet A, Jardin F (2001) Acute cor pulmonale in acute respiratory distress syndrome submitted to protective ventilation: incidence, clinical implications and prognosis. Crit Care Med 29:1551–1555
16. Jardin F (2003) Ventricular interdependence: how does it impact on hemodynamic evaluation in clinical practice? Intensive Care Med 29:361–363
17. Visner MC, Arentzen CE, O'Conner MJ, Larson EV, Anderson RW (1983) Alterations in left ventricular three-dimensional dynamic geometry and systolic function during acute right ventricular hypertension in the conscious dog. Circulation 67:353–365
18. Goto Y, Yamamoto J, Saito M, Haze K, Sumiyoshi T, Fukami K, Hiramori K (1985) Effects of right ventricular ischemia on left ventricular geometry and the end-diastolic pressure-volume relationship in the dog. Circulation 72:1104–1114
19. Renaud E, Karpati P, Mebazaa A (2002) Acute right ventricular failure: physiology and therapy. In: Vincent J-L (ed) 2002 yearbook of intensive care and emergency medicine Springer, Berlin Heidelberg New York, pp 209–218
20. Taylor RR, Covell JYW, Sonnenblick EH, Ross J (1967) Dependence of ventricular distensibility on filling of the opposite ventricle. Am J Physiol 218:711–718
21. Brookes C, Ravn H, White P, Moeldrup U, Oldershaw P, Redington A (1999) Acute right ventricular dilatation in response to ischemia significantly impairs left ventricular systolic performance. Circulation 100:761–767
22. Santamore WP, Gray LA (1996) Left ventricular contributions to right ventricular systolic function during LVAD support. Ann Thorac Surg 61:350–356
23. Gatecel C, Mebazaa A, Kong R, Guinard N, Kermarrec M, Matéo J, Payen D (1995) Inhaled nitric oxide improves hepatic tissue oxygenation in right ventricular failure: value of hepatic venous oxygen saturation monitoring. Anesthesiology 82:588–590
24. Dhainaut JF, Brunet F, Monsallier JF Villemant D, Devaux JY, Konnon M, De Gournay JM, Armaganidis A, Iotti G, Huyghebaert MF, Lanore JJ (1987) Bedside evaluation of right ventricular performance using a rapid computerized thermodilution method. Crit Care Med 15:148–152
25. Jardin F, Gueret P, Dubourg O, Farcot JC, Margairaz A, Bourdarias J-P (1985) Right ventricular volumes by thermodilution in the adult respiratory distress syndrome. A comparative study using two-dimensional echocardiography as a reference method. Chest 88:34–39
26. Zwissler B (2000) Acute right heart failure. Etiology-pathophysiology-diagnosis-therapy. Anaesthetist 49:788–808

27. Bowers TR, O'Neill WW, Grines C, Pica MC, Safian RD, Goldstein JA (1998) Effect of reperfusion on biventricular function and survival after right ventricular infarction. N Engl J Med 338:933–940
28. Potapov EV, Sodian R, Leobe M, Drew T, Dreysse S, Hetzer R (2001) Revascularization of the occluded right coronary artery during left ventricular assist device implantation. J Heart Lung Transplant 20:918–922
29. Mercat A, Kiehl JLK, Meyer G, Teboul JL, Sors H (1999) Hemodynamics effects of fluid loading in acute massive pulmonary embolism. Crit Care Med 27:540–544
30. Sibbald WJ, Driedger AA (1983) Right ventricular function in acute disease states: pathophysiologic considerations. Crit Care Med 11:339–345
31. Bundgaard H, Boesgaard S, Mortensen SA, Arendrup H, Aldershvile J (1997) Effect of nitroglycerin in patients with increased pulmonary vascular resistance undergoing cardiac transplantation Scand Cardiovasc J 31:339–342
32. Vincent JL, Carlier E, Pinsky MR, Goldstein J, Naeije R, Lejeune P, Brimioulle S, Leclerc JL, Kahn RJ, Primo G (1992) Prostaglandin E1 infusion for right ventricular failure after cardiac transplantation. J Thorac Cardiovasc Surg 103:33–39
33. Packer M (1985) Vasodilator therapy for primary pulmonary hypertension. Limitations and hazards. Ann Intern Med 103:258–270
34. Ghofrani HA, Wiedemann R, Rose F, Schermuly RT, Olschewski H, Weissmann N, Gunther A, Walmrath D, Seeger W, Grimminger F (2002) Sildenafil for treatment of lung fibrosis and pulmonary hypertension: a randomised controlled trial. Lancet 360:895–900
35. Langer F, Wendler O, Wilhelm W, Tscholl D, Schafers HJ (2001) Treatment of a case of acute right heart failure by inhalation of iloprost, a long-acting prostacylclin analogue. Eur J Anaestheiol 18:770–773
36. Haraldsson A, Kieler-Jensen N, Ricksten SE (1996) Inhaled prostacyclin for treatment of pulmonary hypertension after cardiac surgery or heart transplantation: a pharmacodynamic study. J Cardiothorac Vasc Anesth 10:864–868
37. Mosquera I, Crespo-Leiro MG, Tabuyo T, Paniagua MJ, Fuente L, Bouzas B, Fojon S, Pastor J, Juffe-Stein A, Castro-Beiras A (2002) Pulmonary hypertension and right ventricular failure after heart transplantation: usefulness of nitric oxide. Transplant Proc 34:166–167
38. Christenson J, Lavoie A, O'Connor M, Bhorade S, Pohlman A, Hall JB (2000) The incidence and pathogenesis of cardiopulmonary deterioration after abrupt withdrawal of inhaled nitric oxide. Am J Respir Crit Care Med 161:1443–1449
39. Borade S, Christenson J, O'Connor M, Lavoie A, Pohlman A, Hall JB (1999) Response to inhaled nitric oxide in patients with acute right heart syndrome. Am J Respir Crit Care Med 159:571–579
40. Palhares DB, Figueiredo CS, Moura AJ (1998) Endotracheal inhalatory sodium nitroprusside in severely hypoxic newborns. J Perinat Med 26:219–224
41. De Backer D, Moures JM, Vachiery JL, Leclerc JL, Kahn RJ, Vincent JL (1996) Oxygenation improvement with nitric oxide in right-to-left shunt without significant effects on pulmonary arterial pressure. Chest 110:1361–1363
42. Cholley BP, Guinard N, Mateo J, Payen D (1998) Improvement of extreme hypoxemia during end-stage congenital heart disease using nasal nitric oxide. Anesthesiology 89:1586–1587
43. Lowson SM, Doctor A, Walsh BK, Doorley PA (2002) Inhaled prostacyclin for the treatment of pulmonary hypertension after cardiac surgery. Crit Care Med 30:2762–2764
44. Lowson SM (2002) Inhaled alternatives to nitric oxide. Anesthesiology 96:1504–1513
45. Hoeper MM, Olschewski H, Ghofrani HA, Wilkens H, Winkler J, Borst MM, Niedermeyer J, Fabel H, Seeger W (2000) A comparison of the acute hemodynamic effects of inhaled nitric oxide and aerosolized iloprost in primary pulmonary hypertension. German PPH study group. J Am Coll Cardiol 36:176–182
46. Curtis JJ, McKenney-Knox CA, Wagner-Mann CC (2002) Postcardiotomy centrifugal assist: a single surgeon's experience. Artif Organs 26:994–997
47. Packer M, Leier CV (1987) Survival in congestive heart failure during treatment with drugs with positive inotropic actions. Circulation 75 (Suppl IV): 55–63
48. Packer M, Carver JR, Rodeheffer RJ, Ivanhoe RJ, DiBianco R, Zeldis SM, Hendrix GH, Bommer WJ, Elkayam U, Kukin ML, Mallis GI, Sollano JA, Shannon J, Tandon PK, DeMets DL for the PROMISE study Research Group (1991) Effect of oral milrinone on mortality in severe chronic heart failure. N Engl J Med 352:1468–1475
49. The Xamoterol in Severe Heart Failure Study Group (1990) Xamoterol in severe heart failure. Lancet 336:1–6
50. O'Connor CM, Gattis WA, Uretsky BF, Adams KF Jr, McNulty SE, Grossman SH, McKenna WJ, Zannad F, Swedberg K, Gheorghiade M, Califf RM (1999) Continuous intravenous dobut-amine is associated with an increased risk of death in patients with advanced heart failure: insights from the Flolan International Randomized Survival Trial (FIRST). Am Heart J 138:78–86
51. Unverferth DA, Blanford M, Kates RE, Leier CV (1980) Tolerance to dobutamine after a 72 hour continuous infusion. Am J Med 69:262–266
52. Haikala H, Nissinen E, Etemadzadeh E, Kevijoki J, Linden I-B (1995) Troponin C-mediated calcium sensitization induced by levosimendan does not impair relaxation. J Cardiovasc Pharmacol 25:794–801
53. Ukkonen H, Saraste M, Akkila J, Knuuti MJ, Karanko M, Iida H, Lehikoinen P, Nagren K, Lehtonen L, Voipio-Pulkki LM (2000) Myocardial efficiency during levosimendan infusion in congestive heart failure. Clin Pharmacol Ther 68:522–531
54. Yokoshiki H, Katsube Y, Sunagawa M, Sperelakis N (1997) Levosimendan, a novel calcium sensitizer, activates the glibenclamide-sensitive K^+ channel in rat arterial myocytes. Eur J Pharmacol 333:249–259
55. Slawsky MT, Colucci WS, Gottlieb SS (2000) Acute hemodynamic and clinical effects of levosimendan in patients with severe heart failure. Circulation 102:2222–2227
56. Follath F, Cleland JG, Just H, Papp JG, Scholz H, Peuhkurinen K, Harjola VP, Mitrovic V, Abdalla M, Sandell EP, Lehtonen L (2002) Efficacy and safety of intravenous levosimendan compared with dobutamine in severe low-output heart failure (the LIDO study): a randomised double-blind trial. Lancet 20:196–202
57. Moiseyev VS, Poder P, Andrejevs N, Ruda MY, Golikov AP, Lazebnik LB, Kobalava ZD, Lehtonen LA, Laine T, Nieminen MS, Lie KI (2002) Safety and efficacy of a novel calcium sensitizer, levosimendan, in patients with left ventricular failure due to an acute myocardial infarction. A randomized, placebo-controlled, double-blind study (RUSSLAN). Eur Heart J 23:1422–1432

58. Kivikko M, Antila S, Eha J, Lehtonen L, Pentikainen PJ (2002) Pharmacokinetics of levosimendan and its metabolites during and after a 24-hour continuous infusion in patients with sever heart failure. Int J Clin Pharmacol Ther 40:465–471
59. Molloy WD, Lee KY, Girling L, Schick U, Prewitt RM (1984) Treatment of shock in a canine model of pulmonary embolism. Am Rev Respir Dis 130:870–874
60. Ghignone M, Girling L, Prewitt RM (1984) Volume expansion versus norepinephrine in treatment of a low cardiac output complicating an acute increase in right ventricular afterload in dogs. Anesthesiology 60:132–135
61. Hirsch LJ, Rooney MW, Wat SS, Kleinmann B, Mathru M (1991) Norepinephrine and phenylephrine effects on right ventricular function in experimental canine pulmonary embolism. Chest 100:796–801

M. Piagnerelli
K. Zouaoui Boudjeltia
M. Vanhaeverbeek
J.-L. Vincent

Red blood cell rheology in sepsis

Abstract Changes in red blood cell (RBC) function can contribute to alterations in microcirculatory blood flow and cellular dysoxia in sepsis. Decreases in RBC and neutrophil deformability impair the passage of these cells through the microcirculation. While the role of leukocytes has been the focus of many studies in sepsis, the role of erythrocyte rheological alterations in this syndrome has only recently been investigated. RBC rheology can be influenced by many factors, including alterations in intracellular calcium and adenosine triphosphate (ATP) concentrations, the effects of nitric oxide, a decrease in some RBC membrane components such as sialic acid, and an increase in others such as 2,3 diphosphoglycerate. Other factors include interactions with white blood cells and their products (reactive oxygen species), or the effects of temperature variations. Understanding the mechanisms of altered RBC rheology in sepsis, and the effects on blood flow and oxygen transport, may lead to improved patient management and reductions in morbidity and mortality.

Keywords Erythrocyte · Deformability · Nitric oxide · Sialic acid · Multiple organ failure · Oxygen transport

Introduction

Severe sepsis and septic shock are the commonest causes of death in intensive care units (ICUs), with associated mortality rates of 30–50% [1]. Sepsis is a complex pathophysiological process that involves both alterations in the microcirculation and changes in the biochemical and physiological characteristics of the blood constituents. Microvascular damage plays a crucial role in the impairment of tissue oxygenation that can contribute to multiple organ failure and death [2].

Microcirculatory alterations include slowing of capillary blood flow as a result of decreased perfusion pressure and local arteriolar constriction [2, 3], viscosity alterations [4, 5], and disturbances of red (RBC) and white (WBC) blood cell rheology [6, 7].

Some recent studies [8, 9, 10] have also defined the RBC as a possible oxygen sensor and regulator of vascular tone, opening new perspectives into the pathophysiology of microcirculatory alterations and, perhaps, the treatment of sepsis.

This review evaluates alterations occurring in RBC rheology during sepsis and possible underlying mechanisms. The potential implications of blood transfusion and erythropoietin administration in sepsis will not be discussed.

Major determinants of RBC rheology

Viscosity

Haemorheology is the study of deformation and flow of blood and blood cells. The prime function of blood is transport by flow, and the most important rheological property of blood is its resistance to flow, or viscosity. The definition of viscosity is explained in Fig. 1. Plasma viscosity is about 1.6 times that of water (normal range 1.15–1.35 mPa/s). Blood is a non-Newtonian fluid and

M.R. Pinsky et al. (eds.), *Applied Physiology in Intensive Care Medicine 2: Physiological Reviews and Editorials*,
DOI 10.1007/978-3-642-28233-1_14, © Springer-Verlag Berlin Heidelberg 2012

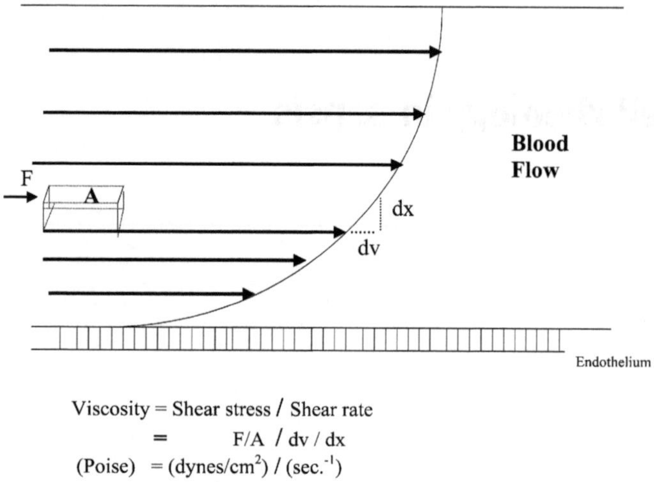

Fig. 1 Blood viscosity. Schematic representation of a vessel lumen. The curved line represents the flow velocity profile in laminar flow. The viscosity (unit: Poise) is expressed as a ratio of shear stress to shear rate, where the shear stress (unit: dynes/cm^2) is the force (*F*) parallel to the direction of flow per unit area of fluid sheared (*A*), and the shear rate (unit: second^{-1}) is the velocity gradient between adjacent layers in laminar flow. [*dv* velocity difference of adjacent fluid laminae, *dx* distance between the fluid laminae (adapted from [5], with permission)]

its viscosity is therefore variable at any given temperature, depending on the shear rate. Haematocrit has a large effect on blood viscosity and blood flow. For example, hyperviscosity syndromes, such as polycythaemia, are associated with profound perfusion problems [11]; in contrast, anaemia favours an increase in cardiac output. In physiological conditions, changes in blood viscosity do not have a pronounced effect on blood flow. However, in low flow states, a reduction in shear rate will cause an increase in viscosity. Blood viscosity, therefore, has the potential to reduce flow under low flow, low shear conditions [3, 4, 5].

When RBCs are added to plasma, blood viscosity increases logarithmically with a linear increase in haematocrit over the range 20–60%. At high shear rates, bulk blood viscosity is low because RBC aggregates are dispersed and deformed into ellipsoids, oriented in parallel with flow streamlines, and with the membrane sliding around its cytoplasm. As shear rates are reduced, blood viscosity rises exponentially. In low flow states, when the shear stress acting on the cell is reduced, the RBC is less deformed; furthermore, the RBCs aggregate to form rouleaux, increasing blood viscosity. In the normal circulation the shear stress is generally sufficient to disperse the rouleaux, allowing RBC deformation and facilitating blood flow [3, 4, 5]. Therefore, the major determinants of whole blood viscosity are shear rate, plasma viscosity, haematocrit, RBC deformability, and RBC aggregation.

It is possible to measure plasma and whole blood viscosity over a wide range of shear rates in a variety of viscometers. Serum viscosity (i.e., plasma viscosity less the effect of fibrinogen) and whole blood viscosity can be measured.

Aggregation

At low shear rates, blood evolves from a low viscosity emulsion to a high viscosity suspension. The electrostatic repulsion of RBC is overcome by the presence of macromolecules which aggregate the cells. In inflammatory states, acute phase proteins (especially fibrinogen and large serum proteins such as a_2 macroglobulin) increase RBC aggregation. Rouleaux of cells bind together in a side-by-side fashion and, together with the continuous uptake of individual cells, networks of larger aggregates are formed.

RBC aggregation is reversible by shear forces. At shear rates of 7–10 s^{-1}, the aggregates in normal blood are dispersed, cells become orientated with flow streamlines, and blood viscosity is reduced as the shear rates increase further. In vitro, this process of aggregation and disaggregation can continue for hours.

In addition to the plasma protein pattern, RBC aggregation is primarily determined by cellular properties; reduction in cell size increases aggregation as does RBC ageing. The haematocrit shows a biphasic effect on red cell aggregation, with a peak effect at around 40–45%.

Conditions of low shear rate in vivo are found primarily in the post-capillary venules. An increase in RBC aggregation would increase blood viscosity at this level [12]. The increased viscosity may promote blood stasis, which may induce local hypoxia and endothelial damage.

There are several methods of estimating RBC aggregation other than low shear rate viscometry, for example, erythrocyte sedimentation rate and direct microscopic observation of aggregation. Microscopic techniques with image analysis have also been developed [13], but the most widely used technique is the light scattering analysis of RBC suspensions that employs light transmission through a RBC suspension to obtain indices of RBC aggregation. This is expressed mainly as the average aggregate size at a certain shear stress.

Deformability

'Cellular deformability' is the term generally used to characterize the RBC's ability to undergo deformation during flow [14]. The deformation response of a RBC to fluid forces is a complex phenomenon that depends on a number of different cell characteristics including membrane material properties [15], cell geometry, and cytoplasmic viscosity [16].

As measures of cellular deformability are dependent on the technique used, quoted values are not comparable.

Methods to measure cellular deformability have been described in detail elsewhere [17, 18]. Briefly, micropipette aspiration provides the most detailed characterization of membrane properties. Single RBCs are aspirated into micropipettes with diameters in the range 1–2 µm; the relationship between the applied negative pressure and the membrane tongue extension is then quantitated. Using ektacytometry, RBCs are subjected to a laminar shear stress field in a cuvette viscometer; the resultant change in cell shape is continuously monitored by laser diffractometry. Unstressed discoid cells generate a circular diffraction pattern. By measuring optical densities at two points along the major and minor axes of the elliptical diffraction pattern, a parameter termed "deformability index" is generated which is a direct measure of cell ellipticity. A numerical value of zero corresponds to non-deformable cells, while increasingly positive values correspond to increasing cellular deformability. The membrane fragmentation assay using the ektacytometer is particularly useful for documenting decreased mechanical integrity of the membrane due to protein defects.

Micropore filtration is limited by the possible occlusion of the filter pores by WBCs [6]. This technique has been replaced by the cell transit analyzer (CTA) as it is insensitive to the presence of WBCs while the passage of individual RBCs are monitored by a computerized system.

Flow cytometry techniques can also be used to appreciate RBC shape, and to study the effect of modifications of osmolality on shape in critically ill patients [19, 20]. The advantage of this technique is that it can provide an easier and more rapid estimation of erythrocyte shape.

RBC Membrane physiology

To undertake oxygen delivery, the RBC must be able to undergo considerable cellular deformation since its diameter (8 µm in humans) far exceeds that of the capillaries (2–3 µm) through which it must pass [14]. The RBC membrane is composed of proteins (52% in weight), lipids (40%), and carbohydrates (8%). Membrane elasticity depends on the structural interactions between the outer plasma membrane and the underlying protein skeleton. The proteins of the RBC membrane are divided into two groups: integral and peripheral (Fig. 2). Integral proteins (glycophorin and Band 3 proteins) are tightly bound to the membrane through hydrophobic interactions lipids in the bilayer [14, 15, 16]. A filamentous network of proteins is anchored to the bilayer by the integral proteins. This network has three principal components: spectrin, actin, and protein 4.1. The peripheral membrane proteins are located on the cytoplasmic surface of the lipid bilayer and can be readily released from the membrane by simple manipulation of the ionic strength of the milieu or variation in the concentrations of other proteins [14].

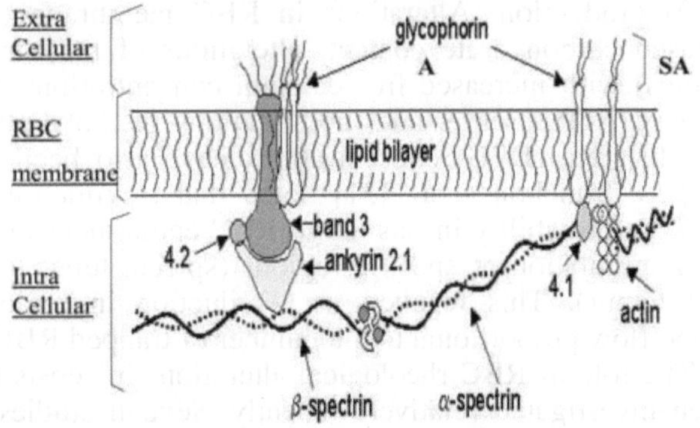

Fig. 2 RBC membrane. Schematic representation of protein orientations in the human RBC. The membrane is composed of a phospholipid membrane bilayer and transmembrane proteins including glycophorin A and Band 3 proteins. Glycophorin A is the major sialoglycoprotein of the RBC. SA bound to glycophorin A is responsible for the negative charge of the RBC membrane. The intracellular compartment (IC) is constituted by spectrin (and subunits), actin, protein 4.1, protein 4.2, and ankyrin

Reversible deformation of the RBC membrane occurs with a change in geometric shape without any change in surface area. With increased deformation, some of the spectrin molecules can attain their maximal linear extension, reaching the limit of reversible deformability [14].

The most abundant and best-studied integral protein of the RBC membrane is glycophorin A. This protein is highly glycosylated, with approximately 60% of its weight being carbohydrate, mostly in the form of 15 O-glycosidically linked tetrasaccharides. The two sialic acid residues (N-acetyl-neuraminic acid; SA) account for the negative electrostatic force on the RBC membrane [14, 15, 16], a necessary feature of the cell's repellent properties. The importance of SA to RBC shape is demonstrated by the observation that neuraminidase-treated cells, which release their membrane SA content, undergo increased aggregation and have a reduced mean curvature [21].

Alterations in microcirculation and blood rheology in sepsis

Sepsis induces profound changes in the microcirculation [2] with loss of capillary density [22], maldistribution of blood flow, increased flow heterogeneity [23], changes in microvascular reactivity [24], and WBC-endothelial cell adhesion and vascular leakage [2].

Microcirculatory dysfunction may be further aggravated by alterations in blood rheology resulting from decreased RBC [2, 6, 12, 25, 26, 27] and WBC deformability [2, 7], RBC aggregation [28, 29] and coagulation disturbances [30]. Interactions with WBCs cause release of oxygen free radicals, stimulating RBC intracellular proteolysis, membrane lipid peroxidation, and nitric oxide

(NO) production. Alterations in RBC membrane (decreased carbohydrate content, alterations of membrane pumps) with increased free calcium concentrations, decreased ATP reserve, and modifications of 2,3 diphosphoglycerate (DPG) concentrations have also been described. Simchon et al. [31] noted that a reduction in RBC deformability in rats led to RBC entrapment in the microcirculation of specific regions (spleen, lung, liver, and femur). This resulted in a reduction in regional blood flow proportional to the number of trapped RBCs.

The role of RBC rheological alterations in sepsis has been investigated relatively recently. Several studies in animals and patients with sepsis have demonstrated decreased RBC deformability, increased aggregation and adhesiveness between WBCs, platelets, and endothelial cells [6, 25, 27, 29, 32]. Moreover, alterations in RBC deformability have been described as an early indicator of infection in trauma patients [33], and as a prognostic factor in canine septic shock [34].

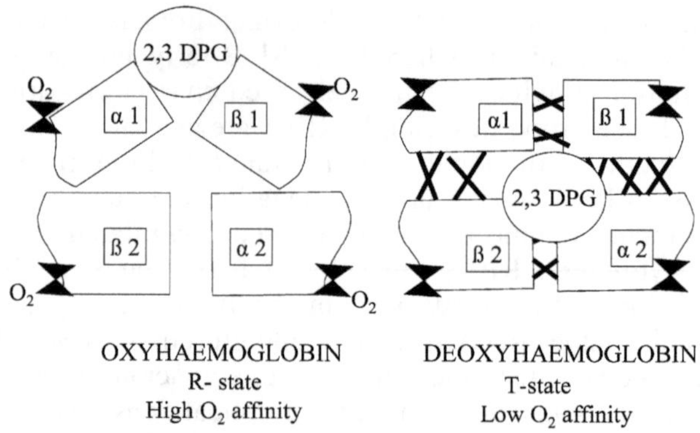

Fig. 3 Role of 2,3 diphosphoglycerate. Diagrammatic representation of the subunit interaction in haemoglobin as O_2 is added. Deoxyhaemoglobin (*right*), with low O_2 affinity, is in the T-state, constrained by salt bridges (*black crosses*) and 2,3 DPG. As O_2 is added in haem (*black double triangles*), the salt bridges are broken (*black dots*), and the 2,3 DPG molecule is expelled, resulting in the R configuration with higher O_2 affinity. As 2,3 DPG lowers the affinity of haemoglobin toward O_2, O_2 transfer from blood to tissues in the microcirculation is increased

Mechanisms underlying alterations in RBC deformability during sepsis

2,3 diphosphoglycerate (2,3 DPG)

2,3 DPG is one of the most important organic phosphates in the RBC (Fig. 3) as it increases oxygen delivery to the tissues by decreasing the interaction between oxygen and haemoglobin. Hypoxaemia stimulates 2,3 DPG production. Han and colleagues [35] reported an increase in 2,3 DPG in critically ill children, even in the absence of hypoxaemia. This may represent a possible response to illness with increased oxygen unloading to the tissues. However, increased 2,3 DPG can also decrease RBC deformability. Suzuki et al. [36] reported that increasing the 2,3-DPG concentration (by incubating human RBCs with inosine and pyruvate) increased intracellular haemoglobin concentrations (MCHC) and ATP content, and decreased intracellular pH. The deformability of 2,3-DPG-enriched RBC was greatly improved when the MCHC (and thus the internal viscosity) was normalized by suspension in a hypotonic solution, but not when the intracellular pH was altered from 6.5 to 7.5, or when the ATP concentration was adjusted by incubation with various concentrations of adenine, inosine, and glucose (0.6–2.1 mM/cells). Hence, decreased RBC deformability is due in part to the increase in internal viscosity, and in part to the increase in membrane viscoelasticity [36].

Nitric oxide (NO)

RBC and modulation of vascular tone via NO

NO is produced by endothelial cells from L-arginine by constitutive (cNOS) or inducible (iNOS) synthase. In physiological conditions, cNOS plays an essential role in producing small amounts of NO, thus maintaining capillary patency. In sepsis, lipopolysaccharide (LPS) and cytokines such as tumour necrosis factor (TNF) and interferon- (INF-) induce iNOS, resulting in the production of much greater quantities of NO. By its action on vascular smooth muscle, NO causes vasodilatation and increased tissue blood flow, but may also lead to arterial hypotension [37]. In the lung, NO rapidly binds to haemoglobin (T-state, 'tense', low oxygen affinity state, partially nitrosylated), forming a relatively stable haemoglobin-NO complex (R-state, 'relaxed', high oxygen affinity state, ligand-bound). Oxyhaemoglobin (R-state) is thus converted to methaemoglobin and nitrate. NO is released by haemoglobin (R-state) in the peripheral circulation, resulting in opening of the microvasculature [38, 39]. Allosteric transition from the R- to the T-state is triggered by oxygen release in the pre-capillary resistance vessels, which is then followed by release of NO. In the lungs, after eliminating carbon dioxide (CO_2) and H^+, haemoglobin (in the T-state) re-captures oxygen and NO and switches back to the R-state [38, 39].

Sprague and colleagues [40, 41] demonstrated this essential role of RBCs on NO release in isolated perfused rabbit lungs. Based on several observations, they showed that ATP is a key mediator for NO release as RBCs contain large amounts of ATP [42] that are released in response to physiological stimuli [8]. Moreover, ATP stimulates endothelial NO synthesis [43], thereby reducing vascular resistance in isolated lungs; this is prevented by the NO synthase inhibitor NG-nitro-L-arginine methyl ester (L-NAME) [40].

In dogs, ATP is also a mediator of NO release. However, in response to mechanical deformation, dog RBCs release much less ATP than rabbit or human RBCs [41]. This may be related to the much lower ATP concentrations found in dog RBCs compared to rabbits and humans [44].

NO is also a modulator of the membrane properties of RBC although the exact mechanism involved is as yet unclear. By an effect on the membrane RBC Ca^{2+}-ATPase channel, NO may increase free intracellular Ca^{2+} and thus decrease RBC deformability. In blood samples from healthy volunteers, endotoxin induced a significant increase in both intracellular Ca^{2+} concentration (evaluated by a fluorescent membrane probe) and membrane viscosity (anisotropy, evaluated by fluorescence spectrophotometry) [45]. Addition of the NO synthase inhibitor N- monomethyl-arginine (NMA) had no effect in control conditions but prevented the changes induced by endotoxin, suggesting that NO plays a role in intracellular Ca^{2+} homeostasis and erythrocyte membrane deformability in sepsis.

RBCs as producers of NO

Several studies have indicated that RBCs have the capacity to synthesize NO under certain conditions [46, 47]. Jubelin et al. [48] suggested that the RBC possesses all the cellular machinery necessary to synthesize its own NO.

Plasmodium falciparum-infected human RBCs can also produce NO, probably by the activation of iNOS [47]. By this means, RBCs may modulate their membrane deformability and oxygen affinity, and perhaps also contribute to the inflammatory host response by reacting with reactive oxygen species (ROS).

Effect of NO on RBC deformability

Korbut and Gryglewski [49] noted that alterations in deformability of isolated rabbit RBCs depended on the WBC concentration; WBCs decreased RBC deformability when the WBC count was below 1.2 10^6 cells/ml, while higher WBC counts abolished this effect. In the presence of a low WBC count, RBC deformability was increased by NO donors, such as sydnonimine (a metabolite of molsidomine; SIN-1) and sodium nitroprusside, but was reduced by the NO synthase inhibitor L-NAME. In endotoxaemic rats, these same authors [50] noted altered RBC deformability (as measured by shear stress laser diffractometry) associated with increased RBC membrane fragility. L-NAME significantly decreased RBC deformability but did not influence fragility. However, L-NAME administration 10 min prior to endotoxin administration also improved endotoxin-induced fragility. This indicates that NO influences RBC deformability and membrane fragility in the first stages of sepsis, probably by stimulation of cNOS [50].

Bateman et al. [51] recently demonstrated that aminoguanidine, an inhibitor of iNOS, prevented the accumulation of NO within the RBC in a rat model of peritonitis, and also prevented the decrease in RBC deformability. Thus, NO may play a role in modulating the mechanical properties of the RBC in vivo. Whether this is a direct action, with NO interfering with cytoskeletal elements, or indirect, via some intermediate such as peroxynitrite oxidizing cellular proteins [52], is unknown.

RBC calcium (Ca^{2+})

RBC membrane fluidity is dependent upon the maintenance of a normal intracellular Ca^{2+} concentration [53]. This is kept within a narrow range (20–30 nM), some 50,000-fold lower than the external free Ca^{2+} concentration, by a membrane-associated ATPase pump mechanism. In human RBCs, as in most cell types, a rise in cytosolic free Ca^{2+} induces a rapid increase in the potassium permeability by activation of a Ca^{2+}-activated K^+ channel, resulting in membrane hyperpolarization [54].

Increased intracellular Ca^{2+} levels in aged RBC may precipitate their removal from the circulation [53]. Sepsis-associated changes in the RBC membrane may alter pump binding sites, inhibit their function, and disrupt intracellular Ca^{2+} homeostasis [55]. Alterations in the RBC Ca^{2+}-ATPase pump in sepsis remain controversial. Todd and Mollitt [56] reported that intracellular (free cytosolic) RBC Ca^{2+} concentrations (determined by fluorescent spectroscopy) are increased in septic surgical patients as in experimental endotoxemia. RBCs incubated with endotoxin had increased intracellular Ca^{2+} concentrations, but these did not correlate with extracellular Ca^{2+} levels. This phenomenon was not prevented by dantrolene, an inhibitor of intracellular Ca^{2+} release, and only partially prevented by calcium-channel blockade, but it was minimized by adenosine or ATP. It was also partially reversed by post-treatment with ATP, but not with adenosine [56]. These same authors [57] noted in an in vitro study that endotoxin increased intracellular free Ca^{2+} within RBCs but only in the presence of WBCs. Pretreatment of these RBCs with allopurinol (xanthine oxidase inhibitor), superoxide dismutase (free radical scavenger), or pentoxifylline (WBC modulator) significantly limited the rise in intracellular Ca^{2+} concentrations induced by endotoxin.

Ca^{2+} channel blockers are unable to influence the deformability of normal RBCs [58, 59]. In diabetic patients, where intracellular Ca^{2+} are increased, some studies have demonstrated a beneficial effect of Ca^{2+} channel blockers on RBC deformability, but at concentrations up to ten times higher than those clinically attainable (10^{-8} mol/l) [59]. Further investigations are necessary to fully define the effects of Ca^{2+}-channel blockers on RBC deformability in sepsis.

ATP

RBCs contain millimolar quantities of ATP [44]. These are produced within the cell by membrane-bound glycolytic pathways, and are used to maintain intracellular hydration and electrolyte composition [42]. ATP content is decreased in old RBCs [42], and this is accompanied by a loss of surface membrane SA, which might be a primary factor in the removal of old RBCs by the reticuloendothelial system.

Bergfeld and Forrester [60] documented that human RBC can release ATP in response to a hypoxic challenge. As ATP binds to receptors on the vascular endothelium, vessel calibre increases and regional blood flow improves [8, 43]. RBCs may act not only as oxygen transporters but also as oxygen sensors able to modify oxygen delivery.

Intracellular RBC ATP levels are decreased in sepsis [56], causing a decrease in energy for the Ca^{2+} RBC membrane pump, thereby increasing RBC intracellular Ca^{2+} and resulting in a decrease in cell deformability. Pretreatment with pentoxifylline may improve RBC deformability through a direct increase in intracellular ATP content [57].

Sialic acid content of the RBC membrane

Decreased RBC SA may be an important mechanism of senescent RBC destruction by the reticulo-endothelial system [61]. Eichelbronner et al. [32] demonstrated that endotoxin promotes adhesion of human RBCs to endothelial cells in vitro, probably by decreasing SA on the RBC membrane, and thereby decreasing the repulsive force between RBCs and the endothelium.

While the effects of SA on RBC aggregation have been well described, the effects of SA on RBC shape remain controversial. We have recently demonstrated a decreased RBC membrane SA content in patients with sepsis that was associated with a modification of RBC shape [62]. Hence, there is a possible link between RBC membrane SA content and RBC shape in sepsis, as is described in other diseases such as diabetes mellitus [63, 64]. Several mechanisms may account for the decrease in SA. There may be increased activity of the SA degrading enzyme, sialidase, either by WBC as has been described in diabetic patients [65], or by the RBC membrane sialidases themselves [66]. Another mechanism could be a direct effect of bacteria upon the RBC [67].

White blood cells (WBC)

Various factors can alter RBC membrane properties including direct contact between RBCs and WBCs [29, 68, 69] or ROS that stimulate intracellular proteolysis and membrane lipid peroxidation [70, 71].

Several studies have reported that WBCs in sepsis have increased rigidity and enhanced aggregation with platelets and RBCs [7, 72, 73]. During inflammation, large numbers of WBCs adhere to or roll along the microvascular endothelium (margination), primarily in the postcapillary venules and only occasionally in the arterioles [13, 29, 74]. In the capillaries, the WBCs usually appear to flow smoothly without rotation. Occasionally, WBCs may impede RBC flow [74]. Berliner et al. [13], using a method involving a slide test and image analysis, demonstrated that both WBC and RBC adhesiveness/aggregation were increased in the peripheral venous blood of septic patients. This phenomenon may impair microvascular flow in sepsis. Moreover, activation of WBCs stimulates multiple mediator networks including the complement, kinin, coagulation and fibrinolytic cascades, along with the release of chemokines, cytokines, soluble receptors, lipid mediators, reactive oxygen species (ROS) and numerous enzymes, including elastase, myeloperoxidase and many proteases [75]. Claster and colleagues [76] demonstrated that ROS released by these activated WBC can attack RBC membranes, causing alterations in lipid and protein structure that may decrease RBC deformability and, ultimately, result in hemolysis. These authors and others also demonstrated a dose-response curve for WBC-mediated lipid peroxidation in RBCs [76, 77].

Reactive oxygen species (ROS)

Sepsis is characterized by increased production of ROS [superoxide anion (O_2^-), hydroxyl radical (OH^-), and hydrogen peroxide H_2O_2)] as well as a decrease in antioxidant defences. Damage occurs when ROS production exceeds the tissues' antioxidant defences [71, 78]. ROS produced by WBCs can also damage haemoglobin and induce haemolysis [76, 77]. Uyesaka et al. [79] demonstrated that RBCs exposed to O_2^- displayed pronounced degradation of membrane proteins (band 3 and spectrin) with formation of new protein bands that can decrease RBC deformability. In sepsis induced by caecal ligation and puncture in rats, Powell et al. [80, 81] demonstrated that the loss of RBC deformability—with increased survival—could be prevented by pre-treatment with the antioxidant a-tocopherol.

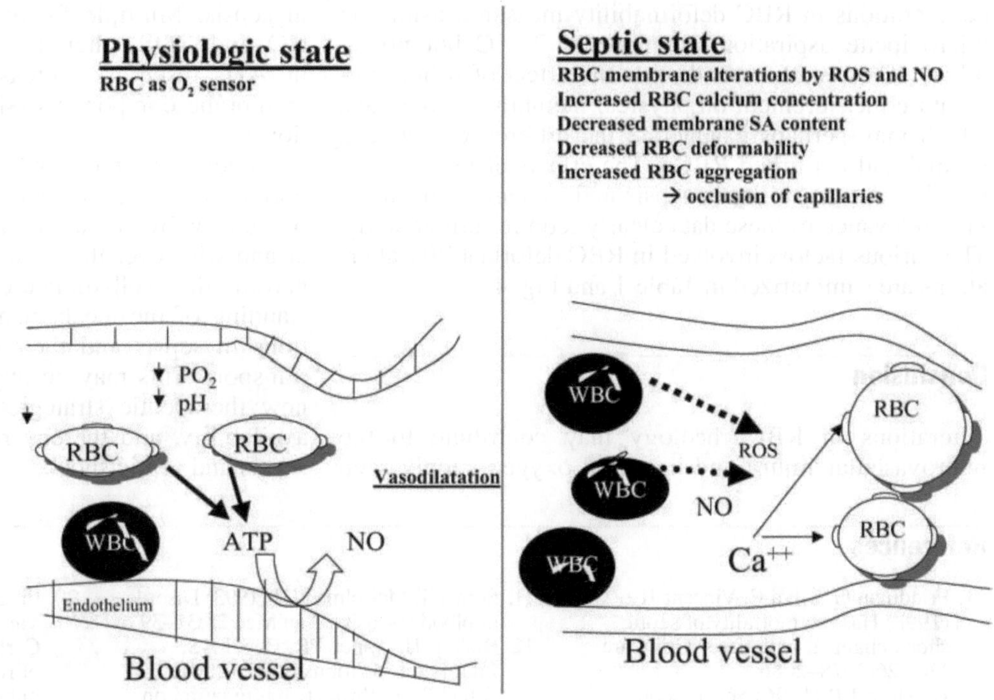

Fig. 4 Schematic relationship between RBCs, WBCs and endothelium. *Left panel:* low PO_2, acidic pH, and decreased RBC deformability lead to ATP liberation from RBCs. These ATP molecules stimulate the endothelial cells to release NO, promoting vasodilatation. *Right panel:* septic conditions with decreased RBC deformability and increased RBC volume with RBC haemolysis. ROS were liberated by the WBC and attack the RBC membrane. The increase in NO induced by sepsis raised the intracellular Ca^{++}. This elevated Ca^{++} impairs the RBC membrane skeleton causing a decline in RBC deformability

Table 1 Some factors influencing RBC deformability

Factor	Potential effects	References
2,3 diphosphoglycerate	Increases tissue O_2 delivery	[35]
	Decreases RBC deformability by increased internal viscosity	[36]
Nitric oxide	Bound by haemoglobin	[37, 38, 39, 40, 41, 42, 43]
	Modulates vascular tone	[39, 40, 41, 43]
	Synthesized by RBC?	[46, 47, 48]
	Modulates RBC membrane properties	[45, 49, 50, 51, 52]
Intracellular calcium	Increased intracellular concentrations by decreased activity of Ca^{++}-ATPase pump	[53, 54, 55, 56, 57]
Adenosine triphosphate	Mediates NO release	[8, 40, 41, 43]
	Maintains intracellular hydration and activity of ionic pumps	[42, 56, 57, 60]
	Released by RBC to improve blood flow	[8, 43, 60]
Sialic acid	Signal recognition for capture by the reticulo-endothelial system.	[61, 64]
	Modifies RBC shape	[62, 63, 64]
	Increases RBC aggregation	[32, 61, 63]
White blood cells	Increase aggregation with RBCs	[7, 13, 29, 68, 69, 72, 73, 74]
	Produce ROS	[70, 71, 75, 76, 77, 79, 80, 81]
Reactive oxygen species (ROS)	Induce degradation of RBC membrane proteins	[71, 76, 77, 78]
	Decrease RBC deformability	[79, 80, 81]
Temperature	Influences in vitro results of RBC deformability	[82, 83, 84, 85]

Effects of temperature

RBC membrane mechanical properties are known to be temperature sensitive. Temperature can have significant effects on RBC deformability. In RBCs from healthy subjects, the elongation index (representing deformability) decreased significantly with a fall in temperature from 37 °C to 5 °C [82]. Artmann and colleagues [83] noted that human RBCs undergo a sudden change from blocking to passing through 1.3±0.2 µm micropipettes at a critical temperature of 36.4±0.3 °C. The authors attributed these findings to an elastomeric transition of haemoglobin from gel-like to fluid, and to an elastomeric transition of membrane proteins such as spectrin [83].

In septic and non-septic rats, Baskurt and Mat [84] noted differences in RBC elongation index only at 37 °C using ektacytometry, while in RBCs from rats incubated with endotoxin (*E. coli*; 75 µg/ml), Jagger et al. [85] noted alterations in RBC deformability measured using the micropipette aspiration technique at 25 °C but not at 37 °C. These authors underline the effect of room temperature measurement on physical membrane properties, which may perhaps exaggerate the differences between normal and perturbed RBCs. The effects of temperature on RBC deformability in sepsis and, in particular, the in vivo relevance of these data clearly require further study. The various factors involved in RBC deformability alterations are summarized in Table 1 and Fig. 4.

Conclusion

Alterations in RBC rheology may contribute to the microvascular injury and impaired oxygen supply seen in sepsis. Multiple factors may be involved including NO and ROS, altered calcium homeostasis, decrease in ATP reserves, increase in intracellular 2,3 DPG, membrane components (sialic acid), and WBC interactions.

Importantly, the RBC is more than an oxygen transporter but also an oxygen sensor and may itself augment blood flow by liberation of ATP and O_2 delivery wherever and whenever the need might arise. New thinking regarding this well-studied cell will lead to a better understanding of the mechanisms of RBC rheological alterations in sepsis and their effect on blood flow and O_2 transport. This may be important in the development of new therapeutic strategies to improve cellular oxygen availability, and thereby reduce organ failure in severe sepsis and septic shock.

References

1. Friedman G, Silva E, Vincent JL (1998) Has the mortality of septic shock changed with time? Crit Care Med 26:2078–2086
2. Hinshaw LB (1996) Sepsis/septic shock: participation of the microcirculation: an abbreviated review. Crit Care Med 24:1072–1078
3. Chien S (1982) Rheology in the microcirculation in normal and low flow states. Adv Shock Res 8:71–80
4. Voerman HJ, Fonk T, Thijs LG (1989) Changes in hemorheology in patients with sepsis or septic shock. Circ Shock 29:219–227
5. Voerman HJ, Groeneveld AB (1989) Blood viscosity and circulatory shock. Intensive Care Med 15:72–78
6. Baskurt OK, Gelmont D, Meiselman HJ (1998) Red blood cell deformability in sepsis. Am J Respir Crit Care Med 157:421–427
7. Yodice PC, Astiz ME, Kurian BM, Lin RY, Rackow EC (1997) Neutrophil rheologic changes in septic shock. Am J Respir Crit Care Med 155:38–42
8. Ellsworth ML, Forrester T, Ellis CG, Dietrich HH (1995) The erythrocyte as a regulator of vascular tone. Am J Physiol 269:H2155–H2161
9. Ellsworth ML (2000) The red blood cell as an oxygen sensor: what is the evidence? Acta Physiol Scand 168:551–559
10. Jagger JE, Bateman RM, Ellsworth ML, Ellis CG (2001) Role of erythrocyte in regulating local O2 delivery mediated by hemoglobin oxygenation. Am J Physiol 280:H2833–H2839
11. Somer T, Meiselman HJ (1993) Disorders of blood viscosity. Ann Med 25:31–39
12. Bishop JJ, Nance PR, Popel AS, Intaglietta M, Johnson PC (2001) Effect of erythrocyte aggregation on velocity profiles in venules. Am J Physiol 280:H222–H236
13. Berliner AS, Shapira I, Rogowski O, Sadees N, Rotstein R, Fusman R, Avitzour D, Cohen S, Arber N, Zeltser D (2000) Combined leukocyte and erythrocyte aggregation in the peripheral venous blood during sepsis. An indication of commonly shared adhesive protein(s). Int J Clin Lab Res 30:27–31
14. Mohandas N (1991) The red blood cell membrane. In: Hoffman R, Benz EJ, Shattil SJ, Furie B, Cohen HJ (eds) Hematology: basis, principles and practice. Churchill-Livingstone, New York, pp 264–269
15. Lux SE (1979) Dissecting the red cell membrane skeleton. Nature 281:426–429
16. Mohandas N, Chasis JA (1993) Red blood cell deformability, membrane material properties and shape: regulation by transmembrane, skeletal and cytosolic proteins and lipids. Semin Hematol 30:171–192
17. Chien S (1977) Principles and techniques for assessing erythrocyte deformability. Blood Cells 3:71–99
18. Mohandas N, Chasis JA, Shohet SB (1983) The influence of membrane skeleton on red cell deformability, membrane material properties, and shape. Semin Hematol 20:225–242
19. Piagnerelli M, Zouaoui Boudjeltia K, Brohee D, Piro P, Vincent JL (2000) Comparison of red cell shape in healthy and septic patients by flow cytometry. Intensive Care Med 26[Suppl 3]: S322 [abstr]
20. Piagnerelli M, Zouaoui Boudjeltia K, Vanhaeverbeek M, Piro P, Vincent JL, Carlier E, Lejeune P (2000) Decrease of red blood cell deformability determined by flow cytometry. Am J Respir Crit Care Med 161:A882 [abstr]
21. Grebe R, Wolff H, Schmid-Schonbein H (1988) Influence of red cell surface charge on red cell membrane curvature. Pflugers Arch 413:77–82
22. Piper RD, Pitt-Hyde M, Li F, Sibbald WJ, Potter RF (1996) Microcirculatory changes in rat skeletal muscle in sepsis. Am J Respir Crit Care Med 154:931–937
23. Lam C, Tyml K, Martin C, Sibbald W (1994) Microvascular perfusion is impaired in a rat model of normotensive sepsis. J Clin Invest 94:2077–2083
24. Tyml K, Yu J, McCormack DG (1998) Capillary and arteriolar responses to local vasodilators are impaired in a rat model of sepsis. J Appl Physiol 84:837–844
25. Astiz ME, DeGent GE, Lin RY, Rackow EC (1995) Microvascular function and rheologic changes in hyperdynamic sepsis. Crit Care Med 23:265–271
26. Powell RJ, Machiedo GW, Rush BFJ (1993) Decreased red blood cell deformability and impaired oxygen utilization during human sepsis. Am Surg 59:65–68
27. Hurd TC, Dasmahapatra KS, Rush BFJ, Machiedo GW (1988) Red blood cell deformability in human and experimental sepsis. Arch Surg 123:217–220

28. Baskurt OK, Temiz A, Meiselman HJ (1997) Red blood cell aggregation in experimental sepsis. J Lab Clin Med 130:183–190
29. Pearson MJ, Lipowsky HH (2000) Influence of erythrocyte aggregation on leukocyte margination in postcapillary venules of rat mesentery. Am J Physiol 279:H1460–H1471
30. Vincent JL (2000) Update on sepsis: pathophysiology and treatment. Acta Clin Belg 55:79–87
31. Simchon S, Jan KM, Chien S (1987) Influence of reduced red cell deformability on regional blood flow. Am J Physiol 253:H898–H903
32. Eichelbronner O, Sielenkamper A, Cepinskas G, Sibbald WJ, Chin-Yee IH (2000) Endotoxin promotes adhesion of human erythrocytes to human vascular endothelial cells under conditions of flow. Crit Care Med 28:1865–1870
33. Langenfeld JE, Livingston DH, Machiedo GW (1991) Red cell deformability is an early indicator of infection. Surgery 110:398–403
34. Chung TW, O'Rear EA, Whitsett TL, Hinshaw LB, Smith MA (1991) Survival factors in a canine septic shock model. Circ Shock 33:178–182
35. Han YY, Murtagh BM, Venkataraman ST (1999) 2,3 diphosphoglycerate increases with critical illness in children. Crit Care Med 27 [Suppl]:A71 [abstr]
36. Suzuki Y, Nakajima T, Shiga T, Maeda N (1990) Influence of 2,3-diphosphoglycerate on the deformability of human erythrocytes. Biochim Biophys Acta 1029:85–90
37. Vincent JL, Zhang H, Szabo C, Preiser JC (2000) Effects of nitric oxide in septic shock. Am J Respir Crit Care Med 161:1781–1785
38. Graf J, Eichelbrönner O, Sibbald WJ (1999) The red blood cell and nitric oxide. In: Vincent JL (ed) Yearbook of intensive care and emergency medicine. Springer, Heidelberg, pp 465–475
39. Jia L, Bonaventura C, Bonaventura J, Stamler JS (1996) S-nitrosohaemoglobin: a dynamic activity of blood involved in vascular control. Nature 380:221–226
40. Sprague RS, Stephenson AH, Dimmitt RA, Weintraub NL, Branch CA, McMurdo L, Lonigro AJ, Weintraub NA (1995) Effect of L-NAME on pressure-flow relationships in isolated rabbit lungs: role of red blood cells. Am J Physiol 269:H1941–H1948
41. Sprague RS, Ellsworth ML, Stephenson AH, Lonigro AJ (1996) ATP: the red blood cell link to NO and local control of the pulmonary circulation. Am J Physiol 271:H2717–H2722
42. Marikovsky Y (1996) The cytoskeleton in ATP-depleted erythrocytes: the effect of shape transformation. Mech Ageing Dev 86:137–144
43. Busse R, Ogilvie A, Pohl U (1988) Vasomotor activity of diadenosine triphosphate and diadenosine tetraphosphate in isolated arteries. Am J Physiol 254:H828–H832
44. Miseta A, Bogner P, Berenyi E, Kellermayer M, Galambos C, Wheatley DN, Cameron IL (1993) Relationship between cellular ATP, potassium, sodium and magnesium concentrations in mammalian and avian erythrocytes. Biochim Biophys Acta 1175:133–139
45. Ismail NH, Cohn EJJ, Mollitt DL (1997) Nitric oxide synthase inhibition negates septic-induced alterations in cytoplasmic calcium homeostasis and membrane dynamics. Am Surg 63:20–23
46. Deliconstantinos G, Villiotou V, Stavrides JC, Salemes N, Gogas J (1995) Nitric oxide and peroxynitrite production by human erythrocytes: a causative factor of toxic anemia in breast cancer patients. Anticancer Res 15:1435–1446
47. Ghigo D, Todde R, Ginsburg H, Costamagna C, Gautret P, Bussolino F, Ulliers D, Giribaldi G, Deharo E, Gabrielli G (1995) Erythrocyte stages of Plasmodium falciparum exhibit a high nitric oxide synthase (NOS) activity and release an NOS-inducing soluble factor. J Exp Med 182:677–688
48. Jubelin BC, Gierman JL (1996) Erythrocytes may synthesize their own nitric oxide. Am J Hypertens 9:1214–1219
49. Korbut R, Gryglewski RJ (1993) Nitric oxide from polymorphonuclear leukocytes modulates red blood cell deformability in vitro. Eur J Pharmacol 234:17–22
50. Starzyk D, Korbut R, Gryglewski RJ (1997) The role of nitric oxide in regulation of deformability of red blood cells in acute phase of endotoxaemia in rats. J Physiol Pharmacol 48:731–735
51. Bateman RM, Jagger JE, Sharpe MD, Ellsworth ML, Mehta S, Ellis CG (2001) Erythrocyte deformability is a nitric oxide-mediated factor in decreased capillary density during sepsis. Am J Physiol 280:H2848–H2856
52. Mallozzi C, Di Stasi AM, Minetti M (1997) Peroxynitrite modulates tyrosine-dependent signal transduction pathway of human erythrocyte band 3. FASEB J 11:1281–1290
53. Shiga T, Sekiya M, Maeda N, Kon K, Okazaki M (1985) Cell age-dependent changes in deformability and calcium accumulation of human erythrocytes. Biochim Biophys Acta 814:289–299
54. Ortiz-Carranza O, Miller ME, Adragna NC, Lauf PK (1997) Alkaline pH and internal calcium increase Na+ and K+ effluxes in LK sheep red blood cells in Cl--free solutions. J Membr Biol 156:287–295
55. Lau YT, Hsieh CC, Liu MS, Hwang TL, Chen MF, Cheng HS (1994) Erythrocyte Ca2+ pump is defective during sepsis. Circ Shock 44:121–125
56. Todd JC, Mollitt DL (1995) Effect of sepsis on erythrocyte intracellular calcium homeostasis. Crit Care Med 23:459–465
57. Todd JC, Mollitt DL (1995) Leukocyte modulation inhibits endotoxin-induced disruption of intracellular calcium homeostasis. J Trauma 39:1148–1151
58. Sowemimo-Coker SO, Debbas NM, Kovacs IB, Turner P (1985) Ex vivo effects of nifedipine, nisoldipine and nitrendipine on filterability of red blood cells from healthy volunteers. Br J Clin Pharmacol 20:152–154
59. Fujita J, Tsuda K, Takeda T, Yu L, Fujimoto S, Kajikawa M, Nishimura M, Mizuno N, Hamamoto Y, Mukai E, Adachi T, Seino Y (1999) Nisoldipine improves the impaired erythrocyte deformability correlating with elevated intracellular free calcium-ion concentration and poor glycaemic control in NIDDM. Br J Clin Pharmacol 47:499–506
60. Bergfeld GR, Forrester T (1992) Release of ATP from human erythrocytes in response to a brief period of hypoxia and hypercapnia. Cardiovasc Res 26:40–47
61. Durocher JR, Payne RC, Conrad ME (1975) Role of sialic acid in erythrocyte survival. Blood 45:11–20
62. Piagnerelli M, Zouaoui Boudjeltia K, Brohee D, Piro P, Carlier E, Vincent JL, Lejeune P, Vanhaeverbeek M (2003) Alterations of red blood cell shape and sialic acid membrane content in septic shock. Crit Care Med (in press)
63. Rogers ME, Williams DT, Niththyananthan R, Rampling MW, Heslop KE, Johnston DG (1992) Decrease in erythrocyte glycophorin sialic acid content is associated with increased erythrocyte aggregation in human diabetes. Clin Sci (Colch) 82:309–313

64. Mazzanti L, Rabini RA, Salvolini E, Tesei M, Martarelli D, Venerando B, Curatola G (1997) Sialic acid, diabetes, and aging: a study on the erythrocyte membrane. Metabolism 46:59–61
65. Chari SN, Nath N (1984) Sialic acid content and sialidase activity of polymorphonuclear leucocytes in diabetes mellitus. Am J Med Sci 288:18–20
66. Chiarini A, Fiorilli A, Di Francesco L, Venerando B, Tettamanti G (1993) Human erythrocyte sialidase is linked to the plasma membrane by a glycosylphosphatidylinositol anchor and partly located on the outer surface. Glycoconj J 10:64–71
67. Milligan TW, Baker CJ, Straus DC, Mattingly SJ (1978) Association of elevated levels of extracellular neuraminidase with clinical isolates of type III group B streptococci. Infect Immun 21:738–746
68. Todd JC, Poulos ND, Davidson LW, Mollitt DL (1993) Role of the leukocyte in endotoxin-induced alterations of the red cell membrane. Second place winner of the Conrad Jobst Award in the Gold Medal paper competition. Am Surg 59:9–12
69. Betticher DC, Keller H, Maly FE, Reinhart WH (1993) The effect of endotoxin and tumour necrosis factor on erythrocyte and leucocyte deformability in vitro. Br J Haematol 83:130–137
70. Machiedo GW, Powell RJ, Rush BFJ, Swislocki NI, Dikdan G (1989) The incidence of decreased red blood cell deformability in sepsis and the association with oxygen free radical damage and multiple-system organ failure. Arch Surg 124:1386–1389
71. Goode HF, Webster NR (1993) Free radicals and antioxidants in sepsis. Crit Care Med 21:1770–1776
72. Drost EM, Kassabian G, Meiselman HJ, Gelmont D, Fisher TC (1999) Increased rigidity and priming of polymorphonuclear leukocytes in sepsis. Am J Respir Crit Care Med 159:1696–1702
73. Kirschenbaum LA, Aziz M, Astiz ME, Saha DC, Rackow EC (2000) Influence of rheologic changes and platelet-neutrophil interactions on cell filtration in sepsis. Am J Respir Crit Care Med 161:1602–1607
74. Schmid-Schonbein GW, Usami S, Skalak R, Chien S (1980) The interaction of leukocytes and erythrocytes in capillary and postcapillary vessels. Microvasc Res 19:45–70
75. Bellingan G (2000) Leukocytes: friend or foe. Intensive Care Med 26[Suppl 1]:S111–S118
76. Claster S, Chiu DT, Quintanilha A, Lubin B (1984) Neutrophils mediate lipid peroxidation in human red cells. Blood 64:1079–1084
77. Davies KJ, Goldberg AL (1987) Oxygen radicals stimulate intracellular proteolysis and lipid peroxidation by independent mechanisms in erythrocytes. J Biol Chem 262:8220–8226
78. Hirayama T, Folmerz P, Hansson R, Jonsson O, Pettersson S, Roberts D, Schersten T (1986) Effect of oxygen free radicals on rabbit and human erythrocytes. Studies on cellular deformability. Scand J Thorac Cardiovasc Surg 20:247–252
79. Uyesaka N, Hasegawa S, Ishioka N, Ishioka R, Shio H, Schechter AN (1992) Effects of superoxide anions on red cell deformability and membrane proteins. Biorheology 29:217–229
80. Powell RJ, Machiedo GW, Rush BFJ, Dikdan G (1991) Oxygen free radicals: effect on red cell deformability in sepsis. Crit Care Med 19:732–735
81. Powell RJ, Machiedo GW, Rush BFJ, Dikdan G (1989) Effect of alpha-tocopherol on red cell deformability and survival in sepsis. Curr Surg 46:380–382
82. Singh M, Stoltz JF (2002) Influence of temperature variation from 5 degrees C to 37 degrees C on aggregation and deformability of erythrocytes. Clin Hemorheol Microcirc 26:1–7
83. Artmann GM, Kelemen C, Porst D, Idt B, Chien S (1998) Temperature transitions of protein properties in human red blood cells. Biophys J 75:3179–3183
84. Baskurt OK, Mat F (2000) Importance of measurement temperature in detecting the alterations of red blood cell aggregation and deformability studied by ektacytometry: a study on experimental sepsis in rats. Clin Hemorheol Microcirc 23:43–49
85. Jagger JE, Ellis CG, Sibbald W, Eichelbrönner O (2001) Measurement temperature plays a pivotal role in the distribution of erythrocyte deformability after LPS. Biorheology 38:439–448

Paul E. Marik
Murugan Raghavan

Stress-hyperglycemia, insulin and immunomodulation in sepsis

Abstract Stress-hyperglycemia and insulin resistance are exceedingly common in critically ill patients, particularly those with sepsis. Multiple pathogenetic mechanisms are responsible for this metabolic syndrome; however, increased release of pro-inflammatory mediators and counter-regulatory hormones may play a pivotal role. Recent data suggests that hyperglycemia may potentiate the pro-inflammatory response while insulin has the opposite effect. Furthermore, emerging evidence suggests that tight glycemic control will improve the outcome of critically ill patients. This paper reviews the pathophysiology of stress hyperglycemia in the critically ill septic patient and outlines a treatment strategy for the management of this disorder.

Keywords Insulin · Glucose · Sepsis · Sepsis syndrome · Critical illness · Insulin resistance · Hyperglycemia

Introduction

In recent decades the reported incidence of sepsis has increased dramatically, largely due to the advancing age of the population, an increased number of invasive procedures being performed and immunosuppressive therapy [1]. In the United States, approximately 750,000 cases of sepsis occur each year, at least 225,000 of which are fatal [2]. Despite the use of antimicrobial agents and advanced life-support care, the case fatality rate for patients with sepsis has remained between 30 and 40% over the past three decades [2, 3].

When the body is challenged by foreign microbial agents homeostatic mechanisms come into play that attempt to rid the body of the foreign agent without damaging the host. This involves the activation of pro- and anti-inflammatory pathways which are tightly controlled and regulated [4]. In most infected persons, the body is able to achieve a balance between pro-inflammatory and anti-inflammatory mediators and homeostasis is restored. In some patients, however, this balance is upset with an excessive pro-inflammatory response resulting in the systemic inflammatory response syndrome (SIRS), multisystem organ dysfunction, and ultimately death [4, 5, 6, 7]. Attempts at down-regulating the pro-inflammatory response with novel agents directed at specific pro-inflammatory mediators has uniformly met with failure [4, 8, 9, 10]. Recent provocative data suggests that tight glycemic control with insulin may the restore the balance between pro-inflammatory and anti-inflammatory mediators and improve the outcome of critically ill patients [11, 12].

In this article we review the physiology of stress hyperglycemia and the immune-modulatory role of insulin in critically ill patients. The reader should be cautioned that many of the studies quoted in our review were performed in non-critically ill patients, many of whom were diabetic. While it is likely that the pathogenetic pathways are similar in both groups of patients, many of these postulates remain unproven in the critical care setting.

M.R. Pinsky et al. (eds.), *Applied Physiology in Intensive Care Medicine 2: Physiological Reviews and Editorials*,
DOI 10.1007/978-3-642-28233-1_15,

Endocrinology of stress

Stress associated with critical illness is characterized by activation of the hypothalamic–pituitary–adrenal (HPA) axis with the release of cortisol from the adrenal gland [13]. Activation of the HPA axis with the release of cortisol is an essential component of the general adaptation to illness and stress and contributes to the maintenance of cellular and organ homeostasis.

In addition to increased cortisol secretion the stress response is characterized by a marked increase in the release of norepinephrine and epinephrine as well as glucagon and growth hormone [14, 15, 16]. Insulin levels are usually normal or decreased, despite peripheral insulin resistance [17, 18, 19]. It has been suggested that insulin release may be suppressed as the result of increased activation of the pancreatic alpha receptors [19]. In addition to causing insulin resistance, interleukin-1 (IL-1) and tumor necrosis factor-α (TNF-α) inhibit insulin release, an effect which appears to be concentration dependent [20]. The low to normal insulin levels together with insulin resistance in the presence of increased secretion of the counter-regulatory hormones results in stress hyperglycemia (see discussion below).

Glucose transporters and the mechanism of insulin action

Glucose is normally taken up across the cellular membranes by a system of carrier-mediated facilitated transport [21]. Five transporter isoforms exists. Three of the isoforms, GLUT 1, GLUT 2, and GLUT 4, are important for glucose uptake [21]. GLUT 1 can be found in many tissues and is responsible for basal uptake. It has a high affinity for glucose and it ensures transport even under the conditions of hypoglycemia. GLUT 2 mediates uptake and release of glucose by hepatocytes and regulation of glucose-stimulated insulin secretion in pancreas. The GLUT2 transporter ensures that the liver is freely permeable to glucose and that glucose transport is not rate-limiting for hepatic glucose uptake. GLUT 4 isoform is involved in glucose transport in tissues where uptake is mediated by insulin which includes skeletal muscle, cardiac muscle, and adipose tissue. Binding of insulin to cell-surface receptors results in autophosphorylation and activation of an intrinsic tyrosine kinase molecule of the insulin receptor (IR) b-subunit. Activated tyrosine kinase subsequently phosphorylates messenger molecular proteins known as insulin receptor substrates (IRS1 and IRS2). The IRS-1 associates with several proteins including the enzyme phosphatidylinositol (PI) 3-kinase. Physiologically insulin increases glucose uptake into the cell by causing translocation of GLUT 4 from intracellular compartments to the plasma membrane. The signaling enzyme molecule PI-3-kinase is essential for insulin stimulated GLUT 4 translocation [22]. PI-3-kinase also mediates many of the metabolic effects of insulin, including activation of glycogen synthase, protein synthesis, lipogenesis, and the regulation of various genes in insulin-responsive cells including inhibition of phosphoenol pyruvate carboxykinase (PEPCK), the key enzyme of gluconeogenesis.

Mechanisms of stress-induced hyperglycemia and insulin resistance in sepsis

The prevalence of stress hyperglycemia in sepsis and critical illness is difficult to establish due to limited data and variations in the definition of hyperglycemia. Stress hyperglycemia has been previously defined as a plasma glucose above 200 mg/dl [23]; however, in view of the results of the Leuven Intensive Insulin Therapy Trial (see below), stress hyperglycemia should be considered in any critically ill patient with a blood glucose in excess of 110 mg/dl [11]. In a study of septic non-diabetic ICU patients 75% had a baseline blood glucose level above 110 mg/dl [24]. In the Leuven Intensive Insulin Therapy Trial, 12% of patients had a baseline blood glucose above 200 mg/dl; however, 74.5% of patients had a baseline blood glucose above 110 mg/dl, with 97.5% having a recorded blood glucose level above 110 mg/dl sometime during their ICU stay [11].

Changes in whole-body glucose uptake and glucose oxidation in sepsis are complex and may depend on the severity of illness and the stage of the disease. Whole-body glucose uptake and glucose oxidation may be increased in the early stages of sepsis and endotoxemia [25, 26]. This may be the result of cytokine-induced increase in non-insulin mediated glucose uptake by tissues rich in mononuclear phagocytes, including the liver, spleen, ileum, and lung [27, 28]. Enhanced non-insulin mediated glucose uptake appears to result from an increase in the synthesis, concentration or activity of the GLUT1 transporter [29, 30]. With the development of insulin resistance (see below) glucose utilization and oxidation may decrease [25, 31, 32]. Exogenous insulin increases glucose utilization and oxidation; however, non-oxidative disposal (storage) remains impaired [25, 31, 32].

The metabolic milieu in which stress-induced hyperglycemia develops in the critically ill in the absence of pre-existing diabetes mellitus is complex. A combination of several factors, including the presence of excessive counter regulatory hormones such as glucagon, growth hormone, catecholamines, glucocorticoids, and cytokines such as IL-1, IL-6, and TNF-α combined with exogenous administration of catecholamines, dextrose, and nutritional support together with relative insulin deficiency, play an important role [23]. Increased gluconeogenesis combined with hepatic insulin resistance are the major factors

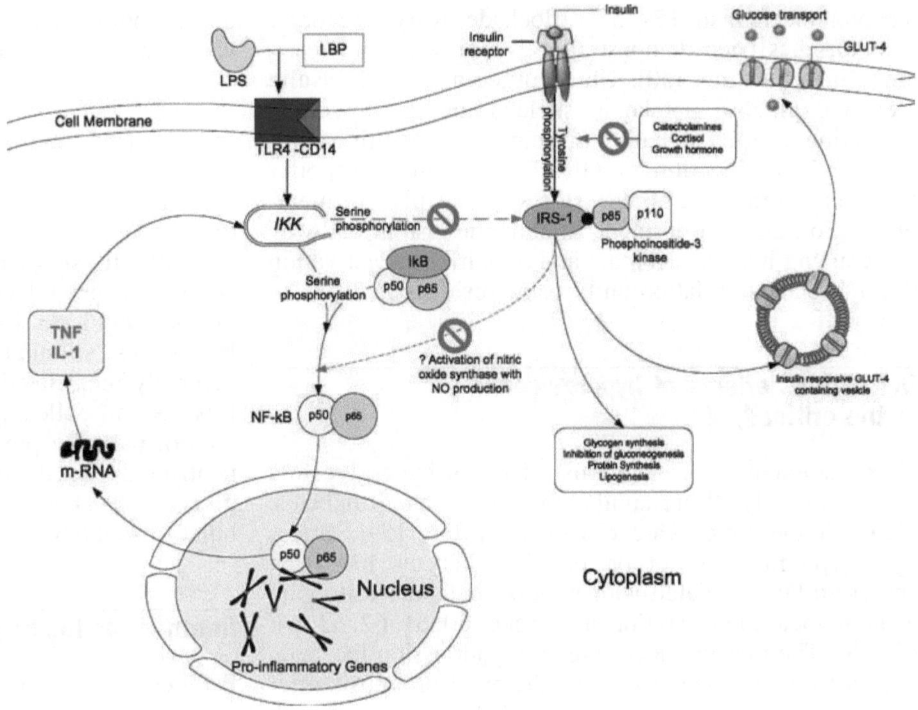

Fig. 1 Postulated interaction between the insulin signaling pathway and activation of the pro-inflammatory cascade in the pathogenesis of stress hyperglycemia of sepsis. *LPS* lipopolysaccharide, *LBP* lipopolysaccharide binding protein, *TLR4* Toll-like receptor 4, *IκB* inhibitor, *IKK* inhibitor κB kinase, *IRS-1*, insulin receptor substrate-1, *IL-1* interleukin-1, *TNF* tumor necrosis factor, *NF-kB* nuclear factor-kappa B

leading to hyperglycemia [33]. Recent human data suggests that hepatic insulin resistence (and PEPCK suppression) remains refractory to intensive insulin therapy [34]. Increased hepatic output of glucose may therefore be more important than peripheral insulin resistance in the genesis of stress hyperglycemia [35]. Gluconeogenic substrates released during stress include lactate, alanine, and glycerol with exogenous glucose failing to suppress gluconeogenesis [16, 36]. Glucagon is the primary hormonal mediator of gluconeogenesis, with septic patients having a significant increase in serum glucagon levels [16]. This effect is mediated by adrenergic stimulation by catecholamines and by cytokines [37]. In addition, cytokines such as TNF-α and IL-1 and catecholamines independently and synergistically promote hepatic glucose production [38, 39].

Sepsis is characterized by marked insulin resistance [19, 25, 31, 32, 40, 41]. The insulin resistance in sepsis is directly proportional to the severity of stress response [19]. During sepsis, insulin induced tyrosine phosphorylation of IRS-1 and subsequent activation of PI-3-kinase is impaired resulting in defective GLUT-4 receptor translocation, diminished glucose uptake, insulin resistance in skeletal muscle, and hepatic insulin resistance [22]. The mechanism whereby sepsis induces these alterations are unknown, but increased levels of TNF-α may play a key role. Aljada and colleagues have demonstrated that in endothelial cells TNF-α causes a reduction of tyrosine phosphorylation and expression of the insulin receptor [42]. TNF-α diminishes insulin-induced IRS-1 tyrosine phosphorylation in hepatocytes and adipocytes and impairs the activation of PI-3 kinase [43, 44, 45, 46]. These alterations of the early steps in insulin action are probably mediated by TNF-α induced IRS-1 serine phosphorylation [43, 46, 47, 48]. Upon serine phosphorylation, IRS1 proteins have a reduced ability to interact with the insulin receptor, to be tyrosine phosphorylated by the insulin receptor and to bind phosphatidylinositol-3 kinase [44, 45].

Recently, Gao and colleagues have demonstrated that activation of the inhibitor κB kinase (IKK) complex is associated with serine phosphorylation of IRS-1 [49]. The IKK is activated by endotoxin via Toll-like receptor 4 (LTR4) as well as by TNF-α and interleukin-1 (IL-1) [50, 51, 52]. The IKK is a serine kinase that controls the activation of nuclear factor-kappa B (NF-κB) a ubiquitous nuclear transcription factor closely associated with the activation of the genes for almost all of the pro-inflammatory mediators [53]. Before activation, NF-κB is bound to inhibitor κB (I κB). This association between I κB and NF-κB results in the cytosolic localiazation of NF-κB. The serine phosphorylation of I κB by the IKK complex results in the degradation of I κB followed by the nuclear translocation of NF κB. The serine phosphorylation of IRS-1 and I κB by IKK may partly explain the insulin resistance noted with activation of the pro-inflammatory cascade (see Fig. 1).

Catecholamines have also been shown to inhibit insulin binding, tyrosine kinase activity, and translocation of GLUT-4 either directly through a receptor or a post-receptor mechanism [54, 55]. Blockade of α_2 adrenergic receptors has been demonstrated to reduce insulin resistance in septic rats [40]. Glucocorticoids impair insulin mediated glucose uptake in skeletal muscle, by down regulating various signaling proteins with resulting inhibition of translocation of GLUT-4 glucose transporter from its internal membrane stores to the plasma membrane [56]. Growth hormone inhibits the insulin pathway by reducing insulin receptors and impairing its activation through phosphorylation on tyrosine residues [57, 58].

Deleterious effects of hyperglycemia in the critically ill

To some extent the deleterious effects of hyperglycemia in the critically ill are similar to that of actual diabetes, although the time scale obviously differs [59]. Stress hyperglycemia but not pre-existing diabetes has been shown to be associated with a worse outcome following acute myocardial infarction and stroke [60, 61, 62, 63, 64, 65, 66]. The plasma glucose level on admission has been shown to be an independent predictor of prognosis after myocardial infarction [60, 61]. In diabetic patients with acute myocardial infarction, therapy to maintain blood glucose at a level below 215 mg/dl improves outcome [62, 63, 64]. The presence of hyperglycemia following an ischemic or hemorrhagic stroke is associated with a two- to threefold increased mortality and significant impairment in functional recovery [65, 66].

Pro-inflammatory effects

Glucose has been shown to be a powerful pro-inflammatory mediator [67], and tight glucose control below 110 mg/dl with insulin has been shown to exert anti-inflammatory effects in the critically ill patient [68]. The oral administration of 75 g of glucose to healthy volunteers increases reactive oxygen species (ROS) generation by polymorphonuclear leukocytes and mononuclear cells [69]. Similarly, an oral glucose load has been demonstrated to increase plasma IL-8 levels [70]. Chettab and coworkers have demonstrated that hyperglycemia upregulates the IL-8 gene [71]. IL-8 is a potent neutrophil chemoattractant, playing an important role in inflammation [72, 73, 74]. Glucose induces an increase in intranuclear NF-κB, a fall in cytosolic I κB, and an increase in I κB kinase in vivo and in vitro which are pro-inflammatory [75, 76, 77]. Glucose also has been shown to exert pro-thrombotic effects and to increase oxidative stress due to increased lipid peroxidation [78, 79]. Glucose increases the expression and plasma concentration of matrix metalloproteinase-2 (MMP-2) and MMP-9, which aid in spread of inflammation [80]. Acute hyperglycemia reduces endothelial nitric oxide levels, causing abnormal vascular reactivity and organ perfusion [81].

Increased susceptibility to infection

In diabetic patients hyperglycemia has long been known to increase the susceptibility to infections [82]. In critically ill surgical and burn patients tight glycemic control has been demonstrated to reduce the risk of septic morbidity [11, 83, 84, 85]. The in vitro responsiveness of leukocytes stimulated by inflammatory mediators is inversely correlated with glycemic control [86, 87]. Rassias and colleagues demonstrated that tight glycemic control partially prevented the postoperative decrease in neutrophil phagocytic activity [88]. In addition, hyperglycemia has been demonstrated to decrease the oxidative burst of leukocytes [89, 90].

Immune-modulatory role of insulin in sepsis

Besides control of hyperglycemia, insulin has potent acute anti-inflammatory effects. In a group of obese subjects, Dandona and colleagues demonstrated that an infusion of insulin was associated with a significant fall of intranuclear NF-κB, and increase in IκB in mononuclear cells [91]. These changes were associated with a fall in the generation of reactive oxygen species and a fall in the serum levels of soluble intercellular adhesion molecule-1 (sICAM-1), monocyte chemoattractant protein-1 (MCP-1), and plasminogen activator inhibitor-1 (PAI-1) [91]. In a similar experiment Aljada et al. demonstrated that insulin decreased expression of the pro-inflammatory transcription factor, early growth response-1 (EGR-1), and this was associated with a significant fall in plasma tissue factor (TF) and PAI-1 levels [92]; thus, while hyperglycemia has pro-thrombotic effects, insulin has anti-thrombotic and fibrinolytic effects by suppressing TF and PAI-1.

One mechanism underlying the anti-inflammatory effect of insulin may be through the release of nitric oxide (NO) from the endothelium. Insulin has been demonstrated to induce an increase in the expression NO synthase (NOS), the enzyme that generates NO [93]. The NO has been demonstrated to down-regulate the expression of endothelial cell adhesion molecules (ECAMs) as well as the pro-inflammatory cytokines [94, 95, 96, 97, 98]. While the anti-inflammatory effects of NO have not been fully delineated, it is thought that NO inhibits the activation of NF-κB. Several authors have demonstrated that NO *S*-nitrosylates a key thiol group in the DNA binding domain of NF-κB p50 and that this is associated with decreased gene transcription and synthesis of NF-κB [96, 99, 100].

NF-κB as a therapeutic target for tight glycemic control

NF-κB is a nuclear transcription factor involved in the regulation of over 150 genes related to inflammation, including TNF-α, IL-1, IL-6, IL-8, cyclooxygenase-2, and inducible nitric oxide synthase [53, 101]. Excessive activation of NF-κB has been identified as a marker of poor prognosis in sepsis [102, 103, 104]. Emerging data suggests that NF-κB may be a therapeutic target for the adjuvant treatment of sepsis [105, 106, 107, 108]. The data cited above suggests that tight glycemic control with insulin may decrease NF-κB activation. This hypothesis is supported by the Leuven Intensive Insulin Therapy Trial in which mannose-binding lectin (MBL) and C-reactive protein (CRP) levels were significantly suppressed by intensive insulin therapy [68].

Intensive insulin therapy in the critically ill

Van Den Berghe et al. in a prospective randomized controlled study involving 1548 patients demonstrated that intensive insulin therapy reduced mortality and morbidity among patients admitted to a surgical critical care unit (the Leuven Intensive Insulin Therapy Trial) [11, 12]. These authors compared an intensive insulin therapy regimen aimed to maintain blood glucose between 80 and 110 mg/dl with conventional treatment in which insulin infusion was only initiated when glucose level was greater than 215 mg/dl and maintenance of glucose between 180 and 200 mg/dl. At 12 months the mortality was 4.6% with the intensive insulin regimen compared with 8.0% in the control group. The benefit was most apparent in patients with greater than 5 days of stay in the intensive care unit. Intensive insulin therapy reduced bloodstream infections by 46%, acute renal failure by 41%, and critical illness poly-neuropathy by 44%. Using multivariate analysis the authors suggested that improved metabolic control, as reflected by normoglycemia, rather than the infused insulin dose per se, was responsible for the beneficial effects of intensive insulin therapy [12]; however, achieving normoglycemia and the administration of insulin are linked, and from the available evidence it appears likely that both factors played a key role in the improved outcome.

The outcome data from the Leuven Intensive Insulin Therapy Trial indicates that there is a dose response curve between the degree of glycemic control and hospital mortality [12] In the long stay patients (>5 days in the ICU) the cumulative hospital mortality was 15% in patients with a mean blood glucose less than 110 mg/dl, 25% in those with a blood glucose between 110 and 150 mg/dl, and 40% in those with a mean blood glucose of greater than 150 mg/dl. In diabetic patients with acute myocardial infarction, therapy to maintain blood glucose at a level below 215 mg/dl improves outcome [62, 63, 64]. This data suggests that even "modest" glycemic control will have an impact on patient outcome. This is very important as in the "real world" it may be very difficult (if not somewhat risky) to attempt to maintain a blood glucose in the range of 80–110 mg/dl. This goal may only be achievable in ICUs with a high nursing-to-patient ratio and close physician supervision. On the other hand, the Leuven study showed that in order to improve morbidity by reducing the incidence of bacteremia, acute renal failure, critical illness polyneuropathy, and transfusion requirements, a blood glucose level of <110 mg/dl was required. Indeed, a blood glucose level of 110–150 mg/dl was not effective on these morbidity measures as compared with >150 mg/d [12]. It is also important to note that in the Leuven Intensive Insulin Therapy Trial all patients received between 200 and 300 g of intravenous glucose on the day of admission followed by parenteral or enteral (or both) nutrition started on the second ICU day. In this study tight early glycemic control was associated with the more rapid improvement of insulin resistance [12]. Based on the results of this study we recommend the initiation of parenteral glucose and enteral nutrition in all ICU patients on the day of ICU admission [109, 110, 111] and the initiation of an insulin infusion in patients with a blood glucose above 150 mg/dl (a threshold of 110 mg/dl may be appropriate in select ICUs). Subcutaneous insulin "sliding scales" are not recommended, at least during the first few days, until the patient's medical condition has stabilized, the blood glucose is well controlled, and the patient has achieved his/her nutritional goal.

Thiazolidinediones are a new class of drugs that are used in the treatment of type-II diabetes mellitus. These drugs reduce insulin resistence through its binding to peroxisome proliferator-activated receptors-λ (PPARλ). Ghanim and colleagues demonstrated that troglitazone caused a significant fall in cellular NF-κB with an increases in I κB in mononuclear cells of diabetic subjects [112]. The changes were associated with a parallel fall in serum levels of TNF-α, sICAM, MCP-1, and PAI-1. While one expects these effects to be useful in chronic situation, it is relevant that these anti-inflammatory were observed within 3–7 days [112, 113]. In an experimental model of acute myocardial infarction, even a single dose of rosiglitazone has been shown to reduce myocardial damage by 50% [114, 115]. Thiazolidinediones may therefore have a role in the metabolic management of patients with sepsis; however, clinical studies are required before these agents can be recommended.

Conclusion

Stress-hyperglycemia and insulin resistance are almost universal findings in patients with sepsis. Multiple pathogenetic mechanisms are responsible for this metabolic syndrome; however, increased release of pro-inflammatory mediators and counter-regulatory hormones may play a pivotal role. Hyperglycemia per se is pro-inflammatory, whereas insulin has anti-inflammatory properties. Emerging evidence suggests that tight glycemic control with insulin will improve the outcome of critically ill patients.

References

1. Martin GS, Mannino DM, Eaton S, Moss M (2003) The epidemiology of sepsis in the nited States from 1979 through 2000. N Engl J Med 348:1546–1554
2. Angus DC, Linde-Zwirble WT, Lidicker J, Clermont G, Carcillo J, Pinsky MR (2001) Epidemiology of severe sepsis in the United States: analysis of incidence, outcome and associated costs of care. Crit Care Med 29:1303–1310
3. Friedman G, Silva E, Vincent JL (1998) Has the mortality of septic shock changed with time? Crit Care Med 26:2078–2086
4. Marik PE, Varon J (2001) Sepsis: state of the art. Dis Mon 47:463–532
5. Bone RC (1996) Sir Isaac Newton, sepsis, SIRS and CARS. Crit Care Med 24:1125–1128
6. Bone RC, Sibbald WJ, Sprung CL (1992) The ACCP-SCCM Consensus Conference on sepsis and organ failure. Chest 101:1481–1483
7. Bone RC, Grodzin CJ, Balk RA (1997) Sepsis: a new hypothesis for pathogenesis of the disease process. Chest 112:235–243
8. Natanson C, Esposito CJ, Banks SM (1998) The sirens' songs of confirmatory sepsis trials: selection bias and sampling error. Crit Care Med 26:1927–1931
9. Eichacker PQ, Parent C, Kalil A, Esposito C, Cui X, Banks SM, Gerstenberger EP, Fitz Y, Danner RL, Natanson C (2002) Risk and the efficacy of antiinflammatory agents: retrospective and confirmatory studies of sepsis. Am J Respir Crit Care Med 166:1197–1205
10. Dellinger RP (1999) Severe sepsis trials: Why have they failed? Minerva Anestesiol 65:340–345
11. van den Berghe G, Wouters P, Weekers F, Verwaest C, Bruyninckx F, Schetz M, Vlasselaers D, Ferdinande P, Lauwers P, Bouillon R (2001) Intensive insulin therapy in critically ill patients. N Engl J Med 345:1359–1367
12. van den Berghe G, Wouters PJ, Bouillon R, Weekers F, Verwaest C, Schetz M, Vlasselaers D, Ferdinande P, Lauwers P (2003) Outcome benefit of intensive insulin therapy in the critically ill: insulin dose versus glycemic control. Crit Care Med 31:359–366
13. Marik PE, Zaloga GP (2002) Adrenal insufficiency in the critically ill: a new look at an old problem. Chest 122:1784–1796
14. Hart BB, Stanford GG, Ziegler MG, Lake CR, Chernow B (1989) Catecholamines: study of interspecies variation. Crit Care Med 17:1203–1218
15. van den Berghe G (2002) Neuroendocrine pathobiology of chronic illness. Crit Care Clin 18:509–528
16. Siegel JH, Cerra FB, Coleman B, Giovannini I, Shetye M, Border JR, McMenamy RH (1979) Physiological and metabolic correlations in human sepsis. Invited commentary. Surgery 86:163–193
17. Clowes GH, Martin H, Walji S, Hirsch E, Gazitua R, Goodfellow R (1978) Blood insulin responses to blood glucose levels in high output sepsis and spetic shock. Am J Surg 135:577–583
18. Dahn MS, Jacobs LA, Smith S, Hans B, Lange MP, Mitchell RA, Kirkpatrick JR (1985) The relationship of insulin production to glucose metabolism in severe sepsis. Arch Surg 120:166–172
19. Mizock BA (2001) Alterations in fuel metabolism in critical illness hyperglycemia. Best Pract Res Clin Endocrinol Metab 15:533–551
20. Mehta VK, Hao W, Brooks-Worrell BM, Palmer JP (1994) Low-dose interleukin 1 and tumor necrosis factor individually stimulate insulin release but in combination cause suppression. Eur J Endocrinol 130:208–214
21. Shepard PR, Kahn BB (1999) Glucose transporters and insulin action. Implications for insulin resistance and diabetes mellitus. N Engl J Med 341:248–257
22. Pessin JE, Saltiel AR (2000) Signaling pathways in insulin action: molecular targets of insulin resistance. J Clin Invest 106:165–169
23. McCowen KC, Malhotra A, Bistrian BR (2001) Stress-induced hyperglycemia. Crit Care Clin 17:107–124
24. Frankenfield DC, Omert LA, Badellino MM, Wiles CE, III, Bagley SM, Goodarzi S, Siegel JH (1994) Correlation between measured energy expenditure and clinically obtained variables in trauma and sepsis patients. J Parenter Enteral Nutr 18:398–403
25. Agwunobi AO, Reid C, Maycock P, Little RA, Carlson GL (2000) Insulin resistance and substrate utilization in human endotoxemia. J Clin Endocrinol Metab 85:3770–3778
26. Gelb AW, Bayona NA, Wilson JX, Cechetto DF (2002) Propofol anesthesia compared to awake reduces infarct size in rats. Anesthesiol 96:1183–1190
27. Sakurai Y, Zhang XJ, Wolfe RR (1996) TNF directly stimulates glucose uptake and leucine oxidation and inhibits FFA flux in conscious dogs. Am J Physiol 270:E864–E872
28. Lang CH, Dobrescu C (1991) Gram-negative infection increases noninsulin-mediated glucose disposal. Endocrinology 128:645–653
29. Meszaros K, Lang CH, Bagby GJ, Spitzer JJ (1987) Tumor necrosis factor increases in vivo glucose utilization of macrophage-rich tissues. Biochem Biophys Res Commun 149:1–6
30. Bird TA, Davies A, Baldwin SA, Saklatvala J (1990) Interleukin 1 stimulates hexose transport in fibroblasts by increasing the expression of glucose transporters. J Biol Chem 265:13578–13583
31. Green CJ, Campbell IT, O'Sullivan E, Underhill S, McLaren DP, Hipkin LJ, MacDonald IA, Russell J (1995) Septic patients in multiple organ failure can oxidize infused glucose, but non-oxidative disposal (storage) is impaired. Clin Sci 89:601–609
32. Saeed M, Carlson GL, Little RA, Irving MH (1999) Selective impairment of glucose storage in human sepsis. Br J Surg 86:813–821
33. Mizock BA (1997) Alterations in fuel metabolism in critical illness. Hyperglycemia. In: Ober KP (ed) Endocrinology of critical disease. Humana Press, Totawa, New Jersey, pp 197–297

34. Mesotten D, Delhanty PJ, Vanderhoydonc F, Hardman KV, Weekers F, Baxter RC, Van den BG (2002) Regulation of insulin-like growth factor binding protein-1 during protracted critical illness. J Clin Endocrinol Metab 87:5516–5523
35. Jeevanandam M, Young DH, Schiller WR (1990) Glucose turnover, oxidation, and indices of recycling in severely traumatized patients. J Trauma 30:582–589
36. Cerra FB (1987) Hypermetabolism, organ failure, and metabolic support. Surgery 101:1–14
37. Wolfe RR (1997) Substrate utilization/insulin resistance in sepsis/trauma. Baillieres Clin Endocrinol Metab 11:645–657
38. Petit F, Bagby GJ, Lang CH (1995) Tumor necrosis factor mediates zymosan-induced increase in glucose flux and insulin resistance. Am J Physiol 268:E219–E228
39. Roh MS, Moldawer LL, Ekman LG, Dinarello CA, Bistrian BR, Jeevanandam M, Brennan MF (1986) Stimulatory effect of interleukin-1 upon hepatic metabolism. Metabolism 35:419–424
40. Lang CH (1992) Sepsis-induced insulin resistance in rats is mediated by a beta-adrenergic mechanism. Am J Physiol 263:E703–E711
41. Chambrier C, Laville M, Rhzioual BK, Odeon M, Bouletreau P, Beylot M (2000) Insulin sensitivity of glucose and fat metabolism in severe sepsis. Clin Sci 99:321–328
42. Aljada A, Ghanim H, Assian E, Dandona P (2002) Tumor necrosis factor-alpha inhibits insulin-induced increase in endothelial nitric oxide synthase and reduces insulin receptor content and phosphorylation in human aortic endothelial cells. Metabolism 51:487–491
43. Hotamisligil GS, Peraldi P, Budavari A, Ellis R, White MF, Spiegelman BM (1996) IRS-1-mediated inhibition of insulin receptor tyrosine kinase activity in TNF-alpha- and obesity-induced insulin resistance. Science 271:665–668
44. Kanety H, Feinstein R, Papa MZ, Hemi R, Karasik A (1995) Tumor necrosis factor alpha-induced phosphorylation of insulin receptor substrate-1 (IRS-1). Possible mechanism for suppression of insulin-stimulated tyrosine phosphorylation of IRS-1. J Biol Chem 270:23780–23784
45. Paz K, Hemi R, LeRoith D, Karasik A, Elhanany E, Kanety H, Zick Y (1997) A molecular basis for insulin resistance. Elevated serine/threonine phosphorylation of IRS-1 and IRS-2 inhibits their binding to the juxtamembrane region of the insulin receptor and impairs their ability to undergo insulin-induced tyrosine phosphorylation. J Biol Chem 272:29911–29918
46. Nunes AL, Carvalheira JB, Carvalho CR, Brenelli SL, Saad MJ (2001) Tissue-specific regulation of early steps in insulin action in septic rats. Life Sci 69:2103–2112
47. Hotamisligil GS, Budavari A, Murray D, Spiegelman BM (1994) Reduced tyrosine kinase activity of the insulin receptor in obesity-diabetes. Central role of tumor necrosis factor-alpha. J Clin Invest 94:1543–9
48. Hotamisligil GS, Murray DL, Choy LN, Spiegelman BM (1994) Tumor necrosis factor alpha inhibits signaling from the insulin receptor. Proc Natl Acad Sci USA 91:4854–4858
49. Gao Z, Hwang D, Bataille F, Lefevre M, York D, Quon MJ, Ye J (2002) Serine phosphorylation of insulin receptor substrate 1 by inhibitor kappa B kinase complex. J Biol Chem 277:48115–48121
50. Gay NJ, Keith FJ (1991) Drosophila Toll and IL-1 receptor. Nature 351:355–356
51. Belvin MP, Anderson KV (1996) A conserved signaling pathway: the Drosophila toll-dorsal pathway. Annu Rev Cell Develop Biol 12:393–416
52. Hoshino K, Takeuchi O, Kawai T, Sanjo H, Ogawa T, Takeda Y, Takeda K, Akira S (1999) Cutting edge: Toll-like receptor 4 (TLR4)-deficient mice are hyporesponsive to lipopolysaccharide: evidence for TLR4 as the Lps gene product. J Immunol 162:3749–3752
53. Barnes PJ, Karin M (1997) Nuclear factor-kB-A pivotal transcription factor in chronic inflammatory diseases. N Engl J Med 336:1066–1071
54. Chiasson JL, Shikama H, Chu DT, Exton JH (1981) Inhibitory effect of epinephrine on insulin-stimulated glucose uptake by rat skeletal muscle. J Clin Invest 68:706–713
55. Haring H, Kirsch D, Obermaier B, Ermel B, Machicao F (1986) Decreased tyrosine kinase activity of insulin receptor isolated from rat adipocytes rendered insulin-resistant by catecholamine treatment in vitro. Biochem J 234:59–66
56. Dimitriadis G, Leighton B, Parry-Billings M, Sasson S, Young M, Krause U, Bevan S, Piva T, Wegener G, Newsholme EA (1997) Effects of glucocorticoid excess on the sensitivity of glucose transport and metabolism to insulin in rat skeletal muscle. Biochem J 321:707–712
57. Smith TR, Elmendorf JS, David TS, Turinsky J (1997) Growth hormone-induced insulin resistance: role of the insulin receptor, IRS-1, GLUT-1, and GLUT-4. Am J Physiol 272:E1071–E1079
58. Dominici FP, Cifone D, Bartke A, Turyn D (1999) Alterations in the early steps of the insulin-signaling system in skeletal muscle of GH-transgenic mice. Am J Physiol 277:E447–E454
59. Khaodhiar L, McCowen K, Bistrian B (1999) Perioperative hyperglycemia, infection or risk? Curr Opin Clin Nutr Metab Care 2:79–82
60. Norhammar AM, Ryden L, Malmberg K (1999) Admission plasma glucose. Independent risk factor for long-term prognosis after myocardial infarction even in nondiabetic patients. Diabetes Care 22:1827–1831
61. Zindrou D, Taylor KM, Bagger JP (2001) Admission plasma glucose: an independent risk factor in nondiabetic women after coronary artery bypass grafting. Diabetes Care 24:1634–1639
62. Malmberg K, Norhammar A, Wedel H, Ryden L (1999) Glycometabolic state at admission: important risk marker of mortality in conventionally treated patients with diabetes mellitus and acute myocardial infarction: long-term results from the Diabetes and Insulin-Glucose Infusion in Acute Myocardial Infarction (DIGAMI) study. Circulation 99:2626–26232
63. Malmberg K (1997) Prospective randomised study of intensive insulin treatment on long-term survival after acute myocardial infarction in patients with diabetes mellitus. DIGAMI (Diabetes Mellitus, Insulin Glucose Infusion in Acute Myocardial Infarction) Study Group. Br Med J 314:1512–1515
64. Malmberg K, Ryden L, Efendic S, Herlitz J, Nicol P, Waldenstrom A, Wedel H, Welin L (1995) Randomized trial of insulin-glucose infusion followed by subcutaneous insulin treatment in diabetic patients with acute myocardial infarction (DIGAMI study): effects on mortality at 1 year. J Am Coll Cardiol 26:57–65

65. Capes SE, Hunt D, Malmberg K, Pathak P, Gerstein HC (2001) Stress hyperglycemia and prognosis of stroke in nondiabetic and diabetic patients: a systematic overview. Stroke 32:2426–2432
66. Woo J, Lam CW, Kay R, Wong AH, Teoh R, Nicholls MG (1990) The influence of hyperglycemia and diabetes mellitus on immediate and 3-month morbidity and mortality after acute stroke. Arch Neurol 47:1174–1177
67. Dandona P, Aljada A, Bandyopadhyay A (2003) The potential therapeutic role of insulin in acute myocardial infarction in patients admitted to intensive care and in those with unspecified hyperglycemia. Diabetes Care 26:516–519
68. Hansen TK, Thiel S, Wouters PJ, Christiansen JS, van den Berghe G (2003) Intensive insulin therapy exerts antiinflammatory effects in critically ill patients and counteracts the adverse effect of low mannose-binding lectin levels. J Clin Endocrinol Metab 88:1082–1088
69. Mohanty P, Hamouda W, Garg R, Aljada A, Ghanim H, Dandona P (2000) Glucose challenge stimulates reactive oxygen species (ROS) generation by leucocytes. J Clin Endocrinol Metab 85:2970–2973
70. Straczkowski M, Dzienis-Straczkowska S, Stepien A, Kowalska I, Szelachowska M, Kinalska I (2002) Plasma interleukin-8 concentrations are increased in obese subjects and related to fat mass and tumor necrosis factor-alpha system. J Clin Endocrinol Metab 87:4602–4606
71. Chettab K, Zibara K, Belaiba SR, McGregor JL (2002) Acute hyperglycaemia induces changes in the transcription levels of 4 major genes in human endothelial cells: macroarrays-based expression analysis. Thromb Haemost 87:141–148
72. Standiford TJ, Kunkel SL, Greenberger MJ, Laichalk LL, Strieter RM (1996) Expression and regulation of chemokines in bacterial pneumonia. J Leukoc Biol 59:24–28
73. Hack CE, Aarden LA, Thijs LG (1997) Role of cytokines in sepsis. Adv Immunol 66:101–195
74. Multz AS, Cohen R (2003) Systemic response to pneumonia in the critically ill patient. Semin Resp Infect 18:68–71
75. Aljada A, Ghanim H, Mohanty P, Hofmeyer D, Tripathy D, Dandona P (2002) Glucose activates nuclear factor kappa B pathway in mononuclear cells (MNC) and induces an increase in p47phox. subunit in MNC membranes [Abstract]. Diabetes 51 (Suppl 2):A537
76. Yorek MA, Dunlap JA (2002) Effect of increased concentration of D-glucose or L-fucose on monocyte adhesion to endothelial cell monolayers and activation of nuclear factor-kappaB. Metabolism 51:225–234
77. Guha M, Bai W, Nadler JL, Natarajan R (2000) Molecular mechanisms of tumor necrosis factor alpha gene expression in monocytic cells via hyperglycemia-induced oxidant stress-dependent and -independent pathways. J Biol Chem 275:17728–17739
78. Ceriello A, Bortolotti N, Motz E, Pieri C, Marra M, Tonutti L, Lizzio S, Feletto F, Catone B, Taboga C (1999) Meal-induced oxidative stress and low-density lipoprotein oxidation in diabetes: the possible role of hyperglycemia. Metabolism 48:1503–1508
79. Ceriello A (1993) Coagulation activation in diabetes mellitus: the role of hyperglycaemia and therapeutic prospects. Diabetologia 36:1119–1125
80. Aljada A, Ghanim H, Mohanty P, Syed T, Dandona P (2003) Glucose intake induces an increase in AP-1 and Egr-1 in mononuclear cells and plasma matrix metalloproteinases and tissue factor (TF) concentrations. J Clin Endocrinol Metab
81. Giugliano D, Marfella R, Coppola L, Verrazzo G, Acampora R, Giunta R, Nappo F, Lucarelli C, D'Onofrio F (1997) Vascular effects of acute hyperglycemia in humans are reversed by L-arginine. Evidence for reduced availability of nitric oxide during hyperglycemia. Circulation 95:1783–1790
82. Pozzilli P, Leslie RD (1994) Infections and diabetes: mechanisms and prospects for prevention. Diabet Med 11:935–941
83. Mowlavi A, Andrews K, Milner S, Herndon DN, Heggers JP (2000) The effects of hyperglycemia on skin graft survival in the burn patient. Ann Plast Surg 45:629–632
84. Furnary AP, Zerr KJ, Grunkemeier GL, Starr A (1999) Continuous intravenous insulin infusion reduces the incidence of deep sternal wound infection in diabetic patients after cardiac surgical procedures. Ann Thorac Surg 67:352–360
85. Zerr KJ, Furnary AP, Grunkemeier GL, Bookin S, Kanhere V, Starr A (1997) Glucose control lowers the risk of wound infection in diabetics after open heart operations. Ann Thorac Surg 63:356–361
86. McManus LM, Bloodworth RC, Prihoda TJ, Blodgett JL, Pinckard RN (2001) Agonist-dependent failure of neutrophil function in diabetes correlates with extent of hyperglycemia. J Leukoc Biol 70:395–404
87. Evans TW (2001) Hemodynamic and metabolic therapy in critically ill patients. N Engl J Med 345:1417–1418
88. Rassias AJ, Marrin CA, Arruda J, Whalen PK, Beach M, Yeager MP (1999) Insulin infusion improves neutrophil function in diabetic cardiac surgery patients. Anesth Analg 88:1011–1016
89. Nielson CP, Hindson DA (1989) Inhibition of polymorphonuclear leukocyte respiratory burst by elevated glucose concentrations in vitro. Diabetes 38:1031–1035
90. Kwoun MO, Ling PR, Lydon E, Imrich A, Qu Z, Palombo J, Bistrian BR (1997) Immunologic effects of acute hyperglycemia in nondiabetic rats. J Parenter Enteral Nutr 21:91–95
91. Dandona P, Aljada A, Mohanty P, Ghanim H, Hamouda W, Assian E, Ahmad S (2001) Insulin inhibits intranuclear nuclear factor kappaB and stimulates IkappaB in mononuclear cells in obese subjects: evidence for an anti-inflammatory effect? J Clin Endocrinol Metab 86:3257–3265
92. Aljada A, Ghanim H, Mohanty P, Kapur N, Dandona P (2002) Insulin inhibits the pro-inflammatory transcription factor early growth response gene-1 (Egr)-1 expression in mononuclear cells (MNC) and reduces plasma tissue factor (TF) and plasminogen activator inhibitor-1 (PAI-1) concentrations. J Clin Endocrinol Metab 87:1419–1422
93. Aljada A, Dandona P (2000) Effect of insulin on human aortic endothelial nitric oxide synthase. Metabolism 49:147–150
94. Peng HB, Spiecker M, Liao JK (1998) Inducible nitric oxide: an autoregulatory feedback inhibitor of vascular inflammation. J Immunol 161:1970–1976
95. Spiecker M, Darius H, Kaboth K, Hubner F, Liao JK (1998) Differential regulation of endothelial cell adhesion molecule expression by nitric oxide donors and antioxidants. J Leukoc Biol 63:732–739

96. Spiecker M, Peng HB, Liao JK (1997) Inhibition of endothelial vascular cell adhesion molecule-1 expression by nitric oxide involves the induction and nuclear translocation of IkappaBalpha. J Biol Chem 272:30969–30974
97. Meldrum DR, McIntyre RC, Sheridan BC, Cleveland JC Jr, Fullerton DA, Harken AH (1997) L-arginine decreases alveolar macrophage proinflammatory monokine production during acute lung injury by a nitric oxide synthase-dependent mechanism. J Trauma 43:888–893
98. Laroux FS, Lefer DJ, Kawachi S, Scalia R, Cockrell AS, Gray L, van der Heyde H, Hoffman JM, Grisham MB (2000) Role of nitric oxide in the regulation of acute and chronic inflammation. Antioxidants Redox Signaling 2:391–396
99. Torre A de la, Schroeder RA, Punzalan C, Kuo PC (1999) Endotoxin-mediated S-nitrosylation of p50 alters NF-kappa B-dependent gene transcription in ANA-1 murine macrophages. J Immunol 162:4101–4108
100. Walley KR, McDonald TE, Higashimoto Y, Hayashi S (1999) Modulation of proinflammatory cytokines by nitric oxide in murine acute lung injury. Am J Respir Crit Care Med 160:698–704
101. Pahl HL (1999) Activators and target genes of rel/NF-kappaB transcription factors. Oncogene 18:6853–6866
102. Bohrer H, Qiu F, Zimmermann T, Zhang Y, Jllmer T, Mannel D, Bottiger BW, Stern DM, Waldherr R, Saeger HD, Ziegler R, Bierhaus A, Martin E, Nawroth PP (1997) Role of NFkappaB in the mortality of sepsis. J Clin Invest 100:972–985
103. Arnalich F, Garcia-Palomero E, Lopez J, Jimenez M, Madero R, Renart J, Vazquez JJ, Montiel C (2000) Predictive value of nuclear factor kappaB activity and plasma cytokine levels in patients with sepsis. Infect Immunol 68:1942–1945
104. Paterson RL, Galley HF, Dhillon JK, Webster NR (2000) Increased nuclear factor kappa B activation in critically ill patients who die. Crit Care Med 28:1047–1051
105. Marik PE (2002) Nuclear factor-kappaB inhibition in sepsis: steroids versus specific nuclear factor-kappaB inhibitors? Crit Care Med 30:2393–2394
106. Christman JW, Lancaster LH, Blackwell TS (1998) Nuclear factor kappa B: a pivotal role in the systemic inflammatory response syndrome and new target for therapy. Intensive Care Med 24:1131–1138
107. Fink MP (2003) Nulcear factor-kB: Is it a therapeutic target for the adjuvant treatment of sepsis. Crit Care Med 31:2400–2402
108. Liu SF, Ye X, Malik AB (1999) Inhibition of NF-kappaB activation by pyrrolidine dithiocarbamate prevents In vivo expression of proinflammatory genes. Circulation 100:1330–1337
109. Marik PE, Zaloga G (2003) Gastric vs post-pyloric feeding? A systematic review. Intensive Care Med
110. Marik PE, Zaloga GP (2001) Early enteral nutrition in acutely ill patients: a systematic review. Crit Care Med 29:2264–2270
111. Marik PE, Pinsky MR (2003) Death by total parenteral nutrition. Intensive Care Med 29:867–869
112. Ghanim H, Garg R, Aljada A, Mohanty P, Kumbkarni Y, Assian E, Hamouda W, Dandona P (2001) Suppression of nuclear factor-kappaB and stimulation of inhibitor kappaB by troglitazone: evidence for an anti-inflammatory effect and a potential antiatherosclerotic effect in the obese. J Clin Endocrinol Metab 86:1306–1312
113. Aljada A, Garg R, Ghanim H, Mohanty P, Hamouda W, Assian E, Dandona P (2001) Nuclear factor-kappaB suppressive and inhibitor-kappaB stimulatory effects of troglitazone in obese patients with type 2 diabetes: evidence of an antiinflammatory action? J Clin Endocrinol Metab 86:3250–3256
114. Yue Tl TL, Chen J, Bao W, Narayanan PK, Bril A, Jiang W, Lysko PG, Gu JL, Boyce R, Zimmerman DM, Hart TK, Buckingham RE, Ohlstein EH (2001) In vivo myocardial protection from ischemia/reperfusion injury by the peroxisome proliferator-activated receptor-gamma agonist rosiglitazone. Circulation 104:2588–2594
115. Wayman NS, Hattori Y, McDonald MC, Mota-Filipe H, Cuzzocrea S, Pisano B, Chatterjee PK, Thiemermann C (2002) Ligands of the peroxisome proliferator-activated receptors (PPAR-gamma and PPAR-alpha) reduce myocardial infarct size. FASEB J 16:1027–1040

Ioanna Dimopoulou
Stylianos Tsagarakis

Hypothalamic-pituitary dysfunction in critically ill patients with traumatic and nontraumatic brain injury

Abstract *Background:* A significant number of studies have shown that critically ill patients with brain injury (BI) frequently exhibit abnormal pituitary hormonal responses during the immediate postinjury period. *Discussion:* The elucidation of endocrine alterations depends on the criteria used, the diagnostic tests applied, and the timing of testing in relation to BI. The pattern of the detected hormonal abnormalities shows considerable variability. Altered endocrine responses are due mostly to hypothalamic changes rather than to pituitary dysfunction. Several studies have examined the correlation between hormonal alterations and BI severity, but the results are inconsistent. Furthermore, it remains currently unclear whether and how pituitary abnormalities adversely affect the clinical course of BI patients during the period of critical illness. On the basis of current knowledge, with the exception of clinically significant relative adrenal deficiency and diabetes insipidus, the other endocrine alterations do not seem to require any therapeutic intervention in severely ill BI patients. It is also uncertain whether hormonal abnormalities detected in the early post-BI period persist for the rest of these patients' lives. *Conclusions:* In view of current evidence indicating a high incidence of pituitary dysfunction even years following BI it is recommended that repetition of endocrine evaluation should be performed during the rehabilitation phase in all patients.

Keywords Brain injury · Critical illness · Endocrine alterations · Treatment · Outcome · Recovery

Introduction

Traumatic brain injury (TBI) is a leading cause of death and disability in young adults [1]. Nontraumatic brain injury (BI) includes ischemic stroke, intracerebral hemorrhage, and aneurysmal subarachnoid hemorrhage (SAH) and constitutes a major public-health burden [2]. Advanced life support in the intensive care unit may be needed in a number of BI patients [3].

Pituitary function is an important regulator of a variety of adaptive responses that allow survival during critical states of any type. The mechanisms regulating pituitary hormone secretion are located within the hypothalamus and the brainstem; consequently acute BI as a result of trauma, stroke, or aneurysmal SAH more than any other type of severe illness might be expected to modify the neuroendocrine responses. Autopsy studies show that more than two-third of patients dying of severe head injury have structural abnormalities in the hypothalamic-pituitary region [4]. Therefore it is not surprising that over the past few years pituitary dysfunction has been increasingly reported in patients with TBI [5, 6, 7].

In this review we first briefly discuss the anatomy of the hypothalamic-pituitary axis and the pathophysiology of pituitary dysfunction along with the endocrinology of the normal stress response. Thereafter we outline the existing data regarding the frequency and pattern of pituitary dysfunction in critically ill patients with TBI and

M.R. Pinsky et al. (eds.), *Applied Physiology in Intensive Care Medicine 2: Physiological Reviews and Editorials*,
DOI 10.1007/978-3-642-28233-1_16,

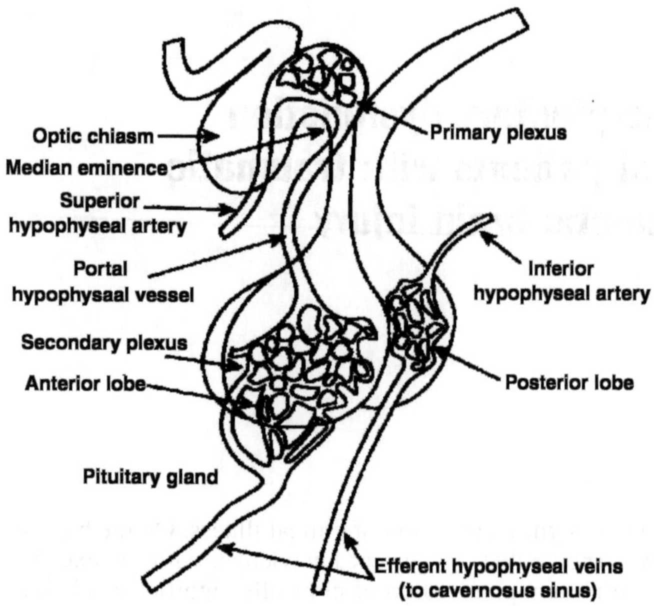

Fig. 1 Anatomy of the hypothalamic-pituitary axis [8]

nontraumatic BI and the clinical relevance of these abnormalities. For this the PubMed search strategy "brain injury and endocrine alterations" was used. Case reports and investigations with a small number of patients (less than five) were excluded.

Anatomy of the hypothalamic-pituitary axis and pathophysiology of pituitary dysfunction following brain injury

The anatomy of the axis is shown in Fig. 1 [8]. The hypothalamus is a structure formed by the anterior and inferior parts of the walls of the third ventricle. It is attached to the pituitary via the stalk, which is derived from the median eminence, a region of the floor of the third ventricle. The median eminence receives the endings of hypothalamic neurons, which produce releasing and inhibiting factors controlling the function of the anterior pituitary lobe. The pituitary is constructed by two parts, the anterior lobe, or adenohypophysis, and the posterior lobe, or neurohypophysis. The adenohypophysis is divided into three regions: (a) the pars distalis, which comprises the major portion of the anterior lobe, (b) the pars intermedia, and (c) the pars tuberalis. The blood supply of the hypothalamus is provided from small branches of all arteries of the circle of Willis. Arterial supply to the anterior pituitary lobe, median eminence, and stalk is derived from paired superior hypophyseal arteries. These arteries form the primary vascular plexus, and converge into venules to form the long and short hypophyseal portal veins. These veins descend to the pars tuberalis and pars distalis of the anterior lobe, where a secondary plexus of sinusoidal capillaries is formed. The long portal veins pass through the diaphragma sella, being thus vulnerable to mechanical compression from brain or pituitary swelling or direct stalk injury. In contrast, the short portal veins originate below the diaphragma sella. Thus the anterior pituitary lobe, particularly its lateral aspects, receives its blood supply indirectly after passage through the median eminence and portal vessels. Consequently any interruption of the portal vessels can result in anterior pituitary dysfunction. In contrast, the neurohypophysis receives a direct arterial blood supply from the inferior hypophyseal arteries.

There are several ways by which BI may adversely affect pituitary function. Direct or indirect (i.e., diffuse brain swelling) mechanical trauma to the hypothalamus, pituitary gland, stalk or vessels is one possible explanation [4, 5, 6]. Functional alterations may also affect pituitary hormone levels. In this context, drugs (opiates, sedatives, antiepileptics, or corticosteroids) have been implicated [9, 10]. During acute BI cytokines, such as tumor necrosis factor α, interleukin 1, and interleukin 6, are produced in large amounts [11]. These may influence hormone levels by exerting stimulatory and/or inhibitory effects [12]. Finally, pituitary dysfunction has been linked to secondary cerebral insults, including hypotension and hypoxemia [13].

Endocrinology of the normal stress response

The endocrinology of the normal stress response is presented in Fig. 2 [14, 15]. The body reacts to hostile conditions by complex physiological and behavioral central nervous system and peripheral adaptive responses. The brain, particularly the hippocampus and amygdala, is intimately involved in the stress response. The stress response is mediated mainly by the sympathoadrenal system (SAS), which includes the sympathetic nervous system (SNS) and the adrenal medulla, and by the hypothalamic-pituitary-adrenal (HPA) axis. The HPA axis and the SAS are functionally related. Activation of SAS results to secretion of epinephrine and norepinephrine from the adrenal medulla and to an increased production of interleukin 6. Activation of the HPA axis involves increased secretion in the hypothalamus of corticotropin-releasing hormone (CRH) and arginine vasopressin, which enhances CRH activity. CRH stimulates the production of corticotropin (ACTH), causing the adrenal cortex to produce more cortisol and dehydroepiadnrosterone; in addition, CRH activates the SAS and SNS. During stress the growth, reproductive and thyroid axes are inhibited at many levels. Glucocorticoids suppress the secretion of growth hormone (GH) and thyroid-stimulating hormone (TSH) and exert an inhibitory effect on the pituitary gonadotrophs and the gonads [16]. These adaptations are initially protective for the human body, how-

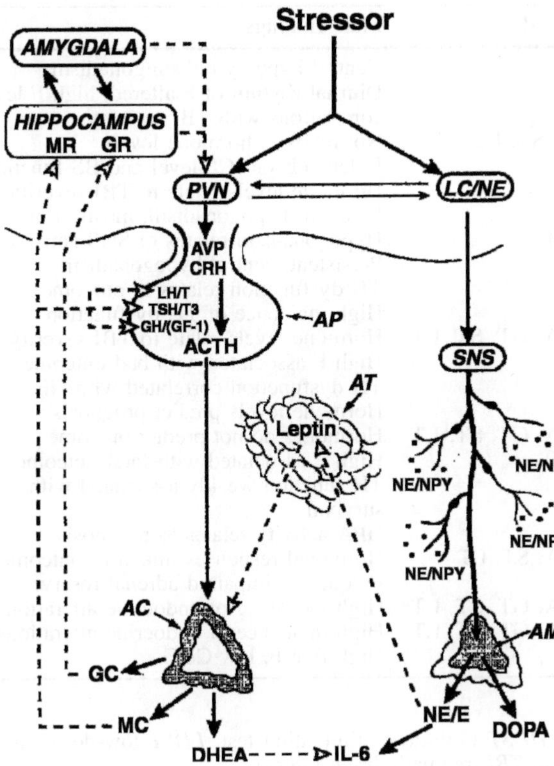

Fig. 2 Endocrinology of the normal stress response. *Straight lines* Stimulation; *dashed lines* inhibition; *PVN* paraventricular nucleus; *AVP* arginine vasopressin; *CRH* corticotropin-releasing hormone; *ACTH* corticotropin; *AP* anterior pituitary; *AC* adrenal cortex; *GC* glucocorticoids; *MC* mineralocorticoids; *DHEA* dehydroepiandrosterone; *LH/T* luteinizing hormone/testosterone; *TSH/T$_3$* thyrotropin/triiodothyronine; *GH/IGF-1* growth hormone/insulin-like growth factor 1; *MR* mineralocorticoid receptors; *GR* glucocorticoid receptors; *LC/NE* locus ceruleus/norepinephrine; *SNS* sympathetic nervous system; *NPY* neuropeptide Y; *AM* adrenal medulla; *E* epinephrine; *IL-6* interleukin-6; *AT* adipose tissue [14, 15]

ever, if inadequate or excessive they may damage health, causing endocrine, metabolic, autoimmune, and psychiatric disturbances [14, 15, 16].

Anterior pituitary dysfunction in brain injury

Anterior pituitary dysfunction in critically ill patients with TBI

In recent years TBI has been increasingly recognized as a cause of neuroendocrine dysfunction [5, 6]. For example, TBI is considered as one of the causes of adult-onset hypopituitarism [7]. Several studies have investigated the anterior pituitary function in TBI patients during the period of critical illness (Table 1) [17, 18, 19, 20, 21, 22, 23, 24, 25, 26, 27, 28, 29, 30, 31, 32, 33, 34, 35, 36, 37, 38, 39].

HPA axis

The HPA axis status is probably the most extensively investigated endocrine function in acute or critically ill TBI patients [18, 20, 27, 31, 32, 34, 35, 36, 37, 38, 39]. Normally patients present with high cortisol levels [18, 20, 28, 32, 34, 35]. These may persist up to 15 days after the trauma [35] and are essential in maintaining vascular tone and endothelial integrity and in potentiating the vasoconstrictor actions of catecholamines [40]. Initially the increase in cortisol is mediated by ACTH [34]. Later other substances, possibly cytokines or catecholamines, act as mediators [12]. The diurnal variation in cortisol may be preserved or abolished [18, 39]. The administration of dexamethasone results in a decrease in plasma cortisol, suggesting an intact negative feedback control mechanism [18].

Studies examining the associations between cortisol dynamics, severity of TBI and outcome prediction have yielded controversial results. Some investigations infer that higher cortisol values are associated with more severe head trauma and with a worse clinical outcome [18, 28, 32, 34], whereas others find lower cortisol values in the most severely injured patients having brainstem dysfunction [20] or in brain-dead victims [41]. Other studies found no correlations between baseline cortisol and TBI severity [35, 37].

The adequacy of cortisol secretion in critical illness, including TBI, remains a diagnostic challenge. This is due mainly to the fact that the normal ranges for baseline or stimulated cortisol levels remain poorly defined. Also, there is much debate on which stimulation test should be used for diagnosis [9, 40]. Assays for serum cortisol measure the total hormone concentration (serum free cortisol plus the protein bound fraction of cortisol). It is believed that free cortisol is responsible for the physiological actions of the hormone. Moreover, it is well known that 90% of circulating cortisol is bound to proteins (corticosteroid-binding globulin and albumin), which both decline in critical illness. Thus in severe illness free cortisol may be a better indicator of adrenal function [42]. On the other hand, measurement of free cortisol is not easily available; thus total cortisol concentration remains the most suitable marker of adrenal function.

Despite the above difficulties some studies have examined relative adrenal dysfunction in critically ill TBI patients (Table 2) [36, 37, 38, 43]. In one of our studies we used the low-dose (1 μg) ACTH stimulation test [43]. This dose of ACTH is similar to the amounts of pituitary ACTH produced under intense stress stimulation [44]. An inadequate adrenal response to this dose indicates that the affected individual is not able to produce adequate amounts of cortisol whenever the need arises. However, the test that we applied indicates adrenal inability to mount a normal cortisol response and does not necessarily

Table 1 Studies on anterior pituitary function in patients with traumatic brain injury during the period of critical illness (*BS* brainstem, *CBG* corticosteroid binding-globulin, *F* cortisol, *GT* gonadotropic, *HPA* hypothalamic pituitary adrenal, *ICP* intracranial pressure, *LT* lactotropic, *NE* norepinephrine, *SNS* sympathetic nervous system, *ST* somatotropic, *TBI* traumatic brain injury, *TH* thyroid)

Reference	*n*	Axes tested	Main findings
Fleischer et al. [17]	15	TH, GT	Central hypothyroidism/gonadism
Steinbock and Thompson [18]	49	HPA	Diurnal rhythm of F altered, high F levels, correlations with TBI severity
King et al. [19]	6	TH, GT, ST, LT	No trends in hormone levels
Feibel et al. [20]	14	HPA	F depends on ICP level and BS function
Matsuura et al. [21]	30	TH, LT	Hormone levels relate to TBI severity
Woolf et al. [22]	54	GT	Frequent hypogonadism, mostly transient
Woolf et al. [23]	31	HPA, GT	Hypogonadism relates to SNS activity
Clark et al. [24]	33	GT, LT	Persistent, central hypogonadism
Woolf et al. [25]	66	TH	TH dysfunction relates to outcome
Chiolero et al. [26]	35	TH	High incidence of TH dysfunction
Chiolero et al. [27]	36	TH, HPA, GT, ST, LT	Hormone levels relate to TBI severity
Woolf et al. [28]	120	HPA	High F associated with bad outcome
Ziegler et al. [29]	23	TH	TH dysfunction correlated with NE
Gottardis et al. [30]	10	TH, ST	Hormone levels predict prognosis
Hackl et al. [31]	21	TH, HPA, GT, ST, LT	Hormones do not predict outcome
Pentelenyi [32]	81	HPA, ST	High F associated with fatal outcome
Mocchegiani et al. [33]	31	TH	TH function weakly associated with survival
Koiv et al. [34]	55	HPA	HPA activity relates to prognosis
Della Corte et al. [35]	22	TH, HPA, ST, LT	Hormonal responses linked to outcome
Hoen et al. [36]	34	HPA	Frequently impaired adrenal reserve
Dimopoulou et al. [37]	34	TH, HPA, GT, ST, LT	High incidence of endocrine alterations
Agha et al. [38]	50	TH, HPA, GT, ST, LT	High incidence of endocrine alterations
Savaridas et al. [39]	9	HPA	High free F, low CBG

Table 2 Results of studies investigating relative adrenal dysfunction in TBI patients during the period of critical illness (*GST* glucagon stimulation test, *hCRH* human corticotrophin-releasing hormone, *HDST* high-dose stimulation test, *LDST* low-dose stimulation test, *TBI* traumatic brain injury)

Reference	*n*	Study entry postinjury	Diagnostic test	Definition of relative adrenal dysfunction	Incidence of relative adrenal dysfunction (%)
Hohen et al. [36]	34	6–63 h	HDST	Increment in cortisol <9 μg/dl	47
Dimopoulou et al. [37]	34	9–60 days	hCRH	Peak cortisol <20 μg/dl	24
Agha et al. [38]	50	7–20 days	GST	Peak cortisol <450 nmol/l	16
Dimopoulou et al. [43]	40	7–60 days	LDST	Peak cortisol <18 μg/dl	15

demonstrate a central defect in the HPA axis. For this reason and to localize the site of HPA axis dysfunction in TBI patients human CRH was applied, and it was found that a subset of patients fail to augment ACTH appropriately in response to human CRH, suggesting a central defect, i.e., hypothalamic-pituitary failure. However, the majority showed increased ACTH after human CRH, indicating primary adrenal dysfunction as the most common cause of inadequate cortisol responses in this clinical setting [43].

Taken together these data indicate that at least on in ten patients with acute TBI develops inadequate HPA function. It seems that in the majority of patients this dysregulation is reminiscent of the relative adrenal insufficiency that presents in a substantial proportion of patients with severe illness. However, it should be mentioned that in a subset of patients HPA dysfunction is centrally mediated. These cases are most likely the result of TBI.

Somatotropic axis

Early after TBI basal plasma GH is within normal limits [30] or high [19, 27, 31]. Insulin-like growth factor 1 has been shown to be normal, or low [37]. However, the adequacy of GH reserve is best investigated by dynamic testing [45]. Agha and coworkers [38] evaluated 50 critically ill TBI patients. The somatotropic axis was assessed by stimulation with glucagon, and the cutoff of 5 ng/ml was selected as a normal response. Nine patients (18%) had GH deficiency. A recent study from our group enrolled 34 TBI patients. GH production was assessed by stimulation with growth hormone releasing hormone (GHRH). We showed that three patients (9%) had partial GH deficiency, defined by a peak GH level between 3 and 5 ng/ml [37].

Some studies have examined the correlation between GH response to provocative tests and prognosis or clinical outcome in the early post-TBI period. However, the reported results are conflicting. For example, it has been shown that the administration of GHRH in comatose TBI

Table 3 Studies on anterior pituitary function in patients with nontraumatic brain injury (*BI*) during the period of critical illness (*CBG* corticosteroid binding-globulin, *HPA* hypothalamic pituitary adrenal, *ICH* itracerebral hemorrhage, *ICP* intracranial pressure, *IS* ischemic stroke, *LT* lactotropic, *SAH* subarachnoid hemorrhage, *TH* thyroid)

References	Type of BI	*n*	Axes tested	Main findings
Feibel et al. [20]	ICH	9	HPA	Cortisol levels depend on ICP and brainstem function
Savaridas et al. [39]	Aneurysmal SAH	6	HPA	High free cortisol, low CBG
Schwarz et al. [47]	IS	22	HPA, TH, LT	Profound endocrine changes, central regulation impaired
Dimopoulou et al. [48]	ICH	3	HPA	High incidence of impaired adrenal reserve, no association with outcome
	IS	17		
	Aneurysmal SAH	4		

survivors entails a significant increase in GH; in contrast, nonsurvivors had no such augmented GH levels [30]. In another investigation a paradoxical rise in GH after glucose loading was observed only in patients with more severe TBI [19]. A subsequent study showed a higher peak GH response to GHRH in patients who had a poor long-term outcome [35].

Gonadotropic-lactotropic axes

TBI produces a profound decrease in testosterone along with low basal follicle-stimulating hormone and luteinizing hormone which develops shortly after injury and deteriorates during the subsequent days [17, 22, 23, 24, 31]. The incidence of hypogonadism in critically ill TBI patients is variable, ranging from 24% to 80% [37, 38]. In a subset of patients testosterone levels normalize within 3–6 months after injury [24]. The magnitude of the decline in testosterone is correlated with head trauma severity in some studies [24, 37, 38] but not in others [22]. The pituitary-ovarian axis is comparably depressed [22].

Several studies attempted to elucidate the mechanisms of hypogonadism in TBI. Clark et al. [46] analyzed the pulse frequency and amplitude of luteinizing hormone in men and found that the former was normal whereas the latter was reduced. The authors concluded that a central dysfunction rather than primary gonadal impairment accounts for hypogonadism after TBI. They suggested that a possible explanation for the reduction in luteinizing hormone pulse amplitude is impaired delivery of gonadotropin-releasing hormone to the anterior pituitary as a consequence of increased intracranial pressure causing stalk compression. The hypothalamic etiology for hypogonadotrophic hypogonadism is further supported by studies showing normal or exaggerated luteinizing hormone and follicle-stimulating hormone responses to releasing factors [17, 22, 31, 37].

Prolactin (PRL) may increase [19, 21, 37, 38], remain normal [35], or decrease [31] in acute TBI. Baseline PRL is correlated with head trauma severity, as expressed by the Glasgow Coma Scale score [38] or the intracranial pressure levels [27]. The PRL responses to GHRH may be of prognostic significance; PRL is higher in TBI patients with a favorable outcome than in those with a poor clinical course [35]. Furthermore, PRL responses to thyrotropin-releasing hormone (TRH) may reflect TBI severity; responses are attenuated in patients with severe head injury [21].

Thyroid axis

Thyroid dysfunction occurs following TBI at an incidence ranging from 4% to 15% [37, 38]. TSH may be normal [19, 26, 33] or low [17, 27, 35], triiodothyronine (T_3) is low [17, 25, 26, 29, 30, 31, 33, 35] and total or free thyroxine (T_4) may be normal [30, 35] or low [17, 25, 26, 29]. Reverse T_3 usually increases [26, 29, 31, 33]. These findings suggest a low T_3 and/or a low T_4 syndrome. Changes in T_3 and reverse T_3 appear immediately after trauma [25] and can persist for at least 2 weeks [35]. Thyroid dysfunction has been shown to be reversible [17]. According to some studies basal thyroidal hormones reflect head trauma severity and predict outcome [17, 25, 26, 33]; thus patients with the greatest neurological dysfunction and a bad ultimate outcome have the lowest T_4 and T_3 levels [25]. However, others have failed to support these associations [35]. Dynamic testing may be of value in predicting clinical outcome; the TSH response after stimulation with TRH has been shown to be absent only in patients having a poor outcome [30, 35].

Anterior pituitary dysfunction in critically ill patients with nontraumatic BI

Pituitary function in critically ill patients with nontraumatic BI has received less systematic attention (Table 3) [20, 39, 47, 48].

Stroke (ischemic stroke and intracerebral hemorrhage)

Evidence that stroke is associated with endocrine dysfunction comes primarily from studies investigating noncritically ill patients with acute stroke. Most research has focused on HPA axis activity showing high cortisol responses [49], disturbed diurnal cortisol rhythm [50], and reduced suppressibility of serum cortisol by dexamethasone [51]. Several other abnormalities have been reported, such as thyroid function suppression [52], hypogonadism [53, 54], and low insulin-like growth factor 1 [55].

Critically ill stroke patients may also experience hormonal dysfunction. A recent study evaluated 22 patients with acute space occupying hemispheric ischemic stroke on admission in the ICU and on days 3, 5, 7, and 9. Plasma levels of PRL, TSH, total and free T_4, total T_3, ACTH, and cortisol were measured; furthermore, on day 3 a TRH stimulation test was performed. The authors found abnormally low cortisol and ACTH concentrations, high PRL, and slightly suppressed thyroid function throughout the observation period. TRH stimulation of plasma TSH and PRL was low. The diurnal rhythm of cortisol was abolished [47]. Our group examined the HPA axis function in 20 critical care patients with stroke. We found that two patients had blunted cortisol responses following dynamic stimulation. Hypoadrenalism was associated with a higher mortality rate, although it did not constitute an independent outcome predictor [48].

Aneurysmal SAH

The concept of SAH-induced hormonal alterations is supported by a study performed in noncritically ill patients with acute SAH. Baseline cortisol was high in all patients, gonadal hormones were within normal ranges, and hyperprolactinemia was present in 14%. Thyroid function abnormalities consisted of high TSH (14%), low T_3 (14%), and low T_4 (6%) [56]. Recent evidence suggests that hormonal abnormalities are frequent in long-term SAH survivors [57, 58, 59, 60], with GH or gonadal deficiencies predominating [57, 58, 60]. This pattern is similar to that in survivors of TBI, suggesting that GH and/or gonadotropin function is more fragile than the other axes, and that the pattern of endocrine abnormalities is unrelated to the type of BI [58, 61].

Data on hormonal changes in critically ill patients with aneurysmal SAH are sparse. A recent study investigated cotisol dynamics in six mechanically ventilated SAH patients. Total cortisol and corticosteroid-binding globulin were measured in the morning and evening, while free cortisol was calculated. In three patients the diurnal variation in total cortisol was abolished. All patients had total cortisol levels within the accepted reference range for nonstressed individuals. However, all patients had low corticosteroid-binding globulin and normal free cortisol. The authors concluded that critically ill SAH patients have no evidence of cortisol depletion [39].

Posterior pituitary dysfunction in brain injury

A normal function of the posterior pituitary is crucial for water homeostasis. Posterior pituitary dysfunction is a well-recognized complication of traumatic BI, but there are only scarce data in patients with SAH [62]. Inadequate antidiuretic hormone (ADH) secretion results in diabetes insipidus (DI). The most reliable data regarding the prevalence and natural course of posttraumatic DI have been published recently by Agha et al. [62]; they reported a prevalence of DI in the immediate period following TBI of 21.6%. In this series the occurrence of DI was related to the severity of the traumatic insult, but it was unrelated to the development of anterior pituitary abnormalities. In most cases posttraumatic DI was transient. A prospective study by Agha et al. [63] reported that 9 of 13 patients who had DI in the acute posttraumatic phase recovered by 6 months, and one additional patient recovered by 12 months. Interestingly, the majority of patients with permanent DI had only partial vasopressin deficiency.

Apart from hypernatremic dehydration induced by ADH deficiency, hyponatremia also develops in a substantial proportion of patients during the acute period of BI due to an inappropriate release of ADH (syndrome of inappropriate antidiuretic hormone, SIADH) as a result of damage to the pituitary stalk or the posterior pituitary. The reported prevalence of this abnormality varies form 2.3% to 36%. As a rule SIADH induced by TBI is transient [63].

Clinical implications of pituitary function alterations in brain injury

It has been stated that the importance of delineating pituitary function during the early phase of traumatic or nontraumatic BI is threefold: (a) to detect abnormalities that hamper recovery of these patients during the critical phase of their illness, (b) to obtain prognostic information for patients' morbidity and mortality rates, and (c) to diagnose pituitary hormone deficiencies that may persist later in life at an early stage.

Pituitary function and impaired recovery

As in other critical states, it is not clear whether hormone deficiencies discovered during the acute phase of BI are adaptive or detrimental [64]. Suppression of the hypothalamic-pituitary-gonadal axis may be appropriate to downregulate the production of anabolic androgens to conserve utilization of metabolic substrates by the less vital organs. On the other hand, loss of the sex steroids with their anabolic properties might be expected to affect wound healing and convalescence [65]. The changes in the thyroid axis have been interpreted as an attempt to reduce energy expenditure and are generally believed to be adaptive for the individual [66]. Although not widely accepted [6, 61], some studies suggest that both gonadal and thyroid endocrine abnormalities are transient in critically ill TBI patients [17, 22, 23, 24]; thus it is questionable whether they should be treated. Similarly, the GH deficiency state observed during the acute phase in some patients with BI does not seem to require medical intervention. A large multicenter study showed that the administration of high doses of GH in critically ill patients, instead of improving outcome, doubled mortality [67]. Thus GH supplementation is not currently recommended during the acute phase of critical illness of any type. However, diminished GH secretion persisting later in life may be harmful since GH is beneficial on the net protein balance, bone mineral density, well-being, and cardiac and immune function [68].

In contrast, independently of its cause, the inability to mount an adequate cortisol response may increase the risk of death during severe illness, especially in patients with multiple organ failure and hemodynamic instability [10, 40]. On the other hand, no strict biochemical criteria for "normal" serum cortisol concentrations in critically ill patients are currently available [9, 10, 69]. Consequently, baseline or stimulated cortisol levels in deciding when to treat patients need further assessment. It should be noted that a recent large, randomized, placebo-control study showed that the early administration of pharmacological doses of methylprednisolone is not beneficial in patients with TBI injury. In fact this treatment was associated with a significant rise in risk of death within 2 weeks [70]. Therefore it is recommended that in the presence of clinically significant functional hypoadrenalism only physiological doses of steroid replacement be applied.

The same is true for posterior pituitary dysfunction occurring as a result of BI. Untreated DI leads to polyuria. Since in the early post-TBI period water intake may be inadequate due to impaired cognition, polyuria can lead to hypernatremic dehydration with increased morbidity and impairment of recovery, a condition that is reversible with appropriate treatment with desmopressin and maintenance of fluid balance. Similarly, recognition and treatment of SIADH is important as hyponatremia increases the risk of cerebral edema and is associated with increased morbidity and mortality in BI patients.

Pituitary function and prognosis

The relevance of pituitary hormonal changes to patients' morbidity and mortality remains controversial. Some studies infer that basal hormones and/or hormonal responses to provocative tests serve as markers of head trauma severity. As a consequence such associations might be useful in establishing early prognosis in TBI patients. However, other studies have failed to confirm these relationships. The relationship between pituitary dysfunction and long-term functional outcome is also controversial; one study showed that a good neurological recovery is more common in patients without hormonal abnormalities [13], while a recent investigation did not support this finding [61].

Early detection of persistent pituitary function abnormalities

A number of recent reports have examined the incidence and type of hormonal deficiencies in short or long-term survivors of BI. These studies suggest that subjects with a history of BI frequently develop pituitary dysfunction. The time-course of these anterior pituitary function abnormalities is currently unclear. One possibility is that these abnormalities occur in the early postinjury period; another possibility is that they appear progressively during the years following the acute insult. However, based on the data presented in this review pituitary dysfunction occurring in the early phase of BI consists of a mixture of pathophysiologically different changes. Thus most hormonal deficiencies observed during the early phase of BI follow the same course as in almost all critical states, and therefore it is difficult to discern a separate effect attributed to structural neuroendocrine damage. Even in those patients presenting with altered pituitary function tests during the early phase it is currently unclear whether these changes are permanent or reversible. Therefore and given the high prevalence of pituitary deficits in BI survivors it is strongly recommended that the management of these patients routinely include a complete neuroendocrine reevaluation at their recovery phase.

Conclusions

In critically ill BI patients abnormal pituitary endocrine responses are due principally to hypothalamic changes. Several studies have examined the correlation between these hormonal alterations and BI severity, but the results are inconsistent. It remains currently unclear whether and how pituitary abnormalities adversely affect the clinical course of BI patients during the period of critical illness. With the exception of clinically significant relative adrenal deficiency and DI, the other endocrine alterations do not seem to require any therapeutic intervention in severely ill BI patients. It is also uncertain whether endocrine abnormalities detected in the early post-BI period persist for the rest of these patients' lives. In view of current evidence indicating a high incidence of pituitary dysfunction even years following BI it is recommended that repetition of endocrine evaluation be performed during the rehabilitation phase in all patients.

References

1. Marik PE, Varon J, Trask T (2002) Management of head trauma. Chest 122:699–711
2. Warlow C, Sudlow C, Dennis M, Wardlaw J, Sandercock P (2003) Stroke. Lancet 362:1211–1224
3. Fahy BG, Sivaraman V (2002) Current concepts in neurocritical care. Anesthesiol Clin North America 20:441–462
4. Crompton MR (1971) Hypothalamic lesions following closed head injury. Brain 94:165–172
5. Edwards OM, Clark JD (1986) Post-traumatic hypopituitarism. Six cases and review of the literature. Medicine (Baltimore) 65:281–290
6. Benvega S, Campenni A, Ruggeri RM, Trimarchi F (2000) Clinical Review 113. Hypopituitarism secondary to head trauma. J Clin Endocrinol Metab 85:1353–1361
7. Lamberts SWJ, de Herder WW, van der Lely AJ (1998) Pituitary insufficiency. Lancet 352:127–134
8. Amar AP, Weiss MH (2003) Pituitary anatomy and physiology. Neurosurg Clin N Am 13:11–23
9. Oelkers W (1996) Adrenal insufficiency. N Engl J Med 335:1206–1212
10. Cooper MS, Stewart PM (2003) Corticosteroid insufficiency in acutely ill patients. N Engl J Med 348:727–734
11. McKeating EG, Andrews PJD (1998) Cytokines and adhesion molecules in acute brain injury. Br J Anaesth 80:77–84
12. Bornstein SR, Chroussos GP (1999) Clinical review 104. Adrenocorticotropin (ACTH)- and non-ACTH-mediated regulation of the adrenal cortex: neural and immune inputs. J Clin Endocrinol Metab 84:1729–1736
13. Kelly DF, Gaw Gonzalo IT, Cohan P, Berman N, Swerdloff R, Wang C (2000) Hypopituitarism following traumatic brain injury and aneurysmal subarachnoid hemorrhage: a preliminary report. J Neurosurg 93:743–752
14. Chroussos GP (2000) The role of stress and the hypothalamic-pituitary-adrenal axis in the pathogenesis of the metabolic syndrome: neuroendocrine and target tissue-related causes. Int J Obes Relat Metab Disord 24:S50–S55
15. Vanltallie TB (2002) Stress: a risk factor for serious illness. Metabolism 51 [Suppl 1]:40–45
16. Charmandari E, Tsigos C, Chrousos G (2005) Endocrinology of the stress response. Annu Rev Physiol 67:259–284
17. Fleischer AS, Rudman DR, Payne NS, Tindall GT (1978) Hypothalamic hypothyroidism and hypogonadism in prolonged traumatic coma. J Neurosurg 49:650–657
18. Steinbok P, Thompson G (1979) Serum cortisol abnormalities after craniocerebral trauma. Neurosurgery 5:559–565
19. King LR, Knowles HC, McLaurin RL, Brielmaier J, Perisutti G, Piziak VK (1981) Pituitary response to head injury. Neurosurgery 9:229–235
20. Feibel J, Kelly M, Lee L, Woolf P (1983) Loss of adrenocortical suppression after acute brain injury: role of increased intracranial pressure and brain stem function. J Clin Endocrinol Metab 57:1245–1250
21. Matsuura H, Nakazawa S, Wakabayashi I (1985) Thyrotropin-releasing hormone provocative release of prolactin and thyrotropin in acute head injury. Neurosurgery 16:791–795
22. Woolf PD, Hamill RW, McDonald JV, Lee LA, Kelly M (1985) Transient hypogonadotropic hypogonadism caused by critical illness. J Clin Endocrinol Metab 60:444–450
23. Woolf PD, Hamill RW, McDonald JV, Lee LA, Kelly M (1986) Transient hypogonadotrophic hypogonadism after head trauma: effects on steroid precursors and correlation with sympathetic nervous system activity. Clin Endocrinol (Oxf) 25:265–274
24. Clark JD, Raggatt PR, Edwards OM (1988) Hypothalamic hypogonadism following major head injury. Clin Endocrinol (Oxf) 29:153–165
25. Woolf PD, Lee LA, Hamill RW, McDonald JV (1988) Thyroid test abnormalities in traumatic brain injury: correlation with neurologic impairment and sympathetic nervous system activation. Am J Med 84:201–208
26. Chiolero RL, Lemarchand-Beraud T, Schutz Y, de Tribolet N, Bayer-Berger M, Freeman J (1988) Thyroid function in severely traumatized patients with or without head injury. Acta Endocrinol (Copenh) 117:80–86
27. Chiolero R, Lemarchand T, Schutz Y, de Tribolet N, Felber JP, Freeman J, Jequier E (1988) Plasma pituitary hormone levels in severe trauma with or without head injury. J Trauma 28:1368–1374
28. Woolf PD, Cox C, Kelly M, Nichols D, McDonald JV, Hamill RW (1990) The adrenocortical response to brain injury: correlation with the severity of neurologic dysfunction, effects of intoxication, and patient outcome. Alcohol Clin Exp Res 14:917–921
29. Ziegler MG, Morrissey EC, Marshall LF (1990) Catecholamine and thyroid hormones in traumatic injury. Crit Care Med 18:253–258
30. Gottardis M, Nigitsch C, Schmutzhard E, Neumann M, Putensen C, Hackl JM, Koller W (1990) The secretion of human growth hormone stimulated by human growth hormone releasing factor following severe cranio-cerebral trauma. Intensive Care Med 16:163–166
31. Hackl JM, Gottardis M, Wieser C, Rumpl E, Stadler C, Schwarz S, Monkayo R (1991) Endocrine abnormalities in severe traumatic brain injury-a cue to prognosis in severe craniocerebral trauma? Intensive Care Med 17:25–29
32. Pentelenyi T (1992) Significance of endocrine studies in the general assessment and prediction of fatal outcome in head injury. Acta Neurochir Suppl 55:21–24
33. Mocchegiani E, Imberti R, Testasecca D, Zandri M, Santarelli L, Fabris N (1995) Thyroid and thymic endocrine function and survival in severely traumatized patients with or without head injury. Intensive Care Med 21:334–341
34. Koiv L, Merisalu E, Zilmer K, Tomberg T, Kaasik AE (1997) Changes of sympatho-adrenal and hypothalamo-pituitary-adrenocortical system in patients with head injury. Acta Neurol Scand 96:52–58
35. Della Corte F, Mancini A, Valle D, Gallizzi F, Carducci P, Mignani V, De Marinis L (1998) Provocative hypothalamopituitary axis tests in severe head injury: correlations with severity and prognosis. Crit Care Med 26:1419–1426
36. Hoen S, Asehnoune K, Brailly-Tabart S, Mazoit JX, Benhamou D, Moine P, Edouard AR (2002) Cortisol response to corticotropin stimulation in trauma patients: influence of hemorrhagic shock. Anesthesiology 97:807–813
37. Dimopoulou I, Tsagarakis S, Theodorakopoulou M, Douka E, Zervou M, Kouyialis AT, Thalassinos N, Roussos C (2004) Endocrine abnormalities in critical care patients with moderate-to-severe head trauma: incidence, pattern and predisposing factors. Intensive Care Med 30:1051–1057
38. Agha A, Rogers B, Mylotte D, Taleb F, Tormey W, Phillips J, Thompson CJ (2004) Neuroendocrine dysfunction in the acute phase of traumatic brain injury. Clin Endocrinol (Oxf) 60:584–591
39. Savaridas T, Andrews PJD, Harris B (2004) Cortisol dynamics following acute severe brain injury. Intensive Care Med 30:1479–1483
40. Lamberts SWJ, Bruining HA, de Jong FH (1997) Drug therapy: corticosteroid therapy in severe illness. N Engl J Med 337:1285–1292

41. Dimopoulou I, Tsagarakis S, Anthi A, Milou E, Ilias I, Stavrakaki K, Charalambidis C, Tzanela M, Orfanos S, Mandragos K, Thalassinos N, Roussos C (2003) High incidence of decreased cortisol reserve in brain-dead potential organ donors. Crit Care Med 31:1113–1117
42. Hamrahian AH, Oseni TS, Arafah B (2004) Measurements of serum free cortisol in critically ill patients. N Engl J Med 350:1629–1638
43. Dimopoulou I, Tsagarakis S, Kouyialis AT, Roussou P, Assithianakis G, Christoforaki M, Ilias I, Sakas DE, Thalassinos N, Roussos C (2004) Hypothalamic-pituitary-adrenal dysfunction in critically ill patients with traumatic brain injury: incidence, pathophysiology, and relationship to vasopressor dependence and peripheral interleukin-6 levels. Crit Care Med 32:404–408
44. Dickstein G, Shechner C, Nicholson WE, Rosner I, Shen-Orr Z, Adawi F, Lahav M (1991) Adrenocorticotropin stimulation test: effects of basal cortisol level, time of day, and suggested new sensitive low dose test. J Clin Endocrinol Metab 72:773–778
45. Stavrou S, Kleinberg DL (2001) Diagnosis and management of growth hormone deficiency in adults. Endocrinol Metab Clin North Am 30:545–563
46. Clark JDA, Raggatt PR, Edwards OM (1992) Abnormalities of the hypothalamo-pituitary-gonadal axis after head injury. Clin Endocrinol (Oxf) 36:481–485
47. Schwarz S, Schwab S, Klinga K, Maser-Gluth C, Bettendorf M (2003) Neuroendocrine changes in patients with acute space occupying ischemic stroke. J Neurol Neurosurg Psychiatry 74:725–727
48. Dimopoulou I, Tsagarakis S, Douka E, Zervou M, Kouyialis AT, Dafni U, Thalassinos N, Roussos C (2004) The low-dose corticotropin stimulation test in acute traumatic and non-traumatic brain injury: incidence of hypo-responsiveness and relationship to outcome. Intensive Care Med 30:1216–1219
49. Fassbender K, Schmidt R, Mossner R, Daffertshofer M, Hennerici M (1994) Pattern of activation of the hypothalamic-pituitary-adrenal axis in acute stroke. Relation to acute confusional state, extent of brain damage, and clinical outcome. Stroke 25:1105–1108
50. Johansson A, Ahren B, Nasman B, Carlstrom K, Olsson T (2000) Cortisol axis abnormalities early after stroke—relationships to cytokines and leptin. J Intern Med 247:179–187
51. Olsson T, Marklund N, Gustafson Y, Nasman B (1992) Abnormalities at different levels of the hypothalamic-pituitary-adrenocortical axis early after stroke. Stroke 23:1573–1576
52. Hagg E, Asplund K, Eriksson S, Lithner F, Strand T, Wester PO (1986) Serum thyroid-stimulating hormone in cerebrovascular disease. Acta Med Scand 219:53–58
53. Pepper GM, Koenigsberg R, Zito JL, Deutsch S (1993) Alterations of serum pituitary hormone levels in postmenopausal women with stroke. Stroke 24:805–808
54. Jeppesen LL, Jorgensen HS, Nakayama H, Raaschou HO, Olsen TS, Winther K (1996) Decreased serum testosterone in men with acute ischemic stroke. Arterioscler Thromb Vasc Biol 16:749–754
55. Schwab S, Spranger M, Krempien S, Hacke W, Bettendorf M (1997) Plasma insulin-like growth factor I and IGF binding protein 3 levels in patients with acute cerebral ischemic injury. Stroke 28:1744–1748
56. Mangieri P, Suzuki K, Ferreira M, Domingues L, Casulari LA (2003) Evaluation of pituitary and thyroid hormones in patients with subarachnoid hemorrhage due to ruptured intracranial aneurysm. Arq Neuropsiquiatr 61:14–19
57. Brandt L, Saveland H, Valdenmarsson S, Sjoholm H, Reinstrup P (2004) Fatigue after aneurysmal subarachnoid hemorrhage evaluated by pituitary function and 3D-CBF. Acta Neurol Scand 109:91–96
58. Aimaretti G, Ambrosio MR, Di Somma C, Fusco A, Cannavo S, Gasperi M, Scaroni C, De Marinis L, Benvega S, Degli Uberti EC, Lombardi G, Mantero F, Martino E, Giordano G, Ghigo E (2004) Traumatic brain injury and subarachnoid haemorrhage are conditions at high risk for hypopituitarism: screening study at 3 months after the brain injury. Clin Endocrinol (Oxf) 61:320–326
59. Kreitschmann-Andermahr I, Hoff C, Saller B, Niggemeier S, Pruemper S, Hutter BO, Rohde V, Gressner A, Matern S, Gilsbach JM (2004) Prevalence of pituitary deficiency in patients after aneurysmal subarachnoid hemorrhage. J Clin Endocrinol Metab 89:4986–4992
60. Dimopoulou I, Kouyialis AT, Tzanella M, Armaganidis A, Thalassinos N, Sakas DE, Tsagarakis S (2004) High incidence of neuroendocrine dysfunction in long-term survivors of aneurysmal subarachnoid hemorrhage. Stroke 35:2884–2889
61. Bondanelli M, De Marinis L, Ambrosio MR, Monesi M, Valle D, Zatelli MC, Fusco A, Bianchi A, Farneti M, Degli Uberti EC (2004) Occurrence of pituitary dysfunction following traumatic brain injury. J Neurotrauma 21:685–696
62. Agha A, Thornton E, O'Kelly P, Tormey W, Phillips J, Thompson CJ (2004) Posterior pituitary dysfunction after traumatic brain injury. J Clin Endocrinol Metab 89:5987–5992
63. Agha A, Sherlock M, Phillips J, Tormey W, Thompson CJ (2005) The natural history of post-traumatic neurohypophysial dysfunction. Eur J Endocrinol 152:371–377
64. Van den Berghe G (2000) Novel insights into the neuroendocrinology of critical illness. Eur J Endocrinol 143: 1–13
65. Spratt DI (2001) Altered gonadal steroidogenesis in critical illness: is treatment with anabolic steroids indicated? Baillieres Best Pract Res Clin Endocrinol Metab 15:479–494
66. Stathatos N, Levetan C, Burman KD, Wartofsky L (2001) The controversy of the treatment of critically ill patients with thyroid hormone. Baillieres Best Pract Res Clin Endocrinol Metab 15:465–478
67. Takala J, Ruokonen E, Webster NR, Nielsen MS, Zandstra DF, Vundelinckx G, Hinds CJ (1999) Increased mortality associated with growth hormone treatment in critically ill adults. N Engl J Med 341:785–792
68. Carroll PV (2001) Treatment with growth hormone and insulin like growth factor-I in critical illness. Baillieres Best Pract Res Clin Endocrinol Metab 15:435–451
69. Ligtenberg JJM, Zijlstra JG (2004) The relative adrenal insufficiency syndrome revisited: which patients will benefit from low-dose steroids? Curr Opin Crit Care 10:456–460
70. CRASH trial collaborators (2204) Effect of intravenous corticosteroids on death within 14 days in 10.008 adults with clinically significant head injury (MRC CRASH trial): randomised placebo-controlled trial. Lancet 364:1321–1328

Pierre Squara

Matching total body oxygen consumption and delivery: a crucial objective?

Abstract The strength of the rationale for incorporating total body oxygen consumption (VO_2) and delivery (DO_2) into our decision making strategies contrasts with the absence of demonstrated benefits of bedside calculations in clinical practice. This situation mandates a careful reappraisal of the theoretical limitations of bedside calculations of DO_2 and VO_2, including a re-evaluation of the clinical situations in which these calculations are valid. Three levels of complexity can be distinguished when analysing a patient's hemodynamic status: 1) simple cases where investigations can be limited to clinical monitoring, including lactate changes over time; 2) intermediate situations requiring invasive investigations in which continuous monitoring of VO_2-related variables such as cardiac output and mixed venous oxygen saturation often provide enough information to guide clinical decision; and 3) complex situations where assessment of VO_2 and VO_2/DO_2 analysis might be recommended. Although studies that support such recommendations are limited they are based on a widely accepted physiological model. VO_2 and DO_2 analysis is also limited by theoretical and technical difficulties. In this article, we discuss the validity of these limitations in the bedside assessment of VO_2 and DO_2, and review data supporting the use of VO_2/DO_2 analysis in the clinical evaluation of complex cases.

Introduction

Regardless of the cause of shock, failure to rapidly restore adequate status leads to impaired mitochondrial O_2 uptake and dysoxia. Significant O_2 uptake due to nonoxidative systems may occur only when dysoxia has resolved, as these systems have lower affinity for oxygen than do oxidative systems [1, 2, 3]. A reasonable assumption therefore is that below a critical level, VO_2 is inversely correlated to the risk of cell dysfunction and to the severity of shock. Once a substantial amount of cell necrosis has occurred, organ function recovery is not always possible even when an adequate VO_2 is restored. In a large population of shock of various origins it has been shown that a VO_2 value below that expected is the one most strongly related to death [4]. Thus early VO_2 adaptation to tissue needs should be the major treatment goal in patients with shock [5, 6]. The contrast between this strong rationale and the lack of consensus that bedside VO_2 assessment is beneficial in practice mandates a careful reappraisal of our means to match VO_2 and needs.

The VO_2/DO_2 relationship

The physiological model

In both isolated cells [7, 8, 9] and whole organisms [10, 11, 12] a biphasic relationship between O_2 use and resources has been established. When DO_2 is higher than a threshold value, VO_2 remains stable (O_2 supply independency) because the O_2 extraction rate of oxygen ($EO_2=VO_2/DO_2$) changes proportionally. When DO_2 falls below this threshold, a proportional increase in EO_2

M.R. Pinsky et al. (eds.), *Applied Physiology in Intensive Care Medicine 2: Physiological Reviews and Editorials*,
DOI 10.1007/978-3-642-28233-1_17, © Springer-Verlag Berlin Heidelberg 2012

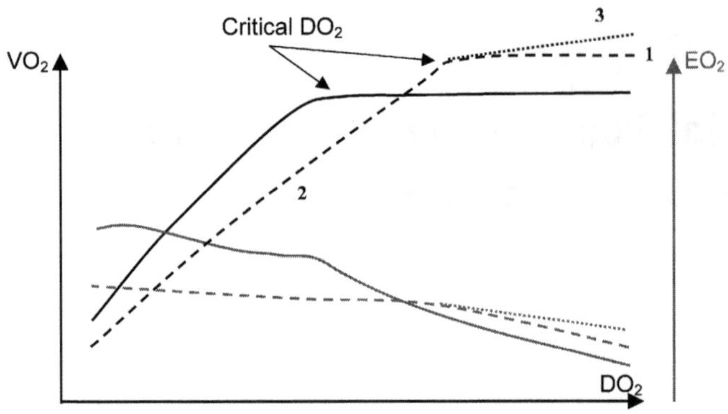

Fig. 1 Pathophysiological changes in the VO_2/DO_2 relationship. *Solid black line* Normal relationship; *dotted lines* abnormal relationships *1* increased VO_2 needs; *2* impaired EO_2; *3* other mechanisms (see text). *Gray curves* Corresponding EO_2/DO_2 relationships

cannot be maintained, and the VO_2 linearly drops to zero (O_2 supply dependency). The inflection point between the two slopes is accepted as indicating the critical level of DO_2 (Fig. 1). The O_2 supply dependency is associated with an increase in blood lactate concentration denoting possible activation of the anaerobic pathway [11, 13, 14, 15].

Assessment of the VO_2/DO_2 relationship is a theoretical means of evaluating the gap between actual VO_2 and needed VO_2. A DO_2 challenge can be performed easily at the bedside by increasing cardiac output (CO) [16], increasing low hemoglobin concentration (Hb) [11, 17], or increasing low SaO_2 [18]. When DO_2 increases, an increase in VO_2 argues for inadequate O_2 supply. In contrast, a stable VO_2 value when DO_2 increases suggests either that VO_2 matches needs when associated with decreasing lactate levels [11, 13, 14, 15], or that VO_2 is limited by other mechanisms than O_2 supply, when associated with increasing lactate levels [19, 20, 21].

Although VO_2 can be calculated by spirometry or indirect calorimetry, the reverse Fick method using a pulmonary artery catheter (PAC) is the most popular method for assessing the VO_2/DO_2 relationship in clinical practice. DO_2 is the arterial oxygen delivery calculated as the product of CO by arterial oxygen content (CaO_2). VO_2 can be calculated as the product of CO by the arteriovenous oxygen difference in oxygen contents ($Ca{-}vO_2=CaO_2-CvO_2$).

"Patho-physiological" changes

Two mechanisms delay achievement of the VO_2 plateau and account for a rightward shift in the critical DO_2 point (Fig. 1). When VO_2 needs are excessive (uncoupling and/or increased metabolic activity), the VO_2 plateau is reached at a higher level of VO_2 [22, 23]. When O_2 tissue diffusion is impaired (impaired microcirculation and/or impaired O_2 mitochondrial use), the slope of the dependent part of the VO_2/DO_2 relationship is decreased [24, 25, 26].

Three other mechanisms result in an increase in VO_2 as DO_2 increases beyond the critical point, so that a slight upward slope, usually of less than 5%, replaces the expected VO_2 plateau. Although more difficult, identification of the critical DO_2 inflection point remains possible when these mechanisms are operative, because the slope of the VO_2/DO_2 dependency segment ranges from 20% to 50% [27]. The first mechanism occurs during a DO_2 challenge involving an increase in CO because the VO_2 needs of kidneys [28], stomach [29], and muscle [30] increase in direct proportion to flow. Furthermore, infusion of inotropic agents increases myocardial O_2 consumption [11, 15, 27]. Another mechanism is additional oxygen uptake due to nonmitochondrial oxidase systems when dysoxia has resolved [1, 31]. The last mechanism, conformance, is a decrease in the cells' metabolic needs in response to a gradual decline in available O_2. Although secondary to a chronic change, this phenomenon has been observed in acute situations [32], and recovery from conformance may account for progressive increase in metabolic needs [33].

The spurious "pathological" supply dependency

A controversy arose in the 1980s from several studies on the acute respiratory distress syndrome and/or sepsis in which the expected VO_2 plateau was not observed in patients who were recovering from shock and had high DO_2 values [34, 35, 36, 37]. This was interpreted as evidence of "pathological O_2 supply dependency" possibly related to a hidden oxygen deficit contributing to multiorgan failure and death. However, increasing DO_2 to supranormal values was beneficial in some studies [38, 39, 40, 41] but not in others [42, 43]. Furthermore, it has been suggested this so-called "pathological supply dependency" results from spurious upsloping of the VO_2/DO_2 relationship due to mathematical coupling of measurement errors when using a PAC because in some studies simultaneous and independent assessments of VO_2 demonstrated a plateau [12, 44, 45, 46].

Methodological limitations of VO_2/DO_2 relationship assessment

The formulas of $VO_2=CO\times[Hb\times1.36\times(SaO_2-SvO_2)]$ and $DO_2=CO\times SaO_2\times Hb\times1.36$, where blood gases are neglected, shows that VO_2 and DO_2 share three variables: Hb, SaO_2, and CO (plus height and weight if CO is indexed). It is therefore necessary to study the impact of these shared variables on the VO_2/DO_2 relationship.

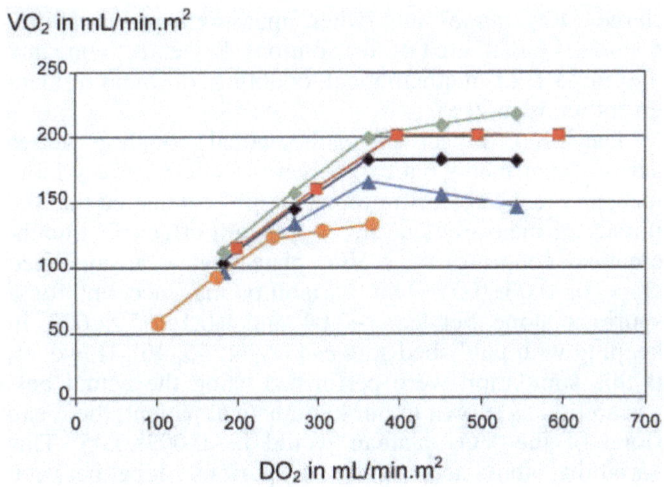

Fig. 2 Effect of systematic errors in the VO_2/DO_2 relationship. *Black curve* A hypothetical patient. The critical DO_2 is reached at the third point. *Red curve* Systematic 10% overestimation of CO, Hb, or $CavO_2$; *blue curve* systematic 10% overestimation of SvO_2 with no error in SaO_2; *green curve* systematic 10% underestimation of SvO_2 with no error in SaO_2; *orange curve* 0.5 l/min absolute underestimation of CO

Systematic measurement errors

Systematic relative errors in Hb, CO, height, or weight measurements do not modify the shape of the curve because all points are changed proportionally (Fig. 2). Even if VO_2 and DO_2 values are over- or underestimated, the critical DO_2 is identified at the same moment during a DO_2 challenge. From the formulae it is easy to understand that the shape of the VO_2/DO_2 relationship can only change when there is an absolute error in CO (with upsloping of the VO_2 plateau when CO is underestimated), or when errors of different magnitude occur in SvO_2 and SaO_2 values (with upsloping of the VO_2 plateau when SvO_2 is selectively underestimated or SaO_2 selectively overestimated).

Most sources of CO error such as tricuspid regurgitation and left-to-right shunting are more likely to create a relative systematic error [47]. The most likely systematic source of absolute underestimation of CO is underestimation of left ventricle output related to the fact that the bronchial circulation is disregarded when DO_2 and VO_2 are calculated from right ventricular output. Bronchial blood flow may increase by 200% in injured lungs [48]. We can speculate that the magnitude of the error is relatively constant and dependent on lung injury severity and on lung oxygen consumption. However, even when lung oxygen consumption reaches 20% of the total VO_2, the spurious slope ranges from 4% to 6%.

Absolute underestimation of SvO_2 as compared to SaO_2 is possible only if venous sampling is repeatedly flawed, which can occur in practice only when HbO_2 saturation is not measured but calculated from PO_2 [49]. Aspiration of capillary blood when mixed venous blood is sampled too quickly or with an inflated balloon leads to CvO_2 overestimation with a downsloping VO_2 plateau.

Random measurement errors

In clinical practice, when all analyzers are properly calibrated, random error is the most likely type of error. Although the combined variability of within-patient, between-patient, between-device, and between-day measurements may be large, it is of no assistance for estimating the effect of random errors on the VO_2/DO_2 relationship determined using one device on one day in one patient. Within-patient variability (S_d) is much smaller. Here we consider the 95% confidence interval (95%CI, which is $\pm 2S_d$) for S_d. The S_d value for hemodynamic variables should be reassessed in the light of recent changes in devices. With current continuous CO calculators, variability is lower than previously reported [44, 50, 51] because there is no manual intervention and because more than three measurements are averaged. We assume a mean error of 0 and a 95%CI of 10% [52]. The 95%CI of hemoglobin measurements can been estimated at 2% [53], and the 95%CI of HbO_2 saturation at 4% [54]. The global impact of these random errors on VO_2 is 18% (range −9 to +9%). This 95%CI obtained using PAC is close to values obtained when VO_2 is assessed by indirect calorimetry (95%CI=10%, range [−7 to +3%] [55]. Then random measurement errors may affect absolute values of variables but the VO_2 plateau starts at the same point of the DO_2 challenge as for exact values (Fig. 3). Therefore the clinical conclusion remains the same.

Mathematical coupling of data

Archie [56] emphasized mathematical coupling of data when the relationship between two variables having one or more common components is being assessed. Caution is required in distinguishing between "mathematical" coupling and "other" couplings. All biological variables coming from the same patient may be dependent on one another due to overt or hidden couplings. Any pertinent information provided by two variables derives exclusively from their (a) mean, (b) variability, and (c) associative function. Thus mathematical coupling, if present, is a classical form of the relationship between two conventional variables. It remains worthwhile to study the relationship between two variables if the underlying medical question makes sense, regardless of whether coupling is clearly present.

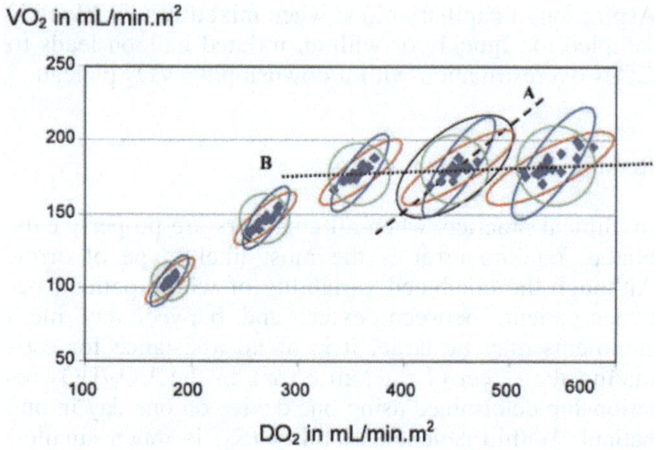

Fig. 3 Mathematical coupling in the VO_2/DO_2 relationship. *Black points* show 20 examples of the effect of random errors in our hypothetical experiment assuming a 95%CI of 10%, 2%, and 4% for CO, Hb, and $SavO_2$ measurements, respectively. The biphasic shape of the curve remains easy to identify. In the *red*, *blue*, and *green* areas the 95%CI of measured values increased to 20% for CO (or Hb), 10% for SaO_2, and 10% for SvO_2, respectively. *A* Global area and slope of mathematical coupling of all random errors. *B* Slope of the VO_2/DO_2 relationship

Mathematical coupling of random measurement errors

In contrast, mathematical coupling of measurement errors supplies no information of interest [6, 46, 57, 58]. When VO_2 and DO_2 are calculated from the same values of CO, Hb, and SaO_2, mathematical coupling of random error for each common variable linearly extends the dispersion of each VO_2/DO_2 point. The slope of each axis of variation depends on the associative functions between variables: 0.33 for CO, 1 for SaO_2, and 0 for SvO_2 because this is not a common variable. The combination of random errors for all components therefore creates an area of dispersion around the correct value that combines all specific variable axes (Fig. 3). Depending on the magnitude of possible error in each common variable, the global slope usually varies from 0.25 to 0.50. This global slope determines the statistical area of dispersion of measured values around the correct value of a single VO_2/DO_2 point (slope A in Fig. 3). It should not be confused with the slope of the plateau joining two consecutive points (slope B in Fig. 3), for which the probabilities of upward shifting and of downward shifting are similar.

These probabilities are similar but not exactly equal because the areas of dispersion around the exact value slope upwards and enlarge when DO_2 increases. Therefore the average B slope of many experiments is expected to be slightly positive. Calculation of a reliability coefficient (R_D) allows appropriate weighting of this slope and recalculation of the true relationship [57, 58]. Figure 3 provides an intuitive understanding of what R_D means. When the distance between two points increases (large DO_2 range) and when measurement variability decreases (small area of distribution), R_D tends to one and the impact of mathematical coupling of measurement errors tends to zero.

The final impact of mathematical coupling varies across experiments but can be very low. Using very large measurement errors, Stratton et al. [58] calculated that the impact of measurement errors (random effect plus mathematical coupling) on a VO_2 plateau gave an averaged slope of 0.06±0.05. This variability may account for a spurious slope between −0.04 and +0.16 [59, 60], in keeping with published studies [12, 44, 45, 46]. However, if this simulation were performed using the actual best variability, as shown in our hypothetical patient, the mean slope of the VO_2 plateau would be 0.007±0.05. This variability may account for a spurious slope between −0.10 and +0.10. The mathematical coupling of error is then negligible compared with the effect of random errors.

The use of empirical regression models

It thus makes sense to plot VO_2 against DO_2 to identify the critical DO_2 value in a specific situation. Obtaining more than two measurements can smooth the curve [59, 60]. However, the use of linear regression to calculate the VO_2/DO_2 slope raises several concerns. It is not possible to use simple models to characterize the VO_2/DO_2 relationship when the well-established physiological model predicts a biphasic curve [37]. Testing two different regression models to identify the biphasic shape of the curve requires that the inflection point be identified. The best pair of equations could be determined by testing all possible pairs of equations for all possible inflection points and by selecting the best pair of equations based on its minimum sum of residual sums of squares [61, 62].

Another concern arises because linear regression analyses are based on the minimum sum of squared residuals. The residual is the difference, for each x value, between observed and calculated y values on the x-axis. Therefore this model assumes that x values are correct (independent variable), or at least that the error on the x-axis is small compared to the error on the y-axis. This prerequisite is not met for the VO_2/DO_2 relationship even when DO_2 and VO_2 are measured independently. This is another source of spurious upsloping (Fig. 4). Because DO_2 is presumed to increase proportionally with time during a DO_2 challenge, using time as the actual independent variable is more appropriate (Figs. 4, 5). Additionally, the error in VO_2 is usually proportional to the VO_2 value; therefore the residuals of the regression line are not randomly distributed. Thus, when analyzing a family of regression lines from several patients, a more appropriate approach is a weighted linear regression model that also allows handling of between-patient variability [44, 63].

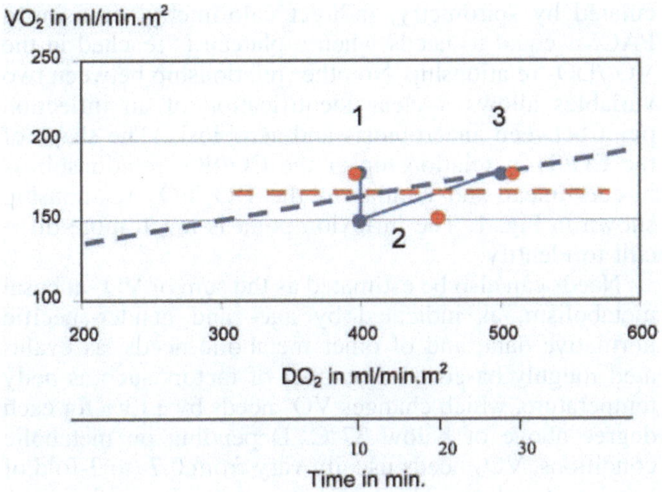

Fig. 4 Spurious upsloping due to an error in DO_2. *Points 1, 2, and 3* Three successive points of a VO_2/DO_2 plateau with a measurement error in point 2. The regression line between these three points shows a positive relationship (*blue dotted line*). This does not take into account the fact that during a DO_2 challenge DO_2 is expected to increase steadily. When time is used as the independent variable, the relationship is flat (*red dotted line*)

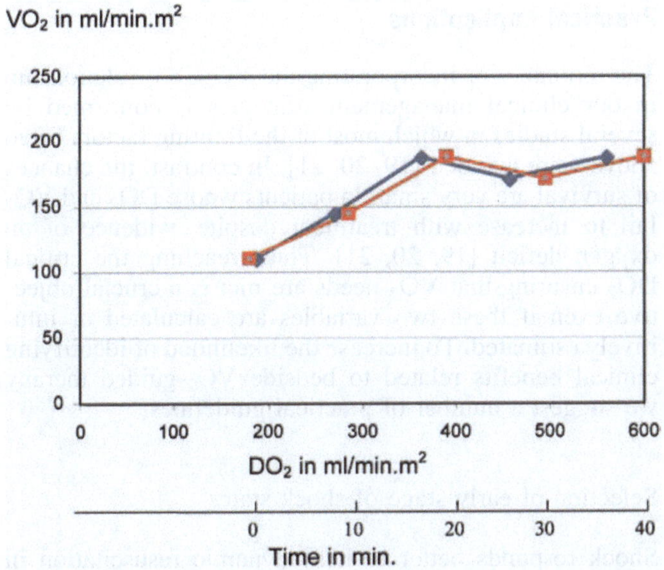

Fig. 5 Combination of the VO_2/DO_2 relationship and of the VO_2/time relationship in one random experiment in our hypothetical model, using the same random errors as in Fig. 3. For this figure DO_2 increased linearly with time. This helps to identify the critical VO_2 point and eliminates the possible effect of mathematical coupling of error

The impact of pooling data

Some studies of goal-oriented strategies for improving DO_2 and VO_2 found no improvement in survival but pooled patients with different disease processes, different metabolic needs, and different stages of shock [42, 43]. In contrast, the strategies were successful in studies investigating only postoperative surgical patients [18, 39, 41, 64, 65, 66, 67, 68], or patients who had a variety of diseases but were all included at the very early stage of shock [23, 69, 70]. Thus, the most conspicuous difference between studies that did and did not find better survival is heterogeneity vs. homogeneity of circulatory disorder characteristics in the study populations [71].

Analysis of the VO_2/DO_2 relationship on pooled data from several patients is also likely to show a spurious positive slope, for three reasons. Firstly, a large increase in mathematical coupling of errors is expected because the coefficient of variation for each measurement increases due to variability across patients, devices, and days [57]. Secondly, pooled data are likely to come from a mix of patients with inadequate resuscitation, adequate resuscitation, and relapsing shock. Thus with pooled data a substantial proportion of patients may have hidden dysoxia with physiological VO_2/DO_2 dependency. Thirdly, pooled data are also likely to come from patients with different metabolic needs. After circulatory shock critical DO_2 may vary from 8 to 21 ml/kg depending on the cause of the shock [22, 62, 72]. Even in comparable patients, differences in oxygen deficits, sedation, and/or activities may account for substantial differences in metabolic needs [73]. Therefore even if all patients are adequately resuscitated, analysis of pooled data from different levels of the VO_2 plateau results in a slope without any relevance. Thus it is more appropriate to average the slopes of each individual patient [44, 46].

Other means for matching VO_2 and needs

Although most of the limitations to the DO_2/VO_2 relationship can be corrected and/or optimized, matching VO_2 and needs by ensuring that a VO_2 plateau has been reached remains difficult. Considerable effort has been expended to develop alternatives. Three levels of clinical complexity can be distinguished.

1. Clinical improvement is a good indicator of adequate resuscitation [74]. In practice, VO_2 needs are usually met by decreasing metabolic needs, optimizing the hematocrit and SaO_2 level, and increasing blood flow empirically, until the clinical status improves. This situation does not require invasive hemodynamic investigations. A clear improvement in blood lactate clearance is also a good, minimally invasive, indicator of adequate resuscitation [74]. The blood lactate concentration alone fails to discriminate between dysoxia and aerobiosis [75, 76]. Although more reliable [4, 74, 77, 78], the time course of lactate levels is not an ideal marker. Lactate limitations have been recently reviewed by De Backer [76]. Diabetus mellitus, liver dysfunction, tissue reperfusion, catecholamine infusion, cellular metabolic alter-

ations, and inhibition of pyruvate dehydrogenase can result in a marked increase in blood lactate concentrations despite an improvement in tissue dysoxia. In these more complex situations where a clear clinical improvement and a normalization of blood lactate cannot be obtained, an evaluation of the adequacy of tissue oxygenation is required.

2) Some investigators have recommended that DO_2 be increased to supranormal values, greater than the usual critical level, without paying much attention to VO_2. This simplification of the method based on the VO_2/DO_2 relationship was associated with favorable outcomes in homogeneous population of high-risk surgery patients [18, 39, 41, 64, 67, 79], cardiogenic shock following myocardial infarction [69], and acute respiratory failure [23, 60] but failed to verify beneficial effects after onset of organ failure [67], or when different causes of shock were pooled [23, 60]. Other studies argue that sequential DO_2 and VO_2 calculations can be advantageously replaced by continuous measurement of CO [80] and/or SvO_2 [81]. More recently a clinical algorithm including $ScvO_2$ monitoring in patients with sepsis was shown to be clinically beneficial [70]. The use of these variables allows continuous comparison between measured values and targeted values.

However, targeting a preestablished value for DO_2, CO, or SvO_2 does not prove that these values meet the needs of an individual patient [22]. These preestablished targets are derived from normal findings or from survivors in selected populations of patients. The determination of the needed value of one given variable must take into consideration the limitation of other variables which are specific to the patient, his past history, the actual pathological event, the delay before onset of shock, and often the recent therapeutic interventions. Intuitive evaluation of the needed value for each variable in each specific case requires considerable expertise. Misinterpretation of PAC-related information and heterogeneity in the medical decision process is frequent [42, 43]. Even for experts the intuitive evaluation of needs may be subject to errors [22]. In some conditions, such as coronary disease, efforts to increase CO to "normalize" the cardiac index to more than 2.5 $l\ min^{-1}\ m^{-2}$ or the SvO_2 value to more than 70% can be harmful. In addition, there is some evidence that an excessive O_2 supply may be deleterious, either via the useless metabolic cost of an excessive increase in DO_2 or via activation of nonoxidative systems. Failure to consider the latter two mechanisms may also explain the poor results obtained in studies targeting nonspecific "supranormal" values of DO_2 in heterogeneous populations of patients [42, 43] Thus treatment efforts should be limited to what is necessary (not less but not more).

3. All hemodynamic variables are interrelated, and the VO_2 value is the final result. Ensuring that VO_2 meets tissue needs is the best means of ensuring that global hemodynamic status is adequate [4]. VO_2, whether calculated by spirometry, indirect calorimetry, or using a PAC, is equal to needs when a plateau is reached in the VO_2/DO_2 relationship. No other relationship between two variables allows a clear identification of an inflection point between anaerobiosis and aerobiosis. The shape of the CO/SvO_2 relationship or the CO/EO_2 relationship is bi-curvilinear and similar to the DO_2/EO_2 relationship shown in Fig. 1. The inflexion point is much more difficult to identify.

Needs can also be estimated as the sum of VO_2 at basal metabolism, as indicated by age- and gender-specific normative data, and of other metabolic needs, as evaluated roughly based on a number of factors such as body temperature, which changes VO_2 needs by ±13% for each degree above or below 37°C. Depending on metabolic conditions, VO_2 needs usually vary from 0.7- to 3-fold of basal metabolism. The two latter methods can be combined. When the VO_2 plateau is reached at a value close to the estimated value, the patient's needs are probably met. Handling the large amount of information required to assess O_2 needs can be difficult [82, 83, 84], and computer assistance may be helpful (http://www.hemodyn.com) [4, 85].

Practical implications

The rationale for incorporating the VO_2/DO_2 relationship in our clinical management strategies is confirmed by several studies in which most of the limiting factors listed above were avoided [19, 20, 21]. In contrast, the chances of survival are very small in patients whose DO_2 and VO_2 fail to increase with treatment despite evidence of an oxygen deficit [19, 20, 21]. Thus, reaching the critical DO_2 ensuring that VO_2 needs are met is a crucial objective even if these two variables are calculated or intuitively estimated. To increase the likelihood of identifying clinical benefits related to bedside VO_2-guided therapy we suggest a number of practical guidelines.

Selection of early stage of shock states

Shock responds better to hemodynamic resuscitation in the early stages [70]. Although the final objective is to provide enough oxygen to each cell, there is some evidence that rapidly achieving a sufficient total body VO_2 is a prerequisite. Late-stage shock is a far more complex situation involving not only the macro- and microcirculation but also cell metabolism and the consequences of cell necrosis, which cannot be corrected by hemodynamic resuscitation alone.

Matching VO_2 with needs is the first objective

In most situations targeting a clinical improvement, a decrease in lactate level, or a preestablished value for CO or SvO_2 or both is an acceptable means of intuitively reaching an adequate VO_2. In complex situations, by plotting VO_2/DO_2 over time during a DO_2 challenge, the critical DO_2 value can be evaluated rapidly as the inflection area on the curve, and resuscitation efforts can then be limited to what is necessary. Because the critical DO_2 value can be determined visually with a 95%CI of 20%, it is reasonable to limit DO_2 to its observed critical value +20%. When lactate remains high despite evidence that a VO_2 plateau has been reached, there is no argument that increasing DO_2 further is beneficial [19, 20, 21]. Continuous efforts to decrease O_2 demand and to improve the microcirculation may be more appropriate [86, 87]. Combined analysis of the VO_2/DO_2 and VO_2/time relationships provide the most useful means of eliminating the effects of mathematical coupling of errors and the theoretical limitations due to DO_2 variability in the regression line derivations. A mild upsloping of the VO_2 plateau (slope <10%) should not be confounded with O_2 dependency. When necessary, the critical DO_2 point can be determined more accurately using the method developed by John-Alder and Bennet [61].

To reach this objective the best compromise must be identified, based on metabolic cost

In the case of persistent O_2 supply dependency the first way to match VO_2 and needs is to decrease the needs. Hyperthermia, acute respiratory failure, and/or pain increase VO_2 needs sharply. Antipyretic drugs [88], sedation [89], and mechanical ventilation [90] often produce a 50% decrease in VO_2 needs. This has exactly the same favorable effect as doubling the CO or doubling the EO_2.

When VO_2 needs have been lowered as much as possible, because $VO_2=EO_2 \times DO_2$, matching VO_2 and needs implies to increase EO_2 or DO_2. Improving EO_2 must be always considered first, although this rarely produces a rapid VO_2 increase. Treating infection, excessive sedation, or excessive water retention, for example, may increase EO_2 [70]. Finally, when the only possibility is to increase DO_2, clinicians must choose among various means that presumably differ in their caloric effects. Arterial vasodilatation improves DO_2 and decreases myocardial O_2 requirements. In contrast, inotropic agents and vasoconstrictors have major caloric effects. Whatever the method used, a metabolic price must be paid for improving VO_2 and DO_2 to the critical values. This metabolic cost (a part of the total VO_2 requirement) must also be limited to what is strictly necessary.

Conclusion

Whereas there is a strong rationale for incorporating VO_2 into our early goal-oriented management strategies, proof that this improves patient survival is lacking. However, this should not lead to discontinuation of bedside VO_2 assessment, because no studies have been designed specifically to evaluate the potential benefits of rapidly increasing VO_2 to the specific value required by each individual patient at a given point in time. The present review is a call for such a study.

Acknowledgements The author thanks Dr. Hervé Mentec, Pr. Jean Daniel Chiche, and Pr. Didier Payen for their critical review of the manuscript.

References

1. Cain SM (1984) Supply dependency of oxygen uptake in ARDS: myth or reality? Am J Med Sci 288:119–124
2. Schumacker P, Cain S (1987) The concept of critical oxygen delivery. Intensive Care Med 13:223–229
3. Cain SM, Curtis SE (1991) Experimental models of pathologic oxygen supply dependency. Crit Care Med 19:603–612
4. Squara P, Journois D, Formela F, Dhainaut J, Sollet JP, Bleichner G (1994) Value of elementary, calculated and modeled hemodynamic variables. J Crit Care 9:223–235
5. Ronco JJ, Fenwick JC, Tweeddale MG, Wiggs BR, Phang PT, Cooper DJ, Cunningham KF, Russell JA, Walley KR (1993) Identification of the critical oxygen delivery for anaerobic metabolism in critically ill septic and nonseptic humans. JAMA 270:1724–1730
6. Russell JA, Phang PT (1994) The oxygen delivery/consumption controversy. Approaches to management of the critically ill. Am J Respir Crit Care Med 149:533–537
7. Kennedy FG, Jones DP (1986) Oxygen dependence of mitochondrial function in isolated rat cardiac myocytes. Am J Physiol 250:C374–C383
8. Vallet B, Curtis SE, Guery B, Mangalaboyi J, Menager P, Cain SM, Chopin C, Dupuis BA (1995) ATP-sensitive K+ channel blockade impairs O2 extraction during progressive ischemia in pig hindlimb. J Appl Physiol 79:2035–2042
9. Guery BP, Mangalaboyi J, Menager P, Mordon S, Vallet B, Chopin C (1999) Redox status of cytochrome a,a3: a noninvasive indicator of dysoxia in regional hypoxic or ischemic hypoxia. Crit Care Med 27:576–582
10. Cain SM (1975) Oxygen delivery and utilization in dogs with a sublethal dose of cobalt chloride. J Appl Physiol 38:20–25

11. Gilbert EM, Haupt MT, Mandanas RY, Huaringa AJ, Carlson RW (1986) The effect of fluid loading, blood transfusion, and catecholamine infusion on oxygen delivery and consumption in patients with sepsis. Am Rev Respir Dis 134:873–878
12. Hanique G, Dugernier T, Laterre PF, Dougnac A, Roeseler J, Reynaert MS (1994) Significance of pathologic oxygen supply dependency in critically ill patients: comparison between measured and calculated methods. Intensive Care Med 20:12–18
13. Haupt MT, Gilbert EM, Carlson RW (1985) Fluid loading increases oxygen consumption in septic patients with lactic acidosis. Am Rev Respir Dis 131:912–916
14. Kruse JA, Haupt MT, Puri VK, Carlson RW (1990) Lactate levels as predictors of the relationship between oxygen delivery and consumption in ARDS. Chest 98:959–962
15. Vincent JL, Roman A, De Backer D, Kahn RJ (1990) Oxygen uptake/supply dependency. Effects of short-term dobutamine infusion. Am Rev Respir Dis 142:2–7
16. De Backer D, Berre J, Moraine JJ, Melot C, Vanfraechem J, Vincent JL (1996) Effects of dobutamine on the relationship between oxygen consumption and delivery in healthy volunteers: comparison with sodium nitroprusside. Clin Sci (Lond) 90:105–111
17. Ronco JJ, Phang PT, Walley KR, Wiggs B, Fenwick JC, Russell JA (1991) Oxygen consumption is independent of changes in oxygen delivery in severe adult respiratory distress syndrome. Am Rev Respir Dis 143:1267–1273
18. Ziegler DW, Wright JG, Choban PS, Flancbaum L (1997) A prospective randomized trial of preoperative "optimization" of cardiac function in patients undergoing elective peripheral vascular surgery. Surgery 122:584–592
19. Ronco JJ, Fenwick JC, Wiggs BR, Phang PT, Russell JA, Tweeddale MG (1993) Oxygen consumption is independent of increases in oxygen delivery by dobutamine in septic patients who have normal or increased plasma lactate. Am Rev Respir Dis 147:25–31
20. Vallet B, Chopin C, Curtis SE, Dupuis BA, Fourrier F, Mehdaoui H, LeRoy B, Rime A, Santre C, Herbecq P et al (1993) Prognostic value of the dobutamine test in patients with sepsis syndrome and normal lactate values: a prospective, multicenter study. Crit Care Med 21:1868–1875
21. Rhodes A, Lamb FJ, Malagon I, Newman PJ, Grounds RM, Bennett ED (1999) A prospective study of the use of a dobutamine stress test to identify outcome in patients with sepsis, severe sepsis, or septic shock. Crit Care Med 27:2361–2366
22. Mohsenifar Z, Goldbach P, Tashkin DP, Campisi DJ (1983) Relationship between O2 delivery and O2 consumption in the adult respiratory distress syndrome. Chest 84:267–271
23. Bihari D, Smithies M, Gimson A, Tinker J (1987) The effects of vasodilation with prostacyclin on oxygen delivery and uptake in critically ill patients. N Engl J Med 317:397–403
24. Nelson DP, Beyer C, Samsel RW, Wood LD, Schumacker PT (1987) Pathological supply dependence of O2 uptake during bacteremia in dogs. J Appl Physiol 63:1487–1492
25. Schumacker PT, Samsel RW (1989) Analysis of oxygen delivery and uptake relationships in the Krogh tissue model. J Appl Physiol 67:1234–1244
26. Gutierrez G, Marini C, Acero AL, Lund N (1990) Skeletal muscle PO2 during hypoxemia and isovolemic anemia. J Appl Physiol 68:2047–2053
27. De Backer D, Moraine JJ, Berre J, Kahn RJ, Vincent JL (1994) Effects of dobutamine on oxygen consumption in septic patients. Direct versus indirect determinations. Am J Respir Crit Care Med 150:95–100
28. Jeppsson A, Ekroth R, Friberg P, Kirno K, Milocco I, Nilsson F, Svensson S (2000) Renal effects of amino acid infusion in cardiac surgery. J Cardiothorac Vasc Anesth 14:51–55
29. Jacobson E (1963) Effects of histamine, acetylcholine, and norepinephrine on gastric vascular resistance. AM J Physiol 204:1013–1017
30. Duran W, Renkin E (1974) Oxygen consumption and blood flow in resting mamalians skeletal muscles. Am J Physiol 226:173–177
31. McCord J (1985) Oxygen-derived free radicals in post ischemic tissue injury. N Engl J Med 312:159–161
32. Schumacker PT, Chandel N, Agusti AG (1993) Oxygen conformance of cellular respiration in hepatocytes. Am J Physiol 265:L395–L402
33. Schumacker PT, Soble JS, Feldman T (1994) Oxygen delivery and uptake relationships in patients with aortic stenosis. Am J Respir Crit Care Med 149:1123–1131
34. Powers SR Jr, Mannal R, Neclerio M, English M, Marr C, Leather R, Ueda H, Williams G, Custead W, Dutton R (1973) Physiologic consequences of positive end-expiratory pressure (PEEP) ventilation. Ann Surg 178:265–272
35. Danek SJ, Lynch JP, Weg JG, Dantzker DR (1980) The dependence of oxygen uptake on oxygen delivery in the adult respiratory distress syndrome. Am Rev Respir Dis 122:387–395
36. Gutierrez G, Pohil RJ (1986) Oxygen consumption is linearly related to O2 supply in critically ill patients. J Crit Care 1:45–53
37. Clarke C, Edwards JD, Nightingale P, Mortimer AJ, Morris J (1991) Persistence of supply dependency of oxygen uptake at high levels of delivery in adult respiratory distress syndrome. Crit Care Med 19:497–502
38. Shoemaker W (1987) Relation of oxygen transport patterns to the pathophysiology and therapy of shock states. Intensive Care Med 13:230–243
39. Shoemaker W, Appel P, Kram H, Waxman K, Lee T (1988) Prospective trial of supranormal values of survivors as therapeutic goals in high-risk surgical patients. Chest 94:1176–1186
40. Shoemaker W (1989) Shock states: pathophysiology, monitoring, outcome, prediction and therapy. In: Shoemaker W (ed) Textbook of critical care. Saunders, Philadelphia, pp 977–993
41. Edwards J, Brown G, Nightingale P, et al (1989) Use of survivors' cardiorespiratory values as therapeutic goals in septic shock. Crit Care Med 17:1098–1103
42. Hayes MA, Timmings AC, Yau EH, Palazzo M, Hinds CJ, Watson D (1994) Elevation of systemic oxygen delivery in the treatment of critically ill patients. N Engl J Med 330:1717–1722
43. Gattinoni L, Brazzi L, Pelozzi P (1995) A trial of goal-oriented hemodynamic therapy in critically ill patients. N Engl J Med 333:1025–1032
44. Phang PT, Cunningham KF, Ronco JJ, Wiggs BR, Russell JA (1994) Mathematical coupling explains dependence of oxygen consumption on oxygen delivery in ARDS. Am J Respir Crit Care Med 150:318–323
45. Mira J, Fabre J, Baigorr iF, Coste J, Annat G, Artigas A, Nitenberg G, Dhainaut J (1994) Lack of oxygen supply dependency in patients with severe sepsis. A study of oxygen delivery increased by military antishock trouser and dobutamine. Chest 106:1524–1531
46. Granton JT, Walley KR, Phang PT, Russell JA, Lichtenstein S (1998) Assessment of three methods to reduce the influence of mathematical coupling on oxygen consumption and delivery relationships. Chest 113:1347–1355
47. Perret C, Tagan D, Feihl F, Marini J (1996) Measuring Cardiac output: sources of error. In: The pulmonary artery catheter in critical care: a concise handbook. Arnette Blackwell, Cambridge p 109

48. Lakshminarayan S, Bernard S, Polissar NL, Glenny RW (1999) Pulmonary and bronchial circulatory responses to segmental lung injury. J Appl Physiol 87:1931–1936
49. Nierman DM, Schechter CB (1994) Mixed venous O2 saturation: measured by co-oximetry versus calculated from PVO2. J Clin Monit 10:39–44
50. Stetz CW, Miller RG, Kelly GE, Raffin TA (1982) Reliability of the thermodilution method in the determination of cardiac output in clinical practice. Am Rev Respir Dis 126:1001–1004
51. Rubini A, Del Monte D, Catena V, Attar I, Cesaro M, Soranzo D, Rattazzi G, Alati GL (1995) Cardiac output measurement by the thermodilution method: an in vitro test of accuracy of three commercially available automatic cardiac output computers. Intensive Care Med 21:154–158
52. Le Tulzo Y, Belghith M, Seguin P, Dall'Ava J, Monchi M, Thomas R, Dhainaut JF (1996) Reproducibility of thermodilution cardiac output determination in critically ill patients: comparison between bolus and continuous method. J Clin Monit 12:379–385
53. Picard F, Gicquel C, Marnet L, Guesnu M, Levy J (1999) Preliminary evaluation of the new hemotology analyser COULTER GEN-S in a university hospital. Clin Chem Lab Med 37 (6)
54. Scuderi PE, MacGregor DA, Bowton DL, Harris LC, Anderson R, James RL (1993) Performance characteristics and interanalyzer variability of PO2 measurements using tonometered human blood. Am Rev Respir Dis 147:1354–1359
55. Ronco J, Phang T (1991) Validation of an indirect calorimeter to measure oxygen consumption in critically ill patients. J Crit Care 6:36–41
56. Archie JP (1981) Mathematic coupling of data. Ann Surg 193:296–303
57. Moreno LF, Stratton HH, Newell JC, Feustel PJ (1986) Mathematical coupling of data: correction of a common error for linear calculations. J Appl Physiol 60:335–343
58. Stratton HH, Feustel PJ, Newell JC (1987) Regression of calculated variables in the presence of shared measurement error. J Appl Physiol 62:2083–2093
59. Dorinsky PM, Costello JL, Gadek JE (1988) Relationships of oxygen uptake and oxygen delivery in respiratory failure not due to the adult respiratory distress syndrome. Chest 93:1013–1019
60. Hankeln K, Gronemeyer R, Held A, Bohmert F (1991) Use of continuous noninvasive measurement of oxygen consumption in patients with adult respiratory distress syndrome following shock of various etiologies. Crit Care Med 19:642–649
61. John-Alder H, Bennet A (1981) Thermal dependence of endurance and locomotory energetics in a lizard. Am J Physiol 241:R342–R349
62. Komatsu T, Shibutani K, Okamoto K, Kumar V, Kubal K, Sanchala V, Lees DE (1987) Critical level of oxygen delivery after cardiopulmonary bypass. Crit Care Med 15:194–197
63. Feldman H (1988) Families of lines: random effects in linear regression analysis. J Appl Physiol 64:1721–1732
64. Boyd O, Grounds RM, Bennett ED (1993) A randomized clinical trial of the effect of deliberate perioperative increase of oxygen delivery on mortality in high-risk surgical patients. JAMA 270:2699–2707
65. Yu M, Burchell S, Hasaniya NW, Takanishi DM, Myers SA, Takiguchi SA (1998) Relationship of mortality to increasing oxygen delivery in patients >or=50 years of age: a prospective, randomized trial. Crit Care Med 26:1011–1019
66. Wilson J, Woods I, Fawcett J, Whall R, Dibb W, Morris C, McManus E (1999) Reducing the risk of major elective surgery: randomised controlled trial of preoperative optimisation of oxygen delivery. BMJ 318:1099–1103
67. Kern JW, Shoemaker WC (2002) Meta-analysis of hemodynamic optimization in high-risk patients. Crit Care Med 30:1686–1692
68. Fenwick E, Wilson J, Sculpher M, Claxton K (2002) Pre-operative optimisation employing dopexamine or adrenaline for patients undergoing major elective surgery: a cost-effectiveness analysis. Intensive Care Med 28:599–608
69. Creamer JE, Edwards JD, Nightingale P (1990) Hemodynamic and oxygen transport variables in cardiogenic shock secondary to acute myocardial infarction, and response to treatment. Am J Cardiol 65:1297–1300
70. Rivers E, Nguyen B, Havstat D, Ressler J, Muzzin A, Knoblish B, Peterson E, Tomlanovitch M (2001) Early goal-directed theraphy in the treatment of severe sepsis and septic shock. N Engl J Med 345:1368–1377
71. Pinsky M (1994) Beyond global oxygen supply-demand relations: in search of measures of dysoxia. Intensive Care Med 20:1–3
72. Shibutani K, Komatsu T, Kubal K, Sanchala V, Kumar V, Bizzarri DV (1983) Critical level of oxygen delivery in anesthetized man. Crit Care Med 11:640–643
73. Weissman C, Kemper M (1991) The oxygen uptake-oxygen delivery relationship during ICU interventions. Chest 99:430–435
74. Bakker J, Coffernils M, Leon M, Gris P, Vincent JL (1991) Blood lactate levels are superior to oxygen-derived variables in predicting outcome in human septic shock. Chest 99:956–962
75. Curtis SE, Cain SM (1992) Regional and systemic oxygen delivery/uptake relations and lactate flux in hyperdynamic, endotoxin-treated dogs. Am Rev Respir Dis 145:348–354
76. De Backer D (2003) Lactic acidosis. Intensive Care Med 29:699–702
77. Vincent J, Dufaye P, Berre J, Leeman M, De Gaute J, Kahn R (1983) Serial lactate determination during circulatory shock. Crit Care Med 11:449–451
78. Bakker J, Gris P, Coffernils M, Kahn RJ, Vincent JL (1996) Serial blood lactate levels can predict the development of multiple organ failure following septic shock. Am J Surg 171:221–226
79. Polonen P, Ruokonen E, Hippelainen M, Poyhonen M, Takala J (2000) A prospective, randomized study of goal-oriented hemodynamic therapy in cardiac surgical patients. Anesth Analg 90:1052–1059
80. Mihm FG, Gettinger A, Hanson CW, 3rd, Gilbert HC, Stover EP, Vender JS, Beerle B, Haddow G (1998) A multicenter evaluation of a new continuous cardiac output pulmonary artery catheter system. Crit Care Med 26:1346–1350
81. Armaganidis A, Dhainaut JF, Billard JL, Klouche K, Mira JP, Brunet F, Dinh-Xuan AT, Dall'Ava-Santucci J (1994) Accuracy assessment for three fiberoptic pulmonary artery catheters for SvO2 monitoring. Intensive Care Med 20:484–488
82. Iberti T, Fischer E, Leibowitz A, Panacek E, Silverstein E, Albertson T (1990) A multicenter study of physician's knowledge of the pulmonary artery catheter. JAMA 12:2933–2940
83. Gnaegi A, Feihl F, Perret C (1997) Intensive care physicians' insufficient knowledge of right heart catheterization at the bedside: time to act? Crit Care Med 25:213–220
84. Squara P, Bennett D, Perret C (2002) Pulmonary artery catheter: does the problem lie in the users? Chest 121:2009–2015

85. Squara P, Dhainaut J, Lamy M, Perret C, Larbuisson R, Poli S, Armaganidis A, de Gournay J, Bleichner G (1989) Computer assistance for hemodynamic evaluation. J Crit Care 4:273–282
86. Kirov MY, Evgenov OV, Evgenov NV, Egorina EM, Sovershaev MA, Sveinbjornsson B, Nedashkovsky EV, Bjertnaes LJ (2001) Infusion of methylene blue in human septic shock: a pilot, randomized, controlled study. Crit Care Med 29:1860–1867
87. Spronk PE, Ince C, Gardien MJ, Mathura KR, Oudemans-van Straaten HM, Zandstra DF (2002) Nitroglycerin in septic shock after intravascular volume resuscitation. Lancet 360:1395–1366
88. Gozzoli V, Treggiari MM, Kleger GR, Roux-Lombard P, Fathi M, Pichard C, Romand JA (2004) Randomized trial of the effect of antipyresis by metamizol, propacetamol or external cooling on metabolism, hemodynamics and inflammatory response. Intensive Care Med 30:401–407
89. Bruder N, Lassegue D, Pelissier D, Graziani N, Francois G (1994) Energy expenditure and withdrawal of sedation in severe head-injured patients. Crit Care Med 22:1114–1119
90. Miwa K, Mitsuoka M, Takamori S, Hayashi A, Shirouzu K (2003) Continuous monitoring of oxygen consumption in patients undergoing weaning from mechanical ventilation. Respiration 70:623–630

Brian P. Kavanagh
L. Joanne Meyer

Normalizing physiological variables in acute illness: five reasons for caution

B.P.K. is funded by the Canadian Institutes of Health Research and the Ontario Ministry of Science and Technology.

Introduction

Acute illness is accompanied by the development of abnormal physiology. The development and severity of illness, as well as recovery, is paralleled by changes in the physiological variables that clinicians commonly monitor. Several factors may prompt clinicians to address and treat the variables in isolation from addressing the underlying disease. This article explores why clinicians may target and attempt to normalize abnormal physiological variables and identifies five reasons why such an approach can be hazardous.

Physiological parameters and illness

The evolution of many illnesses usually follows predictable patterns. For example, septic shock, an acute syndrome that is perhaps emblematic of critical care medicine and has a high mortality, commonly follows a foreseeable trajectory from localized to generalized infection, progressive hemodynamic deterioration, multiple organ dysfunction and, in over 30% of patients, death [1]. The cardiovascular changes associated with this syndrome typically include tachycardia and decreased blood pressure and usually an increase in cardiac output.

There are several reasons why clinicians monitor and attempt to correct such physiological variables in the acutely ill. First, in some highly specific situations this approach appears to work. Indeed, although seriously questioned [2, 3], randomized controlled clinical trials have suggested improvement in survival associated with rigorous control of plasma glucose in postoperative adult cardiac surgical patients [4] or more rapid resuscitation of patients with recently diagnosed septic shock [1]. Second, traditionally physiology has been the basis for assessment and treatment in critically ill patients, where monitoring directs how therapy is applied [5]. Although ongoing developments of molecular medicine and evidence-based medicine may alter how patients are treated in the future, the "physiological" approach, i.e., treatment based on physiological monitoring, has been a cornerstone of teaching in critical care medicine for decades [6]. Third, the extent to which physiological variables differ from normal values indicates how ill the patient is. This is important because clinicians know well that disease severity is an important indicator of ultimate outcome, and the assessment of severity is largely based on the degree to which the measured variables (e.g., perturbations of the cardiovascular, respiratory, and acid-base systems) differ from normal values. Indeed such impressions have been validated by numerous scoring systems that incorporate the extent of physiological derangement and predict outcomes

M.R. Pinsky et al. (eds.), *Applied Physiology in Intensive Care Medicine 2: Physiological Reviews and Editorials*,
DOI 10.1007/978-3-642-28233-1_18, © Springer-Verlag Berlin Heidelberg 2012

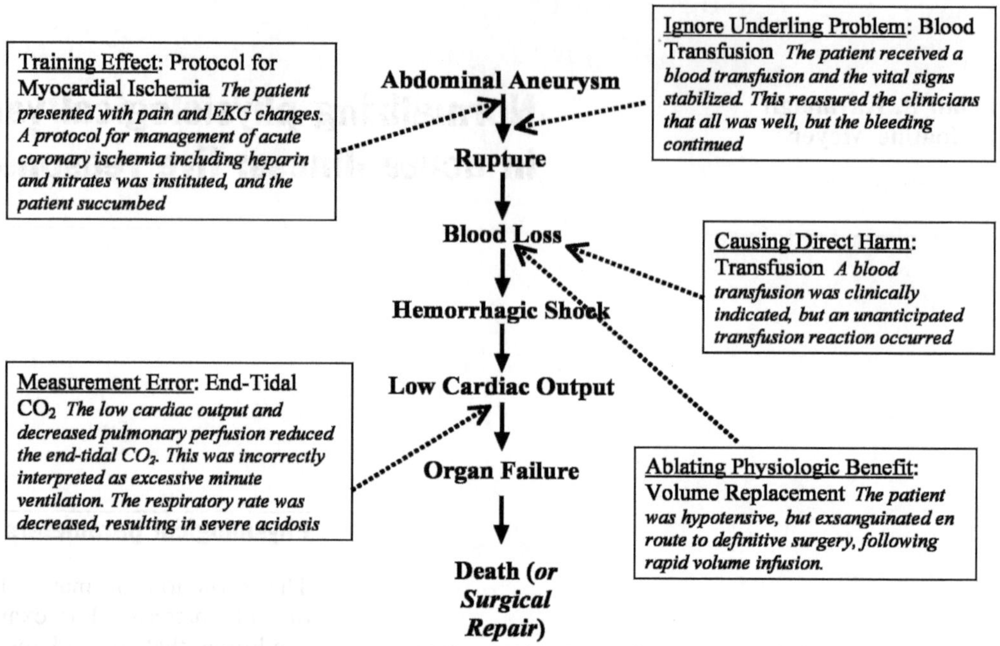

Fig. 1 An example of an acute illness state: hemorrhagic shock resulting from a ruptured abdominal aortic aneurysm. This flowchart illustrates how, using the five identified erroneous approaches, clinicians may intervene but direct therapy inappropriately

in populations of critically ill adults [7, 8] and children [9]. Fourth, beyond linking the initial degree of physiological derangement with severity of illness at the outset, established data have documented a close association between the sequential changes in physiological abnormalities and prognosis from acute illness [10]. Finally, in the same way that increasing deviation of variables from normal values reflects worsening of disease and poor prognosis, the converse is also true; normalization of abnormal variables parallels disease resolution and may be the principal objective evidence that a patient's condition is improving.

Despite this rationale the approach is imperfect and sometimes has disastrous results. A recent randomized controlled trial of nitric oxide synthase inhibition in septic shock was designed with simple pathophysiological rationale [11]; although the drug was effective in correcting the blood pressure and reversing shock [12], mortality was increased, not decreased [11]. Indeed, more comprehensive consideration, including attention to the critical importance of myocardial function in sepsis, might have predicted such a response [13, 14]. This vivid example illustrates the need for reflection about simplistic physiological rationale vs. demonstration of actual outcome benefit, and the potential for error associated with the former.

Normalization as a therapeutic endpoint

Based on the above considerations it is understandable why clinicians would instinctively focus on attempting to normalize abnormal physiological variables in patients who are acutely ill. Although several studies have demonstrated adverse effects of increasing levels of physiological support to supranormal levels (e.g., oxygen delivery [15], endocrine replacement [16]), clinicians may not appreciate dangers that may be associated with adjustment of variables to normal levels. We outline in this contribution five principles by which targeting and attempting to normalize physiological variables in acutely ill patients can lead to harm. These principles are illustrated by published examples and suggest global approaches for avoidance of such complications. An illustrated outline is provided in Fig. 1, focusing on the potential harm associated with correcting variables in a patient with ruptured abdominal aneurysm.

Ignoring the underlying problem

Classical approaches to treating acute illness involve provision of supportive care while at the same time addressing the primary problem. There are clearly some derangements in physiological variables, for example, severe hypoxemia, which are inherently life-threatening and must therefore be immediately treated. However, the clinician cannot be content with the return of measured variables to normal but must consider the underlying cause of the derangement. Failure to do so can result in significant harm to the patient.

Consider a patient presenting with severe hypovolemic shock from a massive gastrointestinal hemorrhage. Initial management may include fluids, blood products, and potentially vasopressors. It is gratifying to see the blood pressure climb to normal levels with the supportive care. It would be catastrophic, however, if one did not continue with definitive management of the bleeding. Similarly, a patient with pyonephrosis from an obstructed ureter could develop septic shock and all the physiological derangements that occur with multiorgan dysfunction. The variables can look much better with usual critical care support (e.g., mechanical ventilation, fluids, vasopressors), but the patient is unlikely to improve overall without appropriate abscess drainage. In both situations it is obvious that the management of the patient requires both supportive care in addition to measures directed at the underlying cause.

Consider also each individual parameter monitored in the critical care unit. Derangements in any variable can have a myriad of causes. For example, pulse oximetry may inform the clinician about a potentially important change in a key physiological parameter, oxygen saturation. Desaturation can have any of numerous underlying causes, each requiring specific therapy. Such concerns are reflected in an editorial commentary on the intraoperative use of pulse oximetry wherein Fairley [17] wrote, "As the blindfolded anesthetist walks unknowingly towards the cliff of hypoxia.... the protective hand of the pulse oximeter sentry stops him from falling over the edge. The oximeter will not tell him why.... or the direction back."

Inducing harm

It has long seemed logical to clinicians that in acutely ill patients the restoration of vital functions to normal levels would result in reduced imposition on the physiological reserve and increase the probability, and the rapidity, of recovery [18]. In terms of transfusion of red blood cells, the rationale—representing conventional thinking up to 5 years ago—was that the increased O_2 delivery to tissues resulting from transfusion would permit greater O_2 consumption at the cellular level, and that this would translate into better outcome. Although simplistic, such concepts have long provided the impetus for "topping up" hemoglobin levels in acutely ill patients [19, 20].

In fact, this specific intervention—red cell transfusion—has been subjected to several important clinical studies, with unexpected results [21, 22]. To test the acute effects of red cell transfusion on tissue oxygenation, Marik and Sibbald [21] transfused patients suffering from systemic sepsis who were mildly anemic. Several important lessons were learned. First, global O_2 consumption was not increased when directly measured, despite indirect estimation suggesting the contrary. Second, at a local tissue level the majority of the transfusions resulted in adverse, not beneficial, changes in the oxygenation status. This was detected using gastric tonometry, a technique that assesses the O_2 supply-demand status of the vulnerable mucosal cells that line the stomach. In addition, the age of the transfused red cells was predictive of the degree of mucosal dysoxia, raising the possibility that storage duration, well within ranges common in North America, resulted in dysfunctional red cells.

While the pathophysiological responses to stored red cells are of mechanistic interest, a subsequent clinical study has provided important outcome data that may mandate changes in practice [22]. This study demonstrated that transfusion, even to a modest hemoglobin concentration, does not improve the status of anemic patients who are acutely ill in the intensive care unit; in fact subgroup analysis suggests that it may increase mortality [22], perhaps due to leukocyte-mediated actions [23] or altered volume status. Other examples exist where treatment aimed at normalizing variables can result in adverse outcome. For example, rapid correction of serum sodium concentration in cases of hyponatremia can result in brainstem destruction from central pontine myelinolysis [24]; conversely, rapid normalization of hyperosmolar states, such a hyperosmolar coma and diabetic ketoacidosis, can result in accelerated cerebral edema, with devastating consequences. In preterm infants the targeting of normal, not high, levels of oxygenation with low amounts of supplemental O_2 was hypothesized to improve neurodevelopment [25]. The hypothesis, although apparently soundly constructed, turned out to be false [25], and the approach instead of helping caused harm, resulting in an increased incidence of chronic lung disease. Finally, it is now apparent that the high tidal volumes associated with frankly lowered $PaCO_2$ towards or below normal levels in patients with acute respiratory distress syndrome (ARDS) are associated with increased mortality [26, 27, 28]; indeed alternative approaches to management of ARDS have been proposed [29, 30].

Ablation of physiological benefit

Whereas abnormal physiological variables always suggest an abnormal milieu or disease state, this does not mean that all abnormal variables are directly causing harm. Indeed, in some situations abnormal variables (e.g., mild hypotension) may benefit the patient.

Resuscitation of trauma victims who have developed hypotension due to blood loss has traditionally followed the "A, B, C" (i.e., airway, breathing, circulation) approach [31, 32]. In this scenario the patient's airway is controlled, breathing assured, and the depleted circulating volume is restored, all in rapid succession. However, the idea that circulating volume should be rapidly restored has undergone reevaluation during the past decade. Indeed, a randomized controlled trial in hypotensive trauma patients suggested that delayed correction of depleted circulating volume, as compared with the traditional immediate correction, leads to superior outcome in terms of survival and duration of hospital stay [33].

How could such an approach be beneficial? The results of that study suggest that hypotension in such a population [33], although reflecting severe depletion of circulating volume, is in fact protective because it reduces the propensity for ongoing bleeding. The idea is supported by direct experimental evidence [34, 35]. Thus although it is not suggested that prolonged or severe hypotension is beneficial per se, or is even sustainable, the data do indicate that rapid volume correction without first attending to the sources of bleeding may be associated with elevated systemic blood pressure, reinitiating or increasing blood loss, and escalating the risk of death from hemorrhage [33]. Thus in this specific context and perhaps in others, for example, ruptured aortic aneurysm, temporary hypotension is protective.

There are other examples whereby an abnormal parameter is protective. It has been suggested that acidemia, the presence of a pH in the extracellular fluid that is lower than normal, may protect against the ongoing production of endogenous organic acids such as lactic and keto acids [36] as well as augmenting release of oxygen from hemoglobin [37, 38]. In diabetic ketoacidosis the standard approach is to provide insulin and careful rehydration, with assiduous attention to osmolality and electrolyte abnormalities. Administration of insulin addresses the generation of ketoacids, the fundamental biochemical disorder in this syndrome, and that as the ketoacids are cleared a major component of the acidemia resolves. In some circumstances clinicians have opted for treating the pH per se by buffering with intravenous bicarbonate. Significant concerns have arisen with this approach, however, with the evolving awareness that bicarbonate therapy may worsen, not improve, cerebral oxygenation in this condition [39]. Indeed, a clinical trial has demonstrated that such therapy does not help in treating the underlying condition; on the contrary, buffering the pH reverses resolution of the underlying ketoacidosis [40]. The same approach to normalizing pH has also been in another acute illness, septic shock [41]. Here the important findings were that buffering the pH did not improve either the cardiovascular performance, or the effectiveness of the vasoactive drugs being used [41].

Although not translated into the clinical setting, several laboratory studies suggest that abnormal physiology may have protective effects (e.g., hyperpyrexia in sepsis [42], and hyperosmolarity [43] and hypercapnia [44] in reperfusion injury). It has recently been suggested that multiple organ dysfunction in the context of critical illness represents a protective adaptive response rather than a set of circumstances to be aggressively prevented or reversed [45]. It was further argued that such organ dysfunction represents an effort on the part of the body to cope with on-going critical illness, and that attempts to correct this pathophysiological state could therefore result in harm [45].

Generation of associated errors

Medical error has been the focus of intense recent interest. In hospitalized patients error is an important source of morbidity and mortality, with 75% of errors being associated with "diagnostic mishaps" and 70% occurring in acute care settings [46]. An important type of error is misinterpretation of data, and when monitoring the acutely ill errors in the acquisition or interpretation of data can certainly mislead. Many examples of errors in monitoring have been described, and in many cases these result in a cascade of events that lead to significant patient harm [47].

We present an example in which experienced clinicians were misled by an incorrectly placed central vascular catheter; in this example, the response to subsequent therapy compounded the misimpression that catheter placement was correct, and that the therapy was effective [48]. The patient was assessed in the emergency room and was noted to be cyanosed, febrile, and hypotensive. The clinicians diagnosed septic shock in a patient with cyanotic cardiac disease, performed a procedure to insert a catheter into the femoral artery for monitoring purposes, and commenced infusion of a vasoconstrictor agent. The initial response, elevation in intravascular pressure in response to the therapy, appeared gratifying. However, the patient deteriorated, and upon placement of an additional central vascular catheter, which was placed in a central artery, it became obvious that the initial catheter had been placed in a vein instead of an artery. The error was detected because the waveforms of the two intravascular pressures were different. However, the error was possible because of the conditions presented. The patient had severe tricuspid valve regurgitation, and in the setting of systemic hypotension and cyanosis this resulted in severely elevated venous pressures being mistaken for arterial pressures. The error was compounded, however, because the response to therapy being sought, elevation in systemic arterial pressure, appeared to be obtained, but in fact the elevation was that of venous pressure. Thus instead of providing cardiovascular support with increased arterial pressure the therapy was compromising the heart, reducing forward flow, and increasing backward regurgitant flow. This is an example in which experienced clinicians were deceived by assumption of correct monitoring placement, a false assumption that was compounded by an apparent beneficial response to administered medication [48].

Training effect

The "science" of medicine involves understanding the processes and mechanisms of sickness. Such insight should enable clinicians to adapt to altered circumstances within the context of an illness and in addition to translate knowledge and techniques from one illness state to another. While we often consider why research findings are "lost in translation" between scientific research and patient benefit [49, 50], we may not consider how appropriate it is to translate findings from one illness context to another. Examples of translation include application of positive airways pressure to sleep apnea instead of its original use in acute respiratory failure [51], the use of a therapy that was originally thought to act on the coagulation pathway (e.g., activated protein C) to treatment of sepsis [52], and high frequency oscillatory ventilation, developed originally for treatment of neonatal respiratory failure, and now being studied in adults with ARDS [53, 54]. Such translation of treatment modalities from one disease state or population to another presupposes that the clinician understands the mechanisms of action in the original disease as well as the mechanisms of action and risk-benefit profile in the subsequent disease. In fact, although physiological insight is continuously evolving and would be necessary to predict successful "knowledge transfer" from one situation to another, there is often a major gap between physiological expectation, as predicted by the clinician, and the results of careful context-specific physiological evaluation. Thus certain interventions that may seem to make sense from past experience may ultimately be detrimental when used in an alternative context.

We present an example of a traditional therapy, hyperventilation, almost certainly highly effective in incipient brainstem herniation but harmful when translated to other patients with brain trauma in the absence of cerebral hyperemia. It has been known for decades that hyperventilation reduces intracranial pressure [55], and in subsequent years it became apparent that this could be used to clinical advantage. In incipient brainstem herniation the intracranial pressure is critically elevated, and the compliance characteristic of the solid cranium and the flexible brain are such that whereas a slight increase in pressure results in herniation and brain death, a slight reduction prevents herniation at that time. Many such patients are the victims of head trauma; indeed, almost all patients with significant head injury serious enough to require intensive care or neurosurgical intervention have at least some degree of elevated intracranial pressure. However, because acute hyperventilation is accepted practice in conditions in which intracranial pressure is most dangerous, it became commonplace to institute the same therapy in the presence of intracranial hypertension, of lesser severity. Unfortunately, this assumed the "benefits" of hyperventilation (i.e., reduction in elevated intracranial pressure, prevention of brainstem herniation) in patients in whom such factors were not important. Conversely, whereas the disadvantages of hyperventilation (i.e., focal ischemia due to vasoconstriction, diminished release of O_2 from circulating hemoglobin, and potentially increased local O_2 demand) appear minimal when weighed against impending death or irreversible brain damage, they may not be minimal when weighed against no benefit. Indeed a randomized controlled trial demonstrated that prophylactic hyperventilation in patients with severe head trauma increased the incidence of long-term CNS disability [56].

Targeting variables: balancing theory, physiology, and outcome

The above account, with examples selected to support the particular points in question, requires balance; while balance is needed, in practice it is difficult. The clinician faces many problems in balancing among the issues he thinks he understands, those he does understand, and those for which he can provide evidence of benefit. Indeed the situation is even more complex because over time the response of some illness states changes. For example, goal-directed therapy in early septic shock may decrease mortality [1], but extending the notion of normalization to pharmacological supranormalization applied in later phases of the same illness can cause harm [15]. In another important condition common in the critically ill, acute respiratory distress syndrome, attempts to recruit lung volume, while successful in early stages of the disease, appear to be far less successful in more established disease [57]. Finally, hyperventilation, while harmful if applied globally to patients with severe head injury [56], may help a small number of patients with intracranial hypertension due to cerebral hyperemia.

The above clinical trials [1, 4, 22, 26, 33] are presented in a simplistic manner. While simplicity has the advantage of clarity, it ignores both the complex nature of the trials and the disease entities involved. Indeed it is important to note that several detailed critiques have generated significant debate about the interpretation and incorporation of clinical studies into practice [2, 30, 58, 59, 60].

Conclusion

Multiple examples of therapies exist in the acute care setting that are based on physiological principles, and that involve monitoring and titrating against physiological endpoints. Many such approaches either have been directly responsible for saving lives in acutely ill patients or have reflected such management strategies. Nonetheless, clinicians recognize that following physiological principles is not the same as normalizing all physiological variables. To illustrate this distinction, and the dangers associated with the latter, we have identified five patterns, with examples of each, whereby such an approach can lead to harm. As knowledge advances, clinicians will integrate evidence-based information, mechanistic knowledge, and evolving error prevention strategies to incorporate advances in monitoring technology for provision of optimal patient care.

Acknowledgements The authors acknowledge Drs. Deborah Cook and Arthur Slutsky for their insightful comments.

References

1. Rivers E, Nguyen B, Havstad S, Ressler J, Muzzin A, Knoblich B, Peterson E, Tomlanovich M (2001) Early goal-directed therapy in the treatment of severe sepsis and septic shock. N Engl J Med 345:1368–1377
2. Finney SJ, Zekveld C, Elia A, Evans TW (2003) Glucose control and mortality in critically ill patients. JAMA 290:2041–2047
3. Natanson C, Danner RL (2002) Early goal-directed therapy reduced mortality and multiorgan dysfunction in severe sepsis or septic shock. ACP J Club 136:90
4. Berghe G van den, Wouters P, Weekers F, Verwaest C, Bruyninckx F, Schetz M, Vlasselaers D, Ferdinande P, Lauwers P, Bouillon R (2001) Intensive insulin therapy in the critically ill patients. N Engl J Med 345:1359–1367
5. Colice GL (1998) A historical perspective on intensive care monitoring. In: Tobin MJ (ed) Principles and practice of intensive care monitoring. McGraw Hill, New York, pp 1–31
6. Ibsen B (1999) Intensive therapy: background and development. A history of critical care and hyperbaric oxygen therapy as documented in the international anesthesiologiy clinics 37:1–14
7. Knaus WA, Draper EA, Wagner DP, Zimmerman JE (1985) APACHE II: a severity of disease classification system. Crit Care Med 13:818–829
8. Peres Bota D, Melot C, Lopes Ferreira F, Nguyen Ba V, Vincent JL (2002) The Multiple Organ Dysfunction Score (MODS) versus the Sequential Organ Failure Assessment (SOFA) score in outcome prediction. Intensive Care Med 28:1619–1624
9. Leteurtre S, Martinot A, Duhamel A, Proulx F, Grandbastien B, Cotting J, Gottesman R, Joffe A, Pfenninger J, Hubert P, Lacroix J, Leclerc F (2003) Validation of the paediatric logistic organ dysfunction (PELOD) score: prospective, observational, multicentre study. Lancet 362:192–197
10. Ferreira FL, Bota DP, Bross A, Melot C, Vincent JL (2001) Serial evaluation of the SOFA score to predict outcome in critically ill patients. JAMA 286:1754–1758
11. Lopez A, Lorente JA, Steingrub J, Bakker J, McLuckie A, Willatts S, Brockway M, Anzueto A, Holzapfel L, Breen D, Silverman MS, Takala J, Donaldson J, Arneson C, Grove G, Grossman S, Grover R (2004) Multiple-center, randomized, placebo-controlled, double-blind study of the nitric oxide synthase inhibitor 546C88: effect on survival in patients with septic shock. Crit Care Med 32:21–30
12. Watson D, Grover R, Anzueto A, Lorente J, Smithies M, Bellomo R, Guntupalli K, Grossman S, Donaldson J, Le Gall JR (2004) Cardiovascular effects of the nitric oxide synthase inhibitor NG-methyl-L-arginine hydrochloride (546C88) in patients with septic shock: results of a randomized, double-blind, placebo-controlled multicenter study (study no. 144-002). Crit Care Med 32:13–20
13. Cohen RI, Shapir Y, Davis A, Loona R, Scharf SM (2000) Comparison between selective and nonselective nitric oxide synthase inhibition and phenylephrine in normal and endotoxic swine. Crit Care Med 28:3257–3267
14. Barrington KJ, Etches PC, Schulz R, Talbot JA, Graham AJ, Pearson RJ, Cheung PY (2000) The hemodynamic effects of inhaled nitric oxide and endogenous nitric oxide synthesis blockade in newborn piglets during infusion of heat-killed group B streptococci. Crit Care Med 28:800–808
15. Hayes MA, Timmins AC, Yau EHS, Palazzo M, Hinds CJ, Watson D (1994) Elevation of systemic oxygen delivery in the treatment of critically ill patients. N Engl J Med 330:1717–1722
16. Takala J, Ruokonen E, Webster NR, Nielsen MS, Zandstra DF, Vundelinckx G, Hinds CJ (1999) Increased mortality associated with growth hormone treatment in critically ill adults. N Engl J Med 341:785–792
17. Fairley HB (1989) Changing perspectives in monitoring oxygenation. Anesthesiology 70:2–4
18. Shoemaker WC, Sullivan MJ, Wo CCJ (2000) Hemodynamic evaluation and management of acute illnesses in the emergency department. Textbook of Critical Care 258–272
19. Czer LS, Shoemaker WC (1978) Optimal hematocrit value in critically ill postoperative patients. Surg Gynecol Obstet 147:363–368
20. Shoemaker WC, Bryan-Brown CW (1973) Resuscitation and immediate care of the critically ill and injured patient. Semin Drug Treat 3:249–267
21. Marik PE, Sibbald WJ (1993) Effect of stored-blood transfusion on oxygen delivery in patients with sepsis. JAMA 269:3024–3029
22. Hebert PC, Wells G, Blajchman MA, Marshall J, Martin C, Pagliarello G, Tweeddale M, Schweitzer I, Yetisir E (1999) A multicenter, randomized, controlled clinical trial of transfusion requirements in critical care. Transfusion Requirements in Critical Care Investigators, Canadian Critical Care Trials Group. N Engl J Med 340:409–417
23. Hebert PC, Fergusson D, Blajchman MA, Wells GA, Kmetic A, Coyle D, Heddle N, Germain M, Goldman M, Toye B, Schweitzer I, vanWalraven C, Devine D, Sher GD (2003) Clinical outcomes following institution of the Canadian universal leukoreduction program for red blood cell transfusions. JAMA 289:1941–1949
24. Lundbom N, Laurila O, Laurila S (1993) Central pontine myelinolysis after correction of chronic hyponatraemia. Lancet 342:247–248
25. Askie LM, Henderson-Smart DJ, Irwig L, Simpson JM (2003) Oxygen-saturation targets and outcomes in extremely preterm infants. N Engl J Med 349:959–967
26. Amato MB, Barbas CS, Medeiros DM, Magaldi RB, Schettino GP, Lorenzi-Fihlo G, Kairalla RA, Deheinzelin D, Munoz C, Oliveira R, Takagaki TY, Carvalho CR (1998) Effect of a protective-ventilation strategy on mortality in the acute respiratory distress syndrome. N Engl J Med 338:347–354
27. Hickling KG, Walsh J, Henderson S, Jackson R (1994) Low mortality rate in adult respiratory distress syndrome using low-volume, pressure-limited ventilation with permissive hypercapnia: a prospective study. Crit. Care Med. 22:1568–1578
28. Hickling KG, Wright T, Laubscher K, Town IG, Tie A, Graham P, Monteath J, A'Court G (1998) Extreme hypoventilation reduces ventilator-induced lung injury during ventilation with low positive end-expiratory pressure in saline-lavaged rabbits. Crit Care Med 26:1690–1697
29. Marini JJ, Gattinoni L (2004) Ventilatory management of acute respiratory distress syndrome: a consensus of two. Crit Care Med 32:250–255
30. Dreyfuss D, Saumon G (2002) Evidence-based medicine or fuzzy logic: what is best for ARDS management? Intensive Care Med 28:230–234
31. Trauma Life Support Committee, National Association of Emergency Medical Technicians in cooperation with Committee on Trauma, American College of Surgeons (1995) Prehospital trauma life support instructors' manual, 3rd edn. Mosby, St. Louis
32. American College of Surgeons (1997) Advanced trauma life support for doctors, 6th edn. American College of Surgeons, Chicago
33. Bickell WH, Wall MJ, Pepe PE, Martin RR, Ginger VF, Allen MK, Mattox KL (1994) Immediate versus delayed fluid resuscitation for hypotensive patients with pentrating torso injuries. N Engl J Med 331:1105–1109

34. Dronen SC, Stern SA, Wang X, Stanley M (1993) A comparison of the response of near-fatal acute hemorrhage models with and without a vascular injury to rapid volume expansion. Am J Emerg Med 11:331–335
35. Stern SA, Dronen SC, Birrer P, Wang X (1993) Effect of blood pressure on hemorrhage volume and survival in a near-fatal hemorrhage model incorporating a vascular injury. Ann Emerg Med 22:155–163
36. Hood VL, Tannen RL (1998) Protection of acid-base balance by pH regulation of acid production. N Engl J Med 339:819–826
37. Laffey JG, Kavanagh BP (2002) Hypocapnia. N Engl J Med 347:43–53
38. Laffey JG, Kavanagh BP (1999) Carbon dioxide and the critically ill—too little of a good thing? (hypothesis paper). Lancet 354:1283–1286
39. Bureau MA, Begin R, Berthiaume Y, Shapcott D, Khoury K, Gagnon N (1980) Cerebral hypoxia from bicarbonate infusion in diabetic acidosis. J Pediatr 96:968–973
40. Okuda Y, Adrogue HJ, Field JB, Nohara H, Yamashita K (1996) Counterproductive effects of sodium bicarbonate in diabetic ketoacidosis. J Clin Endocrinol Metab 81:314–320
41. Cooper DJ, Walley KR, Wiggs BR, Russell JA (1990) Bicarbonate does not improve hemodynamics in critically ill patients who have lactic acidosis. A prospective, controlled clinical study. Ann Intern Med 112:492–498
42. Jiang Q, Cross AS, Singh IS, Chen TT, Viscardi RM, Hasday JD (2000) Febrile core temperature is essential for optimal host defense in bacterial peritonitis. Infect Immun 68:1265–1270
43. Rizoli SB, Kapus A, Parodo J, Rotstein OD (1999) Hypertonicity prevents lipopolysaccharide-stimulated CD11b/CD18 expression in human neutrophils in vitro: role for p38 inhibition. J Trauma 46:794–798
44. Shibata K, Cregg N, Engelberts D, Takeuchi A, Fedorko L, Kavanagh BP (1998) Hypercapnic acidosis may attenuate acute lung injury by inhibition of endogenous xanthine oxidase. Am J Respir Crit Care Med 158:1578–1584
45. Singer M, De Santis V, Vitale D, Jeffcoate W (2004) Multiorgan failure is an adaptive, endocrine-mediated, metabolic response to overwhelming systemic inflammation. Lancet 364:545–548
46. Leape LL, Brennan TA, Laird N, Lawthers AG, Localio AR, Barnes BA, Hebert L, Newhouse JP, Weiler PC, Hiatt H (1991) The nature of adverse events in hospitalized patients. Results of the Harvard Medical Practice Study II. N Engl J Med 324:377–384
47. Deyo RA (2002) Cascade effects of medical technology. Annu Rev Public Health 23:23–44
48. Gilron I, Magder S (1995) Monitoring complication due to a pulsatile femoral vein from tricuspid regurgitation. Can J Anaesth 42:141–143
49. Wolpert HA, Anderson BJ (2001) Metabolic control matters: Why is the message lost in the translation? The need for realistic goal-setting in diabetes care. Diabetes Care 24:1301–1303
50. Lenfant C (2003) Shattuck lecture-clinical research to clinical practice-lost in translation? N Engl J Med 349:868–874
51. Sullivan CE, Issa FG, Berthon-Jones M, Eves L (1981) Reversal of obstructive sleep apnoea by continuous positive airway pressure applied through the nares. Lancet I:862–865
52. Bernard GR, Vincent JL, Laterre PF, LaRosa SP, Dhainaut JF, Lopez-Rodriguez A, Steingrub JS, Garber GE, Helterbrand JD, Ely EW, Fisher CJ Jr (2001) Efficacy and safety of recombinant human activated protein C for severe sepsis. N Engl J Med 344:699–709
53. Derdak S, Mehta S, Stewart TE, Smith T, Rogers M, Buchman TG, Carlin B, Lowson S, Granton J (2002) High-frequency oscillatory ventilation for acute respiratory distress syndrome in adults: a randomized, controlled trial. Am J Respir Crit Care Med 166:801–808
54. Froese AB (1997) High-frequency oscillatory ventilation for adult respiratory distress syndrome: let's get it right this time! Crit Care Med 25:906–908
55. Lundberg N, Kjallquist A, Bien C (1959) Reduction of increased intracranial pressure by hyperventilation. A therapeutic aid in neurological surgery. Acta Psychiatr Scand 34 [Suppl 139]:1–64
56. Muizelaar JP, Marmarou A, Ward JD, Kontos HA, Choi SC, Becker DP, Gruemer H, Young HF (1991) Adverse effects of prolonged hyperventilation in patients with severe head injury: a randomized trial. J. Neurosurg. 75:731–739
57. Grasso S, Mascia L, Del Turco M, Malacarne P, Giunta F, Brochard L, Slutsky AS, Marco Ranieri V (2002) Effects of recruiting maneuvers in patients with acute respiratory distress syndrome ventilated with protective ventilatory strategy. Anesthesiology 96:795–802
58. Silverman HJ, Miller FG (2004) Control group selection in critical care randomized controlled trials evaluating interventional strategies: an ethical assessment. Crit Care Med 32:852–857
59. Miller FG, Silverman HJ (2004) The ethical relevance of the standard of care in the design of clinical trials. Am J Respir Crit Care Med 169:562–564
60. Eichacker PQ, Gerstenberger EP, Banks SM, Cui X, Natanson C (2002) Meta-analysis of acute lung injury and acute respiratory distress syndrome trials testing low tidal volumes. Am J Respir Crit Care Med 166:1510–1514

Shane M. Tibby
Andrew Durward

Interpretation of the echocardiographic pressure gradient across a pulmonary artery band in the setting of a univentricular heart

Introduction

Pulmonary artery (PA) banding has been established as a palliative surgical technique for congenital heart defects for over 50 years [1]. With the advent of earlier corrective surgery, the indications for PA banding have changed over time [2, 3]. Currently these include: (a) limitation of pulmonary blood flow in the setting of an excessive left-to-right shunt; (b) regulation of pulmonary blood flow in the univentricular circulation; and (c) a training procedure for the left ventricle prior to conversion to the systemic pumping chamber (late presentation of D-transposition of the great arteries, or prior to a double-switch procedure with L-transposition).

From a physiological perspective the goals of PA banding in conditions (a) and (b) are threefold:

1. To protect the pulmonary arteries from hypertrophy and the development of irreversible pulmonary vascular disease. This phenomenon is thought to be both pressure- and flow mediated [4].
2. To regulate the pulmonary to systemic flow ratio (Qp:Qs) in the setting of a univentricular heart, and minimize the risk of developing inadequate systemic and coronary blood flow.
3. To prevent the development of congestive heart failure from an excessive total cardiac output (Qp plus Qs).

This article primarily considers PA banding and its interpretation in the setting of a univentricular heart. For simplicity sake, we assume complete mixing of venous return in the systemic ventricle, and an absence of streaming. In addition, we do not discuss limitations in echocardiographic measurements using the Doppler principle or the Bernouilli equation (as these can be found in any major textbook), but instead assume that such measurements are made correctly.

Assessment of the adequacy of banding

The importance of accurate assessment of PA band tightness is highlighted by the fact that undiagnosed loose bands are associated with a higher mortality [5]. The commonest bedside method for assessing the adequacy of a PA band involves echocardiographic estimation of the pressure drop across the band, via the modified Bernoulli equation, in tandem with measurement of arterial oxygen saturations using pulse oximetry [2, 6]. This provides a measure of the degree of protection from pressure effects on the pulmonary vasculature (via the band gradient), and an estimate of Qp:Qs (from the arterial oxygen saturation). Optimal band tightness in the univentricular setting is thought to be represented by an estimated pressure drop of the order of 40–60 mmHg, with arterial oxygen saturations in the range of 75–85% [3, 7]. Several publications have highlighted the value of concurrent assessment of parameters such as acid-base status, arterial blood lactate measurements, urine output and chest X-ray, but this is by no means universal [3, 8].

M.R. Pinsky et al. (eds.), *Applied Physiology in Intensive Care Medicine 2: Physiological Reviews and Editorials*,
DOI 10.1007/978-3-642-28233-1_19, © Springer-Verlag Berlin Heidelberg 2012

Limitations of this method

Unfortunately, this may be an oversimplification, as there are many factors which can confound interpretation of both band gradient and arterial oxygen saturation.

Band gradient

The mean pressure drop across a PA band is a function of the flow through the band and the resistance of the band itself (pressure drop = flow × resistance). This means that a low resistance band receiving high flow may yield the same pressure drop as a high resistance band with low flow; thus, when interpreting a band gradient, it is necessary to consider concurrently *all* factors which contribute to flow through the band, including the following: total cardiac output; the ratio of systemic to pulmonary flow (Qp:Qs); systemic vascular resistance; band resistance; and the resistance of the pulmonary vasculature distal to the band (the latter two may be regarded functionally as being in series). These factors are represented in Fig. 1.

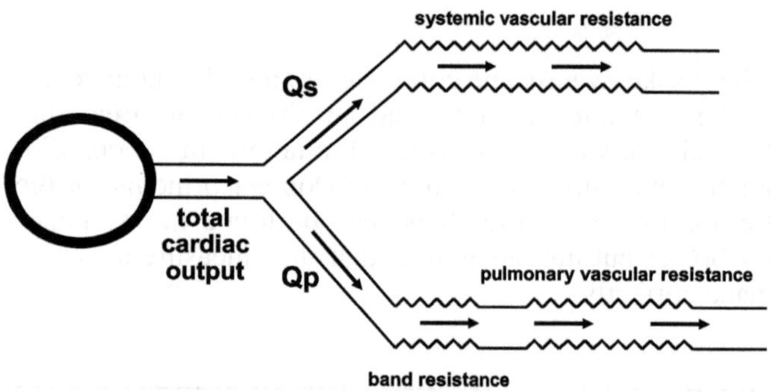

Fig. 1 Variables which influence the pressure gradient across the pulmonary arterial band. *Qp*, pulmonary blood flow; *Qs*, systemic blood flow

Arterial oxygen saturations

For a univentricular heart with common mixing, arterial saturations are a function of both the proportionate inflow from the various venous sources (systemic, pulmonary, coronary and thebesian) and their oxygen saturations. Fig. 2 shows two hypothetical situations that may produce identical arterial oxygen saturations. (For ease of demonstration coronary and thebesian venous blood flow is ignored, and pulmonary venous blood is considered to be fully saturated.) Fig. 2a shows an "ideal" situation with a Qp:Qs of 1:1, resulting in an arterial saturation of 80%. Fig. 2b shows overcirculation, with a Qp:Qs of 3:1. In this setting, inadequate systemic flow has resulted in a reduction in the mixed venous saturation, the net result also yielding an arterial saturation of 80%. The limitation of arterial saturation as an estimate of Qp:Qs is well documented in the intensive care management of patients with hypoplastic left heart syndrome [9–11]. The importance of concurrent measurement of the mixed venous saturation has been highlighted in this setting. Typically this is expressed in terms of the arteriovenous oxygen saturation difference.

Incorporating arteriovenous oxygen saturation difference into band assessment

We suggest that postoperative assessment following PA band placement could be improved by considering the arteriovenous oxygen saturation difference in conjunction with the band gradient. The theoretical relationship between these two variables is shown in Fig. 3, which was constructed by application of the Fick principle, shunt and vascular resistance equations (Table 1) to a hypothetical patient. For simplicity sake, we made several haemodynamic assumptions, including: complete mixing (i. e. a true univentricular heart); absence of intracardiac

Fig. 2 a,b Limitation of the arterial oxygen saturation as an estimate of pulmonary to systemic flow ratio (*Qp:Qs*)

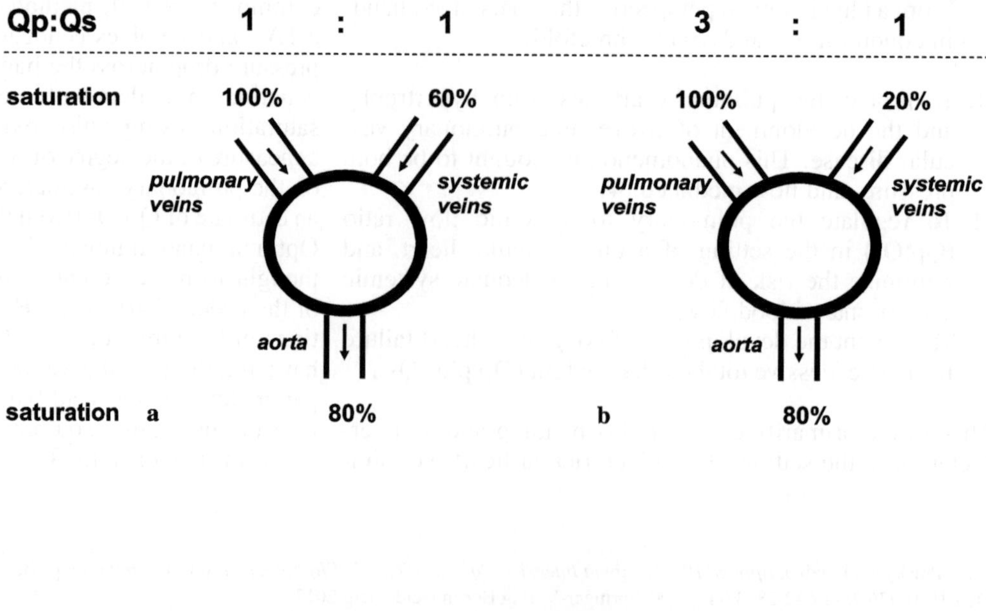

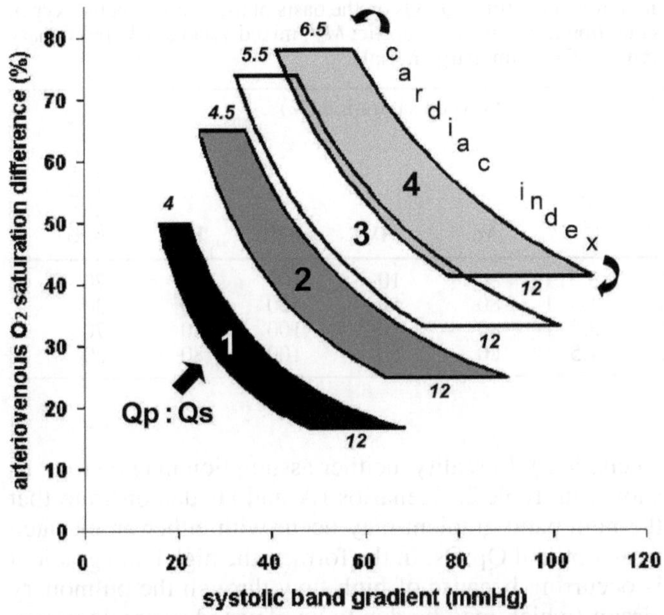

Fig. 3 Theoretical relationship between systolic pressure drop across the pulmonary arterial band and the arteriovenous oxygen saturation difference. Haemodynamic assumptions include: complete intracardiac mixing; oxygen consumption of 160 ml/min m^{-2}; haemoglobin of 120 gm/l; pulmonary venous oxygen saturation of 100%; and constant systemic and pulmonary vascular resistances (the latter being distal to the band). Four regions of "iso-shunt" are shown, with Qp:Qs ranging from 1 to 4. Total cardiac index (systemic plus pulmonary) is measured in litres per minute per square metre, and may vary within each iso-shunt region. Low cardiac index is associated with higher arteriovenous oxygen saturation differences and smaller band gradients occurring towards the top of the iso-shunt blocks, whereas higher cardiac index occurs with smaller arteriovenous oxygen saturation differences and larger band gradients

streaming of blood; oxygen consumption at the lower limit for age (160 ml/min m^{-2}); haemoglobin of 120 g/l; pulmonary venous saturations of 100%; and constant systemic and pulmonary vascular resistances. (Here pulmonary resistance refers to that which is distal to the band.)

Superimposed on the diagram are blocks which represent potential areas of constant shunt (Qp:Qs). The width of these blocks was chosen by considering the upper and lower limits for band resistance that may occur with an error of ± 1 mm when applying the Trussler formula to infants [12]. (If we assume laminar flow, then band resistance is proportional to band radius to the fourth power; and an error of ± 1 mm in the Trussler-derived band circumference will alter the band radius by ± circumference/2π, resulting in a potential variation in resistance of approximately 30% for infants from 2 to 5 kg.) If band resistance is known, we can calculate the mean pressure drop across the PA band for a given cardiac output and Qp:Qs, which is related to the systolic pressure drop by a factor of one third (given that mean blood pressure = diastolic pressure plus one-third pulse pressure, and that diastolic pressure is likely to be equal on either side of the band). Because it is pressure drop that we are estimating, the absolute values for systolic and diastolic pressures in this setting are irrelevant.

This produces a relationship between band gradient and arteriovenous oxygen saturation difference incorporating a variety of shunts and a range of total (pulmonary plus systemic) cardiac output (Fig. 3). Within each iso-shunt block, it can be seen that low total cardiac output occurs towards the upper portion and is associated with a higher arteriovenous difference. Conversely, cardiac output increases, and arteriovenous difference decreases as one progresses towards the lower end of each iso-shunt block.

Limitations of this method

The number of assumptions (and hence unmeasured variables) means that this diagram cannot be used to estimate Qp:Qs in individual patients, as a unique diagram must be constructed for every different combination of oxygen consumption, pulmonary venous oxygen saturation, haemoglobin concentration and systemic and pulmonary

Table 1 Haemodynamic formulae. VO_2, oxygen consumption (ml/min m^{-2}); CaO_2, arterial oxygen content (ml/l); $C_{MV}O_2$, mixed venous oxygen content; *Hgb*, haemoglobin concentration (g/l); SaO_2, arterial oxygen saturation; PaO_2, partial pressure of dissolved oxygen; $S_{Ao}O_2$, aortic oxygen saturation; $S_{MV}O_2$, mixed venous oxygen saturation; $S_{PV}O_2$, pulmonary venous oxygen saturation; $S_{PA}O_2$, pulmonary arterial oxygen saturation

Parameter	Formula
Fick's principle	Cardiac index = $VO_2/(CaO_2 - C_{MV}O_2)$
Oxygen content	$CaO_2 = (1.34 \times Hgb \times SaO_2) + (PaO_2 \times 0.003)$
Pulmonary to systemic flow ratio	$Qp{:}Qs = S_{Ao}O_2 - S_{MV}O_2/S_{PV}O_2 - S_{PA}O_2$
Vascular resistance index	VRI = 79.9 × pressure drop/cardiac index

Units of measurement: cardiac index, l/min m^{-2}; vascular resistance index, dyn-s/cm^5 m^{-2}

Table 2 Hypothetical scenarios demonstrating the inconsistency of the relationship between arterial oxygen saturation, band gradient and degree of shunt (*Qp:Qs*). In this case a high Qp:Qs is differentiated from an optimal Qp:Qs on the basis of the arteriovenous oxygen saturation difference. *Ao*, aortic; *MV*, mixed venous; *PV*, pulmonary venous; *PA*, pulmonary arterial

Scenario	Band resistance dyn-s/cm^5 m^{-2}	Band gradient mean (mm Hg)	Band systolic pressure drop (mm Hg)	Cardiac index (l/min m^{-2})			Qp:Qs	Oxygen saturation (%)				Arteriovenous difference (%)
				Pulmonary	Systemic	Total		Ao	MV	PV	PA	
1 A	428	26.7	80	4.98	1.42	6.40	3.5 : 1	80	10	100	80	70
1 B	428	26.7	80	4.98	3.32	8.29	1.5 : 1	80	50	100	80	30
2 A	161	10.0	30	4.98	1.42	6.40	3.5 : 1	80	10	100	80	70
2 B	161	10.0	30	4.98	3.32	8.29	1.5 : 1	80	50	100	80	30

vascular resistances. In addition, the diagram has been simplified such that the blocks of Qp:Qs ratios represent whole numbers only; inclusion of smaller increments (Qp:Qs of 1.5, 2.5, etc.) would result in a degree of overlap that would render the diagram uninterpretable.

Our calculations utilise oxygen saturations from mixed venous blood, whereas in clinical practice central venous oxygen saturations are usually obtained. Consistent with other authors, we recommend that the superior vena caval site be used, as the haemodynamic assumptions remain valid [13, 14].

Lastly, the calculations refer to placement of a single, central pulmonary artery band, and not to the placement of bilateral (right and left pulmonary artery) banding that is utilised as part of the hybrid procedure for hypoplastic left heart syndrome [15]; however, Fig. 3 does illustrate two important points:

1. For a given band gradient, larger Qp:Qs values are associated with higher arteriovenous oxygen differences.
2. Higher band gradients are likely to be associated with larger shunts, which is counterintuitive to traditional teaching.

This can be illustrated further by considering two typical clinical scenarios. A patient with a measured arterial oxygen saturation of 80% and a systolic band gradient of 80 mmHg is likely to be interpreted as having an adequate band (scenario 1), whereas a patient with the same oxygen saturation but band gradient of 30 mmHg may be interpreted as having a band that is too loose (scenario 2). In reality, neither assumption may be true, as shown in Table 2. Scenarios 1A and 1B demonstrate that the high band gradient may occur with either an elevated or an optimal Qp:Qs. In the former, the high band gradient is occurring because of high flow through the pulmonary circuit (which may be due to an elevated systemic vascular resistance), and the "adequate" arterial saturations of 80% are occurring because the mixed venous saturations are very low (10%). The two situations are readily differentiated by comparing the arteriovenous oxygen saturation differences. In scenario 2, the lower band gradient is a function of decreased band resistance (a looser band). Similar to scenario 1, markedly different Qp:Qs are possible because of an altered ratio of systemic vascular resistance to the pulmonary vascular resistance distal to the band; again, these may manifest identical arterial oxygen saturations but can be differentiated by the arteriovenous oxygen saturation difference.

The requirement for central venous blood sampling means that this technique is not practical for all patients following PA banding. In addition, it may take some time for post-operative haemodynamic equilibrium to be achieved; thus, it may be unwise to interpret adequacy of PA banding with this method in the early post-operative period (0–12 h). However, the technique may be of most benefit (a) in the intermediate post-operative period, (b) for patients who are unable to be successfully weaned from mechanical ventilation and (c) for those with ongoing heart failure. It also underlines the importance of adopting a wider physiological perspective, rather than interpreting a haemodynamic parameters in isolation.

References

1. Muller WH Jr, Danimann JF Jr (1952) The treatment of certain congenital malformations of the heart by the creation of pulmonic stenosis to reduce pulmonary hypertension and excessive pulmonary blood flow; a preliminary report. Surg Gynecol Obstet 95:213–219
2. Corno AF (2005) Pulmonary artery banding. Swiss Med Wkly 135:515–519
3. Plunkett M, Laks H. Pulmonary Artery Banding. E-medicine http://www.emedicine.com/ped/topic2900.htm accessed 28 March 2007
4. Granton JT, Rabinovitch M (2002) Pulmonary arterial hypertension in congenital heart disease. Cardiol Clin 20:441–457
5. Pinho P, von Oppell UO, Brink J, Hewitson J (1997) Pulmonary artery banding: adequacy and long-term outcome. Eur J Cardiothorac Surg 11:105–111
6. Fyfe DA, Currie PJ, Seward JB, Tajik AJ, Reeder GS, Mair DD, Hagler DJ (1984) Continuous-wave Doppler determination of the pressure gradient across pulmonary artery bands: hemodynamic correlation in 20 patients. Mayo Clin Proc 59:744–750
7. Wernovsky G, Bove EL (1998) Single ventricle lesions. In: Chang AC, Hanley FL, Wernovsky G, Wessel DL (eds) Pediatric cardiac intensive care. Lippincott Williams and Wilkins, Philadelphia, pp 275–276
8. Corno AF (2000) Revised pulmonary artery banding. Ann Thorac Surg 69:1295–1296
9. Barnea O, Austin EH, Richman B, Santamore WP (1994) Balancing the circulation: theoretic optimization of pulmonary/systemic flow ratio in hypoplastic left heart syndrome. J Am Coll Cardiol 24:1376–1381
10. Charpie JR, Dekeon MK, Goldberg CS, Mosca RS, Bove EL, Kulik TJ (2001) Postoperative hemodynamics after Norwood palliation for hypoplastic left heart syndrome. Am J Cardiol 87:198–202
11. Taeed R, Schwartz SM, Pearl JM, Raake JL, Beekman RH III, Manning PB, Nelson DP (2001) Unrecognized pulmonary venous desaturation early after Norwood palliation confounds Gp:Gs assessment and compromises oxygen delivery. Circulation 103:2699–2704
12. Albus RA, Trusler GA, Izukawa T, Williams WG (1984) Pulmonary artery banding. J Thorac Cardiovasc Surg 88:645–653
13. Rivers EP, Ander DS, Powell D (2001) Central venous oxygen saturation monitoring in the critically ill patient. Curr Opin Crit Care 7:204–211
14. Li J, Zhang G, McCrindle BW, Holtby H, Humpl T, Cai S, Caldarone CA, Redington AN, Van Arsdell GS (2007) Profiles of hemodynamics and oxygen transport derived by using continuous measured oxygen consumption after the Norwood procedure. J Thorac Cardiovasc Surg 133:441–448
15. Akintuerk H, Michel-Behnke I, Valeske K, Mueller M, Thul J, Bauer J, Hagel KJ, Kreuder J, Vogt P, Schranz D (2003) Stenting of the arterial duct and banding of the pulmonary arteries: basis for combined Norwood stage I and II repair in hypoplastic left heart. Circulation 105:1099–1103

Theodoros Vassilakopoulos

Ventilator-induced diaphragm dysfunction: the clinical relevance of animal models

Abstract Experimental evidence suggests that controlled mechanical ventilation (CMV) can induce dysfunction of the diaphragm, resulting in an early-onset and progressive decrease in diaphragmatic force-generating capacity, called ventilator-induced diaphragmatic dysfunction (VIDD). The mechanisms of VIDD are not fully elucidated, but include muscle atrophy (resulting from lysosomal, calpain, caspase and proteasome activation), oxidative stress, structural injury (disrupted myofibrils, increased numbers of lipid vacuoles, and abnormally small and disrupted mitochondria), myofiber remodeling and mitochondrial dysfunction. The major clinical implication of the VIDD is to limit the use of CMV to the extent possible. Partial (assisted) modes of ventilatory support should be used whenever feasible, since these modes attenuate the deleterious effects of mechanical ventilation on respiratory muscles.

Keywords Mechanical ventilation · Complications · Disuse atrophy · Weaning · Diaphragm

Introduction

Controlled mechanical ventilation (CMV) is a mode of ventilatory support where the respiratory muscles are not contracting and the ventilator takes full responsibility for inflating the respiratory system. Animal studies suggest that CMV can induce dysfunction of the diaphragm, resulting in decreased force-generating capacity, called ventilator-induced diaphragmatic dysfunction (VIDD) [1].

The frequency of CMV use cannot be determined with certainty. The international mechanical ventilation study group reported that 13% of mechanically ventilated patients receive a neuromuscular blocker for 8% of the total days of ventilatory support [2]. In these patients full ventilatory support is mandatory. There are additional patients who are on full ventilator support without receiving neuromuscular blockers (e.g. traumatic brain injury patients, postoperative neurosurgical patients, comatose patients, and patients with status epilepticus on barbiturate coma to suppress seizure activity). Thus, a significant proportion of mechanically ventilated patients are on full ventilator support and could be potentially vulnerable to VIDD.

The mechanisms of this dysfunction and the clinical relevance for mechanically ventilated patients will be the subject of this review.

Evidence from animal models

Diaphragmatic force and endurance following CMV

Measurements in intact animals

Controlled mechanical ventilation leads to decreased diaphragmatic force-generating capacity in various animal species. In the intact diaphragm studied in vivo, transdiaphragmatic pressure (Pdi) generation upon phrenic nerve stimulation declines at all stimulation frequencies (20–100 Hz) (Fig. ESM 1) [3–6]. The decline ensues early (1 day in rabbits [5], 3 days in piglets [4, 6]) and is progressive, Pdi decreasing to 63% of the control value after 1 day of CMV and to 49% of the control value after 3 days of CMV in rabbits [5]. Within a few days (3 days in rabbits, 3–5 days in piglets, 11 days in baboons) the

M.R. Pinsky et al. (eds.), *Applied Physiology in Intensive Care Medicine 2: Physiological Reviews and Editorials*,
DOI 10.1007/978-3-642-28233-1_20, © Springer-Verlag Berlin Heidelberg 2012

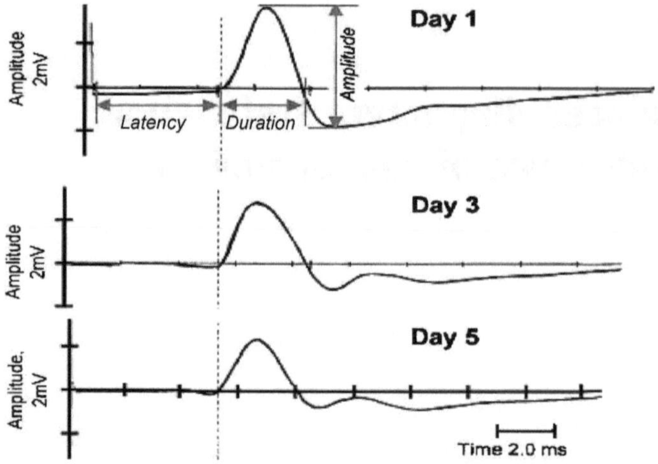

Fig. 1 The evoked compound muscle action potential (*CMAP*) tracings of the diaphragm upon electrical stimulation of the phrenic nerves in vivo from one piglet on days 1, 3 and 5 of CMV. The time from the stimulus to the onset of CMAP (*Latency*) does not change after 3-5 days of CMV, whereas the amplitude of CMAP is progressively reduced. From reference [4] with permission. This indicates that the neural and neuromuscular transmission are not affected when VIDD develops and that the contractile dysfunction resides within the diaphragmatic myofibers

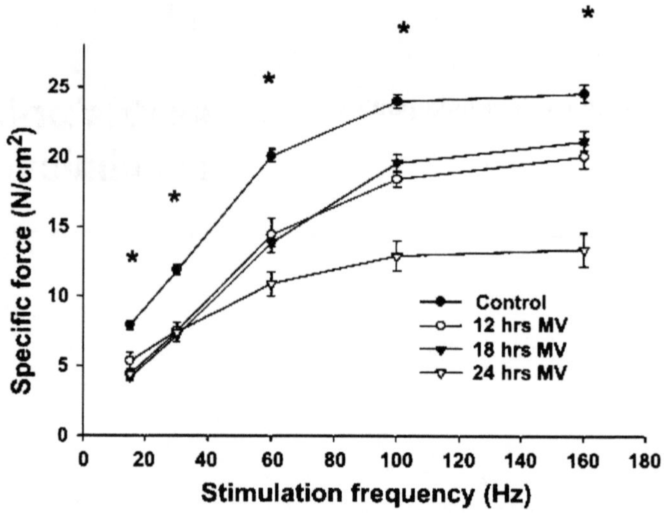

Fig. 2 Effects of prolonged CMV on the diaphragmatic force–frequency response in vitro in rats. Values are means ± SE. Compared with control, CMV (all durations) resulted in a significant ($*p<0.05$) reduction in diaphragmatic specific force production at all stimulation frequencies. From reference [8] with permission. Please note that the decline in force is progressive, worsening as the duration of CMV is prolonged

pressure generating capacity of the diaphragm declines by 35–50%. The endurance of the diaphragm is also compromised [3].

The decreased force-generating capacity ensuing with CMV is not due to changes in lung volume [6] or to changes in abdominal compliance [3, 4]. Neural and neuromuscular transmission remain intact, as evidenced by the lack of changes in phrenic nerve conduction (latency) and the stable response to repetitive stimulation of the phrenic nerve [4] (Fig. 1). In contrast, the compound muscle action potential (CMAP) declines progressively, suggesting that excitation/contraction coupling or membrane depolarization may be involved (Fig. 1) [4]. Thus, the CMV-induced impairment in the diaphragmatic force-generating capacity appears to reside within the myofibers.

In vitro measurements

The isometric (both twitch and tetanic) tension development by isolated diaphragmatic strips in vitro [7–10] confirm the in vivo findings and suggest that the decline in contractility is an early (12 h) and progressive phenomenon (Fig. 2) [8], the isometric force declining by 30–50% after 1–3 days of CMV in rats. The force–velocity relationship of the diaphragm also changes, the maximum shortening velocity increasing after CMV [11] (Fig. ESM 2; for details and implications see the ESM text).

The effects of CMV on diaphragm in vitro fatigability are controversial (see ESM).

Pathophysiology

Muscle atrophy

CMV leads to diaphragmatic atrophy [7, 9, 10, 12]. Ventilator-induced atrophy [13] develops rapidly (as early as 12 h after the institution of CMV [14]) and is more pronounced in the diaphragm, which atrophies earlier than the peripheral skeletal muscles that are also inactive during CMV [7, 9, 12]. Two days of CMV with PEEP (2 cmH_2O) induced atrophy in rabbits [10], whereas 3 days of CMV without PEEP were inadequate to induce atrophy [5], which suggests that the rapidity of atrophy development might be augmented with the use of PEEP. The increased lung volume at the end of expiration with the use of PEEP would put the passive diaphragm in a relatively shortened position, and skeletal muscles atrophy faster in the shortened position [15, 16].

The decreased volume of the cytoplasm (atrophy) was observed in the presence of decreased number of myonuclei (skeletal muscle cells are multinucleated cells and theoretically a single myonucleus can sustain the necessary gene expression for a limited area of the cytoplasm, a relationship known as the myonuclear domain [17]), so that the myonuclear domain remains constant [14]. This decrease in myonuclear content was mediated by caspase-3-dependent increased apoptosis, which was evident as early as 6 h after the onset of CMV [14]. Both the apoptosis and the atrophy were attenuated with caspase-3 inhibition [14].

Atrophy can result from decreased protein synthesis, increased proteolysis or both. Six hours of CMV in rats decreased the in vivo rate of mixed muscle protein synthesis (an average synthesis rate for all muscle proteins) by 30% and the rate of myosin heavy chain protein synthesis by 65%, both of which persisted throughout 18 h of CMV [18]. In addition, 24 h of CMV suppressed the mRNA levels of insulin-like growth factor (IGF)-1, which stimulates protein synthesis [19]. Thus, CMV decreases protein synthesis in the diaphragm.

Increased proteolysis has been documented in diaphragm strips of animals subjected to 18 h of CMV [12]. All systems of proteases that mammalian cells have for intracellular proteolysis (the lysosomal proteases, the calpains, the caspases and the proteasome system) [20]), are activated after CMV [12, 14, 21]. Calpains do not fully degrade, but only partially cleave proteins in vivo (Fig. ESM 3). This renders the proteins amenable to the proteasome [13]. The stimulus for calpain activation in not known, but calcium elevation in the cell is prerequisite. The reduced (mRNA) levels of sarcoplasmatic reticulum calcium ATPase (the enzyme that removes calcium from the sarcoplasm) secondary to 24 h of CMV [22] may contribute to calpain activation. The lysosomal proteases such as cathepsin B are also activated secondary to CMV [21]. Caspases are proteases that can degrade proteins and especially complexes of actin and myosin [20, 23]. Upregulation of caspase-3 expression has been documented in the diaphragm secondary to CMV [14]. Caspase-3 can be activated by oxidative stress, increased intracellular calcium and increased calpain activity [20].

Using the proteasome inhibitor lactacystin, Shanely et al. [12] showed that the proteasome is involved in the augmented proteolysis of the diaphragm strips from CMV animals. The proteasome is a multi-subunit multi-catalytic

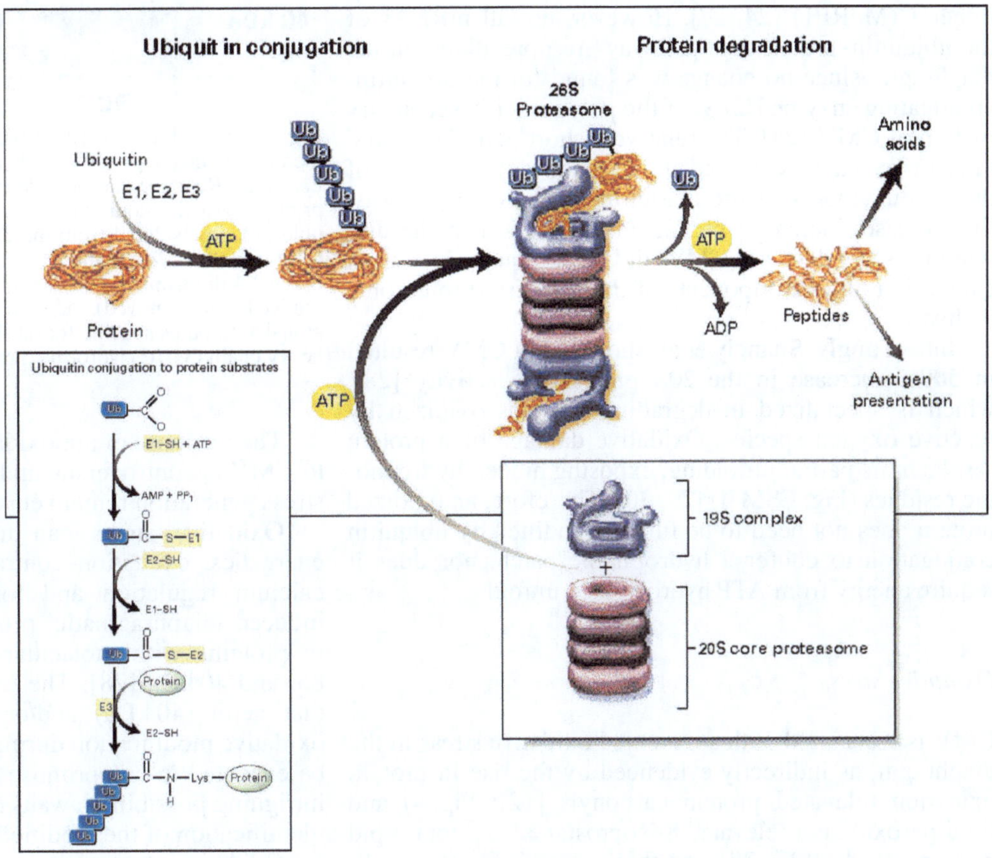

Fig. 3 The ubiquitin–proteasome pathway of proteolysis. Proteins degraded by the ubiquitin–proteasome pathway are first conjugated to ubiquitin (*Ub*). The process of linking ubiquitin to lysine residues in proteins destined for degradation (inlet) involves the activation of ubiquitin by the E1 enzyme in an ATP-dependent reaction. Activated ubiquitin is transferred to an E2 carrier protein and then to the substrate protein, a reaction catalyzed by an E3 enzyme (E3 ligase). This process is repeated as multiple ubiquitin molecules are added to form a ubiquitin chain. In ATP-dependent reactions, ubiquitin-conjugated proteins are recognized and bound by the 19S complex, which releases the ubiquitin chain and catalyzes the entry of the protein into the 20S core proteasome. Degradation occurs in the 26S core proteasome, which contains multiple proteolytic sites within its two central rings. Peptides produced by the proteasome are released and rapidly degraded to amino acids by peptidases in the cytoplasm or transported to the endoplasmic reticulum and used in the presentation of class I antigens. The ubiquitin is not degraded but is released and reused. *SH* denotes sulfhydryl, PP_1 pyrophosphate, and *ATP*, *ADP* adenosine tri- and diphosphate respectively. From reference [25] with permission

complex that exists in two major forms (Fig. 3): the core 20S proteasome can be free or bound to a pair of 19S regulators to form the 26S proteasome, which degrades (in an ATP-dependent manner) proteins covalently bound to a polyubiquitin protein chain (ubiquitinated proteins). The binding of ubiquitin to protein substrates requires the ubiquitin-activating enzyme (E1), which utilizes ATP-derived energy to form a covalent link with a ubiquitin protein, followed by transfer of the active ubiquitin moiety to a ubiquitin-conjugating enzyme (E2) and finally transfer of this ubiquitin to the protein to be degraded via a ubiquitin ligase (E3). Accordingly, CMV increases the level of ubiquitin–protein conjugates in the diaphragm [24] that are the substrates of the 26S proteasome (Fig. 3) [25]. Furthermore, key enzymes involved in the function of ubiquitin–proteasome pathway are upregulated in the diaphragm, such as the skeletal muscle-specific ubiquitin ligases (E3 enzymes) muscle atrophy F-box (MAFbx/Atrogin-1) [24, 26, 27] and muscle ring finger-1 (MuRF1) [24, 27]. However, not all mRNAs of the ubiquitin–proteasome pathway are upregulated in the diaphragm, since no change was found for the ubiquitin-conjugating enzyme $E2_{14k}$, or the polyubiquitin secondary to 12 h of CMV [24]. The relatively short period of CMV (12 h) may have been inadequate for the upregulation of these components of the ubiquitin–proteasome pathway. In any case, increased protein ubiquitination in the diaphragm secondary to CMV did not require increased expression of all components of the ubiquitin-proteasome pathway.

Interestingly, Shanely et al. showed that CMV resulted in 500% increase in the 20S proteasome activity [28], which is specialized in degrading proteins oxidized by reactive oxygen species. Oxidative damage of a protein results in its partial unfolding, exposing hidden hydrophobic residues (Fig. ESM 4) [29, 30]. Therefore, an oxidized protein does not need to be further modified by ubiquitin conjugation to confer a hydrophobic patch, nor does it require energy from ATP hydrolysis to unfold.

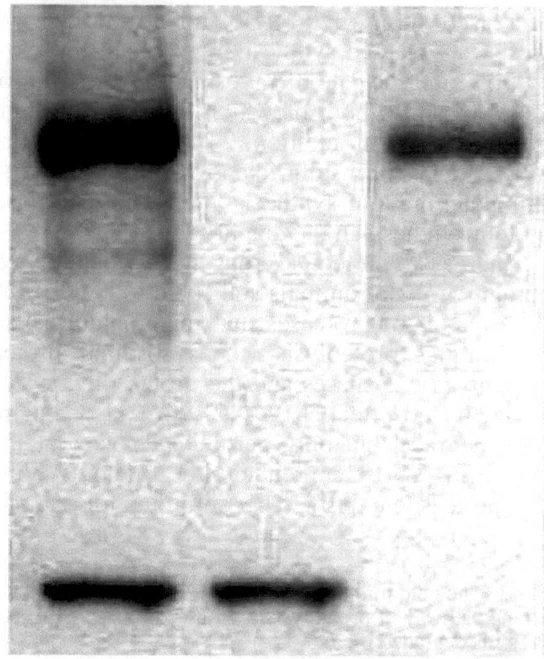

Fig. 4 Illustration of Western blots using monoclonal antibodies to identify oxidized proteins with molecular masses of 200–40 kDa. *Left lane:* Reactive carbonyl derivatives (*RCD*), which are the footprints of protein modifications induced by oxidative stress in insoluble proteins isolated from the diaphragm of an animal exposed to CMV for 18 h. *Middle* and *right lanes:* The same membrane stripped of the 2,4-dinitrophyenylhydrazone antibody (the antibody recognizing RCD was removed) and then sequentially re-probed with monoclonal antibodies specific for rat skeletal muscle actin and all myosin heavy chain (*MHC*) isoforms. From reference [28] with permission

Oxidative stress

CMV is associated with augmented oxidative stress in the diaphragm, as indirectly evidenced by the rise in protein oxidation (elevated protein carbonyls [12]; Fig. 4) and lipid peroxidation (elevated 8-isoprostane [12], total lipid hydroperoxides [27, 28] and thiobarbituric reactive substance content [6]) and directly shown by the increased emissions of dichlorofluorescein (a molecule that fluoresces upon reacting with reactive oxygen species within cells) when diaphragmatic strips from CMV-treated animals are incubated in vitro with the dye [31]. The onset of oxidative injury is rapid, occurring within 6 h after the institution of CMV in rats [28], and is long-lasting, being present after 3 days of CMV in piglets [6].

The response of antioxidant enzymes in the diaphragm to CMV is controversial and the mechanisms of oxidative stress generation remain elusive (for both see ESM).

Oxidative stress can modify proteins involved in energetics, excitation–contraction coupling, intracellular calcium regulation and force generation [32]. CMV-induced diaphragmatic protein oxidation was evident in proteins with molecular masses of about 200, 128, 85, and 40 kDa [28]. These findings raise the possibility that actin (40 kDa) and/or myosin (200 kDa) undergo oxidative modification during CMV (Fig. 4), which would be expected to compromise diaphragm contractility. This intriguing possibility awaits confirmation by more specific identification of the modified proteins.

Oxidative stress and especially the lipid peroxidation product 4-hydroxy-2-nonenal (produced in the diaphragm under conditions such as sepsis or resistive loading [33]) can reduce the activity of plasma membrane calcium ATPase [34]. This would retard calcium removal from the diaphragmatic myofibers and would contribute to calcium accumulation and calpain activation [20]. Oxidative stress could also injure various intracellular structures (organelles).

Structural injury

Structural abnormalities of different subcellular components of diaphragm myofibers progressively develop after 2–3 days of CMV in rabbits (Fig. ESM 5) [5, 11, 35]. The changes consisted of disrupted myofibrils, increased numbers of lipid vacuoles in the sarcoplasm, and abnormally small mitochondria containing focal membrane disruptions. Similar alterations were observed in the external intercostal muscles of ventilated animals [35] but not in the hindlimb muscle [5]. The structural abnormalities have detrimental effects on diaphragmatic contractility. The number of abnormal myofibrils is inversely related to the force output of the diaphragm [5]. The mechanisms of injury have not been elucidated, but may involve activation of calpains, which have the ability to degrade several sarcomeric proteins and direct cellular injury secondary to augmented oxidative stress [1].

Muscle fiber remodeling

Muscle fibers are classified as either slow-twitch (type I) or fast-twitch (type II) based on their myosin heavy chain (MHC) isoform content (in increasing order of maximum shortening velocity, MHC isoforms are I, IIa, IIx and IIb) [36]. Muscles can modify their MHC phenotype in two ways: preferential atrophy/hypertrophy of fibers containing a specific MHC isoform and actual transformation from one fiber type to another. Both short-term [12, 22] and long-term [9] CMV result in significant modifications of the MHC phenotype in rats. Within 12 and 18 h of CMV both type I and II fibers are reduced in size [12, 14], yet type II fibers exhibit much greater reduction [12], and within 24 h of mechanical ventilation the transcript levels of the MHC 2A and 2B isoforms are decreased by ~20% [22], consistent with the preferential atrophy observed in the above-mentioned studies. This modification of the MHC phenotype could contribute to the force decline of the diaphragm, since the force produced by slow fibers is less than the force produced by fast fibers [37], but at the same time could explain the increased fatigue resistance observed [38], (though this result is not uniform in all studies), since type I fibers have higher oxidative capacity and thus endurance than type II fibers. However, prolonged (44–93 h) CMV in rats results in a different pattern of MHC phenotype modification, with decreased number of type I fibers and increases in fast MHC isoforms mainly within hybrid fibers (fibers co-expressing both slow and fast isoforms) [9]. This slow-to-fast transformation does not compromise diaphragmatic contractility per se, but reduces diaphragmatic endurance, since fewer slow-twitch fatigue-resistant fibers are available. The basis of this different response is not known, but may be related to the ventilatory strategy or the duration of CMV (< 24 h vs. 44–93 h). Despite similar respiratory rates, the tidal volume and thus the degree of phasic diaphragmatic shortening was double in the study of Shanely et al. [12] (1 ml/100 g body weight) compared to the tidal volume used by Yang et al. [9] (0.5 ml/100 g body weight). In contrast, the degree of tonic diaphragmatic shortening imposed by positive end-expiratory pressure (PEEP) was much greater in the study of Yang et al. [9] (PEEP = 4 cmH_2O) than in the study of Shanely et al. [12] (PEEP = 1 cmH_2O). Whether different ventilatory patterns result in different fiber type transformations is not known. Interestingly, in limb muscles the duration of inactivity influences the fiber type transformation observed. Whereas short-term inactivity results in fast-to-slow transformation (similar to short-term mechanical ventilation), longer inactivity results in slow-to-fast transformation. Although the duration of inactivity was much longer (6 weeks) in limb muscles, the diaphragm might exhibit much faster adaptation to inactivity, since it is continuously contracting throughout life with much higher duty cycles (duration of contraction relative to relaxation) than the limb muscles. In rabbits, 2 days of CMV resulted in atrophy of the respiratory muscles and in decreased cross-sectional area of type IIa and IIb fibers but not type I fibers (fast-to-slow transformation), with no change in their proportion [10], whereas 3 days of mechanical ventilation did not affect the cross-sectional areas of slow and fast fibers but resulted in a decrease in the proportion of the fast MHC2X isoform (a form of fast-to-slow transformation) [5]. The differences might be attributed to the presence of PEEP (2 cmH_2O in [10], 0 cmH_2O in [5]) or to the episodes of breakthrough diaphragmatic activity observed [5].

Interestingly, 24 h of CMV in rats resulted in changes in the mRNA expression of the myogenic regulatory transcription factors myoD (myogenic determination gene D) (decrease) and myogenin (increase) with a consequent decrease in the myoD/myogenin ratio [22]. These transcription factors bind to the promoter of many skeletal muscle-specific genes and drive myoblast determination and differentiation during embryogenesis, but may also influence fiber type transformation in the adult muscle. The levels of myoD are significantly greater in fast than in slow muscle fibers, myogenin is preferentially located in slow fibers, and their ratio is highly correlated with muscle fiber phenotype. Whether this correlation is causal is debated [39]. In the diaphragm, the deletion of MyoD resulted in a shift in MHC phenotype from MHC IIb toward the slower MHC IIa and IIx (fast to slow transformation), associated with decreased force-generating capacity [40]. Thus, the decreased myoD/myogenin ratio in the diaphragm secondary to 24 h of CMV [22] might contribute to the observed fast-to-slow fiber type transformation.

Remodeling could also lead to reduced optimal diaphragmatic length [7, 9] (see ESM).

Drugs

Anesthetics should be excluded as causes of VIDD, since studies that used appropriate controls (to the extent feasible, i.e. a group of anesthetized spontaneously breathing animals) concluded that the decreased contractility was due to the effects of mechanical ventilation per se (and not to anesthetic use) [5].

Neuromuscular blockers [3, 9] cannot solely account for the decreased contractility secondary to CMV, since decreased contractility was also observed in studies that did not use these drugs [5, 8]. However, the effects of 24 h of CMV and aminosteroidal neuromuscular blockers (rocuronium) are synergistic in depressing diaphragm contractility, in inducing atrophy of type IIx/b fibers and in upregulating the ubiquitin ligase (E3) MuRF1 (but not the E3 MAFbx/Atrogin-1) [27], a synergism not observed with different doses of benzylisoquinoline neuromuscular blockers (cisatracurium) [41].

Metabolic enzymes and mitochondrial function

The changes documented after CMV are not dramatic (see ESM).

Clinical relevance

Evidence for VIDD in humans

Although there is no definite evidence of VIDD in humans, several intriguing data suggest that it is a clinical relevant phenomenon. The twitch transdiaphragmatic pressure elicited by magnetic stimulation of the phrenic nerves was reduced in mechanically ventilated patients [42] and in patients ready to undergo weaning trials [43] compared to normal subjects. This is not specific evidence for the presence of VIDD, since other factors leading to muscle weakness in the ICU may have contributed. Diaphragmatic atrophy was documented (by ultrasound) in a tetraplegic patient after prolonged CMV [44]. However, denervation removes neurotrophic influences for the muscle, which is not the case for VIDD. Retrospective analysis of postmortem data obtained in neonates who received ventilatory assistance for 12 days or more immediately before death documented diffuse diaphragmatic myofiber atrophy (small myofibers with rounded outlines), not present in extradiaphragmatic muscles [45]. Furthermore, preliminary data suggest that brain-dead organ donors (with an intact circulation) who underwent CMV for 18–72 h exhibit reduced cross-sectional area (i.e. atrophy) of both slow and fast diaphragmatic fibers (by 40% and 36% respectively) compared to matched control patients subjected to surgery for resection of solitary pulmonary nodules (receiving CMV for less than 2 h) [46]. The ubiquitin–proteasome pathway was implicated in the development of atrophy, since both the ubiquitin–protein conjugates and the mRNA levels of the E3 ligases MAFbx/Atrogin-1 and MuRF1 were upregulated in the diaphragms of brain-dead patients receiving CMV [47].

Clinical context

VIDD should be suspected in patients who fail to wean after a period of CMV. The weaning failure is related to respiratory muscle weakness. Other causes of respiratory muscle weakness should be ruled out [48]. However, the above-mentioned conditions may coexist with VIDD.

VIDD prevention

Ventilatory strategy

Since data in humans are lacking, suggestions are based on animal models and speculations. The time spent in CMV must be curtailed to the extent possible, especially in older individuals, since the effects of aging and CMV are additive [49]. Although CMV induced similar losses (24%) in diaphragmatic isometric tension in both young and old animals, the combined effects of aging and CMV resulted in a 34% decrement in diaphragmatic isometric tension compared to young control animals.

When feasible, partial support modes should be used. Recent studies raise the possibility of partial support modes in conditions traditionally considered as indications for CMV such as ALI/ARDS [50, 51]. In an animal model, assisted (flow-triggered pressure-limited) mechanical ventilation from the onset of ventilator support resulted in attenuation of the force loss induced by CMV (Fig. 5) [26]. Thus, it stands to reason that preserving diaphragmatic contractions during mechanical ventilation should attenuate the force loss induced by CMV, though other forms of partial ventilatory support (pressure support, SIMV) have not been experimentally tested. It should be stressed that these suggestions may be valid in the absence of sepsis, since during sepsis in rats (albeit of short duration, 4 h), CMV protects the diaphragm from injury [52].

Assisted modes or even noninvasive mechanical ventilation in hypercapnic COPD [53–55] can be an alternative strategy in patients who experience weaning failure after a spontaneous breathing trial or after extubation and who may be ventilated using CMV [56], a strategy based on the premise that respiratory muscle fatigue (requiring rest to recover) is the cause of weaning failure [57, 58]. This is because the load that the respiratory muscles of patients who fail to wean are facing is increased to the range that would predictably produce fatigue of the respiratory muscles [59], if patients were allowed

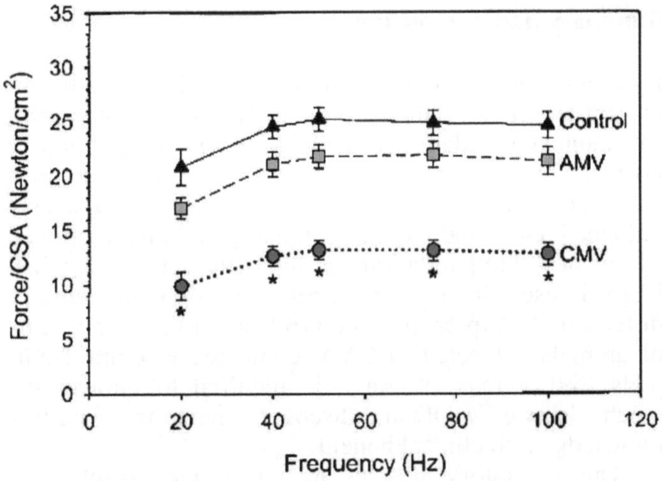

Fig. 5 Diaphragmatic tetanic force at various stimulation frequencies in control circumstances, assisted mechanical ventilation (*AMV*), and controlled mechanical ventilation (*CMV*) in rats. Values are mean ± SE. * $p<0.01$, CMV versus control and AMV. *CSA*, cross-sectional area. From reference [26] with permission

to continue spontaneous breathing without ventilator assistance. Recent evidence, however, does not support the existence of low-frequency fatigue (the type of fatigue that is long-lasting, taking more than 24 h to recover) in patients who fail to wean despite the excessive respiratory muscle load [43]. This is because physicians have adopted criteria of spontaneous breathing trial failure and termination of unassisted breathing, which lead them to put patients back on the ventilator before the development of low-frequency respiratory muscle fatigue. Thus, no reason exists to completely unload the respiratory muscles with CMV for fatigue reversal if weaning is terminated based on predefined criteria [56].

Intermittent diaphragmatic contractions

When CMV is inevitable, short periods of diaphragmatic activity have been suggested as a preventive countermeasure. This could be achieved with either phrenic nerve stimulation or short periods of intermittent spontaneous breathing. Only 30 min of pacing of one hemidiaphragm each day attenuated atrophy in this hemidiaphragm during prolonged CMV in a tetraplegic patient compared to the non-paced hemidiaphragm [44]. In rats subjected to 24 h of CMV, either 5 min or 60 min of spontaneous breathing every 6 h did not preserve diaphragm force. Rats receiving CMV developed reduced cross-sectional areas of type I and type IIx/b diaphragmatic fibers, which was not observed in intermittently spontaneously breathing rats, yet no difference was observed in the cross-sectional areas between the CMV rats and the intermittently spontaneously breathing rats [60]. Whether more frequent or longer intervals of spontaneous breathing might be more effective in preventing VIDD awaits experimental proof.

Pharmacological approaches

Antioxidant supplementation could decrease the oxidative stress and thus could attenuate VIDD. Accordingly, when rats were administered the antioxidant Trolox (an analogue of vitamin E) from the onset of CMV, its detrimental effects on contractility (Fig. 6) and proteolysis were prevented [61].

A similar approach is adopted by nature itself! Various dormant animals immobilized for prolonged periods of time prevent muscle atrophy through a decrease in metabolic rate that reduces formation of reactive oxygen species and through a concomitant rise in antioxidant enzymes [62, 63]. Interestingly, a combination of vitamins E and C administered to critically ill surgical (mostly trauma) patients was effective in reducing the duration of mechanical ventilation compared to nonsupplemented patients [64]. It is tempting to speculate that part of this beneficial effect was mediated by preventing VIDD. Thus, when CMV is used, concurrent administration of antioxidants seems justified, since a recent meta-analysis suggests that they are beneficial in critical care patients [65].

Administration of leupeptin (an inhibitor of lysosomal proteases and calpain) at the beginning of CMV prevented the development of diaphragmatic contractile dysfunction and atrophy [21] in experimental animals. This raises the possibility of future clinical trials of protease inhibitors in patients to prevent VIDD.

Recovery from VIDD

There is no established or experimentally tested therapy for VIDD. Theoretically, resumption of spontaneous

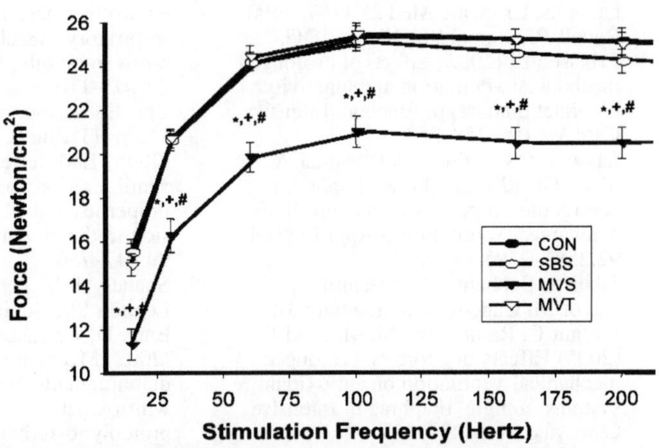

Fig. 6 Force–frequency curves of in vitro diaphragm strips from control rats (*CON*), spontaneously breathing animals (*SBS*), mechanically ventilated animals (*MVS*), and mechanically ventilated animals receiving Trolox (*MVT*). Values represent means ± SEM. * Significantly different from CON group, $p<0.05$; + significantly different from SBS group, $p<0.05$; # significantly different from MVT group, $p<0.05$. From reference [61] with permission

breathing would retrain the respiratory muscles, yet the time course of recovery of normal function is unknown. A major concern is that diaphragm disuse associated with CMV would increase its susceptibility to subsequent contraction-induced injury, once respiratory efforts are resumed, similar to other skeletal muscles [66]. Rats receiving 24 h of CMV exhibited 26% decline in maximal specific diaphragmatic force with no apparent injury to the cell membrane or evidence of inflammation [67]. Resumption of spontaneous breathing for 2 h in these rats did not exacerbate contractile dysfunction or induce membrane injury or macrophage invasion [67]. However, reloading was associated with increased myeloperoxidase activity and neutrophil infiltration in the diaphragm, which is expected to cause injury at a later time point, should reloading be continued [67]. Further studies are needed to elucidate the recovery response of the diaphragm that has developed VIDD to the resumption of spontaneous respiratory muscle activity.

Summary and conclusion

In recent years researchers have discovered that mechanical ventilation can damage previously injured lungs [68]. Mechanical ventilation can also damage the previously normal respiratory muscles. CMV imposes a unique form of skeletal muscle disuse: the diaphragm is simultaneously unloaded, electrically quiescent, and phasically shortened by cyclical lung inflation, or tonically shortened when PEEP is used. Recent microarray analysis identified 354 differentially expressed gene products in the diaphragms of animals subjected to CMV compared to control animals [69]. Intense research is required to unravel the mechanisms of VIDD and discover ways to translate this knowledge into clinical benefit.

The respiratory muscles are not an inert mechanical pump that can be "light-heartedly" substituted by the ventilator. The respiratory muscles should remain active because they are plastic, and vulnerable.

References

1. Vassilakopoulos T, Petrof BJ (2004) Ventilator-induced diaphragmatic dysfunction. Am J Respir Crit Care Med 169:336–341
2. Arroliga A, Frutos-Vivar F, Hall J, Esteban A, Apezteguia C, Soto L, Anzueto A (2005) Use of sedatives and neuromuscular blockers in a cohort of patients receiving mechanical ventilation. Chest 128:496–506
3. Anzueto A, Peters JI, Tobin MJ, de los SR, Seidenfeld JJ, Moore G, Cox WJ, Coalson JJ (1997) Effects of prolonged controlled mechanical ventilation on diaphragmatic function in healthy adult baboons. Crit Care Med 25:1187–1190
4. Radell PJ, Remahl S, Nichols DG, Eriksson LI (2002) Effects of prolonged mechanical ventilation and inactivity on piglet diaphragm function. Intensive Care Med 28:358–364
5. Sassoon CS, Caiozzo VJ, Manka A, Sieck GC (2002) Altered diaphragm contractile properties with controlled mechanical ventilation. J Appl Physiol 92:2585–2595
6. Jaber S, Sebbane M, Koechlin C, Hayot M, Capdevila X, Eledjam JJ, Prefaut C, Ramonatxo M, Matecki S (2005) Effects of short vs. prolonged mechanical ventilation on antioxidant systems in piglet diaphragm. Intensive Care Med 31:1427–1433
7. Le Bourdelles G, Viires N, Boczkowski J, Seta N, Pavlovic D, Aubier M (1994) Effects of mechanical ventilation on diaphragmatic contractile properties in rats. Am J Respir Crit Care Med 149:1539–1544
8. Powers SK, Shanely RA, Coombes JS, Koesterer TJ, McKenzie M, Van Gammeren D, Cicale M, Dodd SL (2002) Mechanical ventilation results in progressive contractile dysfunction in the diaphragm. J Appl Physiol 92:1851–1858
9. Yang L, Luo J, Bourdon J, Lin MC, Gottfried SB, Petrof BJ (2002) Controlled mechanical ventilation leads to remodeling of the rat diaphragm. Am J Respir Crit Care Med 166:1135–1140
10. Capdevila X, Lopez S, Bernard N, Rabischong E, Ramonatxo M, Martinazzo G, Prefaut C (2003) Effects of controlled mechanical ventilation on respiratory muscle contractile properties in rabbits. Intensive Care Med 29:103–110
11. Zhu E, Sassoon CS, Nelson R, Pham HT, Zhu L, Baker MJ, Caiozzo VJ (2005) Early effects of mechanical ventilation on isotonic contractile properties and MAF-box gene expression in the diaphragm. J Appl Physiol 99:747–756
12. Shanely RA, Zergeroglu MA, Lennon SL, Sugiura T, Yimlamai T, Enns D, Belcastro A, Powers SK (2002) Mechanical ventilation-induced diaphragmatic atrophy is associated with oxidative injury and increased proteolytic activity. Am J Respir Crit Care Med 166:1369–1374
13. Hussain SN, Vassilakopoulos T (2002) Ventilator-induced cachexia. Am J Respir Crit Care Med 166:1307–1308
14. McClung JM, Kavazis AN, Deruisseau KC, Falk DJ, Deering MA, Lee Y, Sugiura T, Powers SK (2007) Caspase-3 regulation of diaphragm myonuclear domain during mechanical ventilation-induced atrophy. Am J Respir Crit Care Med 175:150–159
15. Jarvinen MJ, Einola SA, Virtanen EO (1992) Effect of the position of immobilization upon the tensile properties of the rat gastrocnemius muscle. Arch Phys Med Rehabil 73:253–257
16. Jokl P, Konstadt S (1983) The effect of limb immobilization on muscle function and protein composition. Clin Orthop Relat Res 222–229
17. Allen DL, Roy RR, Edgerton VR (1999) Myonuclear domains in muscle adaptation and disease. Muscle Nerve 22:1350–1360
18. Shanely RA, Van Gammeren D, Deruisseau KC, Zergeroglu AM, McKenzie MJ, Yarasheski KE, Powers SK (2004) Mechanical ventilation depresses protein synthesis in the rat diaphragm. Am J Respir Crit Care Med 170:994–999
19. Gayan-Ramirez G, De Paepe K, Cadot P, Decramer M (2003) Detrimental effects of short-term mechanical ventilation on diaphragm function and IGF-I mRNA in rats. Intensive Care Med 29:825–833
20. Powers SK, Kavazis AN, Deruisseau KC (2005) Mechanisms of disuse muscle atrophy: role of oxidative stress. Am J Physiol Regul Integr Comp Physiol 288:R337–R344

21. Maes K, Testelmans D, Powers S, Decramer M, Gayan-Ramirez G (2007) Leupeptin inhibits ventilator-induced diaphragm dysfunction in rats. Am J Respir Crit Care Med 175:1134–1138
22. Racz GZ, Gayan-Ramirez G, Testelmans D, Cadot P, De Paepe K, Zador E, Wuytack F, Decramer M (2003) Early changes in rat diaphragm biology with mechanical ventilation. Am J Respir Crit Care Med 168:297–304
23. Du J, Wang X, Miereles C, Bailey JL, Debigare R, Zheng B, Price SR, Mitch WE (2004) Activation of caspase-3 is an initial step triggering accelerated muscle proteolysis in catabolic conditions. J Clin Invest 113:115–123
24. Deruisseau KC, Kavazis AN, Deering MA, Falk DJ, Van Gammeren D, Yimlamai T, Ordway GA, Powers SK (2005) Mechanical ventilation induces alterations of the ubiquitin–proteasome pathway in the diaphragm. J Appl Physiol 98:1314–1321
25. Mitch WE, Goldberg AL (1996) Mechanisms of muscle wasting. The role of the ubiquitin–proteasome pathway. N Engl J Med 335:1897–1905
26. Sassoon CS, Zhu E, Caiozzo VJ (2004) Assist–control mechanical ventilation attenuates ventilator-induced diaphragmatic dysfunction. Am J Respir Crit Care Med 170:626–632
27. Testelmans D, Maes K, Wouters P, Gosselin N, Deruisseau K, Powers S, Sciot R, Decramer M, Gayan-Ramirez G (2006) Rocuronium exacerbates mechanical ventilation-induced diaphragm dysfunction in rats. Crit Care Med 34:3018–3023
28. Zergeroglu MA, McKenzie MJ, Shanely RA, Van Gammeren D, Deruisseau KC, Powers SK (2003) Mechanical ventilation-induced oxidative stress in the diaphragm. J Appl Physiol 95:1116–1124
29. Shringarpure R, Grune T, Davies KJ (2001) Protein oxidation and 20S proteasome-dependent proteolysis in mammalian cells. Cell Mol Life Sci 58:1442–1450
30. Davies KJ (2001) Degradation of oxidized proteins by the 20S proteasome. Biochimie 83:301–310
31. Falk DJ, Deruisseau KC, Van Gammeren DL, Deering MA, Kavazis AN, Powers SK (2006) Mechanical ventilation promotes redox status alterations in the diaphragm. J Appl Physiol 101:1017–1024
32. Reid MB (2001) Invited Review: Redox modulation of skeletal muscle contraction: what we know and what we don't. J Appl Physiol 90:724–731
33. Hussain SN, Matar G, Barreiro E, Florian M, Divangahi M, Vassilakopoulos T (2006) Modifications of proteins by 4-hydroxy-2-nonenal in the ventilatory muscles of rats. Am J Physiol Lung Cell Mol Physiol 290:L996–1003
34. Siems W, Capuozzo E, Lucano A, Salerno C, Crifo C (2003) High sensitivity of plasma membrane ion transport ATPases from human neutrophils towards 4-hydroxy-2,3-trans-nonenal. Life Sci 73:2583–2590
35. Bernard N, Matecki S, Py G, Lopez S, Mercier J, Capdevila X (2003) Effects of prolonged mechanical ventilation on respiratory muscle ultrastructure and mitochondrial respiration in rabbits. Intensive Care Med 29:111–118
36. Bottinelli R (2001) Functional heterogeneity of mammalian single muscle fibres: do myosin isoforms tell the whole story? Pflugers Arch 443:6–17
37. Geiger PC, Cody MJ, Macken RL, Sieck GC (2000) Maximum specific force depends on myosin heavy chain content in rat diaphragm muscle fibers. J Appl Physiol 89:695–703
38. Shanely RA, Coombes JS, Zergeroglu AM, Webb AI, Powers SK (2003) Short-duration mechanical ventilation enhances diaphragmatic fatigue resistance but impairs force production. Chest 123:195–201
39. Talmadge RJ (2000) Myosin heavy chain isoform expression following reduced neuromuscular activity: potential regulatory mechanisms. Muscle Nerve 23:661–679
40. Staib JL, Swoap SJ, Powers SK (2002) Diaphragm contractile dysfunction in MyoD gene-inactivated mice. Am J Physiol Regul Integr Comp Physiol 283:R583–R590
41. Testelmans D, Maes K, Wouters P, Powers SK, Decramer M, Gayan-Ramirez G (2007) Infusions of rocuronium and cisatracurium exert different effects on rat diaphragm function. Intensive Care Med 33:872–879
42. Watson AC, Hughes PD, Louise HM, Hart N, Ware RJ, Wendon J, Green M, Moxham J (2001) Measurement of twitch transdiaphragmatic, esophageal, and endotracheal tube pressure with bilateral anterolateral magnetic phrenic nerve stimulation in patients in the intensive care unit. Crit Care Med 29:1325–1331
43. Laghi F, Cattapan SE, Jubran A, Parthasarathy S, Warshawsky P, Choi YS, Tobin MJ (2003) Is weaning failure caused by low-frequency fatigue of the diaphragm? Am J Respir Crit Care Med 167:120–127
44. Ayas NT, McCool FD, Gore R, Lieberman SL, Brown R (1999) Prevention of human diaphragm atrophy with short periods of electrical stimulation. Am J Respir Crit Care Med 159:2018–2020
45. Knisely AS, Leal SM, Singer DB (1988) Abnormalities of diaphragmatic muscle in neonates with ventilated lungs. J Pediatr 113:1074–1077
46. Levine S, Nguyen T, BSE, Friscia M, Kaiser LR, Shrager JB (2006) Ventilator-induced atrophy in human diaphragm myofibers. Proc Am Thorac Soc [Abstract] 3:A27
47. Nguyen T, Friscia M, Kaiser LR, Shrager JB, Levine S (2006) Ventilator–induced proteolysis in human diaphragm myofibers. Proc Am Thorac Soc [Abstract] 3:A259
48. Deem S, Lee CM, Curtis JR (2003) Acquired neuromuscular disorders in the intensive care unit. Am J Respir Crit Care Med 168:735–739
49. Criswell DS, Shanely RA, Betters JJ, McKenzie MJ, Sellman JE, Van Gammeren DL, Powers SK (2003) Cumulative effects of aging and mechanical ventilation on in vitro diaphragm function. Chest 124:2302–2308
50. Zakynthinos SG, Vassilakopoulos T, Daniil Z, Zakynthinos E, Koutsoukos E, Katsouyianni K, Roussos C (1997) Pressure support ventilation in adult respiratory distress syndrome: short-term effects of a servocontrolled mode. J Crit Care 12:161–172
51. Putensen C, Zech S, Wrigge H, Zinserling J, Stuber F, Von Spiegel T, Mutz N (2001) Long-term effects of spontaneous breathing during ventilatory support in patients with acute lung injury. Am J Respir Crit Care Med 164:43–49
52. Ebihara S, Hussain SN, Danialou G, Cho WK, Gottfried SB, Petrof BJ (2002) Mechanical ventilation protects against diaphragm injury in sepsis: interaction of oxidative and mechanical stresses. Am J Respir Crit Care Med 165:221–228
53. Nava S, Gregoretti C, Fanfulla F, Squadrone E, Grassi M, Carlucci A, Beltrame F, Navalesi P (2005) Noninvasive ventilation to prevent respiratory failure after extubation in high-risk patients. Crit Care Med 33:2465–2470
54. Ferrer M, Esquinas A, Arancibia F, Bauer TT, Gonzalez G, Carrillo A, Rodriguez-Roisin R, Torres A (2003) Noninvasive ventilation during persistent weaning failure: a randomized controlled trial. Am J Respir Crit Care Med 168:70–76

55. Ferrer M, Valencia M, Nicolas JM, Bernadich O, Badia JR, Torres A (2006) Early noninvasive ventilation averts extubation failure in patients at risk: a randomized trial. Am J Respir Crit Care Med 173:164–170
56. Vassilakopoulos T, Zakynthinos S, Roussos C (2005) Bench-to-bedside review: Weaning failure – should we rest the respiratory muscles with controlled mechanical ventilation? Crit Care 10:204
57. Vassilakopoulos T, Zakynthinos S, Roussos C (1996) Respiratory muscles and weaning failure. Eur Respir J 9:2383–2400
58. Vassilakopoulos T, Roussos C, Zakynthinos S (1999) Weaning from mechanical ventilation. J Crit Care 14:39–62
59. Vassilakopoulos T, Zakynthinos S, Roussos C (1998) The tension-time index and the frequency/tidal volume ratio are the major pathophysiologic determinants of weaning failure and success. Am J Respir Crit Care Med 158:378–385
60. Gayan-Ramirez G, Testelmans D, Maes K, Racz GZ, Cadot P, Zador E, Wuytack F, Decramer M (2005) Intermittent spontaneous breathing protects the rat diaphragm from mechanical ventilation effects. Crit Care Med 33:2804–2809
61. Betters JL, Criswell DS, Shanely RA, Van Gammeren D, Falk D, Deruisseau KC, Deering M, Yimlamai T, Powers SK (2004) Trolox attenuates mechanical ventilation-induced diaphragmatic dysfunction and proteolysis. Am J Respir Crit Care Med 170:1179–1184
62. Grundy JE, Storey KB (1998) Antioxidant defenses and lipid peroxidation damage in estivating toads, *Scaphiopus couchii*. J Comp Physiol [B] 168:132–142
63. Hudson NJ, Franklin CE (2002) Maintaining muscle mass during extended disuse: aestivating frogs as a model species. J Exp Biol 205:2297–2303
64. Nathens AB, Neff MJ, Jurkovich GJ, Klotz P, Farver K, Ruzinski JT, Radella F, Garcia I, Maier RV (2002) Randomized, prospective trial of antioxidant supplementation in critically ill surgical patients. Ann Surg 236:814–822
65. Heyland D (2005) Antioxidant nutrients:a systematic review of trace elements and vitamins in the critically ill patient. Intensive Care Med 31:327–337
66. Vijayan K, Thompson JL, Norenberg KM, Fitts RH, Riley DA (2001) Fiber-type susceptibility to eccentric contraction-induced damage of hindlimb-unloaded rat AL muscles. J Appl Physiol 90:770–776
67. Van Gammeren D, Falk DJ, Deruisseau KC, Sellman JE, Decramer M, Powers SK (2005) Reloading the diaphragm following mechanical ventilation does not promote injury. Chest 127:2204–2210
68. International consensus conferences in intensive care medicine: Ventilator-associated lung injury in ARDS. This official conference report was cosponsored by the American Thoracic Society, The European Society of Intensive Care Medicine, and The Societe de Reanimation de Langue Francaise, and was approved by the ATS Board of Directors, July 1999. Am J Respir Crit Care Med 160:2118–2124
69. Deruisseau KC, Shanely RA, Akunuri N, Hamilton MT, Van Gammeren D, Zergeroglu AM, McKenzie M, Powers SK (2005) Diaphragm unloading via controlled mechanical ventilation alters the gene expression profile. Am J Respir Crit Care Med 172:1267–1275

Caroline Créput
Lionel Galicier
Sophie Buyse
Elie Azoulay

Understanding organ dysfunction in hemophagocytic lymphohistiocytosis

Abstract *Objective:* This review aims to help critical care clinicians maintain a high level of suspicion regarding the diagnosis of Hemophagocytic Histiolymphocytosis (HLH). It describes the clinical and laboratory features of HLH, outlines its pathophysiology and reviews the most frequent etiologies related to HLH. Prognostic factors and therapeutic options are also reported. *Data sources:* Review of the literature. *Results:* The diagnosis of HLH relies on the association of clinical abnormalities and hemophagocytosis in bone marrow, spleen, or lymph node specimens. Liver, pulmonary, renal, cardiac and skin involvement may occur at various degrees possibly leading to multiple organ failure. Three main etiologies can be found, namely infections, lymphoproliferative diseases, or connective tissue diseases. Immune deficiency is often retrieved. Mortality can be as high as 50%. Although clinically mimicking severe sepsis, HLH has a distinct pathophysiology on which specific therapy is based. Early diagnosis and treatment is mandatory to increase the chances of survival. *Conclusion:* The comprehensive management of severe HLH requires the involvement of a multidisciplinary team in order to determine the best therapeutic strategy and to identify the underlying cause.

Keywords Hemophagocytosis · Histiocytosis · Langerhans cells · Th1 Cytokines activation · Cytopenia · Autoimmune disease

Introduction

Hemophagocytosis describes the pathological finding of activated macrophages engulfing erythrocytes, leukocytes, platelets, and their precursor cells. This phenomenon is an important finding in patients with hemophagocytic syndrome, more properly referred to as hemophagocytic lymphohistiocytosis (HLH).

Hemophagocytic lymphohistiocytosis is a distinct clinical entity characterized by fever, pancytopenia, splenomegaly, and the pathological finding of hemophagocytosis in bone marrow and other tissues. The syndrome, also referred to as "histiocytic medullary reticulosis," was first described in 1939 as a condition characterized by a fever, a rapid decline in general health, peripheral lymph node enlargement, pancytopenia, and histiocyte proliferation in the bone marrow with a fatal outcome [1]. Forty years later, Risdall et al. used the term "reactive hemophagocytic syndrome" to designate an inappropriate immune response to viral infection leading to uncontrolled proliferation of benign histiocytes with hemophagocytosis and symptoms matching those described by Scott and Robb-Smith [1]. Subsequently, additional cases related to viral infection were reported [3–5], and hemophagocytic syndrome was described in association with other diseases, including malignancies and systemic connective tissue diseases [6–8].

Hemophagocytic lymphohistiocytosis is a life-threatening condition which may be difficult to distinguish from severe sepsis [9]. A simple clinical approach may be helpful to appraise the diagnosis of HLH. Along this line, autopsy studies suggest that HLH may be underrecognized

M.R. Pinsky et al. (eds.), *Applied Physiology in Intensive Care Medicine 2: Physiological Reviews and Editorials*,
DOI 10.1007/978-3-642-28233-1_21,

Table 1 Diagnostic guidelines for hemophagocytic lymphohistiocytosis. The diagnosis of hemophagocytic lymphohistiocytosis can be established by fulfilling five of the eight criteria. *NK*, natural killer. (From [37])

Clinical criteria
Fever (> 7 days)
Splenomegaly
Laboratory criteria
Bicytopenia without marrow hypoplasia, including:
Hemoglobin < 9 g/l
Platelet count < 100.10×9 mm^3
Neutrophil count < 1.10×9/mm^3
Hypertriglyceridemia (3.0 mmol/l, fasting value)
and/or hypofibrinemia (< 1.5 g/l)
Hyperferritinemia (> 500 ug/l)
Low/absent NK cell activity
Increased soluble CD 25 levels (> 2400 IU/ml)
Histological criteria
Hemophagocytosis

in intensive care unit (ICU) patients [10, 11]. On the other hand, incidence of HLH may be overestimated. Indeed, studies in critically ill septic patients with cytopenia report an incidence of HLH in marrow smears between 0.8 and 4% [10, 12]; however, these studies are often difficult to interpret as no cytological results from relevant control populations are available. Moreover, criteria for the definite diagnosis of HLH were not met, suggesting that although hemophagocytosis was identified, diagnosis of HLH remained doubtful [13].

Several criteria sets have recently been developed for the diagnosis of HLH. In the latest HLH-2004 protocol, a recent revision of diagnostic criteria suggests that HLH diagnosis can be established if five of the eight following diagnostic criteria are fulfilled: (a) fever; (b) splenomegaly; (c) bicytopenia; (d) hypertriglyceridemia (> 3.0 mmol/l fasting value), and/or hypofibrinogenemia (< 1.5 g/l); (e) hemophagocytosis; (f) low or absent natural killer (NK) cell activity; (g) hyperferritinemia (> 500 ug/l); and (h) and increased soluble CD-25 levels (> 2400 IU/ml; Table 1).

This review aims to help critical care clinicians maintain a high level of suspicion regarding the diagnosis of HLH. It describes the clinical and laboratory features of HLH, outlines its pathophysiology, and reviews the most frequent etiologies related to HLH. Prognostic factors and therapeutic options are also reported.

Clinical and laboratory features

The clinical and laboratory features of HLH are nonspecific and may be difficult to separate from those of the underlying disease; however, HLH should be considered routinely in patients with unexplained and atypical multiple organ failure [12]. Diagnosis of HLH relies on clinical, laboratory, and histological findings. Clinical and laboratory manifestations were proposed by the Histiocyte Society and are listed in Table 1. Acute onset with high-grade fever is the rule. Rapid weight loss may occur [14, 15]. Overall, macrophage and T-lymphocyte proliferation and activation in the reticuloendothelial system manifest as peripheral lymphadenopathy (35% of patients) and as enlargement of the liver and spleen (50% of patients) [16, 17]. Clotting disorders may lead to bleeding, and liver involvement may manifest as jaundice and portal hypertension. Pulmonary infiltrates are found in 20–30% of patients [18]. Cardiac or renal involvement may occur. Skin abnormalities are noted in 20% of patients [17], with the most common patterns being rash, erythema, and purpura. Of central nervous system manifestations, encephalopathy, meningitis, and seizures are the most commonly reported [19]. In severe cases, mechanical ventilation is required because of alterations in consciousness. Multiple organ failures may occur. Table 2 reports usual causes in connective-tissue diseases associated with HLH.

Laboratory tests can assist in the diagnosis of HLH. The most prominent laboratory abnormalities noted are cytopenia, which may be profound. Cytopenia results from both hemophagocytosis in the bone marrow and depression of hematopoiesis by cytokines such as interferon-γ (IFN-γ), tumoral necrosis factor-α (TNF-α), and interleukin 1-β (IL-1β) [20]. All patients have anemia, which is usually nonregenerative. Serum chemistry findings may suggest hemolysis, with hyperbilirubinemia and elevation of lactate dehydrogenase. Thrombocytopenia is almost

Table 2 Causes of reactive hemophagocytic lymphohistiocytosis (*HLH*) in published series. (Adapted from [78])

Associated disorders with HLH	Prevalence (%)
Viral infections	29.1
HSV	2.9
EBV	6.9
CMV	10.5
HIV	8.8
Other infections	20.6
Bacteria	31.1
Parasites/fungi	5.2
Mycobacteria	2.3
Lymphoma	19.9
Other hematological malignancies	8.2
Solid cancer	1.6
Systemic disease[a]	7.2
Lupus	
Still's disease	
Rheumatoid arthritis	
Sarcoidosis	
Scleroderma	
Mixed connective tissue disease	
Sjögren's syndrome	
Hereditary	6.2
No identified cause	18.0

Clinical features may be difficult to differentiate from those of the underlying systemic disease
[a] Diseases are set in order of frequency according to Dhote et al. [70]

consistently present, occurs early in the course of the disease, and is usually profound. Leukopenia is less common, less severe, and occurs later in the course of the syndrome. Overall, three of every four patients have pancytopenia and all have bicytopenia. Serum ferritin elevation is the rule [21, 22], the most likely mechanism being IL-1β elevation [23]. Serum ferritin levels may correlate with disease activity and outcome under treatment. Hypertriglyceridemia is an extremely common finding that is ascribable to lipoprotein lipase inhibition by TNF-α [24, 25].

Coagulation disorders are present in most patients. The most common pattern is isolated fibrin deficiency due to liver dysfunction and, above all, plasminogen and factor-X activation by IL-1β [26, 27]. More rarely, disseminated intravascular coagulation (DIC) develops as a result of IFN-γ and TNF-α overproduction. The DIC is associated with high mortality [2, 24]. Liver dysfunction (cytolysis and cholestasis) is frequently reported [28, 29]. IFN-γ contributes to the development of cholestasis [30]. In addition, colony-stimulating factor (CSF), together with Fas/Fas-ligand interaction in response to IFN-γ overproduction, contribute to cause apoptosis and liver damage. IFN-γ elevation also leads to hypoalbuminemia [31].

Renal failure is often reported at the advanced stage of HLH and is related to abnormally high concentrations of nephrotoxic interleukin-6 (IL-6) in serum [32]. Renal biopsy usually shows tiny glomerular lesions [33, 34]. Markers for inflammation are markedly elevated. Many other nonspecific laboratory abnormalities may be found, such as hypo- or hypergammaglobulinemia, a positive Coombs test, or hyponatremia due to syndrome of inappropriate antidiuretic hormone secretion [35].

Cytology and histology

The pathological hallmark of HLH is a proliferation of activated macrophages (histiocytes) engulfing blood cells and their precursors (Fig. 1). This proliferation is found in the reticuloendothelial system (bone marrow, lymph nodes, spleen, and liver) and occasionally affects other sites, such as the skin. Cytological examination of bone marrow smears is the best investigation for confirming HLH, although normal findings, do not rule out the diagnosis. Cellularity is usually normal for all three lines at an early stage. Hypocellularity with reduced granulopoiesis and erythropoiesis may be present [2]. Hyperplasia of the megacaryocyte line with good maturation initially is the rule. Hemophagocytosis in bone marrow occurs not only in HLH, but also in hemolytic diseases and other hematological disorders; therefore, hemophagocytosis does not indicate a diagnosis of HLH unless other clinical and laboratory features of the syndrome are present also [10].

Histological examination of bone marrow biopsies may be less effective in establishing the diagnosis of HLH than examination of bone marrow smears. Nevertheless, bone marrow biopsy may show an underlying hematological disorder or infectious process, as in tuberculosis for example [16]. Liver histology is abnormal in 50% of patients with HLH. Findings may consist of nonspecific histiocytic infiltration of the sinusoid capillaries and portal tracts and/or hepatocyte necrosis [36]. In a study of 30 patients with HLH and liver dysfunction, de Kerguenec and coworkers consistently found sinusoid dilation and hemophagocytosis, with liver biopsy identifying the underlying disease in 50% of cases [28]. Examination of spleen specimens may show red pulp expansion with hemophagocytosis, as well as lymphocyte depletion in white pulp. In HLH, histological examination of spleen sections may also identify the etiology of the process. In lymph node specimens, histiocytic infiltration is more meaningful when found in the sinusoids than in the cortical or paracortical area. Lymphocyte depletion with atrophic germinal centers is an extremely rare pattern. When lymph node architecture

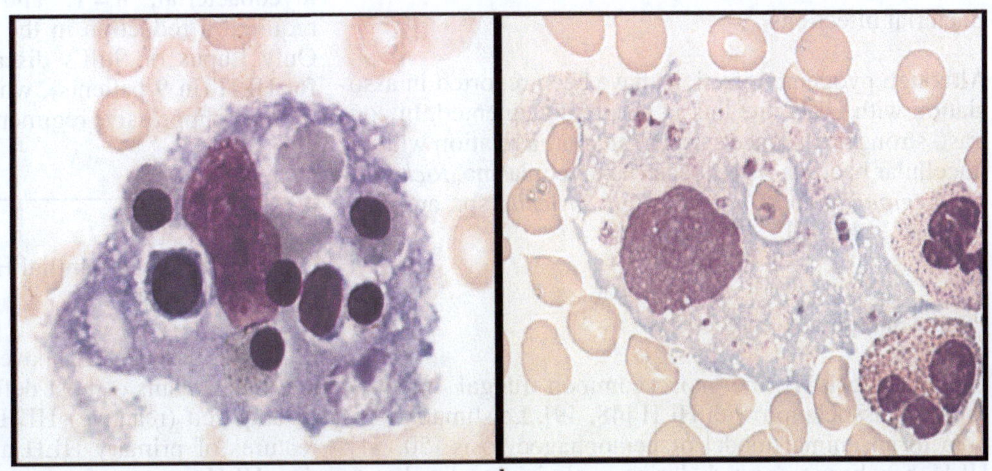

Fig. 1 Evidence of hemophagocytosis on histological samples. Hematoxylin-eosin stain of bone marrow sample shows histiocytes, phagocytosing erythroblasts, and lymphocytes. **a** Hematoxylin-eosin stain of bone marrow sample shows phagocytic cells with engulfed erythrocytes and platelets. **b** Hematoxylin-eosin stain of bone marrow sample shows phagocytic cells with engulfed erythrocytes and platelets

is not invaded by a tumoral proliferation, its structure is usually normal, although vessel proliferation may be present.

Etiologies

Viral infections, other infections, autoimmune disorders, and underlying malignancy are the most common triggers for reactive HLH (Table 2). In adults, acquired (reactive) HLH is commonly associated with immune deficiency, which should be looked for routinely.

Viral infections

Although many viruses can trigger HLH, herpes viruses account for more than 50% of cases of virus-associated HLH [37]. Epstein–Barr virus (EBV) is the most common triggering agent for HLH. The HLH associated with primary EBV infection is more common in young children than in other age groups and may be fatal, most notably in immunocompromised individuals [37]. The diagnosis rests on serology, MNI test, and PCR detection of viral DNA in serum. Cytomegalovirus (CMV) contributes 30–50% of all cases of virus-associated HLH and should be sought routinely, as specific treatment is available [38]. Herpes simplex virus (HSV) [39], and parvovirus [40] are common triggers of HLH. Cases associated with adenovirus [41], hepatitis viruses [42], rubella, respiratory syncytial virus, and coxsackie [43] have been reported. Post-mortem analyses in patients dying after severe avian influenza A (H5N1) infection have also revealed hemophagocytosis [44]. Human immunodeficiency virus (HIV) alone or in the presence of other opportunistic or nonopportunistic infections, or malignancies (e.g., Hodgkin's lymphoma and Castleman's disease), has been associated with hemophagocytic syndrome [45].

Bacterial infections

Although pyogenic infections have been reported in association with HLH, the link is poorly documented. In contrast, stronger evidence exists to support a relation with intracellular bacteria (mycobacteria, mycoplasma, *Rickettsia* sp., *Legionella* sp., *Chlamydia* sp., *Brucella* sp., and *Borrelia* sp.) [46, 47].

Fungal and parasitic infections

Histoplasmosis is the most common fungal infection found in association with HLH [48, 49]. Leishmaniasis is akin to an animal model of hemophagocytosis [50, 51]. HLH has been reported during malaria attacks due to *Plasmodium falciparum* and in *Babesia*-related infections. More rarely, disseminated strongyloidiasis, *Pneumocystis jiroveci* infection [52], aspergillosis [53], toxoplasmosis, cryptococcosis, and candidiasis [54] have been described in association with HLH.

Lymphoproliferative diseases

In non-immunocompromised patients, the first malignancy to be found associated with HLH is T-cell lymphoma [55], above all when the trigger is identified as EBV [56]. Hodgkin's disease is the second malignancy associated with HLH [37, 57, 58]. B-cell lymphoma and intravascular lymphoma may also be associated with HLH, more particularly in Asians [59]. The EBV-induced lymphomas, transplant-recipient lymphomas, and lymphomas in HIV-infected patients are associated with a higher risk of HLH [60]. Human herpes virus 8 (HHV-8) is associated with several distinct lymphoproliferative disorders [61–63]. The HLH triggered by HHV-8 is extremely rare but has been reported in associated lymphoproliferative disorders as well as in immunocompromised patients. Conditions rarely reported in association with HLH include acute T-cell or NK leukemia [64, 65].

Systemic diseases

Occurrence of HLH during connective disease course may be related to the systemic disease activity, to infection, or rarely to lymphoma [66–69]. In a study by Dhote et al. among 26 patients with systemic diseases and HLH, the diagnoses were systemic lupus erythematosus ($n = 14$), Still's disease ($n = 4$), rheumatoid arthritis ($n = 2$), polyarteritis nodosa ($n = 2$), Kawasaki disease ($n = 1$), mixed connective tissue disease ($n = 1$), sarcoidosis ($n = 1$), and Sjögren syndrome ($n = 1$). In 15 patients, HLH was triggered by active infection (viral, $n = 3$; bacterial, $n = 10$; mycobacterial, $n = 1$; and *Aspergillus*, $n = 1$), which required a reduction in the immunosuppressive regimen. Only Lupus or Still's disease were directly responsible for HLH (in 9 patients), which required intensification of immunosuppressive regimens [70].

Pathophysiology

Genetic defects in familial HLH: keys to HLH pathophysiology

Studies of genetic HLH have provided valuable insight into the mechanisms of host defense and the pathophysiology of acquired (reactive) HLH. The clinical and laboratory features of primary HLH are identical to those of reactive HLH, except for occurrence in childhood, greater frequency, and severity of neurological involvement, and higher rates of fatal primary viral infections.

Genetic (primary) HLH is inherited in an autosomal or X-linked manner and can be divided into two subgroups: familial HLH (FHLH), in which the clinical syndrome of HLH is the only manifestation; and the immune deficiencies Chédiak–Higashi syndrome (CHS1), Griscelli syndrome (GS2), and X-linked proliferative syndrome (XLP), which have distinctive clinical features besides the sporadic, though frequent, development of HLH [37].

Since 1999, several genetic loci related to the activity of perforin and granzyme granule have been associated with genetic hemophagocytic syndrome, thus explaining the impaired or absent function of NK cells and cytotoxic T cells characteristic of the disease. The cytotoxic activity of NK cells and of CD8+ T-cell lymphocytes (CTL) is mediated by the release of cytolytic granules (containing large amounts of perforin, granzymes, and other serin-like proteases) via the immunological synapse to the target cell [71]. In genetic HLH, mutations impair the cytotoxic activity of CTL and NK cells without modifying their activation capacity or cytokine secretion. Most of the mutations affect the cytoplasmic granules in cytotoxic cells, altering either the effectors they contain (perforin) or their ability to migrate to the cell membrane [71]. This impairment may remain asymptomatic until the cytokine system is stimulated, when paradoxical inefficient overactivation reveals the illness.

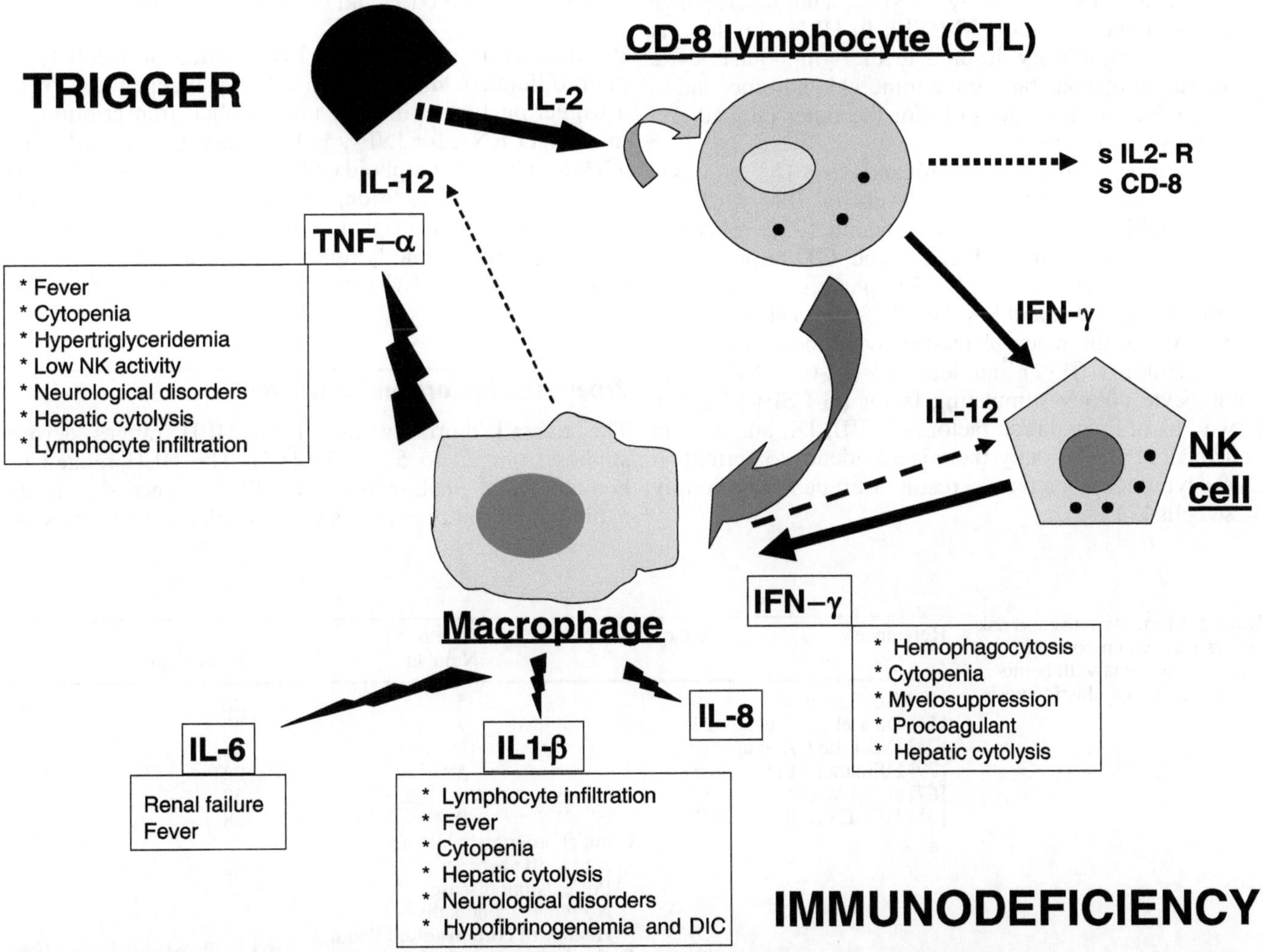

Fig. 2 Immunopathological mechanisms in hemophagocytic lymphohistiocytosis: clinical effects of Th1 activation loop and cytokines production. Activation of CD-8 T lymphocytes results in clonal proliferation and activation of NK cells, with production of high levels of activating cytokines. Elaboration of TNF-α and other cytokines causes fever and systemic illness. TNF-α and IFN-γ production contribute to macrophage activation with resulting hemophagocytosis. *TNF-α*, tumor necrosis factor alpha; *IFN-γ*, interferon-gamma; *IL1-β*, interleukin-1 beta; *IL-2*, interleukin-2; *IL-6*, interleukin-6; *IL-8*, interleukin-8; *IL-12*, interleukin-12; *sCD-8*, soluble cluster of differentiation 8; *NK cell*, natural killer cell

Uncontrolled TH1 response and defective cytotoxic function: key points to reactive HLH pathophysiology

In reactive HLH, there is an overwhelming activation of normal T cells and macrophage which cause clinical and biological alterations: cooperation among triggered histiocytes, macrophages, CTL, and NK cells is at the hub of HLH, where evidence of a cytotoxic response, including Th1 response and cytotoxic cell overactivation, soon becomes apparent (Fig. 2) [72].

Infection with a virus or intracellular pathogen normally induces a Th1 response in which cytotoxic Th1 cells and macrophage cooperate to increase the efficiency of the CTL system and the capacity of macrophage to proliferate. The antigen-presenting cells promote CTL and NK cells expansion and activation via the secretion of interleukin-12 (IL-12) and TNF-α. In turn, the cytotoxic cells release increased amounts of IFN-γ, TNF-α, and macrophage colony-stimulating factor (M-CSF). In HLH, this loop is amplified continuously, leading to the lymphohistiocytic proliferation responsible for the tumoral syndrome, and to the cytokine storm responsible for the other clinical and laboratory features (Fig. 2).

Activation manifests predominantly as a Th1 cytotoxic response with elevated serum levels of IFN-γ, IL-12, IL-2, M-CSF [73, 74], and Fas ligand [75], reflecting the Th1/Th2 imbalance (Fig. 2). The CTL upregulates activation markers such as CD-25 (alpha-chain of the IL-2 receptor), HLA-DR, and Fas [76]. The serum also contains high levels of the macrophage-produced monokines such as interleukin-1 (IL-1), interleukin-6 (IL-6), TNF-α, and granulocyte colony-stimulating factor (G-CSF) [77, 78], as well as of coagulation factors (V, VII, IX, and X) and transferrin. Paradoxically, there is a tendency to peripheral CD8+ lymphocytopenia as a result of tissue infiltration by these cells [74, 79].

Linkage between HLH and infection

The linkage between HLH and infection is complex, as an infection may trigger the development of HLH or complicate the course of HLH. Infection accounts directly for half the deaths in patients with HLH [37]. Clinical immune deficiency complicating HLH results not only from neutropenia, but also from anergy in Th1 cells associated with increased levels of cytokines such as IFN-γ. Infection complicating HLH probably reflects acquired impairments of similar nature. Immune deficiency has been reported in 40–60% of cases of HLH: The main causes of acquired immune deficiency were HIV infection [80] and immunosuppressive treatment for systemic diseases [81] or transplantation [82].

Linkage between HLH and lymphoproliferation

Reactive HLH secondary to EBV-related or T-cell lymphoproliferative disease seems to be independent from a triggering factor. Indeed, uncontrolled transcription of messenger RNA for INF-γ in lymphoid T-cells [83] or of TNF-α in EBV+ lymphoid cells [84] has been documented in such cases. In addition, supernatant from T-EBV cell cultures induce macrophagic differentiation of monocyte lines [56]; thus, some lymphoid proliferations can trigger and perpetuate the Th1 activation and loop via a paracrine effect.

Prognostic factors and mortality

The overall mortality rate from HLH ranges across studies from 22 to 59% (Table 3). The HLH related to hematological malignancies or EBV infection carries a higher mortality rate than cases related to viruses or

Table 3 Mortality rates and risk factors for death reported in studies of patients with hemophagocytic lymphohistiocytosis

Reference	No. of cases	Deaths Number	Percentage
[2] Risdall RJ et al.	19	5	26
[14] Dinarello CA et al.	23	7	30
[24] Dinarello CA et al.	40	18	45
[79] Fujinara F et al.	23	5	22
[67] al Eid W et al.	34	20	59
[55] Jaffe ES et al.	26	10	38
		Clinical prognostic factors	
		Age > 30 years	
		Pre-existing disease	
		No lymphadenopathy	
		History of corticosteroid therapy	
		Biological prognostic factors	
		High bilirubin level	
		High alkaline phosphatase levels	
		High TNF-α concentrations	
		IFN-γ > 30 IU	
		sIL-2-R > 10,000	

intracellular bacteria. In fatal HLH, death usually occurs during the first 4–8 weeks, from multiple organ failure, bleeding, or sepsis. In a retrospective study of 34 cases of HLH, Kaito et al. found that factors predicting death were: (a) age older than 30 years; (b) nature of the underlying disease; (c) hemoglobin level < 10 g/dl; (d) platelet count < 100,000/mm^3; (e) ferritin level > 500 µg/l; or (f) bilirubin or alkaline phosphatase elevation [85]. In adults with active systemic disease and HLH, Dhote et al. did identify the following factors as being associated with death: absence of lymphadenopathy at diagnosis; corticosteroid treatment at diagnosis; and thrombocytopenia [70]; however, some of the prognostic factors identified in both studies are actually considered to be diagnostic criteria. It is thus likely that the outcome of patients with proper HLH was affected in these studies. In some studies, the time of etoposide administration was the main determinant of long-term survival. This effect was particularly marked for EBV-associated HLH. Imashuku et al. reported that survival was 90% in patients given etoposide within the first 4 weeks compared with only 56% in those treated later [86–88].

Therapeutic options

Supportive care

Comprehensive ICU management is needed to support organ function, to apply specific measures aiming to control the symptoms, to identify and treat the underlying cause of HLH, to prevent its recurrence, and also to manage infectious complications. Special attention should be given to correcting coagulation disorders, by transfusing platelets, plasma, and fibrinogen, as appropriate. Fluid and electrolyte balance must be restored and renal replacement therapy given, if needed. Vasoactive drugs may be needed to maintain cardiac function and hemodynamics and assisted ventilation to treat acute respiratory insufficiency. Anemia and neurological disorders may require additional treatment. Antibiotic and antifungal agents should be given as needed to treat infectious complications.

The underlying cause should be treated as soon as it is identified. Antiviral agents have been reported as beneficial in patients with herpes simplex virus, varicella zoster virus, or cytomegalovirus infection [89, 90], but not in HLH associated with EBV, herpes human virus 8, or herpes human virus 6. As soon as infection is ruled out, immediate treatment of lymphoproliferative or systemic disease, along with empiric or prophylactic anti-infectious agents, is essential to control both HLH and its trigger; however, lymphoma may be difficult to detect, as severe hemophagocytosis may develop despite a small tumor burden. The diagnosis may require invasive procedures such as bone marrow or lymph node biopsy, liver biopsy, or splenectomy. In the absence of specific etiological treatment, hemophagocytosis relapses a few days or weeks after the symptomatic treatment.

Measures targeted specifically at HLH

Hemophagocytic lymphohistiocytosis is a highly fatal disease if untreated. Severe HLH should be treated promptly after symptom onset. In less severe forms, investigations for a cause can be performed first, albeit rapidly, as sudden worsening may occur at any time. Life-threatening hyperinflammation, caused by excessive levels of cytokines, can be treated by corticosteroids.

In patients without underlying systemic diseases, etoposide combined with corticosteroid therapy is now the treatment of reference for HLH [86]. Etoposide (VP-16) is a cytotoxic drug that targets the enzyme topoisomerase-2. Although nonspecific, etoposide selectively targets the monocyte line. Etoposide was reported to benefit patients with HLH nearly 10 years ago and was subsequently proven effective in several studies [37, 86]. In patients with severe HLH, etoposide should be administered immediately and acts rapidly, within 24–48 h. Its efficacy far outweighs the risk of secondary leukemia and transient worsening of the neutropenia. Etoposide has been proved superior over intravenous immunoglobulins and cyclosporine in patients with EBV-induced HLH [88, 91]. Moreover, times to treatment was associated with outcome [86]. Once HLH control is achieved, the appropriateness of continuing etoposide therapy must be determined according to the underlying cause.

In patients with infection-related HLH, intravenous immunoglobulin has some chance of success, only if used early [72]; however, intravenous immunoglobulin combined with steroids is thought to be inferior to an etoposide-containing regimen [73].

In case of HLH secondary to lymphoproliferative diseases, treatment should target malignant lymphocytes using combined chemotherapy regimens (which all include corticosteroids). Addition of etoposide in this setting is questionable as it may add some medullar or mucosal toxicity.

In patients with systemic diseases, such as lupus or Still's disease, corticosteroid therapy is the reference [92]. When complementary immunosuppressive treatment is needed, cyclosporine is often the best choice [81, 93, 94]. In patients with Still's disease, TNF-α antagonists (etanercept and infliximab) have generated interest because TNF-α plays a key role in the pathophysiology of both HLH and Still's disease [24, 95].

Conclusion

In conclusion, the diagnosis of HLH relies on the association of clinical abnormalities (fever, splenomegaly, pancytopenia) and hemophagocytosis in bone marrow, spleen, or lymph node specimens. Liver, pulmonary, renal, cardiac, and skin involvement may occur at various degrees possibly leading to multiple organ failure. Three main associated etiologies can be found, namely infections (viral, bacterial, fungal, or parasitic), lymphoproliferative diseases, or connective tissue diseases. Immune deficiency is often retrieved. Although clinically mimicking severe sepsis, HLH has a distinct pathophysiology on which specific therapy is based. The comprehensive management of severe HLH requires the involvement of a multidisciplinary team in order to determine the best therapeutic strategy and to identify the underlying cause. The high mortality in patients with no etiological diagnosis warrants aggressive investigations and treatment. Studies are needed to identify whether early administration of etoposide reverses organ failure and decreases mortality in critically ill patients with HLH.

Acknowledgements. The authors thank M.T. Daniel for her contribution to iconography preparation and A. Wolfe for her help with the manuscript.

References

1. Scott R, Robb-Smith A (1939) Histiocytic medullary reticulosis. Lancet 2:194–198
2. Risdall RJ, McKenna RW, Nesbit ME, Krivit W, Balfour HH Jr, Simmons RL, Brunning RD (1979) Virus-associated hemophagocytic syndrome: a benign histiocytic proliferation distinct from malignant histiocytosis. Cancer 44:993–1002
3. Cohen RA, Hutter JJ Jr, Boxer MA, Goldman DS (1980) Histiocytic medullary reticulosis associated with acute Epstein–Barr (EB) virus infection. Am J Pediatr Hematol Oncol 2:245–248
4. McKenna RW, Risdall RJ, Brunning RD (1981) Virus associated hemophagocytic syndrome. Hum Pathol 12:395–398
5. Wilson ER, Malluh A, Stagno S, Crist WM (1981) Fatal Epstein–Barr virus-associated hemophagocytic syndrome. J Pediatr 98:260–262
6. Ezdinli EZ, Kucuk O, Chedid A, Sinclair TF, Thomas K, Singh S, Sarpel S, Jovanovic L (1986) Hypogammaglobulinemia and hemophagocytic syndrome associated with lymphoproliferative disorders. Cancer 57:1024–1037
7. Liang DC, Chu ML, Shih CC (1986) Reactive histiocytosis in acute lymphoblastic leukemia and non-Hodgkin's lymphoma. Cancer 58:1289–1284
8. March LM, Webb J, Eckstein RP (1986) Cytophagic panniculitis. Aust N Z J Med 16:397–401
9. Gauvin F, Toledano B, Champagne J, Lacroix J (2000) Reactive hemophagocytic syndrome presenting as a component of multiple organ dysfunction syndrome. Crit Care Med 28:3341–3345
10. Strauss R, Neureiter D, Westenburger B, Wehler M, Kirchner T, Hahn EG (2004) Multifactorial risk analysis of bone marrow histiocytic hyperplasia with hemophagocytosis in critically ill medical patients: a postmortem clinicopathologic analysis. Crit Care Med 32:1316–1321
11. Nahum E, Ben-Ari J, Stain J, Schonfeld T (2000) Hemophagocytic lymphohistiocytic syndrome: unrecognized cause of multiple organ failure. Pediatr Crit Care Med 1:51–54
12. Stephan F, Thioliere B, Verdy E, Tulliez M (1997) Role of hemophagocytic histiocytosis in the etiology of thrombocytopenia in patients with sepsis syndrome or septic shock. Clin Infect Dis 25:1159–1164
13. Grom AA (2003) Macrophage activation syndrome and reactive hemophagocytic lymphohistiocytosis: The same entities? Curr Opin Rheumatol 15:587–590
14. Dinarello CA, Wolff SM (1993) The role of interleukin-1 in disease. N Engl J Med 328:106–113
15. Dinarello CA, Cannon JG (1993) Cytokine measurements in septic shock. Ann Intern Med 119:853–854
16. Reiner AP, Spivak JL (1988) Hematophagic histiocytosis. A report of 23 new patients and a review of the literature. Medicine (Baltimore) 67:369–388
17. Shirono K, Tsuda H (1995) Virus-associated haemophagocytic syndrome in previously healthy adults. Eur J Haematol 55:240–244
18. Ohta H, Yumara-Yagi K, Sakata N, Inoue M, Kawa-Ha K (1994) Capillary leak syndrome in patients with hemophagocytic lymphohistiocytosis. Acta Paediatr 83:1113–1114
19. Honig LS, Snipes GJ, Vogel H, Horoupian DS (1991) Sensorimotor neuropathy in hemophagocytosis syndrome. Acta Neurol Scand 84:316–320
20. Hanada T, Ono I, Iinuma S, Nagai Y (1989) Pure red cell aplasia in association with virus associated haemophagocytic syndrome (VAHS). Br J Haematol 73:570–571
21. Koduri PR, Carandang G, DeMarais P, Patel AR (1995) Hyperferritinemia in reactive hemophagocytic syndrome report of four adult cases. Am J Hematol 49:247–249
22. Esumi N, Ikushima S, Todo S, Imashuku S (1987) Hyperferritinemia in malignant histiocytosis and virus-associated hemophagocytic syndrome. N Engl J Med 316:346–347
23. Esumi N, Ikushima S, Hibi S, Todo S, Imashuku S (1988) High serum ferritin level as a marker of malignant histiocytosis and virus-associated hemophagocytic syndrome. Cancer 61:2071–2076
24. Dinarello CA, Gelfand JA, Wolff SM (1993) Anticytokine strategies in the treatment of the systemic inflammatory response syndrome. J Am Med Assoc 269:1829–1835
25. Henter JI, Carlson LA, Soder O, Nilsson-Ehle P, Elinder G (1991) Lipoprotein alterations and plasma lipoprotein lipase reduction in familial hemophagocytic lymphohistiocytosis. Acta Paediatr Scand 80:675–681
26. Ooe K (1992) Pathogenesis and clinical significance of hemophagocytic syndrome: hypothesis. Pediatr Pathol 12:309–312
27. McClure PD, Strachan P, Saunders EF (1974) Hypofibrinogenemia and thrombocytopenia in familial hemophagocytic reticulosis. J Pediatr 85:67–70
28. de Kerguenec C, Hillaire S, Molinie V, Gardin C, Degott C, Erlinger S, Valla D (2001) Hepatic manifestations of hemophagocytic syndrome: a study of 30 cases. Am J Gastroenterol 96:852–857
29. Billiau AD, Roskams T, Van Damme-Lombaerts R, Matthys P, Wouters C (2005) Macrophage activation syndrome: characteristic findings on liver biopsy illustrating the key role of activated, IFN-gamma-producing lymphocytes and IL-6- and TNF-alpha-producing macrophages. Blood 105:1648–1651
30. Whiting JF, Green RM, Rosenbluth AB, Gollan JL (1995) Tumor necrosis factor-alpha decreases hepatocyte bile salt uptake and mediates endotoxin-induced cholestasis. Hepatology 22:1273–1278

31. Iso ON, Hashimoto N, Tanaka A, Sunaga S, Oka T, Kurokawa K, Watanabe T (1998) Cytokine-induced hypoalbuminemia in a patient with hemophagocytic syndrome: direct in vitro evidence for the role of tumor necrosis factor-alpha. Dig Dis Sci 43:67–73
32. Weber J, Yang JC, Topalian SL, Parkinson DR, Schwartzentruber DS, Ettinghausen SE, Gunn H, Mixon A, Kim H, Cole D et al. (1993) Phase I trial of subcutaneous interleukin-6 in patients with advanced malignancies. J Clin Oncol 11:499–506
33. Braun MC, Cohn RA, Kletzel M (1996) Nephrotic syndrome accompanying familial hemophagocytic syndrome. J Pediatr Hematol Oncol 18:195–197
34. Thaunat O, Delahousse M, Fakhouri F, Martinez F, Stephan JL, Noel LH, Karras A (2006) Nephrotic syndrome associated with hemophagocytic syndrome. Kidney Int 69:1892–1898
35. Chubachi A, Miura I, Hatano Y, Ohshima A, Nishinari T, Miura AB (1995) Syndrome of inappropriate secretion of antidiuretic hormone in patients with lymphoma-associated hemophagocytic syndrome. Ann Hematol 70:53–55
36. Favara BE (1996) Histopathology of the liver in histiocytosis syndromes. Pediatr Pathol Lab Med 16:413–433
37. Janka GE (2007) Hemophagocytic syndromes. Blood Rev 21:245–253
38. Danish EH, Dahms BB, Kumar ML (1985) Cytomegalovirus-associated hemophagocytic syndrome. Pediatrics 75:280–283
39. Lasserre M, Huguet C, Terno O (1993) Acute severe herpes simplex hepatitis with virus-associated hemophagocytic syndrome in an immunocompetent adult. J Hepatol 18:256–257
40. Boruchoff SE, Woda BA, Pihan GA, Durbin WA, Burstein D, Blacklow NR (1990) Parvovirus B19-associated hemophagocytic syndrome. Arch Intern Med 150:897–899
41. Morimoto A, Teramura T, Asazuma Y, Mukoyama A, Imashuku S (2003) Hemophagocytic syndrome associated with severe adenoviral pneumonia: usefulness of real-time polymerase chain reaction for diagnosis. Int J Hematol 77:295–298
42. Kyoda K, Nakamura S, Machi T, Kitagawa S, Ohtake S, Matsuda T (1998) Acute hepatitis A virus infection-associated hemophagocytic syndrome. Am J Gastroenterol 93:1187–1188
43. Guerin C, Pozzetto B, Berthoux F (1989) Hemophagocytic syndrome associated with coxsackie virus A 9 infection in a non-immunosuppressed adult. Intensive Care Med 15:547–548
44. Henter JI, Chow CB, Leung CW, Lau YL (2006) Cytotoxic therapy for severe avian influenza A (H5N1) infection. Lancet 367:870–873
45. Chen TL, Wong WW, Chiou TJ (2003) Hemophagocytic syndrome: an unusual manifestation of acute human immunodeficiency virus infection. Int J Hematol 78:450–452
46. Baraldes MA, Domingo P, Gonzalez MJ, Aventin A, Coll P (1998) Tuberculosis-associated hemophagocytic syndrome in patients with acquired immunodeficiency syndrome. Arch Intern Med 158:194–195
47. Yang WK, Fu LS, Lan JL, Shen GH, Chou G, Tseng CF, Chi CS (2003) Mycobacterium avium complex-associated hemophagocytic syndrome in systemic lupus erythematosus patient: report of one case. Lupus 12:312–316
48. Masri K, Mahon N, Rosario A, Mirza I, Keys TF, Ratliff NB, Starling RC (2003) Reactive hemophagocytic syndrome associated with disseminated histoplasmosis in a heart transplant recipient. J Heart Lung Transplant 22:487–491
49. Kumar N, Jain S, Singh ZN (2000) Disseminated histoplasmosis with reactive hemophagocytosis: aspiration cytology findings in two cases. Diagn Cytopathol 23:422–424
50. Kontopoulou T, Tsaousis G, Vaidakis E, Fanourgiakis P, Michalakeas E, Trigoni E, Samarkos M (2002) Hemophagocytic syndrome in association with visceral leishmaniasis. Am J Med 113:439–440
51. Tapisiz A, Belet N, Ciftci E, Ince E, Dogru U (2007) Hemophagocytic lymphohistiocytosis associated with visceral leishmaniasis. J Trop Pediatr 11:11
52. Taillan B, Ferrari E, Heudier P, Fuzibet JG, Dujardin P (1991) Hemophagocytic syndrome in pneumocystosis. Presse Med 20:1456–1457 [in French]
53. Garcia Escudero A, Benitez Moya JM, Lag Asturiano E (2000) Hemophagocytic syndrome and invasive aspergillosis in a patient with Churg-Strauss vasculitis. Med Clin (Barc) 115:598 [in Spanish]
54. Bhatia S, Bauer F, Bilgrami SA (2003) Candidiasis-associated hemophagocytic lymphohistiocytosis in a patient infected with human immunodeficiency virus. Clin Infect Dis 37:e161–e166
55. Jaffe ES, Costa J, Fauci AS, Cossman J, Tsokos M (1983) Malignant lymphoma and erythrophagocytosis simulating malignant histiocytosis. Am J Med 75:741–749
56. Chuang HC, Lay JD, Hsieh WC, Su IJ (2007) Pathogenesis and mechanism of disease progression from hemophagocytic lymphohistiocytosis to Epstein–Barr virus-associated T-cell lymphoma: nuclear factor-kappa B pathway as a potential therapeutic target. Cancer Sci 98:1281–1287
57. Janka G, Imashuku S, Elinder G, Schneider M, Henter JI (1998) Infection- and malignancy-associated hemophagocytic syndromes. Secondary hemophagocytic lymphohistiocytosis. Hematol Oncol Clin North Am 12:435–444
58. Kojima H, Takei N, Mukai Y, Hasegawa Y, Suzukawa K, Nagata M, Noguchi M, Mori N, Nagasawa T (2003) Hemophagocytic syndrome as the primary clinical symptom of Hodgkin's disease. Ann Hematol 82:53–56
59. Aouba A, Lambotte O, Vasiliu V, Divine M, Valensi F, Varet B, Bazarbachi A, Hermine O (2004) Hemophagocytic syndrome as a presenting sign of transformation of smoldering to acute adult T-cell leukemia/lymphoma: efficacy of antiretroviral and interferon therapy. Am J Hematol 76:187–189
60. Srichaikul T, Punyagupta S, Mongkolsritrakul W, Jidpugdeebodin S (2004) EBV and hemophagocytic syndrome: analysis of 3 cases, with speculation on clinical features, therapy and role of EBV. J Med Assoc Thai 87:974–983
61. Fardet L, Blum L, Kerob D, Agbalika F, Galicier L, Dupuy A, Lafaurie M, Meignin V, Morel P, Lebbe C (2003) Human herpesvirus 8-associated hemophagocytic lymphohistiocytosis in human immunodeficiency virus-infected patients. Clin Infect Dis 37:285–291
62. Seliem RM, Griffith RC, Harris NL, Beheshti J, Schiffman FJ, Longtine J, Kutok J, Ferry JA (2007) HHV-8+, EBV+ multicentric plasmablastic microlymphoma in an HIV+ Man: the spectrum of HHV-8+ lymphoproliferative disorders expands. Am J Surg Pathol 31:1439–1445
63. Li CF, Ye H, Liu H, Du MQ, Chuang SS (2006) Fatal HHV-8-associated hemophagocytic syndrome in an HIV-negative immunocompetent patient with plasmablastic variant of multicentric Castleman disease (plasmablastic microlymphoma). Am J Surg Pathol 30:123–127

64. Okuda T, Sakamoto S, Deguchi T, Misawa S, Kashima K, Yoshihara T, Ikushima S, Hibi S, Imashuku S (1991) Hemophagocytic syndrome associated with aggressive natural killer cell leukemia. Am J Hematol 38:321–323
65. Ma L, Bandarchi B, Glusac EJ (2005) Fatal subcutaneous panniculitis-like T-cell lymphoma with interface change and dermal mucin, a dead ringer for lupus erythematosus. J Cutan Pathol 32:360–365
66. Palazzi DL, McClain KL, Kaplan SL (2003) Hemophagocytic syndrome after Kawasaki disease. Pediatr Infect Dis J 22:663–666
67. al-Eid W, al-Jefri A, Bahabri S, al-Mayouf S (2000) Hemophagocytosis complicating Kawasaki disease. Pediatr Hematol Oncol 17:323–329
68. Okada M, Suzuki K, Hidaka T, Shinohara T, Kataharada K, Matsumoto M, Takada K, Ohsuzu F (2001) Hemophagocytic syndrome in systemic lupus erythematosus. Intern Med 40:1263–1264
69. Sekigawa I, Suzuki J, Nawata M, Ikeda K, Koike M, Iida N, Hashimoto H, Oshimi K (2001) Hemophagocytosis in autoimmune disease. Clin Exp Rheumatol 19:333–338
70. Dhote R, Simon J, Papo T, Detournay B, Sailler L, Andre MH, Dupond JL, Larroche C, Piette AM, Mechenstock D, Ziza JM, Arlaud J, Labussiere AS, Desvaux A, Baty V, Blanche P, Schaeffer A, Piette JC, Guillevin L, Boissonnas A, Christoforov B (2003) Reactive hemophagocytic syndrome in adult systemic disease: report of twenty-six cases and literature review. Arthritis Rheum 49:633–639
71. Menasche G, Feldmann J, Fischer A, Basile Gde S (2005) Primary hemophagocytic syndromes point to a direct link between lymphocyte cytotoxicity and homeostasis. Immunol Rev 203:165–179
72. Egeler RM, Shapiro R, Loechelt B, Filipovich A (1996) Characteristic immune abnormalities in hemophagocytic lymphohistiocytosis. J Pediatr Hematol Oncol 18:340–345
73. Osugi Y, Hara J, Tagawa S, Takai K, Hosoi G, Matsuda Y, Ohta H, Fujisaki H, Kobayashi M, Sakata N, Kawa-Ha K, Okada S, Tawa A (1997) Cytokine production regulating Th1 and Th2 cytokines in hemophagocytic lymphohistiocytosis. Blood 89:4100–4103
74. Akashi K, Hayashi S, Gondo H, Mizuno S, Harada M, Tamura K, Yamasaki K, Shibuya T, Uike N, Okamura T et al. (1994) Involvement of interferon-gamma and macrophage colony-stimulating factor in pathogenesis of haemophagocytic lymphohistiocytosis in adults. Br J Haematol 87:243–250
75. Hasegawa D, Kojima S, Tatsumi E, Hayakawa A, Kosaka Y, Nakamura H, Sako M, Osugi Y, Nagata S, Sano K (1998) Elevation of the serum Fas ligand in patients with hemophagocytic syndrome and Diamond-Blackfan anemia. Blood 91:2793–2799
76. Imashuku S, Hibi S, Sako M, Ishida Y, Mugishima H, Chen J, Tsunematsu Y (1995) Soluble interleukin-2 receptor: a useful prognostic factor for patients with hemophagocytic lymphohistiocytosis. Blood 86:4706–4707
77. Imashuku S, Hibi S (1991) Cytokines in hemophagocytic syndrome. Br J Haematol 77:438–440
78. Henter JI, Elinder G, Soder O, Hansson M, Andersson B, Andersson U (1991) Hypercytokinemia in familial hemophagocytic lymphohistiocytosis. Blood 78:2918–2922
79. Fujiwara F, Hibi S, Imashuku S (1993) Hypercytokinemia in hemophagocytic syndrome. Am J Pediatr Hematol Oncol 15:92–98
80. Castilletti C, Preziosi R, Bernardini G, Caterini A, Gomes V, Calcaterra S, Carletti F, Capobianchi MR, Armignacco O (2004) Hemophagocytic syndrome in a patient with acute human immunodeficiency virus infection. Clin Infect Dis 38:1792–1793
81. Lambotte O, Khellaf M, Harmouche H, Bader-Meunier B, Manceron V, Goujard C, Amoura Z, Godeau B, Piette JC, Delfraissy JF (2006) Characteristics and long-term outcome of 15 episodes of systemic lupus erythematosus-associated hemophagocytic syndrome. Medicine (Baltimore) 85:169–182
82. Karras A, Thervet E, Legendre C (2004) Hemophagocytic syndrome in renal transplant recipients: report of 17 cases and review of literature. Transplantation 77:238–243
83. Lin MT, Chang HM, Huang CJ, Chen WL, Lin CY, Lin CY, Chuang SS (2007) Massive expansion of EBV+ monoclonal T cells with CD5 down regulation in EBV-associated haemophagocytic lymphohistiocytosis. J Clin Pathol 60:101–103
84. Chuang HC, Lay JD, Chuang SE, Hsieh WC, Chang Y, Su IJ (2007) Epstein–Barr virus (EBV) latent membrane protein-1 down-regulates tumor necrosis factor-alpha (TNF-alpha) receptor-1 and confers resistance to TNF-alpha-induced apoptosis in T cells: implication for the progression to T-cell lymphoma in EBV-associated hemophagocytic syndrome. Am J Pathol 170:1607–1617
85. Kaito K, Kobayashi M, Katayama T, Otsubo H, Ogasawara Y, Sekita T, Saeki A, Sakamoto M, Nishiwaki K, Masuoka H, Shimada T, Yoshida M, Hosoya T (1997) Prognostic factors of hemophagocytic syndrome in adults: analysis of 34 cases. Eur J Haematol 59:247–253
86. Imashuku S (2000) Advances in the management of hemophagocytic lymphohistiocytosis. Int J Hematol 72:1–11
87. Imashuku S, Hibi S, Tabata Y, Todo S (1999) Hemophagocytic syndrome in five patients with Epstein–Barr virus negative B-cell lymphoma. Cancer 85:2298–2300
88. Imashuku S, Kuriyama K, Sakai R, Nakao Y, Masuda S, Yasuda N, Kawano F, Yakushijin K, Miyagawa A, Nakao T, Teramura T, Tabata Y, Morimoto A, Hibi S (2003) Treatment of Epstein–Barr virus-associated hemophagocytic lymphohistiocytosis (EBV-HLH) in young adults: a report from the HLH study center. Med Pediatr Oncol 41:103–109
89. Hardikar W, Pang K, Al-Hebbi H, Curtis N, Couper R (2006) Successful treatment of cytomegalovirus-associated haemophagocytic syndrome following paediatric orthotopic liver transplantation. J Paediatr Child Health 42:389–391
90. Ramasamy K, Lim ZY, Savvas M, Salisbury JR, Dokal I, Mufti GJ, Pagliuca A (2006) Disseminated herpes virus (HSV-2) infection with rhabdomyolysis and hemophagocytic lymphohistiocytosis in a patient with bone marrow failure syndrome. Ann Hematol 85:629–630
91. Imashuku S, Hibi S, Ohara T, Iwai A, Sako M, Kato M, Arakawa H, Sotomatsu M, Kataoka S, Asami K, Hasegawa D, Kosaka Y, Sano K, Igarashi N, Maruhashi K, Ichimi R, Kawasaki H, Maeda N, Tanizawa A, Arai K, Abe T, Hisakawa H, Miyashita H, Henter JI (1999) Effective control of Epstein–Barr virus-related hemophagocytic lymphohistiocytosis with immunochemotherapy. Histiocyte Society. Blood 93:1869–1874

92. Papo T, Andre MH, Amoura Z, Lortholary O, Tribout B, Guillevin L, Piette JC (1999) The spectrum of reactive hemophagocytic syndrome in systemic lupus erythematosus. J Rheumatol 26:927–930
93. Ravelli A, Viola S, Benedetti F de, Magni-Manzoni S, Tzialla C, Martini A (2001) Dramatic efficacy of cyclosporine A in macrophage activation syndrome. Clin Exp Rheumatol 19:108
94. Ravelli A (2002) Macrophage activation syndrome. Curr Opin Rheumatol 14:548–552
95. Henzan T, Nagafuji K, Tsukamoto H, Miyamoto T, Gondo H, Imashuku S, Harada M (2006) Success with infliximab in treating refractory hemophagocytic lymphohistiocytosis. Am J Hematol 81:59–61

B. L. De Keulenaer
J. J. De Waele
B. Powell
M. L. N. G. Malbrain

What is normal intra-abdominal pressure and how is it affected by positioning, body mass and positive end-expiratory pressure?

Abstract *Purpose:* To describe what is defined as normal intra-abdominal pressure (IAP) and how body positioning, body mass index (BMI) and positive end-expiratory pressure (PEEP) affect IAP monitoring. *Methods:* A review of different databases was made (Pubmed, MEDLINE (January 1966–June 2007) and EMBASE.com (January 1966–June 2007)) using the search terms of "IAP", "intra-abdominal hypertension" (IAH), "abdominal compartment syndrome" (ACS), "body positioning", "prone positioning", "PEEP" and "acute respiratory distress syndrome" (ARDS). Prior to 1966, we selected older articles by looking at the reference lists displayed in the more recent papers. *Results:* This review focuses on the concept that the abdomen truly behaves as a hydraulic system. The definitions of a normal IAP in the general patient population and morbidly obese patients are reviewed. Subsequently, factors that affect the accuracy of IAP monitoring, i.e., body position (head of bed elevation, lateral decubitus and prone position) and PEEP, are explored. *Conclusion:* The abdomen behaves as a hydraulic system with a normal IAP of about 5–7 mmHg, and with higher baseline levels in morbidly obese patients of about 9–14 mmHg. Measuring IAP via the bladder in the supine position is still the accepted standard method, but in patients in the semi-recumbent position (head of the bed elevated to 30° and 45°), the IAP on average is 4 and 9 mmHg, respectively, higher. Future research should be focused on developing and validating predictive equations to correct for supine IAP towards the semi-recumbent position. Small increases in IAP in stable patients without IAH, turned prone, have no detrimental effects. The role of prone positioning in the unstable patient with or without IAH still needs to be established.

Keywords Intra-abdominal hypertension · Abdominal compartment syndrome · Body positioning · Prone positioning · PEEP and ARDS

Introduction

Intra-abdominal hypertension (IAH) and abdominal compartment syndrome (ACS) are associated with significant morbidity and mortality [1, 2]. Risk factors for developing IAH and ACS have gradually been established, culminating in the publications of the World Society of Abdominal Compartment Syndrome (WSACS, www.wsacs.org) recommendations relating to the assessment and management of patients with IAH and ACS [3–6]. It is clear that clinical assessment of the abdomen for elevated intra-abdominal pressure (IAP) is

M.R. Pinsky et al. (eds.), *Applied Physiology in Intensive Care Medicine 2: Physiological Reviews and Editorials*,
DOI 10.1007/978-3-642-28233-1_22, © Springer-Verlag Berlin Heidelberg 2012

neither sensitive nor specific and therefore it is important to measure the IAP intermittently [4, 7, 8]. Direct IAP measurement is impractical in most situations and the most common method is an indirect measurement via the bladder, a technique that has been validated [9–12] and which correlates well with IAP [3, 4]. This review will only focus on bladder pressure measurements in different body positions. Other routes for IAP measurement, e.g., intragastric, rectal, intravaginal and inferior vena cava pressure monitoring, are described elsewhere in the literature [13].

Ideally, the IAP should be expressed in mmHg and measured at end-expiration in a completely supine position, ensuring that abdominal muscle contractions are absent and with the transducer zeroed at the level of the mid-axillary line [3, 4]. However, most patients in the ICU are nursed with the head of the bed (HOB) elevated to 30° or 45°. This is because there is evidence that patients in a semi-recumbent position (HOB elevation) have a decreased incidence of ventilator-associated pneumonia (VAP) [14, 15] and that this position, in combination with pressure reducing devices, reduces the incidence of pressure ulcers and decubitus [16–18].

This review will focus on the effect different body positions can have on the accuracy and reproducibility of the measured IAP via the standard bladder technique recommended by the WSACS. Further, we will discuss what is considered a normal IAP in the general patient population and the morbidly obese and if the abdomen truly behaves as a hydraulic system. Finally, we will look at the effects of applied PEEP on IAP values.

Methods

A review of different databases was made (Pubmed, MEDLINE (January 1966–June 2007) and EMBASE.com (January 1966–June 2007)) using the search terms of "IAP", "intra-abdominal hypertension" (IAH), "abdominal compartment syndrome" (ACS), "body positioning", "prone positioning", "PEEP" and "acute respiratory distress syndrome" (ARDS). Prior to 1966, we selected older articles by looking at the reference lists displayed in the more recent papers. The search was limited to English, Dutch and French language publications.

Does the abdomen behave as a hydraulic system?

Pressures in the abdomen were recognized to be atmospheric or positive when Rushmer showed that the magnitude of pressure at various levels in the abdomen were related to the height of the hydrostatic column of the abdominal contents above the point of measurement [19]. Prior to 1911, the IAP was considered to be positive or negative depending on the method used to measure it and there was no consensus about this discrepancy [20–22]. In other words, it was recognized that the abdomen behaved as a hydraulic system and the pressures within were hydrostatic in nature.

Rushmer's findings were later challenged by Decramer et al. [23] who reported that gastric pressure swings in dogs were not simply hydrostatic. This study found that the abdomen does not behave as a hydraulic system or a liquid-filled container. Interestingly, the IAP differences observed in the dogs disappeared when the abdominal cavity was filled with 2 L of saline. These rather conflicting results were re-explored by Loring et al. [24], who measured pressures in the abdomen near the ventral abdominal wall and within the stomach of anesthetized dogs. This study concluded that there were three factors that affected IAP: gravity, uniform compression and shear deformation. Uniform compression, i.e., abdominal contraction, diaphragmatic contraction, mechanical ventilation, rib cage excursions and abdominal binding, result in spatially homogeneous changes in pressure that can be superimposed on the gravitational gradients (Fig. 1). Shear deformation, however, which is dependent on the shape stability of the tissue and the degree of deformation, is associated with spatially diverse pressure gradients. It is the relative importance of these individual factors that will determine ultimately if the abdomen behaves as a liquid-filled container. Therefore, the authors concluded that at times the abdomen behaves as a hydraulic system when the viscera are not subjected to shearing forces. All these data, however, are based on animal studies. In 1996, Tzelepis et al. [25] re-established the concept that the

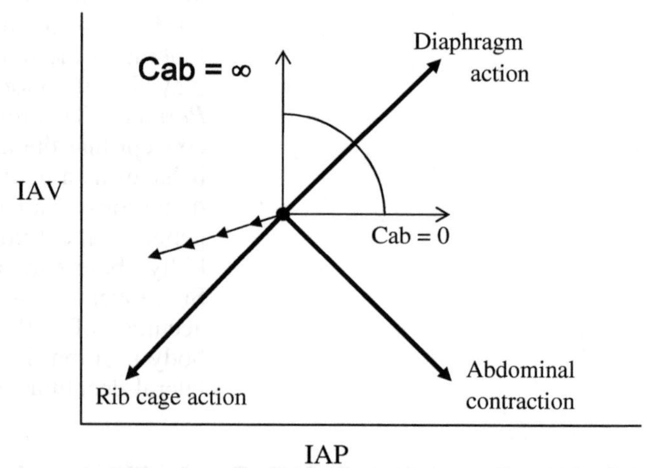

Fig. 1 Relationship between intra-abdominal volume, abdominal wall compliance and intra-abdominal pressure. Intra-abdominal volume (IAV) versus intra-abdominal pressure (IAP). The direction of the movement associated with the sole action of the rib cage inspiratory muscles, abdominal expiratory muscles and the diaphragm is shown. The direction of the latter depends on abdominal compliance (*Cab*) but is constrained within the sector shown

Table 1 Elective intra-abdominal pressure measurement in the general non-obese patient population

	Patient population	Number	IAP (mean ± SD)
Sugerman [31]	UC	5	5.1 ± 1.2
Sanchez [30]	S-NS	27	5.0 ± 2.9
Chionh [29][a]	S-NS	58	7.0 (0.7–13.2)
Lambert [32]	ELS	4	0.0 ± 1.5
Arfvidsson [33]	GS	4	6.2 ± 1.2

[a] Data expressed as median ± range
UC ulcerative colitis, *ELS* elective laparoscopic surgery, *GS* groin surgery, *S-NS* surgical-non-surgical

abdomen behaves as a hydraulic system . Based on the available data, we hypothesize that the impact of shear deformation on the measurement of IAP is probably not significant in the fully sedated, mechanically ventilated patient with sepsis, capillary leak and a positive fluid balance, with or without neuromuscular blocking agents.

What is normal intra-abdominal pressure?

As mentioned before, IAP was originally considered to be positive or negative, based on the methodology used to measure it. In animal studies, sub-atmospheric pressures were often reported [26, 27]. In 1984, Kron et al. [28] published their data suggesting that IAP after abdominal surgery varied between 3 and 15 mmHg, indicating that it was more likely that IAP in humans was positive and not sub-atmospheric. To determine normal values for IAP in the general patient population, several trials measured and compared IAP in non-obese surgical or non-surgical patients [29–33](Table 1).

Based on this data, the WSACS defined that a normal IAP in the general patient population lies between 5 and 7 mmHg. However, in an obese patient the baseline value can be significantly higher (Table 2). Sugerman et al. [31, 34, 35] reported a positive correlation between bladder pressures and the sagittal abdominal diameter (SAD) and found that surgical patients with a mean BMI of 52 ± 1 kg/m^2 had an IAP of 13.2 ± 0.5 mmHg versus surgical patients with a BMI of 24 ± 2 kg/m^2, where the IAP was significantly lower at 5.1 ± 1.2 mmHg. The close correlation between IAP and SAD suggests a link between IAP and visceral fat. Hence, they postulated that increased IAP can contribute to the health risks associated with severe obesity such as pulmonary or arterial hypertension, proteinuria, idiopathic intracranial hypertension, type 2 diabetes, increased cardiac filling and hepatic venous pressures, reflux oesophagitis, hypoventilation and venous stasis [36]. Similar results of elevated IAP have been reported by Sanchez [30] where IAP was higher in patients with a high BMI. The mean IAP for patients with a BMI of 25.0–29.9 kg/m^2 and 30–39.9 kg/m^2 was 6.3 ± 2.9 and 8.9 ± 3.5 mmHg, respectively. A recent multicenter study also identified BMI as an independent predictor of intra-abdominal hypertension (IAH) 2]. Some have even suggested that chronic IAH in patients with central obesity could be responsible for syndrome X [31]. Although it is difficult to draw any conclusions based on the above data, due to differences in measurement techniques and the amount of volume instilled into the bladder during the trials, we suggest that the normal values of IAP in the obese patients should be considered as between 7 and 14 mmHg. A possible explanation for higher pressures in the obese is that there could be a direct effect from the intra-abdominal adipose tissue itself on the measurement of IAP.

In literature, there is also some controversy with regard to the effect of mechanical ventilation and the use of PEEP on IAP. Sussman [37] was the first to look at the effects of PEEP on IAP and showed in their experiment that increasing PEEP to 15 cm of H_2O did not affect the IAP. This was confirmed by Guimaraes and animal data [38–40]. However, on increasing PEEP to 15 cm of H_2O, others have found only a mild increase in IAP in patients with a baseline IAP below 12 mmHg [41–43]. Further, in

Table 2 Comparison of IAP among different weight groups

Study characteristics		IAP (mean + SD) according to BMI			
	N (observations)	Normal	Overweight[a]	Obese[b]	Morbidly obese[c]
Sanchez [30]	77 (231)[d]	5.0 ± 2.9	6.3 ± 2.9	8.9 ± 3.5	8.4 ± 2.5
Sugerman [31]	84 (84)	5.1 ± 1.2	NA	NA	13.2 ± 0.5
Sugerman [59]	15 (15)	NA	NA	7.4 ± 0.7	NA
Lambert [32]	45 (45)	0 ± 1.5	NA	NA	8.8 ± 0.6
Vasquez [47][e]	45 (675)	6.5 (4.5–8.5)	11.2 (7.7–14.6)	13.7 (11.4–16.0)	NA
Arfvidsson [33]	15 (15)	6.2 ± 1.2	NA	NA	14 ± 3
Sugerman [34]	6 (6)	NA	NA	12.5	16.2 ± 2.2

[a] BMI 25.0–29.9 kg/m^2
[b] BMI 30.0-39.9 kg/m^2
[c] BMI > 40
[d] IAP observations
[e] Data expressed as mean with 95% CI

Table 3 Effect of PEEP on IAP

	N	PEEPBL	PEEPset	DeltaPEEPa	DeltaPEEPb	IAP BL	IAP PEEP	Delta PEEP	TAI (%)
Sussman [37]	15	0	15	15	11	10.8	11.7	0.9	8.1
Gattinoni [44]	21	0	15	15	11	10.6 ± 6.0	11.8 ± 6.3	1.4 ± 1.3	12.7
Malbrain [42]	27	15	0	15	11	11.3 ± 4.3	10.3 ± 2.9	1.5 ± 1.2	13.6
Malbrain [42]	27	0	15	15	11	17 ± 3.9	18.3 ± 4.1	1.3 ± 1.1	11.8
Jaber[a]	30	0	12	12	8.8	11.7 ± 4.5	15.2 ± 5.8	3.5 ± 1.7	39.6
Ferrer [43]	12	5	15	15	11	9.5 ± 2.7	11.1 ± 2.8	1.6 ± 0.9	14.5

PEEPBL PEEP baseline, *DeltaPEEPa* PEEP expressed in cm H_2O, *deltaPEEPb* PEEP expressed in mmHg, *TAI* (thoraco-abdominal index) deltaIAP/deltaPEEPb, *MA* midaxillary, *delta IAP* IAP PEEP minus IAP BL

[a] Personal communication

patients with a baseline IAP above 12 mmHg, the effect of PEEP seems to be more pronounced [44]. Table 3 shows the effects of PEEP on IAP.

Head of bed elevation/body positioning

Most patients in the ICU are nursed with an HOB elevation of 30-45° to reduce the risk of VAP and pressure ulcers [14, 16–18]. IAH and ACS, as mentioned before, are associated with increased morbidity and mortality. Therefore, patients at risk of developing IAH or ACS should have their IAP measured every 4 h [4]. It is a common practice to measure IAP in the supine position via the bladder after a maximum of 20 ml of normal saline had been instilled into the bladder with the mid-axillary line at the level of the superior iliac crest as the zero reference point [3, 4].

McBeth et al. [45] showed that IAP varied significantly between different HOB elevations. A total of 37 patients with an 18-Fr triple lumen bladder catheter had their IAP measured intermittently and continuously with the pressure transducer zeroed at the level where the mid-axillary line crossed the iliac crest. Pressures were measured in the supine position and at different HOB elevations. A total of 300 measurements were done showing an IAP difference of 1.2, 2.9, 5.0 and 7.4 mmHg at 10°, 20°, 30° and 45°, respectively. Based on the recent grading classifications of IAH [3, 4], this means that IAH would be over-diagnosed when the HOB is elevated (IAP at 45° would overestimate the pressure by two full grades). They also found in addition to HOB elevation that BMI, PEEP and body temperature correlated with the increase in IAP.

Cheatham et al. [46] conducted a similar, but larger, prospective multi-center trial looking at the effect of different body positions on IAP. A total of 132 patients were included in the trial. IAP was measured via the intermittent transvesical technique with only 20 ml of normal saline instilled and using the same zero reference point as in the previous study. They found similar effects with a mean IAP difference of 1.5 mmHg at 15° and 3.6 mmHg at 30°. Interestingly, this pressure difference was less impressive with IAP equal or above 20 mmHg (0.2 mmHg at 15° and 2.7 mmHg at 30°). This suggests that in patients with impending ACS, IAP could be measured in the semi-recumbent position at 30°. This finding is yet to be confirmed in a larger multi-center trial.

Vasquez et al. [47] measured IAP in 45 trauma patients, comparing the supine position with different HOB elevations as well as the reverse trendelenburg position. The zero reference point was not defined and the authors used 50 ml of normal saline to measure IAP. There was no information about the reverse trendelenburg position and the way the transducer was zero referenced. Nevertheless, overall there was a significant increase in the mean IAP in patients in the supine position compared with those at HOB 45° (10.2 versus 16.7 mmHg). Although the difference in IAP measured in the supine and at 30° with 15° HOB was the highest, a systematic error could have occurred on tilting the bed and potentially changing the zero reference point. Vasquez et al. [47] also found that the BMI was responsible for 25–36% of the total variance in IAP. Similar results were reported by Malbrain where the effect of the upright position (HOB 45°) versus the supine was more significant in patients with higher BMI (10.1 ± 4.4 versus 6.8 ± 3.3 mmHg). The reversed trendelenburg position of the patients increased the IAP by 4.5 mmHg (8.8 ± 3.9 versus 13.3 ± 4.8) [48].

Chionh et al. [29] studied IAP values in three different positions (supine, 30° and 45°) in 58 awake patients who were not receiving mechanical ventilation . They used a portable water manometry, infusing 50–100 ml of normal saline into the bladder with the symphysis pubis as the zero reference point. The median IAP difference in supine versus both upright positions was statistically significant (7.0 versus 8.5 and 10.3 mmHg) and there was a trend toward higher IAP in men versus women. Finally, Cobb et al. [49] measured the IAP in healthy volunteers in different positions and after performing several tasks such as coughing, Valsalva maneuver, standing, jumping or other exercises. They found an average pressure of 16.7 in

Table 4 Effect of body positioning on intra-abdominal pressure measurements

	N (observations)	Supine	HOB 15	HOB 30	HOB 45	Lateral	Reverse trendelenberg	Prone
Malbrain [13][a]	37 (79)	8.8 ± 3.9	NA	NA	17.1 ± 6.1	6.6 ± 2.9	13.3 ± 4.8	
Chionh [29][b]	58 (174)	7 (0.7–13.2)	NA	8.5 (2.2–14)	10.3 (2.9-16.2)	NA	NA	
McBeth [45][a]	37 (300)	13.4 ± 4.2	NA	18.4 ± 4.8	21.5 ± 5.0	NA	NA	
Vasquez [47][c]	45 (675)	10.2 (8.7–11.8)	12.4 (10.7–14.1)	14.0 (12.3–15.8)	16.7 (14.8–18.5)	NA	19.3 (16.8–21.8)	
Cheatham [46][d]	132 (396)	11.8 (11.4–12.2)	13.3 (12.8–13.8)	15.4 (14.9–15.9)	NA	NA	NA	
De Keulenaer [58][a]	10 (60)	6.6 ± 2.9	NA	NA	NA	11.2 ± 3.3	NA	
Cobb [49][a]	20 (180)	1.8 ± 2.0	NA	NA	16.7	NA	NA	
Chiomello [55][a]	11 (60)	8.8 ± 2.1	NA	NA	NA	NA	NA	10.7 ± 2.5
Hering [53][a]	12 (24)	10 ± 3	NA	NA	NA	NA	NA	13 ± 4 12 (15–7)

[a] Data are expressed as means ± SD
[b] Data expressed as median ± range
[c] Data expressed as means with 95% CI
[d] Data expressed as means ± range

the sitting position with a significant correlation between increasing IAP and BMI.

These data, summarized in Table 4, confirm that variation in bladder pressure is a function of body position and that HOB elevation significantly increases IAP. This effect is more pronounced in patients with higher BMI. If we accept that the abdomen behaves as a hydraulic system, then perhaps the descent of intra-abdominal contents by HOB elevation may exert external pressure on the bladder, hence increasing the IAP indirectly when measured via the bladder. Although it is generally accepted that IAP should be measured in the supine position throughout the day, the patient in the ICU will be nursed predominantly in the semi-recumbent position [3, 4]. Thus, patients who have a high risk of developing IAH and ACS could in theory already experience a grade 3 or 4 IAH or even ACS in the elevated position. Whether the increased pressure in that position is an accurate pressure measurement still remains subject to debate. If the abdomen behaves as a liquid-filled container, the pressure we measure (Pascal's law) is a true pressure and therefore should be interpreted according to the above data. We have published a case report of a patient on non-invasive positive pressure ventilation experiencing a cardiac arrest while he was placed in the semi-recumbent position, which instantly increased his IAP and led to ACS [50]. This is an important observation as most ICU patients will be nursed in a semi-recumbent to lateral position, rather than supine, causing an underestimation of the measured IAP that could be significant in the critically ill patient.

It is difficult to make any recommendations with regard to the semi-recumbent position due to differences in methodology, data expression, patient population studied and differences in the degree of the head of bed elevation in all the trials presented here. But based on the available trials [45–48], we conclude that the IAP in the semi-recumbent position at HOB 30° and 45° on average is 4 and 9 mmHg, respectively, higher than the standard bladder pressure measurement in the supine position and that in patients with impending ACS or grade 3–4 IAH this should be taken into account.

Prone positioning

Turning patients to the prone position to improve gas exchange is still a common practice in many ICUs for patients with acute respiratory distress syndrome (ARDS) and acute lung injury (ALI). Yet, the restriction of the abdomen during that position is associated with an increase in IAP in both humans and animals [51, 52]. Hering [53] showed that the IAP increased in patients with ALI, who were mechanically ventilated in the prone position, but there was no effect on systemic blood flow, renal perfusion, hepato-splanchnic function or gastric mucosal-arterial PCO2 gradients . Kiefer et al. [54] demonstrated that in nearly 50% of their prone patients with abdominal sepsis, there was an increase in IAP (intragastric) by more than 3 mmHg and simultaneously an increase in the gastric mucosal–arterial PCO2 gradient. Overall, there was no significant change in the mean intragastric pressure. Finally, Chiumello et al. [55] found an increase in both gastric and bladder pressures in patients with ALI/ARDS when turned to the prone position with or without thoraco-pelvic support. This data contrasted with others where the prone position did not result in a change in IAP. Martejovc et al. [56] studied the effects of proning on hepato-splanchnic hemodynamics in acute lung injury patients and found no change in IAP, hepato-splanchnic blood flow or gastric mucosal–arterial PCO2 gradient. Michelet [57] did not find an increase in IAP in patients who were in the prone position on an air-cushioned mattress. However, the IAP was increased and the plasma disappearance rate of indocyanine green was reduced when foam mattresses were used, probably due to restriction of abdominal movement. Therefore, the type of mattress used is important, but most trials do not specify which device is used. Although this was an interesting finding, it did not influence extravascular lung water and cardiovascular parameters such as cardiac index and mean arterial pressure or oxygenation. Most of these trials, however, did not include patients who were hemodynamically compromised or who at baseline had IAH. Based on the current literature, prone positioning is not significantly detrimental to hepato-splanchnic perfusion or gut mucosal energy balance in patients who are cardiovascularly stable without IAH; however, special precautions should be taken allowing the abdomen to hang free. The relevance of increased IAP in prone positioning still needs to be established.

Lateral position

It is still a common practice in many ICUs to nurse patients every 2–4 h in the left or right lateral semi-recumbent position (interval turning). Turning is generally considered to be another important and effective way of preventing pressure ulcers. There is little evidence describing how the lateral position affects IAP. We conducted a small trial [58] designed to evaluate if the IAP was influenced by lateral decubitus compared to the standard supine position. Ten patients were included and the mean IAP at different time intervals (morning, afternoon and evening) in the lateral and supine positions were 10.9 ± 2.0 versus 6.6 ± 3.2 mmHg (SD with $P < 0.001$), 11.0 ± 4.0 versus 5.4 ± 2.2 ($P < 0.0005$) and 11.6 ± 3.8 versus 7.8 ± 3.0. From these data, we concluded that measuring the IAP in the lateral position can lead to falsely elevated readings (depending on the position of the zero reference) and therefore cannot be recommended for current practice.

Conclusion

The abdomen behaves as a hydraulic system with normal IAP of about 5–7 mmHg and with higher baseline levels in morbidly obese patients of about 9–14 mmHg. Measuring IAP via the bladder in the supine position is still the accepted standard method, but in patients in the semi-recumbent position (HOB 30° and 45°) the IAP on average is 4 and 9 mmHg higher. Future research should be focused on developing and validating predictive equations to correct for supine IAP towards the semi-recumbent position. Small increases in IAP in stable patients without IAH, turned prone, have no detrimental effects.

References

1. Malbrain ML, Chiumello D, Pelosi P, Bihari D, Innes R, Ranieri VM, Del Turco M, Wilmer A, Brienza N, Malcangi V, Cohen J, Japiassu A, De Keulenaer BL, Daelemans R, Jacquet L, Laterre PF, Frank G, de Souza P, Cesana B, Gattinoni L, Malbrain MLNG, Chiumello D, Pelosi P, Bihari D, Innes R, Ranieri VM, Del Turco M, Wilmer A, Brienza N, Malcangi V, Cohen J, Japiassu A, De Keulenaer BL, Daelemans R, Jacquet L, Laterre P-F, Frank G, de Souza P, Cesana B, Gattinoni L (2005) Incidence and prognosis of intraabdominal hypertension in a mixed population of critically ill patients: a multiple-center epidemiological study. Crit Care Med 33:315–322 Comment in: Crit Care Med 2005 Sep;33(9):2150; author reply 2150–2153, Crit Care Med 2005 Feb;33(2):447–449
2. Malbrain ML, Chiumello D, Pelosi P, Wilmer A, Brienza N, Malcangi V, Bihari D, Innes R, Cohen J, Singer P, Japiassu A, Kurtop E, De Keulenaer BL, Daelemans R, Del Turco M, Cosimini P, Ranieri M, Jacquet L, Laterre PF, Gattinoni L, Malbrain MLNG, Chiumello D, Pelosi P, Wilmer A, Brienza N, Malcangi V, Bihari D, Innes R, Cohen J, Singer P, Japiassu A, Kurtop E, De Keulenaer BL, Daelemans R, Del Turco M, Ranieri M, Jacquet L, Laterre P-F, Gattinoni L (2004) Prevalence of intra-abdominal hypertension in critically ill patients: a multicentre epidemiological study. Intensive Care Med 30:822–829
3. Malbrain ML, Cheatham ML, Kirkpatrick A, Sugrue M, Parr M, De Waele J, Balogh Z, Leppaniemi A, Olvera C, Ivatury R, D'Amours S, Wendon J, Hillman K, Johansson K, Kolkman K, Wilmer A, Malbrain MLNG, Cheatham ML, Kirkpatrick A, Sugrue M, Parr M, De Waele J, Balogh Z, Leppaniemi A, Olvera C, Ivatury R, D'Amours S, Wendon J, Hillman K, Johansson K, Kolkman K, Wilmer A (2006) Results from the International Conference of Experts on Intra-abdominal Hypertension and Abdominal Compartment Syndrome. I. Definitions. Intensive Care Med 32:1722–1732
4. Cheatham ML, Malbrain ML, Kirkpatrick A, Sugrue M, Parr M, De Waele J, Balogh Z, Leppaniemi A, Olvera C, Ivatury R, D'Amours S, Wendon J, Hillman K, Wilmer A (2007) Results from the International Conference of Experts on Intra-abdominal Hypertension and Abdominal Compartment Syndrome. II. Recommendations. Intensive Care Med 33:951–962

5. Malbrain ML, De Laet I, Cheatham M (2007) Consensus conference definitions and recommendations on intra-abdominal hypertension (IAH) and the abdominal compartment syndrome (ACS): the long road to the final publications, how did we get there? Acta Clin Belg Suppl 62:44–59
6. Malbrain ML, Vidts W, Ravyts M, De Laet I (2008) Acute intensitinal distress sydrome: the importnace of intra-abdminal pressure. Minerva Anesthesiol 74:657–673
7. Kirkpatrick AW, Brenneman FD, McLean RF, Rapanos T, Boulanger BR (2000) Is clinical examination an accurate indicator of raised intra-abdominal pressure in critically injured patients? Can J Surg 43:207–211 [see comment]
8. Sugrue M, Bauman A, Jones F, Bishop G, Flabouris A, Parr M, Stewart A, Hillman K, Deane SA (2002) Clinical examination is an inaccurate predictor of intraabdominal pressure. World J Surg 26:1428–1431
9. Fusco MA, Martin RS, Chang MC (2001) Estimation of intra-abdominal pressure by bladder pressure measurement: validity and methodology. J Trauma 50:297–302
10. Iberti TJ, Lieber CE, Benjamin E (1989) Determination of intra-abdominal pressure using a transurethral bladder catheter: clinical validation of the technique. Anesthesiology 70:47–50
11. Yol S, Kartal A, Tavli S, Tatkan Y (1998) Is urinary bladder pressure a sensitive indicator of intra-abdominal pressure? Endoscopy 30:778–780
12. Iberti TJ, Kelly KM, Gentili DR, Hirsch S, Benjamin E (1987) A simple technique to accurately determine intra-abdominal pressure. Crit Care Med 15:1140–1142
13. Malbrain ML (2004) Different techniques to measure intra-abdominal pressure (IAP): time for a critical re-appraisal. Intensive Care Med 30:357–371 [see comment]
14. Chastre J, Fagon JY (2002) Ventilator-associated pneumonia. Am J Respir Crit Care Med 165:867–903
15. Bonten MJ, Kollef MH, Hall JB (2004) Risk factors for ventilator-associated pneumonia: from epidemiology to patient management. Clin Infect Dis 38:1141–1149
16. Fowler G (1900) Diffuse septic peritonitis, with special reference to a new method of treatment, namely, the elevated head and trunk posture, to facilitate drainage into the pelvis, with a report of nine consecutive cases of recovery. The Medical Record, New York, pp 617–623
17. Defloor T, De Bacquer D, Grypdonck MH (2005) The effect of various combinations of turning and pressure reducing devices on the incidence of pressure ulcers. Int J Nurs Stud 42:37–46
18. Knox DM, Anderson TM, Anderson PS (1994) Effects of different turn intervals on skin of healthy older adults. Adv Wound Care 7(1):48–52, 54–56
19. Rushmer R (1946) The nature of intraperitoneal and intrarectal pressure. Am J Physiol:242–249
20. Duomarco JLRR (1947) La pression intra-abdominal en el hombre. El Ateneo, Buenos Aires
21. Campbell EJ, Green JH (1953) The variations in intra-abdominal pressure and the activity of the abdominal muscles during breathing: a study in man. J Physiol (Lond) 122:282–290
22. Mills JN (1950) The pressures developed in abdomen and thorax during the Flack tests. J Physiol (Lond) 111:368–375
23. Decramer M, De Troyer A, Kelly S, Zocchi L, Macklem PT (1984) Regional differences in abdominal pressure swings in dogs. J Appl Physiol 57:1682–1687
24. Loring SH, Yoshino K, Kimball WR, Barnas GM (1994) Gravitational and shear-associated pressure gradients in the abdomen. J Appl Physiol 77:1375–1382
25. Tzelepis GE, Nasiff L, McCool FD, Hammond J (1996) Transmission of pressure within the abdomen. J Appl Physiol 81:1111–1114
26. Wagoner G (1926) Studies on intra-abdominal pressure. Am J Med Sci 171:697–707
27. Overholt R (1931) Intraperitoneal pressure. Arch Surg 22:691–700
28. Kron IL, Harman PK, Nolan SP (1984) The measurement of intra-abdominal pressure as a criterion for abdominal re-exploration. Ann Surg 199:28–30
29. Chionh JJ, Wei BP, Martin JA, Opdam HI (2006) Determining normal values for intra-abdominal pressure. ANZ J Surg 76:1106–1109
30. Sanchez NC, Tenofsky PL, Dort JM, Shen LY, Helmer SD, Smith RS (2001) What is normal intra-abdominal pressure? Am Surg 67:243–248
31. Sugerman H, Windsor A, Bessos M, Wolfe L (1997) Intra-abdominal pressure, sagittal abdominal diameter and obesity comorbidity. J Intern Med 241:71–79
32. Lambert DM, Marceau S, Forse RA, Lambert DM, Marceau S, Forse RA (2005) Intra-abdominal pressure in the morbidly obese. Obes Surg 15:1225–1232
33. Arfvidsson B, Eklof B, Balfour J (2005) Iliofemoral venous pressure correlates with intraabdominal pressure in morbidly obese patients. Vasc Endovascular Surg 39:505–509
34. Sugerman HJ, DeMaria EJ, Felton WL 3rd, Nakatsuka M, Sismanis A (1997) Increased intra-abdominal pressure and cardiac filling pressures in obesity-associated pseudotumor cerebri. Neurology 49:507–511
35. Sugerman HJ Effects of increased intra-abdominal pressure in severe obesity. Surg Clin North Am 81:1063-1075
36. Mullens W, Abrahams Z, Skouri HN, Francis GS, Taylor DO, Starling RC, Paganini E, Tang WH (2008) Elevated intra-abdominal pressure in acute decompensated heart failure: a potential contributor to worsening renal function? J Am Coll Cardiol 51:300–306
37. Sussman AM, Boyd CR, Williams JS, DiBenedetto RJ (1991) Effect of positive end-expiratory pressure on intra-abdominal pressure. South Med J 84:697–700
38. Hazebroek EJ, Haitsma JJ, Lachmann B, Steyerberg EW, de Bruin RW, Bouvy ND, Bonjer HJ (2002) Impact of carbon dioxide and helium insufflation on cardiorespiratory function during prolonged pneumoperitoneum in an experimental rat model 16:1073–1078
39. Kotzampassi K, Paramythiotis D, Eleftheriadis E (2000) Deterioration of visceral perfusion caused by intra-abdominal hypertension in pigs ventilated with positive end-expiratory pressure. Surg Today 30:987–992
40. Guimaraes HPSA, Leal PHR, Barcelos GK, Resque Ap, Amaral JL (2003) Influence of the increase of positive end-expiratory pressure (PEEP) on the intra-abdominal pressure. Intensive Care Med 29:S55
41. Ashraf A, Conil JM, Georges B et al (2008) Relation between ventilatory pressures and intra-abdominal pressure. Crit Care 12:P324
42. Malbrain MDY, Bertieaux S (2000) Effect of abdominal compression and decompression on cardiorespiratory function and regional perfusion. Intensive Care Med 26:S264
43. Ferrer CPE, Molina E (2008) Higher PEEP levels result in small increases in intraabdominal pressure in critical care patients. Intensive Care Med 34:S140
44. Gattinoni L, Pelosi P, Suter PM, Pedoto A, Vercesi P, Lissoni A (1998) Acute respiratory distress syndrome caused by pulmonary and extrapulmonary disease. Different syndromes? Am J Respir Crit Care Med 158:3–11 [see comment]

45. McBeth PBZD, Widder S, Cheatham M, Zengerink I, Glowa J, Kirkpatrick AW (2007) Effect of patient postioining on intraabdominal pressure monitoring. Am J Surg 193:644–647
46. Cheatham MLDWJ, De Keulenaer B, Widder S, Kirkpatrick A, Creswell B, Malbrain M, Bodnar Z, Meija J, Reis R, Parr M, Schulze R, Compano S, the WSACS Clinical Trials Group (2007) Effect of body position on intra-abdominal pressure measurement: a multicenter analysis. Acta Clin Belgica 62:246
47. Vasquez DG, Berg-Copas GM, Wetta-Hall R, Vasquez DG, Berg-Copas GM, Wetta-Hall R (2007) Influence of semi-recumbent position on intra-abdominal pressure as measured by bladder pressure. J Surg Res 139:280–285
48. Malbrain MVMN, Verbrugghe W, Daelemans R, Lins R (2003) Effects of different body positions on intra-abdominal pressure and dynamic respiratory compliance. Crit Care 29:1177–1181
49. Cobb WS, Burns JM, Kercher KW, Matthews BD, James Norton H, Todd Heniford B (2005) Normal intraabdominal pressure in healthy adults. J Surg Res 129:231–235
50. De Keulenaer BL, De Backer A, Schepens DR, Daelemans R, Wilmer A, Malbrain ML (2003) Abdominal compartment syndrome related to noninvasive ventilation. Intensive Care Med 29:1177–1181
51. Douglas WWRK, Froukje MB, Sessler AD, Marsh HM (1973) Improved oxygenation in patients with acute respiratory distress syndrome. Am Rev Respir Dis 115:559–566
52. Takata M, Wise RA, Robotham JL (1990) Effects of abdominal pressure on venous return: abdominal vascular zone conditions. J Appl Physiol 69:1961–1972
53. Hering R, Vorwerk R, Wrigge H, Zinserling J, Schroder S, von Spiegel T, Hoeft A, Putensen C (2002) Prone positioning, systemic hemodynamics, hepatic indocyanine green kinetics, and gastric intramucosal energy balance in patients with acute lung injury. Intensive Care Med 28:53–58
54. Kiefer P, Morin A, Putzke C, Wiedeck H, Georgieff M, Radermacher P (2001) Influence of prone position on gastric mucosal–arterial PCO2 gradients. Intensive Care Med 27:1227–1230
55. Chiumello D, Cressoni M, Racagni M, Landi L, Li Bassi G, Polli F, Carlesso E, Gattinoni L (2006) Effects of thoraco-pelvic supports during prone position in patients with acute lung injury/acute respiratory distress syndrome: a physiological study. Crit Care 10:R87
56. Matejovic M, Rokyta R Jr, Radermacher P, Krouzecky A, Sramek V, Novak I (2002) Effect of prone position on hepato-splanchnic hemodynamics in acute lung injury. Intensive Care Med 28:1750–1755
57. Michelet P, Roch A, Gainnier M, Sainty JM, Auffray JP, Papazian L (2005) Influence of support on intra-abdominal pressure, hepatic kinetics of indocyanine green, extravascular lung water during prone positioning in patients with ARDS: a randomized crossover study. Crit Care 9:R251–R257 [see comment; erratum appears in Crit Care. 2005 Aug;9(4):308]
58. De Keulenaer BLCG, Maddox I, Powell B, Jenkins I (2007) Intraabdominal pressure measurements in lateral decubitus and supine position. Acta Clin Belg Suppl 62:269
59. Sugerman H, Windsor A, Bessos M, Kellum J, Reines H, DeMaria E (1998) Effects of surgically induced weight loss on urinary bladder pressure, sagittal abdominal diameter and obesity co-morbidity. Int J Obes Relat Metab Disord 22:230–235

Robb W. Glenny

Determinants of regional ventilation and blood flow in the lung

Abstract The principles of ventilation and perfusion distribution in the lung form the foundation of pulmonary physiology and remain cornerstones in caring for critically ill patients. Due to improved imaging technologies with greater spatial resolution, our understanding of the determinants of local ventilation and blood flow have evolved over the past five decades. This review provides a brief history of how the concepts governing regional ventilation and perfusion have developed and presents the most recent studies that are shaping new perspectives on the determinants of ventilation and perfusion. How these new principles apply to acute lung injury and gas exchange in the intensive care unit (ICU) are reviewed.

Keywords Gravity · Pulmonary blood flow · Ventilation · Supine · Prone

Introduction

The lung has a number of unique properties that influence the regional distribution of blood flow and ventilation. It is the largest organ in the body and consequently has large intravascular hydrostatic and pleural pressure gradients down the lung. Its vascular system is a low-pressure circuit with local blood flow being influenced by both the hydrostatic vascular pressures and the surrounding alveolar pressures. In addition, the lung is highly deformable, expanding and compressing under its own weight from top to bottom.

The geometries of the pulmonary vascular and airway trees also influence the local distribution of blood flow and ventilation, respectively. The resultant distribution of blood flow is therefore determined by a combination of local hydrostatic pressures, alveolar pressures, and vascular resistances. Regional ventilation is determined by pleural hydrostatic gradients, regional compliances, and airway geometries.

Newer imaging methods, with improved spatial resolution, have demonstrated that regional perfusion and ventilation are quite heterogeneous but highly correlated. The mechanisms responsible for this tight matching of local ventilation and perfusion in the normal lung remain unresolved.

The principles of ventilation and perfusion distribution in the lung form the foundation of pulmonary physiology and remain cornerstones in caring for critically ill patients. Our understanding of the determinants of local ventilation and blood flow has been in evolution over the past five decades. This review provides a brief history of the concepts governing regional ventilation and perfusion and presents the most recent studies that are shaping a new perspective on the determinants of ventilation and perfusion. How these new principles

M.R. Pinsky et al. (eds.), *Applied Physiology in Intensive Care Medicine 2: Physiological Reviews and Editorials*,
DOI 10.1007/978-3-642-28233-1_23, © Springer-Verlag Berlin Heidelberg 2012

apply to acute lung injury and gas exchange in the ICU will be reviewed.

Brief historical review

Prior to the 1950s, the lung was thought to have uniform function throughout. Using measures of regional gas exchange, a number of investigators [1, 2] determined that ventilation and perfusion were not uniformly distributed in animal models and humans. With the advent of radioactive gases, physiologists began investigating regional lung function and, by studying subjects in different postures, concluded that gravity influenced the distribution of ventilation and perfusion.

Perfusion

The initial studies in the 1960s focused on the vertical distribution of blood flow. Using inert gases that were either inhaled or injected intravenously, external scintillation counters demonstrated that blood flow tended to be greatest at the lung bases and least at the lung apexes (Fig. 1) [3–6]. These methods, while providing the first insights into regional distributions of perfusion, had relatively poor spatial resolution by today's standards. The data from these studies represented regional perfusion that were averaged within horizontal planes and were not able to detect heterogeneity of blood flow within isogravitational planes.

Bannister and Torrance were the first to suggest that regional alveolar and vascular pressures interact as Starling resistors to impose a nonuniform distribution of perfusion [7]. Based on these and other observations, West et al. created a model in which blood flow progressively increased down the lung [8]. They proposed that the lung has three vertically stacked zones in which blood flow is determined by the relationships between alveolar pressure (P_A), arterial pressure (P_a), and venous pressure (P_v) (Fig. 2). A fourth zone, where blood flow decreased due to mechanical compression, was proposed to exist in the most dependent lung [6]. The conventional wisdom that gravity plays a dominant role in perfusion distribution in the lung has influenced the interpretations of experimental observations and has been taught to generations of medical students [9].

Using imaging methods with higher spatial resolution in the 1970s, a number of investigators demonstrated variations in regional blood flow that could not be accounted for by hydrostatic differences or zonal conditions. Reed and Wood [10] found large differences in regional blood flow within horizontal planes of the lung. In studies conducted by Beck and Rehder [11], regional blood flow and vascular conductances were determined in different lung regions of canines. They observed that, regardless of posture and lung volume, vascular conductance was always highest in the dorsal regions of the lung. These were the first studies to suggest that the structure of the pulmonary vascular tree may also play a role in blood flow distribution.

Ventilation

In a history parallel to the experimentation in blood flow distribution, regional differences in gas exchange suggested that ventilation was greater in the lung bases than in the apices [1, 2]. Using inert radioactive gases, a

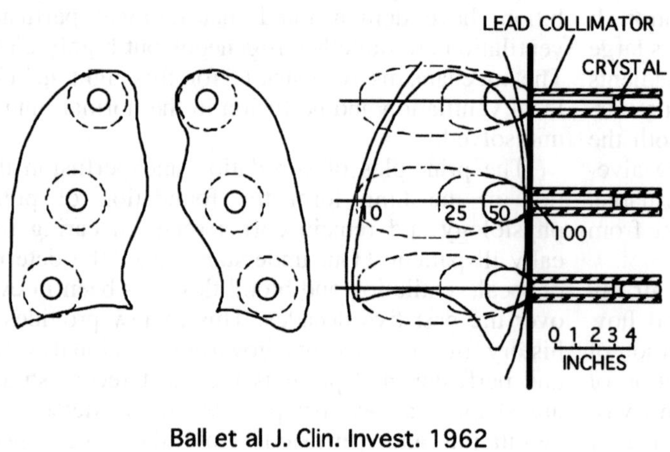

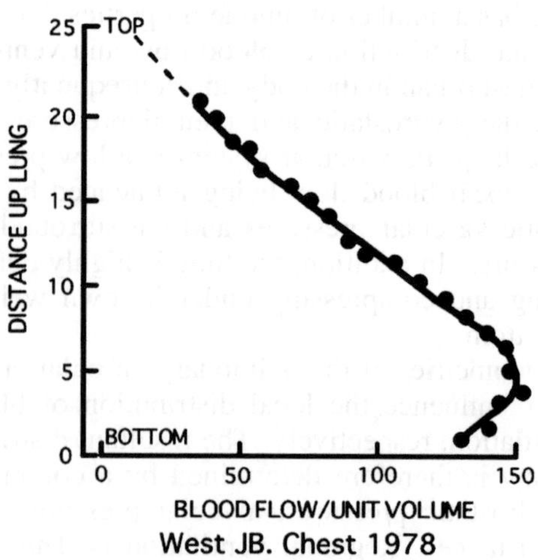

Fig. 1 Initial studies used external scintillation counters on the chest wall to estimate regional blood flow and ventilation. *Leftt* these external counters averaged flow within isogravitational planes. Adapted from Ball et al. [4]. *Right* these studies revealed a vertical distribution of both ventilation and perfusion with increasing flows down the lung. Adapted from West [8]

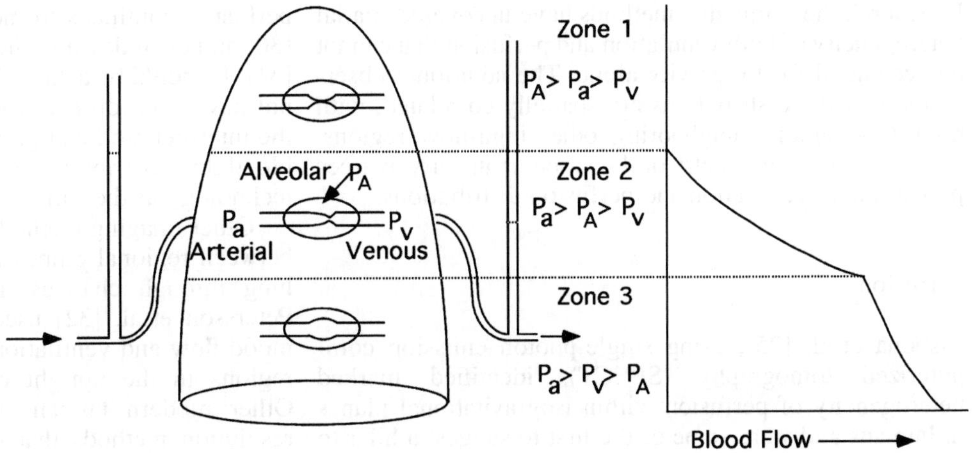

Fig. 2 The three-zone model of pulmonary perfusion proposed by West et al. Note that the zones have been traditionally thought to be vertically stacked but could very well exist within horizontal planes (see text). Adapted from West [8]

number of investigators confirmed this large-scale variation in ventilation [12–14]. The proposed mechanism for this vertical distribution of ventilation was regional differences in lung compliance induced by a vertical gradient in lung compression that others have termed a "Slinky" effect [15]. The lung is suspended at its apex by a negative pleural pressure and its base rests on the diaphragm. As the lung is elastic and compressible, alveolar volumes tend to be greatest at the apices and decrease in size down the lung. The smaller alveoli expand more readily because they are on the more compliant portion of their pressure–volume curve, and ventilation is consequently greater at the lung bases. This idea was applied to other postures with the general concept being that ventilation is greatest in the most dependent lung regions.

Olson and Rodarte [16] measured regional differences in lung compliance of excised dog lungs and found nonuniformity of regional ventilation within small regions at the same vertical height. Using high-resolution computed tomography (CT) scanners, studies performed by Hubmayr et al. [17] explored the determinants of regional ventilation. Their findings were not consistent with the classic model of regional ventilation and concluded that the distribution of ventilation is determined by a complex interaction of lung and chest wall shapes and by the motion of the lobes relative to each other. Rodarte et al. [18] also demonstrated large variations in the regional distribution of ventilation that appeared to be more dependent on the shape of the thoracic cavity rather than on the effect of gravity.

Matching of ventilation and perfusion

Despite the observed regional variability in ventilation and perfusion, gas exchange was noted to be quite efficient, indicating that ventilation and perfusion must be tightly matched. West [19] proposed that the shared effect of gravity accounted for the matching of ventilation and perfusion since they both increased down the lung. He also noted that the rate at which ventilation and perfusion increased were different, creating regions of higher ventilation/perfusion in the apices and regions of lower ventilation/perfusion at the bases [19]. These differences in ventilation/perfusion ratios predicted regional variations in partial pressures of gases. While the model was validated by its ability to account for the observed difference between arterial and alveolar oxygen partial pressures at the whole-lung level, it was purely theoretical and had no regional measurements of gas pressures in the lung to confirm the hypotheses. Michels and West [20] tested the gravitational model of ventilation, perfusion, and their matching through studies performed on humans during parabolic flights that produced transient periods of weightlessness. Indirect measures of ventilation and perfusion heterogeneity were obtained from exhaled gas profiles and they concluded that "virtually all the topographical inequality of ventilation, blood flow, and lung volume seen under 1-G conditions are abolished during short periods of 0 G." [20].

Imaging methods with increased spatial resolution of ventilation and perfusion demonstrated that both were heterogeneous within isogravitational planes and provided the first clues that gravity could not be the only mechanism accounting for matching of regional ventilation and perfusion. This realization was reinforced when astronauts spending time in microgravity maintained normal gas exchange despite not having the shared effect of gravity to match regional ventilation and perfusion.

Modern studies of ventilation and perfusion distributions

Significant advances have been made in imaging modalities in the lung. These new approaches and their application to lung physiology have been recently reviewed [21–24].

In general, these imaging methods have uncovered spatial heterogeneity of both ventilation and perfusion that cannot be accounted for by gravity alone. The additional observation that the distributions are spatially correlated, with high-flow regions neighboring other high-flow regions, suggests that the geometry of the vascular and airway trees play a role in ventilation and perfusion distributions.

Perfusion

Lisbona et al. [25], using single-photon emission computerized tomography (SPECT), identified marked heterogeneity of perfusion within isogravitational planes in humans and were some of the first to suggest a hilar to peripheral gradient in blood flow. Melsom et al. [26] confirmed the observations of isogravitational perfusion heterogeneity using microsphere methods [24] in goats. Glenny et al. [27] also used microsphere methods to measure regional blood flow in dogs while in supine and prone postures. They found that (1) blood flow is nearly as variable within an isogravitational plane as it is across gravitational planes; (2) high-flow regions remain high-flow and low-flow regions remain low-flow, regardless of posture; and (3) blood flow is greater centrally than peripherally. While microsphere methods cannot be used in humans, studies performed in primates yield observations similar to those of prior studies in humans confirming the observed relationship between pulmonary blood flow and height up the lung (Fig. 3) [28, 29]. The primary advantage of the microsphere method is the increased spatial resolution compared with the external counters of older studies. When the data are viewed at the highest spatial resolution, it becomes apparent that there is a great deal of heterogeneity within isogravitational planes and that height up the lung accounts for only a minority of the total variability in regional perfusion. At even finer resolutions, the observed heterogeneity of perfusion continues to increase down to the acinar level [30] and even down to the level of the alveolar capillaries [31]. It should be acknowledged that this variability could not have been observed with prior imaging methods and the interpretation that gravity was the sole determinant of blood flow distribution in the lung was plausible given the technology at the time.

Other imaging methods have explored the relationship between regional pulmonary perfusion and height up the lung through changes in posture. A recent study by Petersson et al. [32] used SPECT to confirm that both blood flow and ventilation redistribute to dependent lung regions in the upright compared with supine posture. Other modern human studies have used high-spatial-resolution methods that can be corrected for the vertical compression of lung tissue. All of these studies have demonstrated a small vertical distribution of blood flow and considerable perfusion heterogeneity within horizontal planes. Using electron-beam computed tomography, Jones et al. [33] found that vertical height accounted for 21–41% of perfusion distribution in supine and prone humans. Hopkins et al. [15] used magnetic resonance imaging in supine humans and found that between 4% and 13% of perfusion heterogeneity was explained by height up the lung. Modeling studies, using high-resolution measurements of the human pulmonary vascular tree, also predict that gravity should play a small role in determining regional blood flow [34].

In addition to imaging methods, indirect measures can be used in human subjects to assess blood flow distributions. While there is no spatial information in these measures, temporal differences in exhaled gas profiles are attributed to topological differences in the lung. Under conditions of sustained microgravity, Prisk et al. [35] estimated that perfusion heterogeneity was reduced to approximately 60% of that on Earth, indicating that the majority of perfusion heterogeneity persists in the absence of gravity. Montmerle et al. [36] found that more than

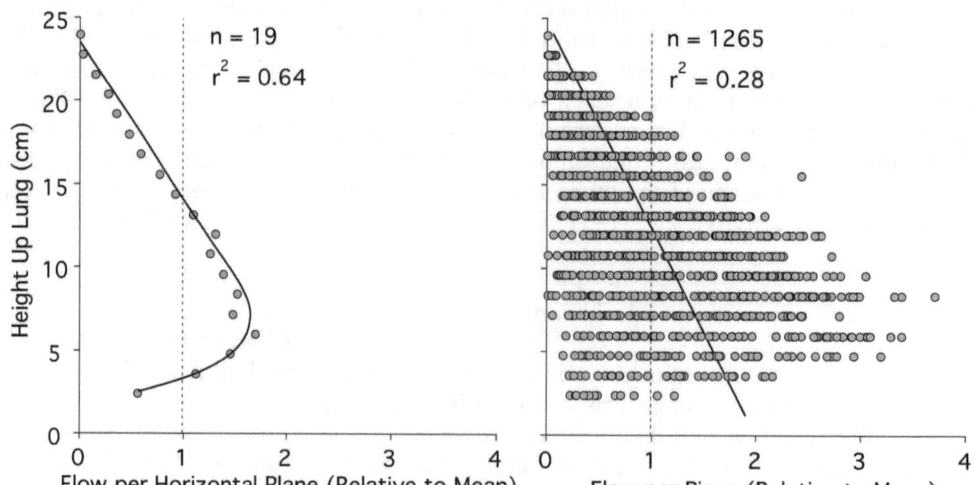

Fig. 3 Microsphere studies of pulmonary blood flow in upright primates confirm the vertical distribution of blood flow. *Left* when the data are averaged within horizontal planes to simulate the spatial resolution of earlier studies, there is a strong relationship between vertical height and blood flow. *Right* however, when the data are viewed at higher spatial resolution, heterogeneity within horizontal planes is evident and the relationship between height and local perfusion is much less strong. From [28]

one-half of indices of perfusion heterogeneity at 1 G are caused by nongravitational mechanisms.

Nearly all studies on the vertical distribution of blood flow have altered the relative direction of gravity by changes in posture to infer the effects of gravity on perfusion distributions. The results and interpretations of these studies are confounded by the ubiquitous presence of gravity and shifting of lung parenchyma between postures [37]. The only way to cleanly study the contribution of gravity to perfusion distribution is to transiently remove gravity. This was accomplished by using microspheres to measure regional blood flow in swine during parabolic flight that produced 25 s of 0-G conditions [38]. Regional blood flow to each lung piece changed little despite alterations in posture and gravitational forces. Using multiple stepwise linear regressions, the contributions of gravity and vascular structure to regional perfusion were separated and it was estimated that height up the lung accounted for 1–4% of variability in blood flow. The contribution of gravity to the spatial distribution of pulmonary perfusion would likely be greater in upright humans due to the greater vertical distance and hydrostatic differences.

A new perspective was obtained when Glenny et al. [39] determined that blood flow is not randomly distributed within isogravitational planes but rather is spatially correlated, with high-flow regions neighboring other high-flow regions and low-flow regions being next to other low-flow regions (Fig. 4). This observation suggested that the geometry of the pulmonary vascular tree produced heterogeneous but spatially correlated flows. A fractal model was proposed in which a dichotomously branching tree structure is created by a recursive mechanism where the tree begins as a main pulmonary artery and bifurcates asymmetrically through successive branches. Branching at the distal tips occurs in a similar pattern until an entire vascular tree is constructed. Such a tree has a number of theoretical advantages [40]. It delivers blood flow throughout the lung using the least amount of biological material to construct the tree. A fractal structure minimizes the amount of blood within the vascular tree. It also minimizes the work required by the heart to pump blood through the lung. Finally, it reduces the amount of genetic code to construct the vascular tree.

Subsequent studies have shown that patterns of perfusion distribution created by the pulmonary vascular tree are stable over days [41] and with growth [42]. Most recently, it has been demonstrated that the geometry of the pulmonary vascular tree and its perfusion pattern is predominantly genetically determined [43]. The observation that perfusion is determined by the geometry of the pulmonary vascular tree also provides a new perspective with respect to "zones" of perfusion. The zones, traditionally thought to be vertically stacked, are more likely to be distributed within isogravitational planes [44, 45], such that there are more regions of zone I in nondependent planes and more zone III regions in dependent planes.

Ventilation

A number of methods for measuring regional ventilation at higher spatial resolutions have been developed recently [21, 23, 24], providing new insights into mechanisms of ventilation distribution. Melsom et al. [46] used radiolabeled and fluorescent aerosols to characterize the distribution of ventilation in awake laboratory animals. They found a large heterogeneity of ventilation within horizontal planes and concluded that factors other than vertical height up the lung must determine regional ventilation. Altemeier et al. [47] used aerosolized fluorescent microspheres in laboratory animals to demonstrate that regional ventilation is both heterogeneous and spatially correlated, with high-ventilation regions near other high-ventilation regions and low-ventilation regions neighboring other low-ventilation regions. This observation

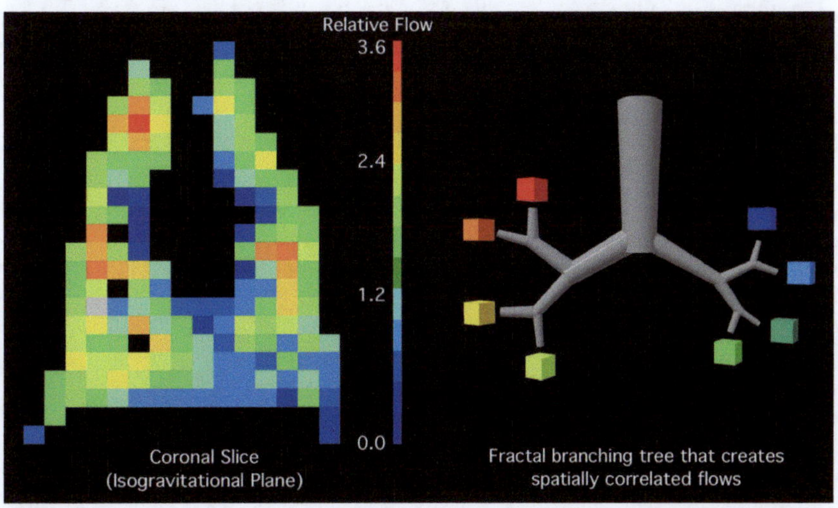

Fig. 4 *Left* blood flow distribution within a horizontal plane. Note that the distribution is not random in space, but rather that high-flow regions are near other high-flow regions and low-flow areas neighbor other low-flow areas. *Right* a dichotomously branching vascular tree with slight asymmetry of resistance at each branch creates heterogeneous blood flow distributions that are spatially correlated

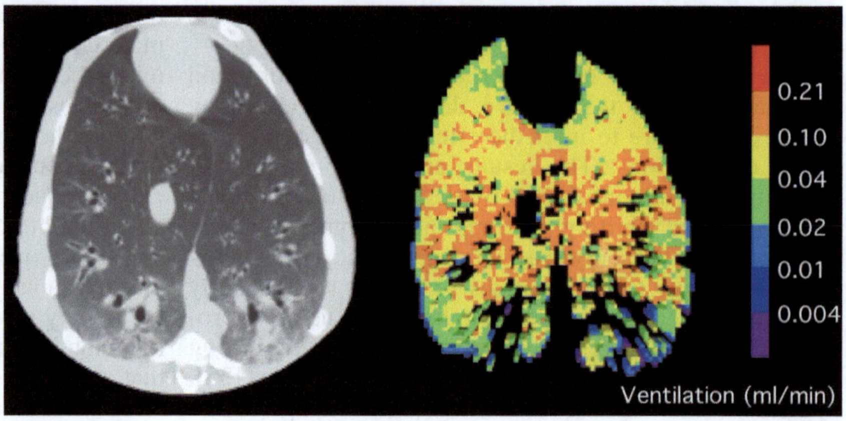

Fig. 5 Regional Xe–CT analysis of ventilation to 16 mm^3 voxels in the lower lobes of a sheep. *Left*, original *gray-scale* image of transverse slice. *Right*, *color maps* of regional ventilation in ml/min to each voxel. Note the heterogeneity of ventilation as well as the spatial correlation. Adapted from Kreck et al. [51]

suggests that regional ventilation may be distributed by a fractal mechanism similar to perfusion [48]. Treppo et al. [49] used positron emission tomography (PET) methods to estimate the spatial heterogeneity of ventilation in dogs. They found a significant vertical gradient in the supine but not the prone posture. They estimated that height up the lung accounted for 24% of the heterogeneity in regional ventilation when supine. More recently, Marcucci and Simon [50] used xenon inhalation with computerized tomography (CT) to explore the spatial distribution of ventilation in dogs and found that ventilation has a vertical distribution in the supine posture but that vertical height only explained a fraction of the heterogeneity in ventilation (37% when supine and 6% when prone). Kreck et al. [51] also used xenon to measure regional ventilation in large laboratory animals and noted both heterogeneity and spatial correlation (Fig. 5). Musch et al. [52] used PET to study ventilation in human subjects and found that a vertical gradient accounted for only 8% of the heterogeneity in ventilation.

Estimates of ventilation distributions have been studied in humans using SPECT [53] and positron emission tomography [52]. By having subjects inhale technigas in one posture and then imaging in alternate postures, Petersson et al. [37] were able to separate out the redistribution of lung parenchyma and ventilation in supine and prone humans. They were unable to detect a vertical gradient in the isotope distribution. Musch et al. [52] confirmed that only a small fraction of ventilation heterogeneity could be explained by a vertical gradient and the residual nongravitational heterogeneity of ventilation is significant.

Matching of ventilation and perfusion

Efficient gas exchange in the lungs can only occur through intimate matching of regional ventilation and perfusion. This has been demonstrated using microsphere methods in large laboratory animals [46, 54] where regional perfusion is tightly matched to ventilation under normal conditions (Fig. 6). Altemeier found that ventilation and perfusion were matched with an average correlation coefficient (*r*) of 0.89, and Melsom observed an average correlation of 0.71. The role of gravity in matching ventilation and perfusion has been studied during sustained weightless conditions in space using indirect measures of gas exchange [55]. Prisk et al. demonstrated that ventilation-perfusion matching changed very little from 1 G to microgravity. They did however observe that ventilation and perfusion matching was slightly better under normal gravitational conditions,

Fig. 6 *Left* despite the heterogeneous distributions of ventilation and perfusion, there is tight correlation between them. *Right* this tight correlation results in a narrow distribution of ventilation/perfusion ratios and efficient gas exchange

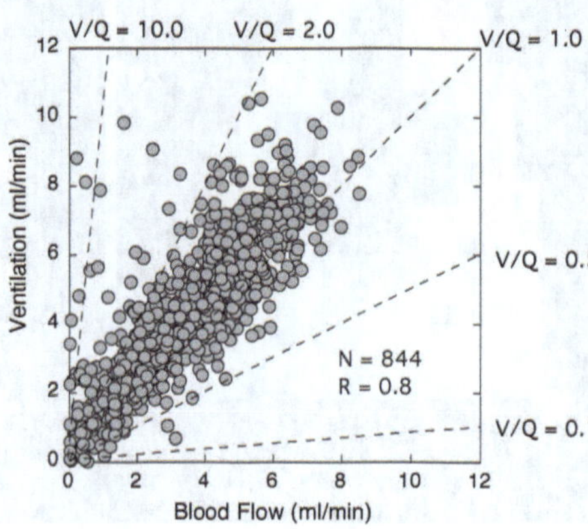

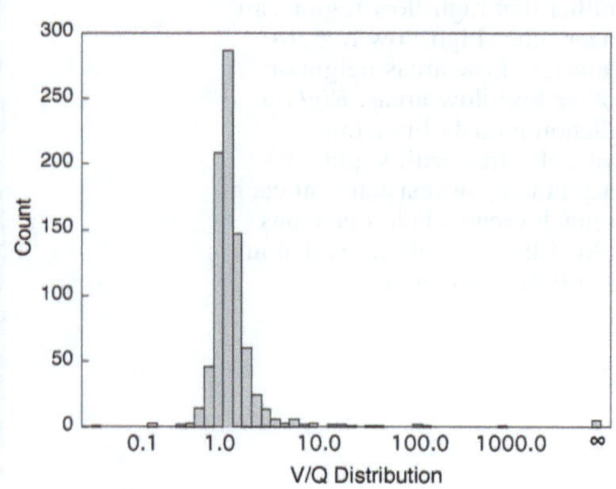

suggesting that gravity does play a role in coordinating the two.

What then is the primary mechanism by which ventilation and perfusion are matched in the normal lung? While hypoxic pulmonary vasoconstriction (HPV) can be invoked in abnormal lung regions, it is not clear that HPV is important in matching ventilation and perfusion in the normal lung. Glenny et al. [56] infused prostacyclin, a potent pulmonary vasodilator, into normal upright primates. Gas exchange, as measured by the A-aO_2 difference, did not change and the distributions of blood flow were not altered with vasodilatation in the normal lung. Melsom et al. [57] measured regional ventilation and perfusion distributions in awake, standing sheep at baseline breathing ambient air, during endogenous NO blockade, breathing NO free air, and breathing 30 ppm NO. They found no change in gas exchange or the distributions of ventilation or perfusion under any of the conditions. The same group also studied the effects of hypoxia and hyperoxia on ventilation and perfusion matching and found that acute changes in alveolar oxygen tensions can alter ventilation and perfusion matching but there was little effect with extended exposures to hypoxia or hyperoxia. A recent study in humans confirmed that various fractions of inhaled oxygen do not influence the heterogeneity of pulmonary perfusion [58]. Numerous studies in humans [59–62] have confirmed that inhaled NO or other vasodilators does not change pulmonary vascular resistance or gas exchange under normal conditions. The combined animal and human data strongly suggest that there is not an active mechanism matching regional ventilation and perfusion in the normal lung.

Although speculative, the simplest explanation is that the lung is constructed anatomically to match regional ventilation and perfusion. Evidence supporting this hypothesis is that airways and pulmonary arteries branch in union with each other [63]. This relationship arises during embryology when the primordial airways signal formation of adjacent endothelial cells into pulmonary arteries [64]. This makes the most sense from an engineering perspective because a system that does not require an active feedback loop to function is more robust and less likely to break down. If the geometries of the vascular and airway trees were similar and were the primary determinants of ventilation and blood flow, it is easy to imagine how ventilation and perfusion could be well matched despite having heterogeneous distributions. The argument against this hypothesis is that regional lung compliance is more important than airway caliber in determining regional ventilation. The potential rebuttal is that regional compliance and airway geometry may be closely linked through a concept of symmorphosis, developed by Weibel [65], where structural design is matched to functional demand. Weibel has noted that diameters of airways are grossly proportional to the size of the peripheral lung supplied by a given branch [66].

Clinical implications

The normal distributions of ventilation and blood flow change dramatically under pathological conditions and during mechanical ventilation. In these settings, the shared geometries of the airway and vascular trees cannot be the primary determinants of ventilation and perfusion matching. The result is less efficient gas exchange. A detailed review of these interactions is beyond the scope of this manuscript. However, an introductory outline is presented as a springboard to further reading and investigations.

Regional hypoxia, due to ventilation and perfusion mismatching, invokes hypoxic pulmonary vasoconstriction (HPV), thereby decreasing blood flow to hypoxic regions. The magnitude of the HPV response varies across the lung [67], is impaired during sepsis [68, 69], and can be greatly decreased with inhalational anesthetics [70] and vasodilators [71].

Mechanical ventilation, in and of itself, does not appear to alter the distribution of blood flow unless positive end expiratory pressure (PEEP) is applied [72, 73]. PEEP tends to create more zone I and II regions within the lung and may therefore increase the vertical gradient of perfusion [74]. Regional ventilation is redistributed with mechanical ventilation and induction of general anesthesia due to changes in diaphragmatic and chest wall motion. Froese and Bryan [75] demonstrated that, during spontaneous breathing, the major motion of the diaphragm is in dependent regions whereas during mechanical ventilation (with anesthesia and paralysis) the primary diaphragmatic motion shifts to the nondependent lung region. This change in diaphragmatic motion induces changes in regional ventilation [76]. Atelectasis occurs with mechanical ventilation and anesthesia [77], resulting in abnormal gas exchange unless HPV and mechanical compression of pulmonary vasculature divert blood flow away from these areas [72]. Lung protective strategies with low tidal volumes will compound this effect.

While pulmonary embolism has long been known to cause hypoxemia, the mechanism of ventilation and perfusion mismatching was not appreciated until recently [54]. By measuring regional blood flow and ventilation before and after the embolization of inert beads, Altemeier et al. demonstrated that, at baseline, high-blood-flow regions are matched with high-ventilation regions and low-blood-flow regions are matched with low-ventilation regions. The embolized beads distributed preferentially to high-blood-flow regions, redistributing blood to previously low-blood-flow regions. Because regional ventilation did not change, new regions with low ventilation/perfusion ratio were created, producing hypoxemia.

Regional lung compliance changes markedly with focal or diffuse lung injury, and consequently, regional ventilation will be altered. In adult respiratory distress syndrome (ARDS), regional lung injury is patchy, resulting in regions of both normal and abnormal compliance. This heterogeneity has lead to the concept of the "baby lung" [78] where much of the tidal volume is distributed to small regions of the lung that have better compliance. The relatively large tidal volumes that are distributed to the compliant lung regions are thought to be a potential mechanism for continued lung injury when normal tidal volumes are applied to the entire lung.

There has been increased interest in the effect of posture on gas exchange in critically ill patients [79, 80]. Although the mechanism by which the prone posture improves oxygenation has been extensively investigated, only speculative answers exist. In the normal lungs of large laboratory animals, ventilation is more evenly distributed and the correlation between regional ventilation and perfusion is greater in the prone compared with the supine posture [81]. This results in a narrower ventilation/perfusion distribution and improved gas exchange. Studies in humans using PET have demonstrated similar findings [52], although much of the redistribution observed may reflect changes in lung parenchyma rather than blood flow or ventilation [37]. As regional ventilation is determined by a combination of local compliance and airway geometry, a more uniform pleural pressure gradient in the prone posture may shift this balance towards airway geometry having a greater influence, improving the inherent matching between ventilation and blood flow.

The mechanism by which the prone posture improves gas exchange in the injured lung is equally speculative. A recent study by Richter et al. [82] used an ovine saline-lavage model of lung injury. They demonstrated that, in the supine posture, shunt occurs because perfusion is greatest in the dependent (dorsal) regions where lung is consolidated due to edema and atelectasis. With a change to the prone posture, the nondependent (dorsal) regions become better aerated while blood flow continues to be greatest in the nondependent (dorsal) region, leading to less shunt and improved gas exchange. This study nicely demonstrates the importance of the pulmonary arterial tree in determining blood flow distribution independent of gravity.

New perspective

Initial studies using external imaging methods identified vertical gradients of ventilation and perfusion in the lung, and gravity was invoked as the mechanism responsible for these distributions. As the spatial resolution of imaging methods improved, variability of perfusion and ventilation were identified within isogravitational planes. The observed heterogeneity was thought to be a random process imposed on the vertical gradient due to gravity. With the observation that this isogravitational heterogeneity was not random but correlated both spatially (similar among neighbors) and temporally (remains similar over time), the geometry of the vascular and airway trees was proposed as another determinant of perfusion and ventilation distributions. This perspective is comparable to other organs such as the heart and kidney where regional perfusion is almost solely dependent on the geometry of the vascular trees. Most physiologists would now agree that the regional distributions of blood flow and ventilation in the lung are determined by both hydrostatic gradients due to gravity and the geometry of the vascular and airway trees. The most important implication of this changing perspective is that it opens the door to new scientific questions that have not been fully considered, such as the mechanisms responsible for matching regional ventilation and perfusion in the normal lung. One speculation is that the shared geometries of the airway and vascular trees may provide some matching of ventilation and perfusion that does not require an active mechanism. In the diseased lung, regional hypoxia and altered lung compliance disrupt the inherent matching of ventilation and perfusion, leading to inefficient gas exchange.

References

1. Martin C, Cline F, Marshall H (1953) Lobar alveolar gas concentrations: effect of body position. J Clin Invest 32:617–621
2. Rahn H, Sadoul P, Farhi L, Shapiro J (1956) Distribution of ventilation and perfusion in the lobes of the dog's lung in the supine and erect position. J Appl Physiol 8:417–426
3. Anthonisen NR, Milic-Emili J (1966) Distribution of pulmonary perfusion in erect man. J Appl Physiol 21:760–766
4. Ball WC Jr, Stewart PB, Newsham LG, Bates DV (1962) Regional pulmonary function studied with xenon 133. J Clin Invest 41:519–531
5. Bryan AC, Bentivoglio LG, Beerel F, Macleish H, Zidulka A, Bates DV (1964) Factors affecting regional distribution of ventilation and perfusion in the lung. J Appl Physiol 19:395–402
6. Hughes JM, Glazier JB, Maloney JE, West JB (1968) Effect of lung volume on the distribution of pulmonary blood flow in man. Respir Physiol 4:58–72

7. Banister J, Torrance RW (1960) The effects of the tracheal pressure upon flow: pressure relations in the vascular bed of isolated lungs. Q J Exp Physiol Cogn Med Sci 45:352–367
8. West JB (1978) Regional differences in the lung. Chest 74:426–437
9. West JB (1977) Respiratory physiology: the essentials. Lippincott Williams & Wilkins, Baltimore
10. Reed JH Jr, Wood EH (1970) Effect of body position on vertical distribution of pulmonary blood flow. J Appl Physiol 28:303–311
11. Beck KC, Rehder K (1986) Differences in regional vascular conductances in isolated dog lungs. J Appl Physiol 61:530–538
12. Amis TC, Heather JD, Hughes JM, Jones HA, Rhodes CG (1979) Regional distribution of pulmonary ventilation and perfusion in the conscious dog [proceedings]. J Physiol 295:40P
13. Bryan AC, Milic-Emili J, Pengelly D (1966) Effect of gravity on the distribution of pulmonary ventilation. J Appl Physiol 21:778–784
14. Glaister DH (1970) Distribution of pulmonary blood flow and ventilation during forward (plus Gx) acceleration. J Appl Physiol 29:432–439
15. Hopkins SR, Henderson AC, Levin DL, Yamada K, Arai T, Buxton RB, Prisk GK (2007) Vertical gradients in regional lung density and perfusion in the supine human lung: the Slinky effect. J Appl Physiol 103:240–248
16. Olson LE, Rodarte JR (1984) Regional differences in expansion in excised dog lung lobes. J Appl Physiol 57:1710–1714
17. Hubmayr RD, Rodarte JR, Walters BJ, Tonelli FM (1987) Regional ventilation during spontaneous breathing and mechanical ventilation in dogs. J Appl Physiol 63:2467–2475
18. Sprung J, Deschamps C, Hubmayr RD, Walters BJ, Rodarte JR (1989) In vivo regional diaphragm function in dogs. J Appl Physiol 67:655–662
19. West JB (1962) Regional differences in gas exchange in the lung of erect man. J Appl Physiol 17:893–898
20. Michels DB, West JB (1978) Distribution of pulmonary ventilation and perfusion during short periods of weightlessness. J Appl Physiol 45:987–998
21. Harris RS, Schuster DP (2007) Visualizing lung function with positron emission tomography. J Appl Physiol 102:448–458
22. Hopkins SR, Levin DL, Emami K, Kadlecek S, Yu J, Ishii M, Rizi RR (2007) Advances in magnetic resonance imaging of lung physiology. J Appl Physiol 102:1244–1254
23. Petersson J, Sanchez-Crespo A, Larsson SA, Mure M (2007) Physiological imaging of the lung: single-photon-emission computed tomography (SPECT). J Appl Physiol 102:468–476
24. Robertson HT, Hlastala MP (2007) Microsphere maps of regional blood flow and regional ventilation. J Appl Physiol 102:1265–1272
25. Lisbona R, Dean GW, Hakim TS (1987) Observations with SPECT on the normal regional distribution of pulmonary blood flow in gravity independent planes. J Nucl Med 28:1758–1762
26. Melsom MN, Flatebo T, Kramer-Johansen J, Aulie A, Sjaastad OV, Iversen PO, Nicolaysen G (1995) Both gravity and non-gravity dependent factors determine regional blood flow within the goat lung. Acta Physiol Scand 153:343–353
27. Glenny RW, Lamm WJ, Albert RK, Robertson HT (1991) Gravity is a minor determinant of pulmonary blood flow distribution. J Appl Physiol 71:620–629
28. Glenny R (2008) Counterpoint: gravity is not the major factor determining the distribution of blood flow in the healthy human lung. J Appl Physiol 104:1533–1535; discussion 1535–1536
29. Glenny RW, Bernard S, Robertson HT, Hlastala MP (1999) Gravity is an important but secondary determinant of regional pulmonary blood flow in upright primates. J Appl Physiol 86:623–632
30. Glenny RW, Bernard SL, Robertson HT (2000) Pulmonary blood flow remains fractal down to the level of gas exchange. J Appl Physiol 89:742–748
31. Wagner WW Jr, Todoran TM, Tanabe N, Wagner TM, Tanner JA, Glenny RW, Presson RG Jr (1999) Pulmonary capillary perfusion: intra-alveolar fractal patterns and interalveolar independence. J Appl Physiol 86:825–831
32. Petersson J, Rohdin M, Sanchez-Crespo A, Nyren S, Jacobsson H, Larsson SA, Lindahl SG, Linnarsson D, Neradilek B, Polissar NL, Glenny RW, Mure M (2009) Regional lung blood flow and ventilation in upright humans studied with quantitative SPECT. Respir Physiol Neurobiol 166:54–60
33. Jones AT, Hansell DM, Evans TW (2001) Pulmonary perfusion in supine and prone positions: an electron-beam computed tomography study. J Appl Physiol 90:1342–1348
34. Burrowes KS, Tawhai MH (2006) Computational predictions of pulmonary blood flow gradients: gravity versus structure. Respir Physiol Neurobiol 154:515–523
35. Prisk GK, Guy HJ, Elliott AR, West JB (1994) Inhomogeneity of pulmonary perfusion during sustained microgravity on SLS-1. J Appl Physiol 76:1730–1738
36. Montmerle S, Sundblad P, Linnarsson D (2005) Residual heterogeneity of intra- and interregional pulmonary perfusion in short-term microgravity. J Appl Physiol 98:2268–2277
37. Petersson J, Rohdin M, Sanchez-Crespo A, Nyren S, Jacobsson H, Larsson SA, Lindahl SG, Linnarsson D, Neradilek B, Polissar NL, Glenny RW, Mure M (2007) Posture primarily affects lung tissue distribution with minor effect on blood flow and ventilation. Respir Physiol Neurobiol 156:293–303
38. Glenny RW, Lamm WJ, Bernard SL, An D, Chornuk M, Pool SL, Wagner WW Jr, Hlastala MP, Robertson HT (2000) Selected contribution: redistribution of pulmonary perfusion during weightlessness and increased gravity. J Appl Physiol 89:1239–1248
39. Glenny RW (1992) Spatial correlation of regional pulmonary perfusion. J Appl Physiol 72:2378–2386
40. West GB, Brown JH, Enquist BJ (1999) The fourth dimension of life: fractal geometry and allometric scaling of organisms. Science 284:1677–1679
41. Glenny RW, McKinney S, Robertson HT (1997) Spatial pattern of pulmonary blood flow distribution is stable over days. J Appl Physiol 82:902–907
42. Glenny RW, Bernard SL, Luchtel DL, Neradilek B, Polissar NL (2007) The spatial–temporal redistribution of pulmonary blood flow with postnatal growth. J Appl Physiol 102:1281–1288
43. Glenny R, Bernard S, Neradilek B, Polissar N (2007) Quantifying the genetic influence on mammalian vascular tree structure. Proc Natl Acad Sci USA 104:6858–6863
44. Glenny RW, Robertson HT (1998) Regional differences in the lung: a changing perspective on blood flow distribution. In: Hlastala MP, Robertson HT (eds) Complexity in structure and function of the lung. Dekker, New York, pp 461–481
45. Wagner WW Jr (2008) Point:Counterpoint: gravity is/is not the major factor determining the distribution of blood flow in the human lung. J Appl Physiol 104:1537
46. Melsom MN, Kramer-Johansen J, Flatebo T, Muller C, Nicolaysen G (1997) Distribution of pulmonary ventilation and perfusion measured simultaneously in awake goats. Acta Physiol Scand 159:199–208
47. Altemeier WA, McKinney S, Glenny RW (2000) Fractal nature of regional ventilation distribution. J Appl Physiol 88:1551–1557

48. Weibel ER (1991) Fractal geometry: a design principle for living organisms. Am J Physiol 261:L361–L369
49. Treppo S, Mijailovich SM, Venegas JG (1997) Contributions of pulmonary perfusion and ventilation to heterogeneity in V(A)/Q measured by PET. J Appl Physiol 82:1163–1176
50. Marcucci C, Nyhan D, Simon BA (2001) Distribution of pulmonary ventilation using Xe-enhanced computed tomography in prone and supine dogs. J Appl Physiol 90:421–430
51. Kreck TC, Krueger MA, Altemeier WA, Sinclair SE, Robertson HT, Shade ED, Hildebrandt J, Lamm WJ, Frazer DA, Polissar NL, Hlastala MP (2001) Determination of regional ventilation and perfusion in the lung using xenon and computed tomography. J Appl Physiol 91:1741–1749
52. Musch G, Layfield JD, Harris RS, Melo MF, Winkler T, Callahan RJ, Fischman AJ, Venegas JG (2002) Topographical distribution of pulmonary perfusion and ventilation, assessed by PET in supine and prone humans. J Appl Physiol 93:1841–1851
53. Petersson J, Sanchez-Crespo A, Rohdin M, Montmerle S, Nyren S, Jacobsson H, Larsson SA, Lindahl SG, Linnarsson D, Glenny RW, Mure M (2004) Physiological evaluation of a new quantitative SPECT method measuring regional ventilation and perfusion. J Appl Physiol 96:1127–1136
54. Altemeier WA, Robertson HT, Glenny RW (1998) Pulmonary gas-exchange analysis by using simultaneous deposition of aerosolized and injected microspheres. J Appl Physiol 85:2344–2351
55. Prisk GK, Fine JM, Cooper TK, West JB (2006) Vital capacity, respiratory muscle strength, and pulmonary gas exchange during long-duration exposure to microgravity. J Appl Physiol 101:439–447
56. Glenny RW, Robertson HT, Hlastala MP (2000) Vasomotor tone does not affect perfusion heterogeneity and gas exchange in normal primate lungs during normoxia. J Appl Physiol 89:2263–2267
57. Melsom MN, Flatebo T, Nicolaysen G (2000) No apparent effect of nitric oxide on the local matching of pulmonary perfusion and ventilation in awake sheep. Acta Physiol Scand 168:361–370
58. Arai TJ, Henderson AC, Dubowitz DJ, Levin DL, Friedman PJ, Buxton RB, Prisk GK, Hopkins SR (2008) Hypoxic pulmonary vasoconstriction does not contribute to pulmonary blood flow heterogeneity in normoxia in normal supine humans. J Appl Physiol 106:1034–1035
59. Brett SJ, Chambers J, Bush A, Rosenthal M, Evans TW (1998) Pulmonary response of normal human subjects to inhaled vasodilator substances. Clin Sci (Lond) 95:621–627
60. Frostell CG, Blomqvist H, Hedenstierna G, Lundberg J, Zapol WM (1993) Inhaled nitric oxide selectively reverses human hypoxic pulmonary vasoconstriction without causing systemic vasodilation. Anesthesiology 78:427–435
61. Rocca GD, Passariello M, Coccia C, Costa MG, Di Marco P, Venuta F, Rendina EA, Pietropaoli P (2001) Inhaled nitric oxide administration during one-lung ventilation in patients undergoing thoracic surgery. J Cardiothorac Vasc Anesth 15:218–223
62. Wilson WC, Kapelanski DP, Benumof JL, Newhart JW 2nd, Johnson FW, Channick RN (1997) Inhaled nitric oxide (40 ppm) during one-lung ventilation, in the lateral decubitus position, does not decrease pulmonary vascular resistance or improve oxygenation in normal patients. J Cardiothorac Vasc Anesth 11:172–176
63. Weibel E, Taylor C (1998) Functional design of the human lung for gas exchange. In: Fishman A (ed) Fishman's pulmonary diseaes and disorders. McGraw-Hill, New York, pp 21–61
64. Hislop A (2005) Developmental biology of the pulmonary circulation. Paediatr Respir Rev 6:35–43
65. Weibel ER, Taylor CR, Hoppeler H (1991) The concept of symmorphosis: a testable hypothesis of structure–function relationship. Proc Natl Acad Sci USA 88:10357–10361
66. Weibel ER, Sapoval B, Filoche M (2005) Design of peripheral airways for efficient gas exchange. Respir Physiol Neurobiol 148:3–21
67. Hlastala MP, Lamm WJ, Karp A, Polissar NL, Starr IR, Glenny RW (2004) Spatial distribution of hypoxic pulmonary vasoconstriction in the supine pig. J Appl Physiol 96:1589–1599
68. Frank DU, Lowson SM, Roos CM, Rich GF (1996) Endotoxin alters hypoxic pulmonary vasoconstriction in isolated rat lungs. J Appl Physiol 81:1316–1322
69. Ullrich R, Bloch KD, Ichinose F, Steudel W, Zapol WM (1999) Hypoxic pulmonary blood flow redistribution and arterial oxygenation in endotoxin-challenged NOS2-deficient mice. J Clin Invest 104:1421–1429
70. Marshall BE (1989) Effects of anesthetics on pulmonary gas exchange. In: Stanley T, Sperry R (eds) Anesthesia and the lung. Kluwer, London, pp 117–125
71. Marshall BE, Hanson CW, Frasch F, Marshall C (1994) Role of hypoxic pulmonary vasoconstriction in pulmonary gas exchange and blood flow distribution. 2. Pathophysiology. Intensive Care Med 20:379–389
72. Tokics L, Hedenstierna G, Strandberg A, Brismar B, Lundquist H (1987) Lung collapse and gas exchange during general anesthesia: effects of spontaneous breathing, muscle paralysis, and positive end-expiratory pressure. Anesthesiology 66:157–167
73. Walther SM, Domino KB, Glenny RW, Hlastala MP (1997) Pulmonary blood flow distribution in sheep: effects of anesthesia, mechanical ventilation, and change in posture. Anesthesiology 87:335–342
74. Walther SM, Domino KB, Glenny RW, Hlastala MP (1999) Positive end-expiratory pressure redistributes perfusion to dependent lung regions in supine but not in prone lambs. Crit Care Med 27:37–45
75. Froese AB, Bryan AC (1974) Effects of anesthesia and paralysis on diaphragmatic mechanics in man. Anesthesiology 41:242–255
76. Rehder K, Sessler AD, Rodarte JR (1977) Regional intrapulmonary gas distribution in awake and anesthetized-paralyzed man. J Appl Physiol 42:391–402
77. Reber A, Engberg G, Sporre B, Kviele L, Rothen HU, Wegenius G, Nylund U, Hedenstierna G (1996) Volumetric analysis of aeration in the lungs during general anaesthesia. Br J Anaesth 76:760–766
78. Gattinoni L, Pesenti A (2005) The concept of "baby lung". Intensive Care Med 31:776–784
79. Alsaghir AH, Martin CM (2008) Effect of prone positioning in patients with acute respiratory distress syndrome: a meta-analysis. Crit Care Med 36:603–609
80. Sud S, Sud M, Friedrich JO, Adhikari NK (2008) Effect of mechanical ventilation in the prone position on clinical outcomes in patients with acute hypoxemic respiratory failure: a systematic review and meta-analysis. CMAJ 178:1153–1161
81. Mure M, Domino KB, Lindahl SG, Hlastala MP, Altemeier WA, Glenny RW (2000) Regional ventilation-perfusion distribution is more uniform in the prone position. J Appl Physiol 88:1076–1083
82. Richter T, Bellani G, Scott Harris R, Vidal Melo MF, Winkler T, Venegas JG, Musch G (2005) Effect of prone position on regional shunt, aeration, and perfusion in experimental acute lung injury. Am J Respir Crit Care Med 172:480–487

H. Ait-Oufella
E. Maury
S. Lehoux
B. Guidet
G. Offenstadt

The endothelium: physiological functions and role in microcirculatory failure during severe sepsis

Abstract The endothelium is a highly dynamic cell layer that is involved in a multitude of physiological functions, including the control of vascular tone, the movement of cells and nutrients, the maintenance of blood fluidity and the growth of new vessels. During severe sepsis, the endothelium becomes proadhesive, procoagulant, antifibrinolytic and is characterized by alterations of vasomotor regulation. Most of these functions have been discovered using in vitro and animal models, but in vivo exploration of endothelium in patients remains difficult. New tools to analyze endothelial dysfunction at bedside have to be developed.

Keywords Endothelium · Sepsis · Coagulation · Cytokines

Introduction

The endothelium consists of a single cell layer lining all vessels, from their origin at the exit of the heart to their finest ramifications, the capillaries. In spite of being both widespread and functionally complex, the importance of this structure was long disregarded. Originally described by Harvey in the seventeenth century and further characterized by Malpighi, the cardiovascular system was considered as a simple pump and tubing device designed to convey oxygen and nutriments to peripheral organs. It does not help that the clinical setting had no telltale signs by which to identify endothelial health or disease. Nowhere in the classical triad of "palpation-auscultation-percussion" would endothelial state appear, no jaundice to give away hepatic distress or crackles pointing to left ventricular insufficiency. And when tools that could be used to explore endothelial functionality finally appeared, they were mainly confined to the research world and failed to greatly impact clinical practice. In spite of all these difficulties, the endothelium has grown in regard and appreciation, on its way to being recognized as an individual organ. As of today, the endothelium figures as a main topic in more than 80,000 publications cited in PubMed.

In this review, we will describe the main functions of the endothelium in an attempt to demonstrate its importance and complexity. We will describe both its physiological properties (see Table 1) and its anomalies in pathological states. We will give special notice to

M.R. Pinsky et al. (eds.), *Applied Physiology in Intensive Care Medicine 2: Physiological Reviews and Editorials*,
DOI 10.1007/978-3-642-28233-1_24, © Springer-Verlag Berlin Heidelberg 2012

Table 1 Examples of endothelial marker distribution according to EC location

Markers	Vascular territories
Von Willebrand factor	Veins > arteries, absent in hepatic sinusoids
t-PA	Abundant in the brain and lung circulation, but not in the pulmonary circulation
TFPI	Microvascular endothelium
Protein C receptor	Vessels of large diameter
Thrombomodulin	Absent in the brain
Endothelial NOS	Arteries > veins
VCAM-1	Abundant in the heart, present in the brain and the small intestine
P-selectin	Abundant in the lung, low expression in the muscle and the brain
CD36	Low expression in the brain

sepsis, a condition where endothelial distress is extreme, and a daily preoccupation in the intensive care units.

Histological description

The endothelium is composed of a single layer of cells that lines the interior surface of all blood vessels. It is estimated to comprise around 10^{13} cells, representing a weight of 1.5 kg and covering 4,000–7,000 m^2, equivalent to six football fields [1, 2].

Endothelial cells (EC) lie at the interface of the circulating blood and the vessel wall. They are flattened cells, having a thickness of about 0.5 μm, and are 100 μm long by 10 μm wide. Their lozenge shapes are juxtaposed in a mosaic such that their long axis is oriented in the direction of blood flow. They are attached to a basal membrane rich in collagen and glycoproteins, forming a complex interface between the circulation and the platelet-activating, pro-coagulant vascular matrix.

EC appositions can be quite variable from one vascular bed to the next, ranging from juxtaposition to overlapping, allowing for an intricate regulation of protein permeability across the endothelium. At one or many points along the intercellular space, neighboring membranes form tight junctions or gap junctions. The former is multifocal membrane fusions that are perfectly tight, whereas the latter consist of a joining of two close cellular membranes around a central channel that allows the exchange of ions, various metabolites and regulatory factors.

At their surface, ECs are lined with a very fine and fragile layer called the glycocalyx. First identified in the 1960s thanks to electronic microscopy [3], it consists of glycoproteins, glycosaminoglycans and proteoglycans [4]. There are five types of glycosaminoglycans including heparan sulfate, a cofactor for antithrombin III that amplifies its anti-thrombotic properties, and dermatan sulfate, which interacts with heparin cofactor II [5]. Globally, the glycocalyx provides an anticoagulant layer because of its negative electrical charge that repels circulating platelets and that allows it to interact with and catalyze the interactions of vitamin K-dependent coagulation factors.

In forming a dense and intermeshed network, the glycocalyx provides a first-line barrier, regulating the cellular and macromolecular traffic at the forefront of the endothelium [6]. Numerous animal studies have demonstrated that destruction of the glycocalyx, using enzymatic approaches, for example, leads to increased capillary permeability [7]. In vivo, degradation of the glycocalyx with heparinase favors tight contacts between circulating leukocytes and the endothelium, through denudation of the protective barrier that normally prevents this [8].

Electronic microscopy recently revealed two characteristic elements of endothelial cells: pinocytic vesicles and Weibel-Palade bodies. Pinocytic vesicles consist of transcellular transport vesicles that shuttle from the apical to the basolateral aspect of endothelial cells. Weibel-Palade bodies are protein-stocking vesicles that appear as plentiful dense bodies, typically containing von Willebrand factor and P selectin.

Endothelial plasticity

At the interface between a liquid phase, blood plasma, and a solid structure, basal membrane, endothelial cells are highly influenced by their environment. They can rapidly modulate their structure and function in response to chemical or physical stimuli, such as a change in blood flow. For example, ECs cultured in vitro have a characteristic cobblestone morphology. However, if cells are placed in a perfusion chamber and exposed to a shear stress that mimics the frictional force of blood flow, they quickly align in the direction of flow, owing to a rearrangement in cytoskeletal proteins [9]. The same elongated morphology is observed in vivo in ECs lining arteries, where shear stress is 30–50 times greater than in veins. In fact, this effect is manifest in coronary bypass grafts in humans. The ECs from saphenous veins, once placed in the arterial context, quickly elongate in the direction of the long axis, parallel to blood flow [10]. Numerous receptors responsible for this response to shear stress, termed mechanosensors, have been identified: tyrosine kinase receptors, integrins, ion channels, G protein-coupled receptors and NADPH oxidases [11].

At the abluminal aspect, the endothelium is affixed to and interacts with the extracellular matrix constituents of the basal membrane, such that the nature of this matrix influences the form and the function of ECs [12]. Jalali et al. [13] showed that ECs grown on fibronectin- or vitronectin-coated surfaces respond differently to shear stress; surface expression of integrins differed both in terms of quantity and distribution from one matrix to the next. ECs adapt very quickly to changes in their environment. In humans, it was shown by RT-PCR of postoperative amygdala that the genetic programming of ECs removed from their native environment changes within a few hours [14]. This should be heeded as a cautionary tale when considering the interpretation of studies using endothelial cells cultured ex vivo or in vitro.

Physiological functions of the endothelium

Primary hemostasis comprises a series of events that occur as a result of a vascular lesion and terminate with the formation of a stable platelet-rich blood clot, paving the way for tissue repair mechanisms that will be followed by fibrinolysis [15]. Endothelial cells play a role in each step of this process since they participate in platelet activation and produce factors involved in the coagulation cascade and in the fibrinolytic system.

When a vascular lesion occurs, an immediate vascular constriction occurs, which reduces blood flow locally and concentrates the repair mechanisms. This is quickly followed by platelet adhesion to the vascular wall [16]. The endothelium, focally destroyed, leaves exposed in its place to the underlying matrix rich in collagen and von Willebrand factor, to which the platelets attach through membrane glycoproteins. The glycoproteins GPIa and VI quickly and reversibly interact with collagen, whereas GPIb-IX-V binds von Willebrand factor. In the veins, where shear stress is much lower, platelets can adhere more readily to damaged endothelium via $\alpha 2\beta 3$ integrins [15]. Adherent platelets become activated, shifting from an oblong morphology to an irregular shape with multiple pseudopods, expressing adhesion receptors at their surface (P-selectin and integrins) and shedding their granulocyte contents [adenosine diphosphate (ADP), serotonin] into the extracellular space. These combined effects result in the attraction and activation of circulating platelets, conglomerating into a dense mass reinforced by a fibrin network. But ECs also oppose primary hemostasis by liberating vasodilator substances [prostacyclin, nitric oxide (NO)] and ADPases that catabolize ADP, one of the most potent platelet activators.

Any deficit in molecules involved in platelet adhesion, such as Bernard-Soulier's disease (GPIb-IX-V deficit/dysfunction) or Glanzman's thrombasthenia ($\alpha 2\beta 3$ deficit/dysfunction), is characterized by facilitated bleeding episodes, either spontaneous or elicited by minor traumas.

Anticoagulant properties

The anticoagulant activity of the endothelium is geared at restricting the generation of thrombin. Several factors are implicated in this process. Heparan sulfate and dermatan sulfate, two glycocalyx glycosaminoglycans, potentiate the activity of two anticoagulant enzymes, antithrombin III (by a factor of 100) [17, 18] and heparin cofactor II, respectively [19]. The endothelium produces tissue factor pathway inhibitor (TFPI), which binds to activated factor X and then inhibits the tissue factor-activated factor VII complex [20]. ECs produce thrombomodulin (TM) that is either attached to the membrane or released into the circulation. Its plasma levels are increased in a number of pathologies where the endothelium is injured (see sepsis). TM binds to the surface of protein C and increases its anticoagulant activity by associating with its specific cofactor, protein S [21]. Finally, the endothelium accelerates activation of protein C by expressing on its surface another receptor, endothelial protein C receptor (EPCR) [22]. Protein C, when activated by all its cofactors, inhibits factors V and VIII. Finally, TM has its own intrinsic anticoagulant activity since several works have demonstrated its ability to bind and directly inhibit activated factor X [23].

Procoagulant properties

The major step in the acquisition by the endothelium of a procoagulant phenotype involves the expression of factor tissue (TF). In vitro, TF is induced by several mediators such as thrombin, endotoxin, cytokines, shear stress, hypoxia or oxidized lipids [24, 25]. Its procoagulant activity is accentuated in the presence of anionic phospholipids that are exposed by apoptotic cells [26, 27]. In the presence of agonists, the levels of TF protein and messenger RNA decline rapidly, presumably to avoid too rapid fibrin extension. Despite these in vitro findings, it remains difficult to show an actual endothelial expression of TF.

Once expressed, TF binds and activates factor VII. The TF-VIIa complex in turn mainly activates factors IX and X. These factors are anchored by their gammacarboxic residues to the membrane phospholipids of platelets and endothelial cells. This latter precision serves to remind us that reactions of the coagulation cascade do not take place in the liquid plasma phase, but rather in the solid phase, usually on cellular membranes or developing clots. Given its position and surface area, the endothelium is the main surface on which the coagulation reaction takes place.

The contact between coagulation factors and the vascular wall occurs either via non-specific physical interactions or through specific receptors synthesized by ECs. Thrombin binds a surface receptor called protease-activating factor (PAR-1) and influences the formation of fibrin and amplifies the coagulation cascade. The PAR-1 receptor is itself activated and induces the expression of different genes (TF, NO, endothelin) [28], illustrating the complex entanglement of the multiple functions of EC, namely coagulation, regulation of vasomotor tone and leukocyte adhesion. Other thrombin receptors such as PAR-2 [29] and PAR-3 [30], which are expressed by ECs and other cell types (platelets, bone marrow precursors), have been described.

Role in fibrinolysis

The endothelium also has physiological profibrinolytic effects. Tissue plasminogen activator (t-PA), the main activator of intravascular fibrinolysis, is a protease released by ECs that transforms plasminogen into plasmin. This reaction occurs either on the endothelial cell surface or on a platelet clot. The plasmin degrades fibrin and releases degradation products of fibrin or D-dimers into the circulation. In vitro, fibrinolytic properties have been documented in different types of ECs, and the ability to express t-PA was therefore ascribed to the endothelium as a whole. However, the in vivo situation is less straightforward. Immunohistochemistry and in situ hybridization studies have detected t-PA solely in the microcirculation, and only in certain territories [31]. Another plasminogen activator, urinary type plasminogen activator (u-PA), was located exclusively at the renal level [32]; it is expressed only in tissue repair processes and during angiogenesis, suggesting that it plays an important role in cell migration and tissue remodeling. Nonetheless, u-PA has a role in vascular homeostasis and the fight against infections since u-PA knockout mice show an exaggerated response to lipopolysaccharide (LPS) injection, characterized by widespread parietal inflammation [33] and extended thrombosis [34].

Two inhibitors control the fibrinolytic system: $\alpha 2$ antiplasmin (a plasmin inhibitor) and plasminogen activation inhibitor (PAI-1, PAI-2 and PAI-3). PAI-1, produced by the liver and activated endothelium, is the most studied inhibitor, and it seems to have the greatest affinity for plasminogen activator. PAI-1 also plays a major role in inflammation through several mechanisms, including induction of lymphocyte and neutrophil recruitment, activation of neutrophils (through Toll-like receptor 4) and clearance of apoptotic cells [35].

Regulation of vasomotor tone

The endothelium is a significant contributor to the regulation of vasomotor tone, under the influence of physical and chemical factors originating from the vascular lumen or the surrounding tissues. ECs produce and release vasodilator substances such as NO and prostacyclin, and vasoconstrictor mediators such as endothelin and platelet-activating factor (PAF). The production of NO by the endothelium is constitutive and modulated by different stimuli, whereas the synthesis of other mediators (prostacyclin, endothelin and PAF) is inducible.

NO is the most important vasodilator arising from the endothelium [36]. It is produced from L-arginine by the constitutive endothelial NO synthase (eNOS), which is activated by increased intracellular calcium and phosphorylation [37]. Agents capable of stimulating eNOS through specific receptors include ADP, bradykinin, substance P and muscarinic agonists, as well as physical forces (shear stress and pulsatile tensile strain). For example, the rise in blood flow during physical exercise increases shear stress, activating eNOS, which allows for vasodilatation [38]. There are two other forms of NOS: the calcium-dependent neuronal NOS (nNOS) and the calcium-independent inducible NOS (iNOS), which is activated mainly by pro-inflammatory cytokines. Regarding endothelium-dependent vasodilatation, tribute should be made to the discovery by Furchgott and Zawadzki, published in 1980 in *Nature*. The authors found that in precontracted vessels, acetylcholine was a vasodilator in the presence of endothelium, whereas after endothelial denudation acetylcholine had no effect. The end point of this process was the production of NO in the endothelium, which diffuses in the media and activates soluble guanylate cyclase, responsible for production of cyclic GMP in smooth muscle cells (SMC), which in turn activates protein kinase G. The latter enzyme reduces the stock of free cytosolic calcium and inhibits the contraction of SMCs by myosin dephosphorylation [39]. Finally, NO has other functions. It inhibits the activation and adherence of platelets to the endothelium, and it promotes disaggregation platelets during the formation of the hemostatic plug [40].

Endothelin (ET) is produced by the endothelium uniquely in response to stimuli such as hypoxia or shear stress [41]. As is the case for NO, ET diffuses in depth and binds to its specific receptor present at the surface of SMCs. This G protein-coupled receptor promotes the release of calcium from the endoplasmic reticulum and induces vasoconstriction. This effect persists long after the dissociation of ET from its receptor by maintenance of a high intracytoplasmic calcium concentration.

Prostacyclin is an eicosanoid derived from arachidonic acid that acts as a paracrine factor. It causes vasodilatation and inhibits platelet aggregation.

Platelet-activating factor (PAF) is a phospholipid that is also derived from the metabolism of arachidonic acid. It causes vasoconstriction and stimulates the adhesion of leukocytes to the endothelium [42, 43].

Leukocyte interactions

When there is a need to quickly eliminate a pathogen or to clean a necrotic area, ECs express adhesion molecules that regulate leukocyte trafficking between the circulating blood and the surrounding tissue. The interaction between leukocytes and ECs follows a conventional set of steps that include short contacts, more prolonged contacts, then leukocyte rolling and strong adhesion before transendothelial migration. Different adhesion molecules intervene at each stage of this process. The selectins (E-and L-selectin) mediate the first phase, as they resist the forces of shear stress and bind (and release) very quickly [44]. The integrins $\alpha 4\beta 7$ and $\alpha 4\beta 1$ are involved in the adhesion of monocytes and polynuclear neutrophils. The subsequent rolling and firm adhesion involve the molecules of the superfamily of immunoglobulins [intercellular adhesion molecule (ICAM-1, ICAM-2) and vascular adhesion molecule (VCAM)] [45, 46], joined by platelet endothelial cell adhesion molecule (PECAM) at the time of diapedesis [47]. This latter process is a complex phenomenon involving the separation of cadherins at tight junctions [48].

In addition to its participation in the innate immune response, the endothelium participates in the adaptive response involving T lymphocytes [49]. ECs in culture express major histocompatibility complex class I (MHC I) and can present antigen to CD8+ cytotoxic T lymphocytes. Furthermore, after stimulation by interferon gamma, they express MHC class II and can interact with CD4+ lymphocytes [50]. ECs can also express LFA-3 (CD58) or B7.2 (CD86) costimulation molecules at their surface, molecules common to other antigen-presenting cells (dendritic cells, macrophages, B lymphocytes) [51]. Moreover, it is now accepted that the ECs are involved in the pathophysiology of graft rejection [52].

Table 2 Endothelial cell implication in various physiological processes through secretion or expression of different molecules

Hemostasis	
Primary hemostasis	
Activation	Von Willebrand factor
Inhibition	Nitric oxide
Coagulation cascade	
Activation	Tissue factor
Inhibition	Tissue factor pathway inhibitor, endothelial protein C receptor, thrombomodulin, heparan/dermatan sulfate
Fibrinolysis	
Activation	Tissue plasminogen activator, urinary plasminogen activator
Inhibition	Plasminogen activator inhibitor
Vasomotor tone regulation	
Dilation	Nitric oxide, prostacyclin
Constriction	Endothelin, thomboxane A_2, platelet-activating factor
Inflammation	
Adhesion	E-selectin, VCAM, ICAM
Co-stimulation	LFA-3, CD80/86
Chemokines	MIP-1 (and -2), MCP-1
Cytokines	IL-1, IL-6, IL-8, TNFα

Endothelial heterogeneity

All ECs share common properties, but also distinct features, that are expressed both during physiological processes and in adverse conditions. This complexity, called endothelial heterogeneity, is so important that we should use the plural form, endothelia (see Table 2). This concept was first brought up by histologists, who distinguished, for example, the continuous endothelium of the brain from the fenestrated endothelium of endocrine glands. The clinicians then showed that ECs were differentially affected by various pathologies; diabetes disturbs the renal and retinal microcirculation especially [53], whereas veno-occlusive liver disease targets vessels of the hepatic sinusoids [54], and thrombotic microangiopathies affect the entire microcirculation with the exception of liver and lungs [55]. That structural differences distinguish endothelial cells according to organ function was then confirmed experimentally. Electron microscopy highlighted differences in the location of the nucleus within the cell or the composition of cytoplasm depending on the site at which ECs are found. Accordingly, in the frog the intracellular volume occupied by Weibel-Palade bodies gradually diminishes from the aortic root to the microcirculation (8% of the cytoplasm in the thoracic aorta versus 0.3% in the capillaries) [56].

This heterogeneity exists for all endothelial functions, and to ignore it exposes us to errors of interpretation. For example, a decrease in the endothelial expression of TM was shown in biopsies of purpuric lesions in children with meningococcal disease [57]. In the brain, ECs do not express TM [58]. Does this mean that the cerebral endothelium was in a state of continuous activation? Of course not. The most likely explanation is that TM is not involved in the hemostatic balance of the brain.

EC heterogeneity also concerns the intensity of the endothelial response to stimuli and endothelial response cannot be likened to a simple on/off switch but rather to a dimmer switch where, for a given gene activation cascade, the expression of a protein can vary between two extremes [59]. What is most challenging is to assess this expression level and deduce the endothelial status: inactivated, activated or abnormally active (dysfunctional). Such distinctions are subtle, and unfortunately limited by the current lack of tools that allow for precise assessment of endothelial function.

Endothelial dysfunction during sepsis

The endothelium is actively involved in defending the body against pathogens by recruiting the leukocytes to infected sites, releasing inflammatory mediators and promoting local coagulation to prevent the spread of blood-borne infection. However, this normally focused adaptative response can become generalized and amplified during sepsis, causing tissue damage. This is referred to as endothelial dysfunction.

Endothelial denudation

Sepsis is accompanied by morphological changes of the endothelium. The injection of LPS in animals induces a detachment of ECs from the basal membrane and causes sub-endothelial edema [60, 61]. Cell lesions include nuclear vacuolation, protrusion and cytoplasmic fragmentation. The time of onset varies from a few minutes, after LPS injection [62], to several hours, in the model of cecal ligation/perforation [63]. This phenomenon has also been observed in humans [64]. Using a double-tagged cell (Von Willebrand factor receptor and EGF), Mutunga et al. showed that the number of circulating ECs was higher in septic patients than in healthy subjects, and even higher in cases of septic shock. Inflammatory mediators released by leucocytes (TNF, IL1, interferon, oxygen free radicals) and hypoxia increase EC apoptosis [65–67]. Apoptotic ECs in turn express adhesion molecules (ICAM-1, VCAM) and release oxygen free radicals, and in doing so amplify the recruitment of white blood cells. Apoptotic ECs also externalize negatively charged phosphatidylserine on the cell membrane and thus expose the circulating blood to a procoagulant surface [26]. Membrane charge asymmetry coupled with the activity of certain enzymes (floppase, scramblase, etc.) allows for the budding and release of membrane microparticles in the circulation [68]. These microparticles, a combination of phospholipid membrane fragments and surface proteins (TF), are involved in spreading endothelial dysfunction [69] and participate in the disseminated intravascular coagulation [70].

Endothelial barrier impairment favors the passage of cells, inflammatory mediators and plasma into the interstitial compartment. The rapid increase in vascular permeability to albumin, which occurs within 6 h of the insult, affects the pulmonary and systemic circulation heterogeneously [71]. In terms of skin and muscles, the injection of endotoxin induces an increase in vascular permeability irrespective of oncotic and hydrostatic pressure, indicating abnormalities of the cell membrane [72].

Pro-adhesive properties

Increased expression of endothelial adhesion molecules either at the membrane level or in the plasma typify the different models of sepsis [73]. In vitro incubation of ECs with bacterial LPS induces the rapid expression of ICAM-1 and E-selectin mRNA. The same effect is obtained by replacing LPS with the plasma of healthy volunteers treated with very low doses of LPS. In this latter experiment, the addition of antibodies blocking TNFα and/or IL-1β at the same time as human plasma inhibits the transcription of mRNA, illustrating the fact that cytokines released by endotoxemia induce in turn the expression of E-selectin and ICAM-1 [74]. Moreover, there is a close relationship between plasma levels of adhesion molecules and consequences of sepsis [75]. In human sepsis, a study has shown that the higher the plasma levels of ICAM-1, the greater the number of organs damaged and the mortality. In animals, the genetic or pharmacological blockade of ICAM-1 protects against endotoxin shock [76].

As regards E-selectin, several human studies have also shown an increase in its soluble form in healthy volunteers receiving an injection of LPS [77] or in patients hospitalized for sepsis [78]. The level of E-selectin in the plasma is positively correlated with the severity of sepsis in patients, evaluated by the SAPSII score or the multiple organ failure (MOF) score [79]. Increased plasma adhesion molecules reflect an increase in the endothelial membrane expression of the proteins and can be directly related to activation and/or dysfunction of the endothelium. It promotes rolling and firm adherence of neutrophils, and ultimately results in their accumulation in organs. This accumulation is in part beneficial, eliminating infectious agents, but it may also exacerbate tissue damage through the production of inflammatory mediators such as cytokines, proteases and oxygen free radicals [80]. A recently published study illustrated this paradigm. Ye et al. [81] selectively inhibited NF-κB activity in the endothelium of adult mice. After LPS injection, these animals were characterized by a decrease in endothelial adhesion molecule expression (ICAM-1, E-selectin), a decrease of neutrophil infiltration in several organs (lung, liver, kidney) and a decrease in tissue damage. In fine, selective endothelial NF-κB inhibition improved survival in endotoxinemic mice. Platelets also contribute to the recruitment of neutrophils, illustrating the complex entanglement between inflammation and coagulation that regulates the pathophysiology of septic shock. Using a perfusion chamber model lined with ECs, where leukocytes circulate in a closed system, Blanks et al. [82] showed that the simultaneous infusion of platelets significantly increases EC-neutrophil interaction. They showed that the binding of platelet P-selectin to its receptor P-selectin glycoprotein ligand 1 (PSGL-1) on polymorphonuclear leukocytes induced the expression of VLA-4, another molecule responsible for adhesion to the endothelium. The relevance of this interaction in vivo has been documented in the cecal ligation and puncture model of sepsis in mice, where platelet depletion reduced leukocyte infiltration in the lung and lesion edema [83].

Pro-coagulant properties

Different studies undertaken in animals and humans have shown that severe sepsis is characterized by a pro-coagulant state [84]. The injection of LPS in healthy volunteers induces the rapid expression of TF by circulating monocytes [85]. Similar results were observed in patients with meningococcemia, with additive prognostic value since the cellular expression of TF was higher among patients who died [86]. The production of endothelial TF is more difficult to document. In infected animals, TF was located at the endothelium of tissue sections [87]. However, such direct evidence is scarce in humans. By analogy, one can cite the example of patients with sickle cell disease, in whom Solovey et al. [88] identified circulating endothelial cells expressing TF.

The TF expressed during sepsis activates coagulation and leads to the formation of thrombin (see Fig. 1). In parallel, counter-regulatory systems (involving the endothelium) such as protein C and TFPI are defective, maintaining intravascular coagulation. The decrease in activated plasma protein C (aPC) in sepsis is partly due to decreased hepatic synthesis of protein C and increased systemic consumption of the protein. Adding to this are complex enzymatic alterations that affect thrombomodulin (TM), whose primary function is to amplify the activation of protein C. In vitro, TNF-α and IL-1 decrease endothelial expression of TM. Moreover, the granulocytes recruited at the inflammatory site release elastases that cleave and inactivate endothelial TM [89, 90]. These experimental results have been corroborated by a study in children with purpura fulminans. From skin biopsies, Faust et al. [57] showed a decreased expression of endothelial TM and endothelial cell protein receptor. In the blood, the levels of protein C, protein S and antithrombin III were also reduced. Moreover, in another study on adults with sepsis, a low rate of aPC was identified as a factor of poor prognosis [91]. The accumulated evidence on the beneficial role of aPC in sepsis has led to serious therapeutic studies. After encouraging results in animals [92] a multicenter international study was conducted. The PROWESS study, published in 2001, showed

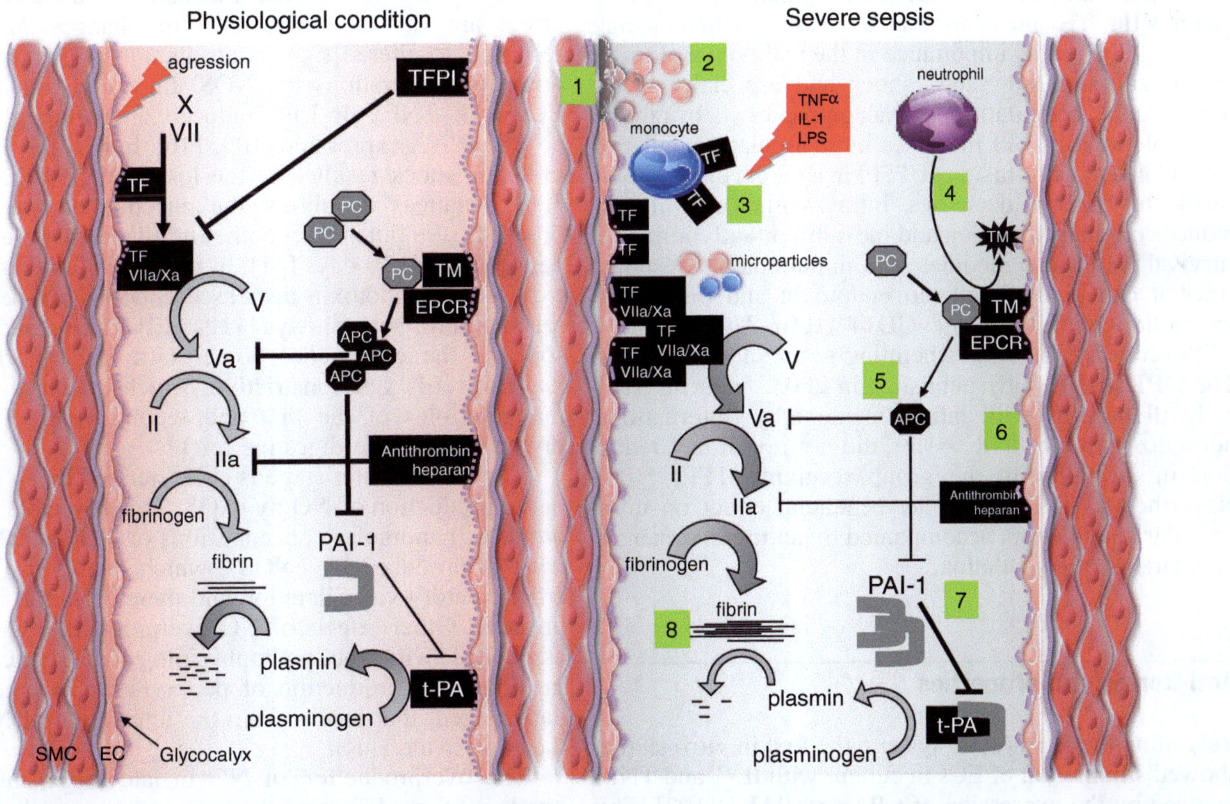

Fig. 1 Physiologically, after vascular aggression, endothelial cells express TF and initiate the coagulation cascade that leads to thrombin activation and fibrin deposition. At the same time, anticoagulant pathways and fibrinolysis are activated to avoid disseminated coagulation and limit fibrin accumulation. In severe sepsis, several disorders occur: endothelial cell apoptosis (*1*), microparticle shedding (*2*), procoagulant phenotype switch with TF expression (ECs, monocytes and microparticles) (*3*) and activation of the coagulation cascade. Alteration of anticoagulant pathways involve: TM degradation by neutrophil elastase (*4*), decreased APC levels (*5*), glycocalyx degradation (*6*), alteration of fibrinolytic pathways with increased PAI-1 activity (*7*) and consecutive fibrin accumulation (*8*)

in a cohort of 1,690 patients that administration of aPC in septic patients with at least two visceral failures reduced the relative mortality by 20% at 28 days [93]. Unfortunately, secondary studies have been disappointing. The ADDRESS study, which evaluated the role of aPC in septic patients with only one organ failure, provided no evidence of benefit in terms of survival and was stopped for "futility" [94]. The RESOLVE study in children with meningococcemia was also negative on composite criteria measuring the resolution of organ failure [95]. A number of limitations have been advanced to explain these negative results, and the controversy regarding the place of aPC in the treatment of severe sepsis remains. Patient selection provides a major point of argument because secondary analysis of the PROWESS trial showed that aPC improved survival in the more severe patients [96, 97]. It is important to note that aPC has other beneficial functions apart from its role in coagulation. In experimental models, aPC mediates anti-apoptotic effects, reduces endothelial barrier permeability and decreases pro-inflammatory cytokine production [98]. For all these reasons, the relationship between aPC and severe sepsis remains relevant.

TFPI is another powerful anticoagulant that binds to factor VIIa, TF and factor Xa. Several lines of evidence have highlighted its importance in the pathophysiology of organ failure during septic shock and especially in the intravascular coagulation that accompanies it. In rabbits, the depletion of TFPI increases intravascular coagulation [99]. Conversely, infusion of TFPI in a model of endotoxin shock in baboon decreases intravascular coagulation, reduces organ dysfunction and most importantly improves survival. TFPI also modulates the inflammatory response since it can bind directly to endotoxin and prevent its interaction with leukocyte CD14 [100]. Unfortunately, TFPI proved to be underwhelming in the clinical setting. The OPTIMIST study published in 2003, featuring critically ill patients with mild coagulopathy (international normalized ration, INR > 1.2), did not reveal any reduction in mortality in the group receiving TFPI [101]. Nevertheless, TFPI had a net beneficial effect on intravascular coagulation, accompanied by an improvement in the markers of coagulation.

Anti-fibrinolytic properties

Regarding the fibrinolytic system, the first in vitro studies showed stimulation of ECs in culture with IL-1 and TNFα induced by the expression of t-PA and PAI-1 [102]. This orientation towards an anti-fibrinolytic phenotype has been difficult to confirm in humans. Some studies have shown increased levels of PAI-1 in the blood of septic patients (both adults and children) [103, 104], and PAI-1 levels are positively related to unfavorable outcomes [105]. Some gene polymorphisms of PAI-1 have been demonstrated to affect the risk of death during meningococcal infection [106]. The final result is heterogenous fibrin deposition, which exacerbates local ischemia [107]. For example, injection of LPS in mice induced deposition fibrin in the kidney, liver and heart, but not in the lung. In the baboon, the injection of lethal doses of *Escherichia coli* induced fibrin deposition in the spleen, hepatic sinusoids and renal glomeruli, but had little effect on the brain, heart and aorta.

Impaired regulation of vasomotor tone

In severe infectious states, emergency care is sought primarily to restore hemodynamic stability due to an imbalance in vasomotor tone and interstitial plasma leakage. Endothelial dysfunction and especially disturbances in NO production are the main causes of circulatory insufficiency.

Disrupted production of NO in the course of sepsis is complex and evolves over time. The first stage, called nitrosopenia, is characterized by decreased production of NO by eNOS [108]. The mechanisms underlying this effect are diverse, ranging from changes in surface receptors to altered signal transduction to quantitative or qualitative alterations in eNOS. In vitro, stimulation of ECs with TNFα or LPS induced a downregulation of eNOS mRNA expression [109, 110]. In rats, the induction of septic shock resulted in the loss of endothelial eNOS [111], whereas in rabbits, the injection of a non-lethal dose of LPS altered endothelium-dependent relaxation between 5 and 20 days [61]. In healthy volunteers, a brief exposure to endotoxin decreased endothelium-dependent relaxation for several days [112, 113]. During early nitrosopenia, the endothelial homeostatic balance therefore leans towards vasoconstriction, which affects the proximal arterioles of the first and second order of certain organs such as the digestive tract.

The second, later stage is characterized by an increase in the production of NO by iNOS. This inducible enzyme produces nanomolar concentrations of NO (1,000-fold of what is produced by eNOS), which causes diffuse microcirculatory vasodilatation and therefore a fall in blood pressure. Other effects of NO overproduction have been associated with the pathophysiology of septic shock, including the production of peroxynitrite, a potent oxidative agent that results from the interaction of NO with the superoxide anion.

The overproduction of NO in late sepsis inspired a number of studies aimed at assessing the therapeutic potential of NOS inhibition. However, results in animals have been contradictory, in part because different models of sepsis were used, coupled with diverse treatments and inhibitors [114–116]. In humans, the first attempts at blocking NOS appeared encouraging, with improved hemodynamic parameters (but no effect on mortality)

[117, 118]. Finally, a large international multi-center study was carried out in 2004. Seven hundred ninety-seven patients suffering from severe sepsis were treated with either a placebo or a non-selective blocker of NOS, L-NAME. The phase III trial was stopped prematurely because despite an improvement in circulatory parameters, administration of L-NAME was accompanied by excess mortality [119]. After the failure of this approach, several studies investigated the beneficial properties of NO. This led to the notion that it is not NO that is responsible for the circulatory failure in sepsis, but rather by its overproduction by iNOS. Therefore new research avenues today are targeting the activation of iNOS [109].

Finally, it is important to remember that advancements in the field of resuscitation are mainly based on experimental animal studies. Disappointing results obtained in the clinical trials could be partially due to significant physiopathological differences between species. At present, the tools available for the assessment of endothelial function in humans are limited and difficult to use in the bedside setting. Orthogonal polarized spectral (OPS) imaging in the sublingual area is an interesting technique that provides information about capillary density, the proportion of perfused capillaries [120] or glycocalyx size [121]. Topical application of pharmacological agents such as acetylcholine improves specific analysis of endothelial function. However, analysis of OPS data requires time and computer assistance and cannot yet help clinicians at the bedside.

Vascular oxidative stress

During severe sepsis, reactive oxygen species (ROS) such as superoxide (O_2^-) are produced in large amounts [122]. Neutrophils are the main source of ROS, but endothelial cells also synthesize ROS in response to oxidative agents or cytokines. For example, in vitro LPS/IFNγ-stimulated ECs produce superoxide within 2 h through the NADPH oxidase pathway. ROS accumulate in ECs and are modified; dismutation of superoxide forms hydrogen peroxide (H_2O_2) and nitration of superoxide forms peroxynitrite ($ONOO^-$). Both products are toxic for proteins and DNA, and could participate in endothelial cell damage [123]. ROS decrease NO availability through peroxynitrite formation and eNOS inhibition, and ultimatly affect vascular tone, platelet adhesion [124] and permeability [125]. These modifications lead to vascular occlusion and exacerbate organ hypoperfusion. Finally, to illustrate entanglement of complex phenomena in severe sepsis, experimental studies have shown that ROS could activate NF-κB, a major transcription factor for genes involved in inflammation [126], and could induce TF expression [127].

Beneficial effects of antioxidants in sepsis have been reported. In mice, vitamin C injections prevent LPS-induced edema and hypotension [128]. In a randomized, prospective, double-blind, placebo-controlled trial with 226 critically ill patients, 28-day survival was increased in the patients that received a combination of vitamin C and E. These data represent a new field of study and warrant further investigation [129].

Conclusion

After a long period in the dark, the endothelium is finally arousing interest among clinicians. Despite both its imposing dimensions and the importance of its functions, the endothelium remains difficult to grasp, as it exhibits a large degree of plasticity and heterogeneity. ECs play a role in primary hemostasis, coagulation, fibrinolysis and regulation of vasomotor tone. More recently, their role in adaptive immunity has also been demonstrated. During sepsis, most endothelial functions are disrupted, leading to a procoagulant, antifibrinolytic and proadhesive state. Production of NO decreases at first, but then it increases unduly because of the induction of iNOS. To the difficulties linked with the variability of endothelial cells, one can also add the practical complications confronted when attempting to assess them; we are not, at the bedside, properly equipped to explore endothelial function. Advances in understanding and treatment of diseases involving the endothelium will require the development of more refined tools.

Acknowledgments Stephanie Lehoux, PhD, is funded by the Canadian Institutes of Health Research (CIHR).

References

1. Wolinsky H, Katz D, Markle R, Mills J, Brem S, Wassertheil-Smoller S (1980) Hydrolase activities in the rat aorta. IV. Relation between clearance rates of circulating 125I-labeled low-density lipoproteins and levels of tissue hydrolase activity. Circ Res 47:433–442
2. Augustin HG, Kozian DH, Johnson RC (1994) Differentiation of endothelial cells: analysis of the constitutive and activated endothelial cell phenotypes. Bioessays 16:901–906
3. Luft JH (1966) Fine structures of capillary and endocapillary layer as revealed by ruthenium red. Fed Proc 25:1773–1783

4. Reitsma S, Slaaf DW, Vink H, van Zandvoort MA, oude Egbrink MG (2007) The endothelial glycocalyx: composition, functions, and visualization. Pflugers Arch 454:345–359
5. Sugahara K, Mikami T, Uyama T, Mizuguchi S, Nomura K, Kitagawa H (2003) Recent advances in the structural biology of chondroitin sulfate and dermatan sulfate. Curr Opin Struct Biol 13:612–620
6. Henry CB, Duling BR (1999) Permeation of the luminal capillary glycocalyx is determined by hyaluronan. Am J Physiol 277:H508–H514
7. Jacob M, Bruegger D, Rehm M, Welsch U, Conzen P, Becker BF (2006) Contrasting effects of colloid and crystalloid resuscitation fluids on cardiac vascular permeability. Anesthesiology 104:1223–1231
8. Constantinescu AA, Vink H, Spaan JA (2003) Endothelial cell glycocalyx modulates immobilization of leukocytes at the endothelial surface. Arterioscler Thromb Vasc Biol 23:1541–1547
9. Davies PF (1995) Flow-mediated endothelial mechanotransduction. Physiol Rev 75:519–560
10. Allaire E, Clowes AW (1997) Endothelial cell injury in cardiovascular surgery: the intimal hyperplastic response. Ann Thorac Surg 63:582–591
11. Lehoux S (2006) Redox signalling in vascular responses to shear and stretch. Cardiovasc Res 71:269–279
12. Aird WC, Edelberg JM, Weiler-Guettler H, Simmons WW, Smith TW, Rosenberg RD (1997) Vascular bed-specific expression of an endothelial cell gene is programmed by the tissue microenvironment. J Cell Biol 138:1117–1124
13. Jalali S, del Pozo MA, Chen K, Miao H, Li Y, Schwartz MA, Shyy JY, Chien S (2001) Integrin-mediated mechanotransduction requires its dynamic interaction with specific extracellular matrix (ECM) ligands. Proc Natl Acad Sci USA 98:1042–1046
14. Lacorre DA, Baekkevold ES, Garrido I, Brandtzaeg P, Haraldsen G, Amalric F, Girard JP (2004) Plasticity of endothelial cells: rapid dedifferentiation of freshly isolated high endothelial venule endothelial cells outside the lymphoid tissue microenvironment. Blood 103:4164–4172
15. Jackson SP, Mistry N, Yuan Y (2000) Platelets and the injured vessel wall—"rolling into action": focus on glycoprotein Ib/V/IX and the platelet cytoskeleton. Trends Cardiovasc Med 10:192–197
16. Roth GJ (1992) Platelets and blood vessels: the adhesion event. Immunol Today 13:100–105
17. Rosenberg RD (1989) Biochemistry of heparin antithrombin interactions, and the physiologic role of this natural anticoagulant mechanism. Am J Med 87:2S–9S
18. Rosenberg RD, Rosenberg JS (1984) Natural anticoagulant mechanisms. J Clin Invest 74:1–6
19. Tollefsen DM, Pestka CA (1985) Heparin cofactor II activity in patients with disseminated intravascular coagulation and hepatic failure. Blood 66:769–774
20. Broze GJ Jr (1995) Tissue factor pathway inhibitor. Thromb Haemost 74:90–93
21. Esmon CT (2001) Protein C anticoagulant pathway and its role in controlling microvascular thrombosis and inflammation. Crit Care Med 29:S48–S51 discussion 51–42
22. Fukudome K, Kurosawa S, Stearns-Kurosawa DJ, He X, Rezaie AR, Esmon CT (1996) The endothelial cell protein C receptor. Cell surface expression and direct ligand binding by the soluble receptor. J Biol Chem 271:17491–17498
23. Thompson EA, Salem HH (1986) Inhibition by human thrombomodulin of factor Xa-mediated cleavage of prothrombin. J Clin Invest 78:13–17
24. Moore KL, Andreoli SP, Esmon NL, Esmon CT, Bang NU (1987) Endotoxin enhances tissue factor and suppresses thrombomodulin expression of human vascular endothelium in vitro. J Clin Invest 79:124–130
25. Bevilacqua MP, Pober JS, Majeau GR, Fiers W, Cotran RS, Gimbrone MA Jr (1986) Recombinant tumor necrosis factor induces procoagulant activity in cultured human vascular endothelium: characterization and comparison with the actions of interleukin 1. Proc Natl Acad Sci USA 83:4533–4537
26. Bombeli T, Karsan A, Tait JF, Harlan JM (1997) Apoptotic vascular endothelial cells become procoagulant. Blood 89:2429–2442
27. Combes V, Simon AC, Grau GE, Arnoux D, Camoin L, Sabatier F, Mutin M, Sanmarco M, Sampol J, Dignat-George F (1999) In vitro generation of endothelial microparticles and possible prothrombotic activity in patients with lupus anticoagulant. J Clin Invest 104:93–102
28. Woolkalis MJ, DeMelfi TM Jr, Blanchard N, Hoxie JA, Brass LF (1995) Regulation of thrombin receptors on human umbilical vein endothelial cells. J Biol Chem 270:9868–9875
29. Mirza H, Yatsula V, Bahou WF (1996) The proteinase activated receptor-2 (PAR-2) mediates mitogenic responses in human vascular endothelial cells. J Clin Invest 97:1705–1714
30. Ishihara H, Connolly AJ, Zeng D, Kahn ML, Zheng YW, Timmons C, Tram T, Coughlin SR (1997) Protease-activated receptor 3 is a second thrombin receptor in humans. Nature 386:502–506
31. Todd AS (1959) The histological localisation of fibrinolysin activator. J Pathol Bacteriol 78:281–283
32. Barnathan ES, Kuo A, Kariko K, Rosenfeld L, Murray SC, Behrendt N, Ronne E, Weiner D, Henkin J, Cines DB (1990) Characterization of human endothelial cell urokinase-type plasminogen activator receptor protein and messenger RNA. Blood 76:1795–1806
33. Carmeliet P, Schoonjans L, Kieckens L, Ream B, Degen J, Bronson R, De Vos R, van den Oord JJ, Collen D, Mulligan RC (1994) Physiological consequences of loss of plasminogen activator gene function in mice. Nature 368:419–424
34. Yamamoto K, Loskutoff DJ (1996) Fibrin deposition in tissues from endotoxin-treated mice correlates with decreases in the expression of urokinase-type but not tissue-type plasminogen activator. J Clin Invest 97:2440–2451
35. Wang L, Bastarache JA, Ware LB (2008) The coagulation cascade in sepsis. Curr Pharm Des 14:1860–1869
36. Furchgott RF, Zawadzki JV (1980) The obligatory role of endothelial cells in the relaxation of arterial smooth muscle by acetylcholine. Nature 288:373–376
37. Stamler JS, Singel DJ, Loscalzo J (1992) Biochemistry of nitric oxide and its redox-activated forms. Science 258:1898–1902
38. Loscalzo J, Vita JA (1994) Ischemia, hyperemia, exercise, and nitric oxide. Complex physiology and complex molecular adaptations. Circulation 90:2556–2559
39. Moncada S, Palmer RM, Higgs EA (1991) Nitric oxide: physiology, pathophysiology, and pharmacology. Pharmacol Rev 43:109–142
40. Pacher P, Beckman JS, Liaudet L (2007) Nitric oxide and peroxynitrite in health and disease. Physiol Rev 87:315–424

41. Levin ER (1995) Endothelins. N Engl J Med 333:356–363
42. Imaizumi TA, Stafforini DM, Yamada Y, McIntyre TM, Prescott SM, Zimmerman GA (1995) Platelet-activating factor: a mediator for clinicians. J Intern Med 238:5–20
43. Lorant DE, Zimmerman GA, McIntyre TM, Prescott SM (1995) Platelet-activating factor mediates procoagulant activity on the surface of endothelial cells by promoting leukocyte adhesion. Semin Cell Biol 6:295–303
44. McEver RP, Moore KL, Cummings RD (1995) Leukocyte trafficking mediated by selectin–carbohydrate interactions. J Biol Chem 270:11025–11028
45. Springer TA (1995) Traffic signals on endothelium for lymphocyte recirculation and leukocyte emigration. Annu Rev Physiol 57:827–872
46. Languino LR, Plescia J, Duperray A, Brian AA, Plow EF, Geltosky JE, Altieri DC (1993) Fibrinogen mediates leukocyte adhesion to vascular endothelium through an ICAM-1-dependent pathway. Cell 73:1423–1434
47. Muller WA, Weigl SA (1992) Monocyte-selective transendothelial migration: dissection of the binding and transmigration phases by an in vitro assay. J Exp Med 176:819–828
48. Dejana E, Corada M, Lampugnani MG (1995) Endothelial cell-to-cell junctions. FASEB J 9:910–918
49. Pober JS, Orosz CG, Rose ML, Savage CO (1996) Can graft endothelial cells initiate a host anti-graft immune response? Transplantation 61:343–349
50. Marelli-Berg FM, Hargreaves RE, Carmichael P, Dorling A, Lombardi G, Lechler RI (1996) Major histocompatibility complex class II-expressing endothelial cells induce allospecific nonresponsiveness in naive T cells. J Exp Med 183:1603–1612
51. Ait-Oufella H, Salomon BL, Potteaux S, Robertson AK, Gourdy P, Zoll J, Merval R, Esposito B, Cohen JL, Fisson S, Flavell RA, Hansson GK, Klatzmann D, Tedgui A, Mallat Z (2006) Natural regulatory T cells control the development of atherosclerosis in mice. Nat Med 12:178–180
52. Murray AG, Khodadoust MM, Pober JS, Bothwell AL (1994) Porcine aortic endothelial cells activate human T cells: direct presentation of MHC antigens and costimulation by ligands for human CD2 and CD28. Immunity 1:57–63
53. Cooper ME, Bonnet F, Oldfield M, Jandeleit-Dahm K (2001) Mechanisms of diabetic vasculopathy: an overview. Am J Hypertens 14:475–486
54. Bearman SI (2000) Veno-occlusive disease of the liver. Curr Opin Oncol 12:103–109
55. Tsai HM (2003) Advances in the pathogenesis, diagnosis, and treatment of thrombotic thrombocytopenic purpura. J Am Soc Nephrol 14:1072–1081
56. Steinsiepe KF, Weibel ER (1970) Electron microscopic studies on specific organelles of endothelial cells in the frog (*Rana temporaria*). Z Zellforsch Mikrosk Anat 108:105–126
57. Faust SN, Levin M, Harrison OB, Goldin RD, Lockhart MS, Kondaveeti S, Laszik Z, Esmon CT, Heyderman RS (2001) Dysfunction of endothelial protein C activation in severe meningococcal sepsis. N Engl J Med 345:408–416
58. Ishii H, Salem HH, Bell CE, Laposata EA, Majerus PW (1986) Thrombomodulin, an endothelial anticoagulant protein, is absent from the human brain. Blood 67:362–365
59. Aird WC (2003) Endothelial cell heterogeneity. Crit Care Med 31:S221–S230
60. Reidy MA, Schwartz SM (1983) Endothelial injury and regeneration. IV. Endotoxin: a nondenuding injury to aortic endothelium. Lab Invest 48:25–34
61. Leclerc J, Pu Q, Corseaux D, Haddad E, Decoene C, Bordet R, Six I, Jude B, Vallet B (2000) A single endotoxin injection in the rabbit causes prolonged blood vessel dysfunction and a procoagulant state. Crit Care Med 28:3672–3678
62. Lee MM, Schuessler GB, Chien S (1988) Time-dependent effects of endotoxin on the ultrastructure of aortic endothelium. Artery 15:71–89
63. Wang P, Wood TJ, Zhou M, Ba ZF, Chaudry IH (1996) Inhibition of the biologic activity of tumor necrosis factor maintains vascular endothelial cell function during hyperdynamic sepsis. J Trauma 40:694–700
64. Mutunga M, Fulton B, Bullock R, Batchelor A, Gascoigne A, Gillespie JI, Baudouin SV (2001) Circulating endothelial cells in patients with septic shock. Am J Respir Crit Care Med 163:195–200
65. Polunovsky VA, Wendt CH, Ingbar DH, Peterson MS, Bitterman PB (1994) Induction of endothelial cell apoptosis by TNF alpha: modulation by inhibitors of protein synthesis. Exp Cell Res 214:584–594
66. Messmer UK, Briner VA, Pfeilschifter J (1999) Tumor necrosis factor-alpha and lipopolysaccharide induce apoptotic cell death in bovine glomerular endothelial cells. Kidney Int 55:2322–2337
67. Stefanec T (2000) Endothelial apoptosis: could it have a role in the pathogenesis and treatment of disease? Chest 117:841–854
68. Piccin A, Murphy WG, Smith OP (2007) Circulating microparticles: pathophysiology and clinical implications. Blood Rev 21:157–171
69. Soriano AO, Jy W, Chirinos JA, Valdivia MA, Velasquez HS, Jimenez JJ, Horstman LL, Kett DH, Schein RM, Ahn YS (2005) Levels of endothelial and platelet microparticles and their interactions with leukocytes negatively correlate with organ dysfunction and predict mortality in severe sepsis. Crit Care Med 33:2540–2546
70. Levi M, Ten Cate H (1999) Disseminated intravascular coagulation. N Engl J Med 341:586–592
71. Heckel K, Kiefmann R, Dorger M, Stoeckelhuber M, Goetz AE (2004) Colloidal gold particles as a new in vivo marker of early acute lung injury. Am J Physiol Lung Cell Mol Physiol 287:L867–L878
72. Parrillo JE (1993) Pathogenetic mechanisms of septic shock. N Engl J Med 328:1471–1477
73. Shapiro NI, Yano K, Sorasaki M, Fischer C, Shih SC, Aird WC (2009) Skin biopsies demonstrate site-specific endothelial activation in mouse models of sepsis. J Vasc Res 46:495–502
74. Nooteboom A, van der Linden CJ, Hendriks T (2004) Modulation of adhesion molecule expression on endothelial cells after induction by lipopolysaccharide-stimulated whole blood. Scand J Immunol 59:440–448
75. Sessler CN, Windsor AC, Schwartz M, Watson L, Fisher BJ, Sugerman HJ, Fowler AA 3rd (1995) Circulating ICAM-1 is increased in septic shock. Am J Respir Crit Care Med 151:1420–1427
76. Xu H, Gonzalo JA, St Pierre Y, Williams IR, Kupper TS, Cotran RS, Springer TA, Gutierrez-Ramos JC (1994) Leukocytosis and resistance to septic shock in intercellular adhesion molecule 1-deficient mice. J Exp Med 180:95–109
77. Kuhns DB, Alvord WG, Gallin JI (1995) Increased circulating cytokines, cytokine antagonists, and E-selectin after intravenous administration of endotoxin in humans. J Infect Dis 171:145–152

78. Boldt J, Muller M, Kuhn D, Linke LC, Hempelmann G (1996) Circulating adhesion molecules in the critically ill: a comparison between trauma and sepsis patients. Intensive Care Med 22:122–128
79. Kayal S, Jais JP, Aguini N, Chaudiere J, Labrousse J (1998) Elevated circulating E-selectin, intercellular adhesion molecule 1, and von Willebrand factor in patients with severe infection. Am J Respir Crit Care Med 157:776–784
80. Harlan JM, Winn RK (2002) Leukocyte-endothelial interactions: clinical trials of anti-adhesion therapy. Crit Care Med 30:S214–S219
81. Ye X, Ding J, Zhou X, Chen G, Liu SF (2008) Divergent roles of endothelial NF-kappaB in multiple organ injury and bacterial clearance in mouse models of sepsis. J Exp Med 205:1303–1315
82. Blanks JE, Moll T, Eytner R, Vestweber D (1998) Stimulation of P-selectin glycoprotein ligand-1 on mouse neutrophils activates beta 2-integrin mediated cell attachment to ICAM-1. Eur J Immunol 28:433–443
83. Asaduzzaman M, Lavasani S, Rahman M, Zhang S, Braun OO, Jeppsson B, Thorlacius H (2009) Platelets support pulmonary recruitment of neutrophils in abdominal sepsis. Crit Care Med 37:1389–1396
84. Aird WC (2001) Vascular bed-specific hemostasis: role of endothelium in sepsis pathogenesis. Crit Care Med 29:S28–S34 discussion S34–25
85. Franco RF, de Jonge E, Dekkers PE, Timmerman JJ, Spek CA, van Deventer SJ, van Deursen P, van Kerkhoff L, van Gemen B, ten Cate H, van der Poll T, Reitsma PH (2000) The in vivo kinetics of tissue factor messenger RNA expression during human endotoxemia: relationship with activation of coagulation. Blood 96:554–559
86. Osterud B, Flaegstad T (1983) Increased tissue thromboplastin activity in monocytes of patients with meningococcal infection: related to an unfavourable prognosis. Thromb Haemost 49:5–7
87. Lupu C, Westmuckett AD, Peer G, Ivanciu L, Zhu H, Taylor FB Jr, Lupu F (2005) Tissue factor-dependent coagulation is preferentially up-regulated within arterial branching areas in a baboon model of Escherichia coli sepsis. Am J Pathol 167:1161–1172
88. Solovey A, Gui L, Key NS, Hebbel RP (1998) Tissue factor expression by endothelial cells in sickle cell anemia. J Clin Invest 101:1899–1904
89. Moore KL, Esmon CT, Esmon NL (1989) Tumor necrosis factor leads to the internalization and degradation of thrombomodulin from the surface of bovine aortic endothelial cells in culture. Blood 73:159–165
90. Nawroth PP, Stern DM (1986) Modulation of endothelial cell hemostatic properties by tumor necrosis factor. J Exp Med 163:740–745
91. Mesters RM, Helterbrand J, Utterback BG, Yan B, Chao YB, Fernandez JA, Griffin JH, Hartman DL (2000) Prognostic value of protein C concentrations in neutropenic patients at high risk of severe septic complications. Crit Care Med 28:2209–2216
92. Taylor FB Jr, Chang A, Esmon CT, D'Angelo A, Vigano-D'Angelo S, Blick KE (1987) Protein C prevents the coagulopathic and lethal effects of Escherichia coli infusion in the baboon. J Clin Invest 79:918–925
93. Bernard GR, Vincent JL, Laterre PF, LaRosa SP, Dhainaut JF, Lopez-Rodriguez A, Steingrub JS, Garber GE, Helterbrand JD, Ely EW, Fisher CJ Jr (2001) Efficacy and safety of recombinant human activated protein C for severe sepsis. N Engl J Med 344:699–709
94. Abraham E, Laterre PF, Garg R, Levy H, Talwar D, Trzaskoma BL, Francois B, Guy JS, Bruckmann M, Rea-Neto A, Rossaint R, Perrotin D, Sablotzki A, Arkins N, Utterback BG, Macias WL (2005) Drotrecogin alfa (activated) for adults with severe sepsis and a low risk of death. N Engl J Med 353:1332–1341
95. Nadel S, Goldstein B, Williams MD, Dalton H, Peters M, Macias WL, Abd-Allah SA, Levy H, Angle R, Wang D, Sundin DP, Giroir B (2007) Drotrecogin alfa (activated) in children with severe sepsis: a multicentre phase III randomised controlled trial. Lancet 369:836–843
96. Ely EW, Laterre PF, Angus DC, Helterbrand JD, Levy H, Dhainaut JF, Vincent JL, Macias WL, Bernard GR (2003) Drotrecogin alfa (activated) administration across clinically important subgroups of patients with severe sepsis. Crit Care Med 31:12–19
97. Toussaint S, Gerlach H (2009) Activated protein C for sepsis. N Engl J Med 361:2646–2652
98. Sarangi PP, Lee HW, Kim M (2009) Activated protein C action in inflammation. Br J Haematol [Epub ahead of print]
99. Sandset PM, Warn-Cramer BJ, Rao LV, Maki SL, Rapaport SI (1991) Depletion of extrinsic pathway inhibitor (EPI) sensitizes rabbits to disseminated intravascular coagulation induced with tissue factor: evidence supporting a physiologic role for EPI as a natural anticoagulant. Proc Natl Acad Sci USA 88:708–712
100. Creasey AA, Chang AC, Feigen L, Wun TC, Taylor FB Jr, Hinshaw LB (1993) Tissue factor pathway inhibitor reduces mortality from *Escherichia coli* septic shock. J Clin Invest 91:2850–2860
101. Abraham E, Reinhart K, Opal S, Demeyer I, Doig C, Rodriguez AL, Beale R, Svoboda P, Laterre PF, Simon S, Light B, Spapen H, Stone J, Seibert A, Peckelsen C, De Deyne C, Postier R, Pettila V, Artigas A, Percell SR, Shu V, Zwingelstein C, Tobias J, Poole L, Stolzenbach JC, Creasey AA (2003) Efficacy and safety of tifacogin (recombinant tissue factor pathway inhibitor) in severe sepsis: a randomized controlled trial. JAMA 290:238–247
102. Levin EG, Marotti KR, Santell L (1989) Protein kinase C and the stimulation of tissue plasminogen activator release from human endothelial cells. Dependence on the elevation of messenger RNA. J Biol Chem 264:16030–16036
103. Green J, Doughty L, Kaplan SS, Sasser H, Carcillo JA (2002) The tissue factor and plasminogen activator inhibitor type-1 response in pediatric sepsis-induced multiple organ failure. Thromb Haemost 87:218–223
104. Mavrommatis AC, Theodoridis T, Economou M, Kotanidou A, El Ali M, Christopoulou-Kokkinou V, Zakynthinos SG (2001) Activation of the fibrinolytic system and utilization of the coagulation inhibitors in sepsis: comparison with severe sepsis and septic shock. Intensive Care Med 27:1853–1859
105. Prabhakaran P, Ware LB, White KE, Cross MT, Matthay MA, Olman MA (2003) Elevated levels of plasminogen activator inhibitor-1 in pulmonary edema fluid are associated with mortality in acute lung injury. Am J Physiol Lung Cell Mol Physiol 285:L20–L28
106. Hermans PW, Hazelzet JA (2005) Plasminogen activator inhibitor type 1 gene polymorphism and sepsis. Clin Infect Dis 41(Suppl 7):S453–S458
107. Regoeczi E, Brain MC (1969) Organ distribution of fibrin in disseminated intravascular coagulation. Br J Haematol 17:73–81

108. Salzman AL, Wang H, Wollert PS, Vandermeer TJ, Compton CC, Denenberg AG, Fink MP (1994) Endotoxin-induced ileal mucosal hyperpermeability in pigs: role of tissue acidosis. Am J Physiol 266:G633–G646
109. Wiel E, Pu Q, Corseaux D, Robin E, Bordet R, Lund N, Jude B, Vallet B (2000) Effect of L-arginine on endothelial injury and hemostasis in rabbit endotoxin shock. J Appl Physiol 89:1811–1818
110. Wiel E, Pu Q, Leclerc J, Corseaux D, Bordet R, Lund N, Jude B, Vallet B (2004) Effects of the angiotensin-converting enzyme inhibitor perindopril on endothelial injury and hemostasis in rabbit endotoxic shock. Intensive Care Med 30:1652–1659
111. Zhou M, Wang P, Chaudry IH (1997) Endothelial nitric oxide synthase is downregulated during hyperdynamic sepsis. Biochim Biophys Acta 1335:182–190
112. Bhagat K, Collier J, Vallance P (1996) Local venous responses to endotoxin in humans. Circulation 94:490–497
113. Bhagat K, Moss R, Collier J, Vallance P (1996) Endothelial "stunning" following a brief exposure to endotoxin: a mechanism to link infection and infarction? Cardiovasc Res 32:822–829
114. Cobb JP, Natanson C, Quezado ZM, Hoffman WD, Koev CA, Banks S, Correa R, Levi R, Elin RJ, Hosseini JM et al (1995) Differential hemodynamic effects of L-NMMA in endotoxemic and normal dogs. Am J Physiol 268:H1634–H1642
115. Jourdain M, Tournoys A, Leroy X, Mangalaboyi J, Fourrier F, Goudemand J, Gosselin B, Vallet B, Chopin C (1997) Effects of N omega-nitro-L-arginine methyl ester on the endotoxin-induced disseminated intravascular coagulation in porcine septic shock. Crit Care Med 25:452–459
116. Walker TA, Curtis SE, King-VanVlack CE, Chapler CK, Vallet B, Cain SM (1995) Effects of nitric oxide synthase inhibition on regional hemodynamics and oxygen transport in endotoxic dogs. Shock 4:415–420
117. Grover R, Zaccardelli D, Colice G, Guntupalli K, Watson D, Vincent JL (1999) An open-label dose escalation study of the nitric oxide synthase inhibitor, N(G)-methyl-L-arginine hydrochloride (546C88), in patients with septic shock. Glaxo Wellcome International Septic Shock Study Group. Crit Care Med 27:913–922
118. Vincent JL, Zhang H, Szabo C, Preiser JC (2000) Effects of nitric oxide in septic shock. Am J Respir Crit Care Med 161:1781–1785
119. Lopez A, Lorente JA, Steingrub J, Bakker J, McLuckie A, Willatts S, Brockway M, Anzueto A, Holzapfel L, Breen D, Silverman MS, Takala J, Donaldson J, Arneson C, Grove G, Grossman S, Grover R (2004) Multiple-center, randomized, placebo-controlled, double-blind study of the nitric oxide synthase inhibitor 546C88: effect on survival in patients with septic shock. Crit Care Med 32:21–30
120. De Backer D, Creteur J, Preiser JC, Dubois MJ, Vincent JL (2002) Microvascular blood flow is altered in patients with sepsis. Am J Respir Crit Care Med 166:98–104
121. Nieuwdorp M, Meuwese MC, Mooij HL, Ince C, Broekhuizen LN, Kastelein JJ, Stroes ES, Vink H (2008) Measuring endothelial glycocalyx dimensions in humans: a potential novel tool to monitor vascular vulnerability. J Appl Physiol 104:845–852
122. Li JM, Shah AM (2004) Endothelial cell superoxide generation: regulation and relevance for cardiovascular pathophysiology. Am J Physiol Regul Integr Comp Physiol 287:R1014–R1030
123. Marechal X, Favory R, Joulin O, Montaigne D, Hassoun S, Decoster B, Zerimech F, Neviere R (2008) Endothelial glycocalyx damage during endotoxemia coincides with microcirculatory dysfunction and vascular oxidative stress. Shock 29:572–576
124. Cerwinka WH, Cooper D, Krieglstein CF, Feelisch M, Granger DN (2002) Nitric oxide modulates endotoxin-induced platelet-endothelial cell adhesion in intestinal venules. Am J Physiol Heart Circ Physiol 282:H1111–H1117
125. Cepinskas G, Wilson JX (2008) Inflammatory response in microvascular endothelium in sepsis: role of oxidants. J Clin Biochem Nutr 42:175–184
126. Lush CW, Cepinskas G, Kvietys PR (2003) Regulation of intestinal nuclear factor-kappaB activity and E-selectin expression during sepsis: a role for peroxynitrite. Gastroenterology 124:118–128
127. Steffel J, Luscher TF, Tanner FC (2006) Tissue factor in cardiovascular diseases: molecular mechanisms and clinical implications. Circulation 113:722–731
128. Shen KP, Lo YC, Yang RC, Liu HW, Chen IJ, Wu BN (2005) Antioxidant eugenosedin-A protects against lipopolysaccharide-induced hypotension, hyperglycaemia and cytokine immunoreactivity in rats and mice. J Pharm Pharmacol 57:117–125
129. Crimi E, Liguori A, Condorelli M, Cioffi M, Astuto M, Bontempo P, Pignalosa O, Vietri MT, Molinari AM, Sica V, Della Corte F, Napoli C (2004) The beneficial effects of antioxidant supplementation in enteral feeding in critically ill patients: a prospective, randomized, double-blind, placebo-controlled trial. Anesth Analg 99:857–863

B. Levy
S. Collin
N. Sennoun
N. Ducrocq
A. Kimmoun
P. Asfar
P. Perez
F. Meziani

Vascular hyporesponsiveness to vasopressors in septic shock: from bench to bedside

Abstract *Purpose:* To delineate some of the characteristics of septic vascular hypotension, to assess the most commonly cited and reported underlying mechanisms of vascular hyporesponsiveness to vasoconstrictors in sepsis, and to briefly outline current therapeutic strategies and possible future approaches. *Methods:* Source data were obtained from a PubMed search of the medical literature with the following MeSH terms: Muscle, smooth, vascular/physiopathology; hypotension/etiology; shock/physiopathology; vasodilation/physiology; shock/therapy; vasoconstrictor agents. *Results:* Nitric oxide (NO) and peroxynitrite are crucial components implicated in vasoplegia and vascular hyporeactivity. Vascular ATP-sensitive and calcium-activated potassium channels are activated during shock and participate in hypotension. In addition, shock state is characterized by inappropriately low plasma glucocorticoid and vasopressin concentrations, a dysfunction and desensitization of alpha-receptors, and an inactivation of catecholamines by oxidation. Numerous other mechanisms have been individualized in animal models, the great majority of which involve NO: MEK1/2–ERK1/2 pathway, H_2S, hyperglycemia, and cytoskeleton dysregulation associated with decreased actin expression. *Conclusions:* Many therapeutic approaches have proven their efficiency in animal models, especially therapies directed against one particular compound, but have otherwise failed when used in human shock. Nevertheless, high doses of catecholamines, vasopressin and terlipressin, hydrocortisone, activated protein C, and non-specific shock treatment have demonstrated a partial efficiency in reversing sepsis-induced hypotension.

Keywords Septic shock · Vasopressor · Nitric oxide · Potassium channels · Catecholamine

Introduction

Septic shock is the primary cause of death in critical care units [1]. Shock states are primarily characterized by acute circulatory failure leading to tissue hypoperfusion, and potentially resulting in multi-organ failure. Observed hypotension can be the consequence of three major hemodynamic disorders: hypovolemia, vascular failure, and heart failure [2]. Vascular dysfunction [3] is characterized by: (1) microvascular dysfunction, (2) endothelial dysfunction, and (3) a decrease in vasoconstrictor tone as well as vascular hyporesponsiveness along with a lesser sensitivity to vasopressor agents such as catecholamine but also vasopressin, angiotensin II,

DOI 10.1007/978-3-642-28233-1_25,

and serotonin [4]. The outcome of the last of these characteristics is vasopressor-refractory arterial hypotension which can ultimately lead to patient death. The purpose of the present review is to assess the most commonly cited and reported underlying mechanisms of decreased responsiveness to vasoconstrictors in sepsis, to summarize their relevance and clinical applicability, and to briefly outline current therapeutic strategies and possible future approaches. This review is not intended to be all-inclusive.

Definition(s) of vascular hyporesponsiveness to vasopressor agents

Vascular hyporeactivity to vasopressor agents is defined by a decreased effect of a vasopressor agent when compared to the normal response due to failure of vascular smooth muscle to constrict [4]. Vascular hyporeactivity can most often be observed either experimentally in organ chambers by exposing segments of isolated vessels to vasopressor agents, or in clinical practice by establishing dose–response curves to a pure alpha-adrenergic agonist such as phenylephrine. In this case, vascular hyporesponsiveness is defined by a smaller increase in arterial blood pressure (in patients) for a similar dose of vasopressor agent (healthy volunteers) [5]. This latter technique also incorporates other regulatory mechanisms, such as cardiac adaptation and baroreflex.

Hypotension associated with vascular hyporeactivity is clearly related, both significantly and independently, to mortality [6]. The extent of this vascular hyporesponsiveness can be assessed clinically by the measure of vasopressor dosage necessary to maintain mean arterial blood pressure [7] and by the drop in diastolic blood pressure reflecting vasoplegia [8, 9].

Physiology

Vasoconstriction is the result of increased intracellular calcium in vascular smooth muscle cells (VSMCs) and involves two mutually dependent and synergistic processes. On the one hand, the increase in intracytoplasmic calcium can result from the action of neural or hormonal ligands such as angiotensin II or norepinephrine via their specific membrane receptors on the VSMC (G protein-coupled receptors). Alternatively, the increase in intracytoplasmic calcium can also be generated by a change in membrane potential. The normal membrane potential of smooth muscle cells varies between −45 and −70 mV. A depolarization of the membrane (to a potential approaching 0 mV) induces the opening of voltage-gated calcium channels and thus the influx of extracellular calcium into the VSMC.

Relaxation of the VSMC results from the decrease in the concentration of cytoplasmic calcium, either by expulsion of calcium to the extracellular space or by its reuptake into the sarcoplasmic reticulum. Again, several mechanisms may be involved.

Certain mediators such as nitric oxide, the atrial natriuretic peptide, as well as acetylcholine, serotonin, and histamine are known vasorelaxant agents. These mediators bring about an increase in cyclic guanosine monophosphate and cyclic adenosine monophosphate (cGMP and cAMP) through the action of guanylate cyclase and adenylyl cyclase respectively.

Clinical evidence of vascular hyporesponsiveness in septic shock

Clinical evidence has confirmed vascular hyporesponsiveness in septic shock, since volume-resuscitated septic shock patients remain hypotensive despite elevated levels of endogenous and exogenous catecholamines [10] and a maximum activation of the renin-angiotensin system. Administration of large doses of catecholamines is hence necessary to increase arterial pressure. In an experimental study, Bellissant and Annane [5] compared 20 patients with septic shock with 12 healthy subjects. Dose–response curves to phenylephrine, a pure alpha-adrenergic agonist, were established and ultimately showed a decreased response to alpha-adrenergic stimulation in the septic shock patients.

Mechanisms involved

Vascular hyporesponsiveness to vasopressor during sepsis is probably multifactorial. Nevertheless, it is important to identify individual contributing factors and mechanisms in order to select meaningful therapeutic targets. As a consequence, a vast array of mechanisms, pathways, and disruptions in cellular homeostasis have been examined in septic vessels [11] (Figs. 1, 2, 3).

Nitric oxide

Nitric oxide (NO) is an omnipresent intercellular messenger found in all vertebrates, notably regulating blood flow, coagulation, and neural activity. Physiologically, NO is produced in picomolar concentrations from L-arginine by nitric oxide synthase (NOS), an enzyme constitutively present in endothelial cells and termed endothelial constitutive NOS (cNOS). According to a few recent studies, a mitochondrial isoform of NOS (mtNOS) may also represent a significant source of NO during

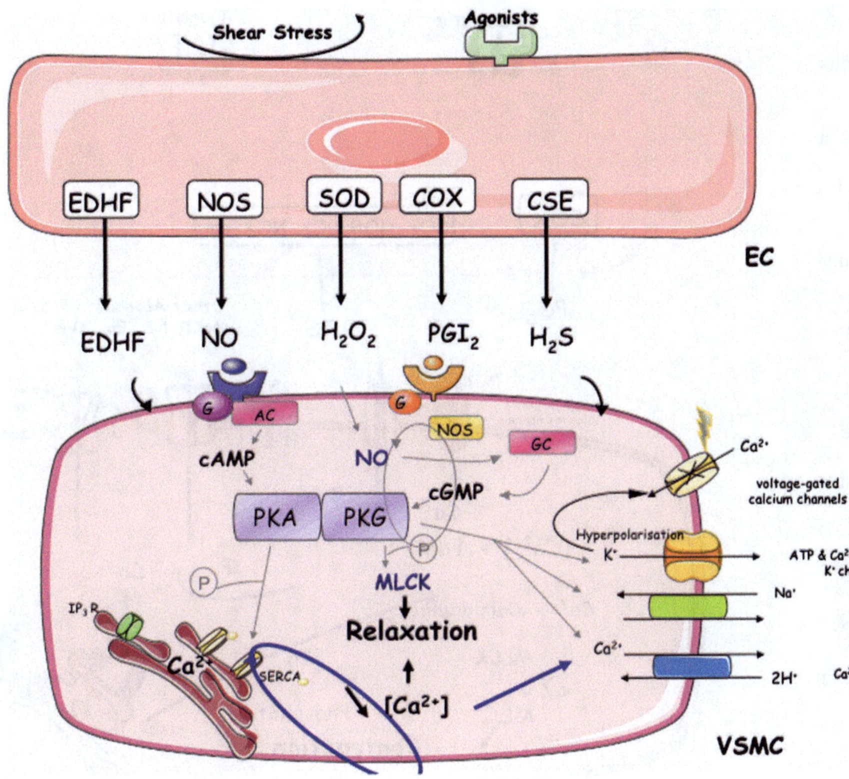

Fig. 1 Endothelium-dependent relaxation. Multiplicity of mechanisms leading to endothelium relaxation such as shear stress and vasorelaxant agonists; ECs synthesize and release various vasorelaxation factors that can diffuse towards the VSMCs and produce relaxation. *EC* endothelial cell, *VSMC* vascular smooth muscle cell, *EDHF* endothelium-derived hyperpolarizing factor, *NOS* nitric oxide synthase, *SOD* superoxide dismutases, *COX* cyclooxygenase, *CSE* cystathionine γ-lyase, *NO* nitric oxide, H_2O_2 hydrogen peroxide, PGI_2 prostacyclin, H_2S hydrogen sulfide; *G* protein G, *AC* adenylyl cyclase, *NO* nitric oxide, *GC* guanylate cyclase, *cAMP* cyclic adenosine monophosphate, *cGMP* cyclic guanosine monophosphate, *PKA* protein kinase A, *PKG* protein kinase G, *MLCK* myosin light-chain kinase, *SERCA* sarcoplasmic/endoplasmic reticulum Ca^{2+}-ATPases, *ATP* adenosine triphosphate, *IP3R* inositol-1,4,5-trisphosphate-receptor, *P* phosphate

circulatory shock [12]. A non-enzymatic source of NO has also been described related to the reduction of nitrites under acidic and reducing conditions, as can occur in ischemic tissues [13]. NO diffuses into the underlying vascular smooth muscle and induces vasorelaxation via stimulation of soluble guanylate cyclase and resulting increase in cGMP concentration [14].

In the mid-1980s, it became apparent that inhibitors of NOS were able to restore, to a large extent, this contractile response to vasoconstrictor agents [15]. These effects were maintained in vessel models ex vivo, even in the absence of endothelium, thereby suggesting that inflammation and sepsis lead to the expression of an inducible NOS (iNOS) in vessel wall smooth muscle. Excessive production of NO (nanomolar concentrations) by iNOS hence resulted in an altered contractile response. Authors thus concluded that the results (1) were consistent with the pathophysiology observed, both experimental and clinical, during sepsis, and (2) may explain the profound vasoplegia and limited response to stimuli that normally regulate blood flow and tissue perfusion. High circulating levels of nitrites/nitrates (stable molecules generated from NO) found in patients with septic shock and associated with decreased vascular tone suggested that NO was clearly implicated in the pathophysiology of septic shock [16].

The above observations led to the initial use of non-selective inhibitors of NOS such as N^G-nitro-L-arginine methyl ester (L-NAME) in LPS models [17]. L-NAME increases blood pressure and vascular resistance along with a decrease in cardiac output. It is important to note, however, that these treatments did not improve survival in an animal model of endotoxemia [18]. Unfortunately, a phase III study was halted due to the emergence of a significant over-mortality in the treated group [19]. It was proposed that the use of a more selective inhibitor of iNOS would provide greater benefit to the patients. Some positive experimental results have since been reported with specific molecules such as *S*-methylisothiourea, L-canavanine [20], and aminoguanidine, but none have been tested to date in clinical trials. However, blocking the production of NO may cause other deleterious effects [21] such as:

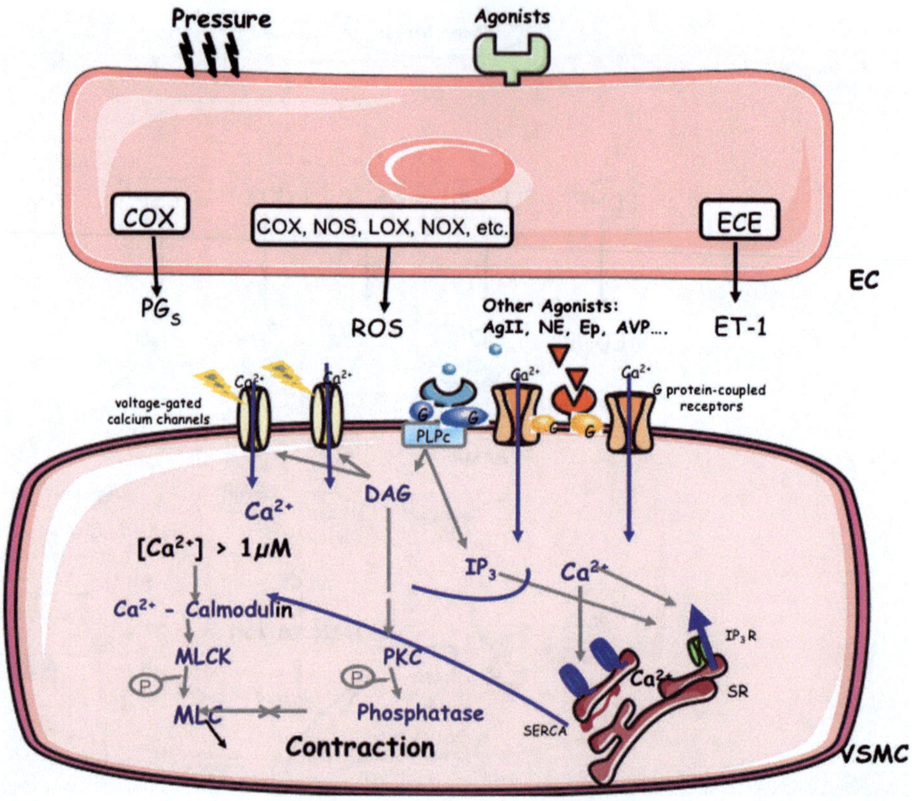

Fig. 2 Mechanisms of contractions. Under certain conditions, the endothelial cells, when activated by neurohumoral mediators or subjected to pressure, release a vasoconstrictor substance(s), which diffuses to the underlying vascular smooth muscle and initiates its contraction. *EC* endothelial cell, *VSMC* vascular smooth muscle cell, *COX* cyclooxygenase, *LOX* lipoxygenase, *NOX* NADPH oxidase, *NOS* nitric oxide synthase, *ECE* endothelin-converting enzyme, *PGs* prostaglandins, *ROS* reactive oxygen species, *ET-1* endothelin-1, *AgII* angiotensin II, *NE* norepinephrine, *Ep* epinephrine, *PLPc* phospholipase C, *DAG* diacylglycerol, *IP3* inositol trisphosphate, *PKC* protein kinase C, *IP3R* inositol-1,4,5-trisphosphate-receptor, *PKC* protein kinase C, *MLCK* myosin light-chain kinase, *SERCA* sarcoplasmic/endoplasmic reticulum Ca^{2+}-ATPases

- Altered microcirculatory flow
- A decrease in NO-dependent bactericidal activity
- A decrease in neutralizing activity of oxygen-derived species
- A decrease in the modulation of blood coagulation
- An increase in oxygen demand by improving mitochondrial respiration in tissues in which perfusion, and hence oxygen delivery, remains precarious, thereby exacerbating the oxygen supply/demand balance

Thus, the current paradigm that NO and soluble guanylate cyclase (sGC) contribute to organ damage and death associated with septic shock may be challenged. For example, Cauwels et al. [22] recently demonstrated that nitrite treatment protects against morbidity and mortality in lipopolysaccharide (LPS)-induced shock in a soluble guanylate cyclase-dependent manner.

To summarize, excess production of NO seems to be a major and central actor in sepsis-induced vascular hyporeactivity. Nevertheless, inhibition through non-selective iNOS inhibitor increased mortality in septic shock.

Prostacyclin and COX-2 pathways

Prostacyclin (PGI_2) is a major product of arachidonic acid metabolism formed in the vascular endothelium by the action of the enzymes cyclooxygenase (COX) and prostacyclin synthase (PGIS). PGI_2 mediates its effects through a G_s protein-coupled receptor (IP), which is located on VSMCs. Stimulation of IP by PGI_2 leads to an increase in cAMP, which likely mediates relaxation of VSMCs. Increased levels of PGI_2 have been reported to occur in patients under septic shock and in animals treated with LPS or proinflammatory cytokines [23]. Recent evidence suggests that the inducible isoform of COX, COX-2, is the enzyme mainly responsible for the increased production of PGI_2 in VSMCs [24]. In keeping with this observation, it has been shown that inhibition of COX-2 attenuates the fall in blood pressure or improves vascular endothelial dysfunction in endotoxemic animals. Recently, Höcherl et al. [25] demonstrated that the selective inhibition of the receptor for prostacyclin attenuated the cardiovascular dysfunction induced by LPS without altering cytokine levels or NOx products, thus evoking a specific role for prostacyclin and/or the receptor for prostacyclin in the development of LPS-induced vascular failure.

Similarly to iNOS inhibitors, the non-selective inhibition of prostaglandin synthesis with ibuprofen failed to improve mortality in septic shock [26].

Free radicals: the peroxynitrite ion and superoxide anion

Free radicals are molecules or portions thereof which possess one or more unpaired electrons in their outer orbital, a state

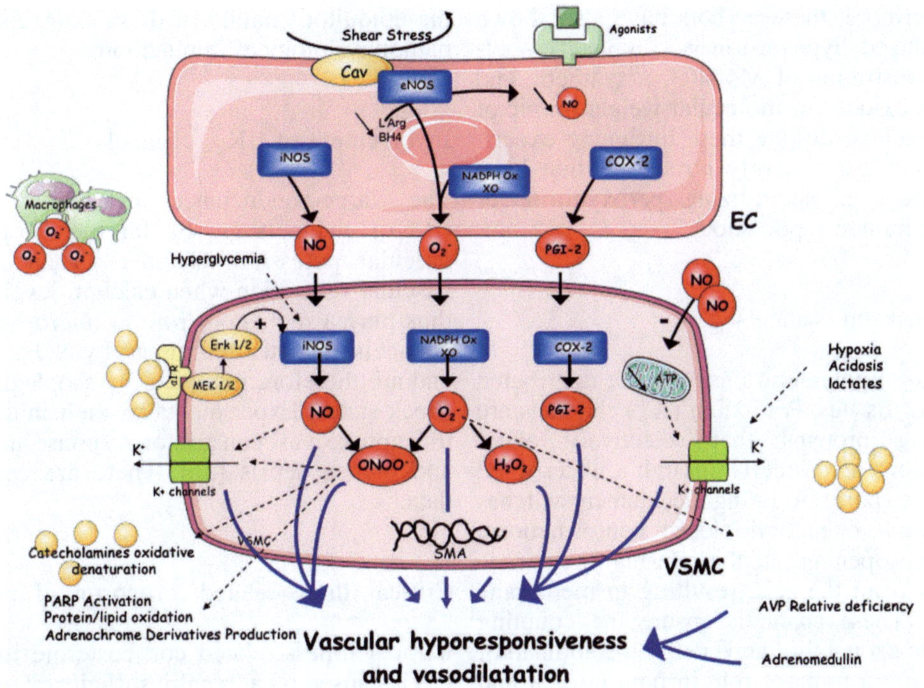

Fig. 3 Mechanisms of vascular dysfunction in sepsis. When the infectious agent invades the bloodstream, systemic activation of inflammation leads to cytokine release and endothelial activation and dysfunction. Multiple cascades of intracellular signaling reactions are initiated and induce vascular hyporesponsiveness and vasodilatation. A functional impairment of ECs and VSMCs contributes to endothelial and vascular dysfunction. Both cells synthesize and release various factors of oxidative stress and vasodilatation, which subsequently react with many products, receptors, and channels to induce their oxidation. *EC* endothelial cell, *VSMC* vascular smooth muscle cell, *eNOS* endothelial nitric oxide synthase, *BH4* 5,6,7,8-tetrahydrobiopterine, *Cav* caveolin-1, *L-Arg* L-arginine, *iNOS* inducible nitric oxide synthase, *COX-2* cyclooxygenase-2, *NADPH Ox* oxy nicotinamide adenine dinucleotide phosphate, *XO* xanthine oxidase O_2^- superoxide anions, *PGI-2* prostacyclin, *NO* nitric oxide, *ONOO*$^-$ peroxynitrite, H_2O_2 hydrogen peroxide, *Erk* extracellular signal-regulated kinases, *MEK 1/2* mitogen-activated protein kinase kinases 1/2, *Erk 1/2* extracellular signal-regulated kinases 1/2, *AVP* arginin vasopressin

that greatly increases their reactivity. The best-known reactive species generated from oxygen include superoxide anion, hydroxyl radical, and peroxynitrite.

It should be emphasized that every time NO and superoxide anion molecules collide, they spontaneously interact to form peroxynitrite [27]. This reaction does not require any enzymatic intervention. As a result, it is possible that the majority of the biological effects attributed to NO are rather due to peroxynitrite.

A state of shock constitutes a propitious environment for the production of peroxynitrite since NO and superoxide are both produced in large quantities and in the same tissues. The upregulated production of superoxide arises from the reactions catalyzed by NAPDH oxidase present in leukocytes and endothelial cells, by the conversion of xanthine dehydrogenase into xanthine oxidase, by the partial reduction of molecular oxygen within mitochondria, and finally by the uncoupling of NOS in conditions of L-arginine or tetrahydrobiopterin deficiency [27]. Formation of peroxynitrite has been demonstrated by using LPS as the inducer of shock with a time course similar to that of iNOS expression in muscle and aorta [28]. In endotoxic and hemorrhagic shock models, it has been shown that inhibitors of peroxynitrite formation and genetic suppression of nicotinamide adenine dinucleotide phosphate (NADPH) are able to reduce the amount of aortic peroxynitrite and reverse vascular hyporesponsiveness. Conversely, the increase in endogenous production of peroxynitrite by inducing a depletion of endogenous glutathione stores aggravates vascular hyporeactivity. Numerous studies have shown that the final effector of the deleterious effect of peroxynitrite on vascular responsiveness is linked to the activation of poly (ADP-ribose) polymerases (PARP), which are proteins involved in many cellular processes such as DNA repair and apoptosis [13].

Superoxide anion per se has also been implicated in vascular hyporeactivity. Superoxide is enzymatically reduced to hydrogen peroxide in the presence of superoxide dismutase (SOD). However, in many disease states such as shock, there is an imbalance between the amount of superoxide formed and the ability of SOD enzyme to remove the former, hence leading to superoxide-driven damage. Macarthur et al. [29] have published experimental evidence suggesting that hyporeactivity to exogenous norepinephrine results from its deactivation by superoxide. Furthermore, these authors have also shown that endotoxin-induced hypotension is completely abolished by the administration of M40403, a synthetic and selective (for superoxide) low molecular weight mimic of SOD [30]. Nevertheless, despite these intriguing experimental results, there are currently no studies that have assessed the effects of neutralizing peroxynitrite or superoxide during human septic shock.

ATP-sensitive potassium channels

ATP-sensitive (K_{ATP}) potassium channels are distributed in a wide variety of tissues. Potassium (K^+) channels are membrane-spanning proteins that selectively allow movement of K^+ ions across cells through a water-filled permeation pathway (pore). A gating mechanism switches the channel between open and closed conformations. Normally, channel opening at the plasma membrane promotes K^+ loss from the cell, resulting in membrane hyperpolarization. These channels ensure the coupling between membrane excitability and energy metabolism of the cell, thus playing a primary role in both normal and pathological situations. Excessive activation of K^+ channels leads to membrane hyperpolarization and inhibition of voltage-sensitive calcium channels, inducing cell relaxation, vasodilation, and finally leading to hypotension and vascular hyporeactivity.

Various pathological situations such as increased NO and peroxynitrite production, ATP depletion, hypoxia, acidosis, and hyperlactatemia present during shock states can activate vascular K_{ATP} channels and induce membrane hyperpolarization, thereby inducing cellular relaxation and vasorelaxation [11].

Experimental evidence for the involvement of K_{ATP} channels was first established by Landry and Oliver [31] who demonstrated in an experimental model of endotoxic shock and hypoxic lactic acidosis that the injection of glibenclamide (a sulfonylurea inhibitor of K_{ATP} channels) restored arterial pressure and responsiveness to catecholamines, both of which are largely reduced during these types of shock. Several experimental studies [32] of endotoxic shock have since confirmed these data, while subsequent studies have highlighted a decrease in contractile function in response to vasoconstrictors in rat arteries incubated in the presence of endotoxin. This hypocontractility is in turn partly restored in the presence of glibenclamide [32].

To date, two studies [33, 34] have studied the effects of glibenclamide versus placebo administration in patients with septic shock. Both studies showed no significant reduction in vasoconstrictor dose requirements or any significant improvement in arterial blood pressure in patients treated with glibenclamide. At the present time, the therapeutic perspectives for the use of potassium channel inhibitors in humans remain disappointing given the ubiquitous nature of these channels and their diverse pathophysiological implications.

Involvement of BK_{Ca} channels

The large-conductance calcium-activated potassium (BK_{Ca}) channels are by far the most abundant of the vascular potassium channels. Their role is to induce vascular relaxation when calcium levels are elevated and thus play a regulatory role in microvascular flow. These channels are activated in part by NO and by peroxynitrite and are therefore involved in vasoplegia observed during shock states. Experimentally, their inhibition enables one to improve vasoconstrictor response in both animal [35] and human sepsis [36]. There are currently no human data.

Critical illness-related corticosteroid insufficiency

Critical illness-related corticosteroid insufficiency (CIRCI) is caused by adrenal insufficiency together with tissue corticosteroid resistance and is characterized by an exaggerated and protracted proinflammatory response [37]. CIRCI should be suspected in hypotensive patients who respond poorly to fluids and vasopressor agents, particularly in the setting of sepsis. In a study recently published by Annane et al. [38], the prevalence of adrenal insufficiency (as determined by metyrapone testing) in patients with severe sepsis and septic shock was reported to be 60%. Nevertheless, using an electrochemiluminescence immunoassay, data stemming from the Corticus Study [39, 40] demonstrated that there was a high inter-assay variation of total serum cortisol. Comparisons with a reference method revealed both over- and underestimations of true cortisol levels. These inter-assay variations in samples of patients with septic shock complicate the diagnosis of corticosteroid insufficiency.

The major effect of adrenal insufficiency in the critically ill patient is manifested through alterations in systemic inflammatory response and cardiovascular function. The use of glucocorticoids in septic shock is discussed in section “Therapeutics”.

Modifications of catecholamine signaling

The regulation of adrenergic receptors during sepsis has been studied at greater length for myocardial beta-receptors than for vascular alpha-receptors. At the heart level, Wu et al. [41] demonstrated that alpha-1 adrenergic receptors in the rat heart were externalized from light vesicles to the sarcolemma during the early hypercardiodynamic phase as opposed to being internalized from surface membranes to intracellular compartments during the late hypocardiodynamic phase of sepsis. The liver is the most studied organ, albeit with the difficulty in correlating the observed modifications with those presumably occurring at the vessel level. For example, McMillan et al. [42] observed a reduction in the number of hepatic alpha-1 adrenergic receptors in a rat model of chronic sepsis. Conversely, Hwang et al. [43] noted that alpha-1 adrenergic receptors in human liver plasma membranes undergo dynamic changes during the development of sepsis; that is, receptor number increased in mild sepsis, returned to normal levels in moderate sepsis, and finally decreased in severe sepsis. This desensitization has no univocal explanation and involves a decrease in the number of receptors (downregulation) and/or an uncoupling of receptors and their intracellular messengers.

The use of beta-blockers in septic shock has been investigated in normotensive rodent models but not in human septic shock [44].

Hyperglycemia and insulin

As part of the stress response, shock patients become hyperglycemic. Clearly, hyperglycemia is associated with adverse outcome and normalizing blood glucose by intensive insulin therapy improves mortality and morbidity. Pacheco et al. [45] demonstrated in healthy rats that high glucose increases iNOS induction and subsequent NO production by activating the protein kinase C-beta II. Glycemic control may affect regional NO bioavailability by changing NOS activity, NOS transcription, NOS substrate availability, or the endogenous NOS inhibitor asymmetric dimethylarginine (ADMA) levels [46].

Although promising in animal models [47], intensive insulin therapy did not improve in-hospital mortality in patients treated with hydrocortisone for septic shock [48].

Vasodilation is heterogeneous

During shock state and especially in sepsis, there are marked differences in vasopressor responses according to the vessel under investigation. Resistance arteries such as those present in the mesenteric vascular bed play a major role in blood pressure maintenance. On the other hand, conductance arteries such as the aorta only make a small contribution to systemic vascular resistance. The majority of in vitro investigations into mechanisms of vascular hyporeactivity have used rodent aortic tissues [15]. In contrast, inducing hyporeactivity in smaller rodent blood vessels has proven to be difficult [49]. Moreover, in septic shock patients, Stoclet et al. [50] found that contractile responses of small omental arteries from septic patients were not significantly altered ex vivo. This observation is certainly intriguing since the arteries were removed from patients whose peripheral resistance and blood pressure were dramatically reduced. Moreover, contraction experiments performed in the presence of either L-NAME or indomethacin unmasked enhanced responses to low concentrations of NE in arteries from septic patients. The mechanisms of this hyperactivity are unknown but highlight the potential opposite behavior between resistive and conductive arteries during sepsis.

From a clinical standpoint, we must keep in mind that arterial pressure during shock is measured in a conductive artery. Thus, the titration of vasopressor may be inadequate in increasing arterial pressure more than is needed for the microcirculation. This latter point is illustrated by the fact that the use of an NO donor such as nitroglycerin in hemodynamically resuscitated septic patients can open the microcirculation and thereby perfuse weak microcirculatory units [51].

Therapeutics

Catecholamines

After volume resuscitation, the use of catecholamine is considered to be the cornerstone of septic shock hemodynamic treatment [52]. Currently, dopamine and above all norepinephrine are the most used agents without any differences in terms of mortality [53]. It is generally considered that vasopressor agents must be titrated to increase mean arterial pressure to about 65–70 mmHg [54]. The pharmacodynamic effects of catecholamines are characterized by the existence of a concentration threshold at which the expected effect is observable (in the order of 100 pg/ml for adrenalin and 1,000 pg/ml for norepinephrine), followed by a linear increase in effect as a function of the logarithm of concentrations [55]. The maximum effect is usually achieved at doses ranging from 100 to 1,000 times the threshold dose, which largely surpasses the standard dosage range used in clinical practice. This type of dose–response curve explains why for threshold doses that differ by only 1 μg/kg/min from one patient to another, an identical pharmacodynamic effect on the dose–response curve will require dosages that differ by 10 μg/kg/min [56]. The obvious conclusion is therefore not to hesitate in transiently increasing the dosage of catecholamines if the patient is vasoplegic and hyperkinetic (although this remains experimental) or to use alternative therapies [57]. In this particular case, which is associated with a dramatic prognosis, other agents such as vasopressin or terlipressin [58], methylene blue [59], high volume hemofiltration [60], or plasmapheresis [61] have demonstrated their efficiency in case report studies or small series.

Vasopressin and terlipressin for catecholamine-resistant septic shock

Vasopressin (AVP), better known as antidiuretic hormone, is a nonapeptide produced by the supraoptic and paraventricular nuclei of the hypothalamus. AVP is synthesized in response to hyperosmolarity and arterial hypotension. As a result, its levels are extremely high in cardiogenic or hypovolemic shock. Paradoxically, in a study by Landry et al. [62] in which AVP levels in patients with cardiogenic shock were compared with that of patients with severe septic shock with both having similar arterial pressure values, sepsis was shown to induce a relative deficiency in AVP (22.7 vs. 3.1 pg/ml). Indeed, the neurohypophysis of a patient in septic shock is virtually depleted in AVP, as confirmed by the absence of T1-weighted hypersignal in magnetic resonance imaging [63]. AVP, by binding to its V1a or V1R receptor, located primarily on blood vessel smooth muscle cells, induces vasoconstriction. In clinical practice, vasopressin increases arterial blood pressure without any change in heart rate while generally decreasing cardiac index. However, some patients remain refractory to the doses of AVP used. It is probable that this lack of effectiveness is likely linked to a decreased vascular responsiveness to vasopressin as previously demonstrated [64]. Although effective in the weaning of vasopressors and for improving renal function, vasopressin treatment is potentially dangerous because of possible intense vasoconstriction if the obtained arterial pressure is too high. The VASST study [65], in which vasopressin was used in substitutive doses (less than 0.04 U/min), showed no overall improvement in mortality. However, in a post hoc study, patients with less severe septic shock (i.e., less than 15 μg/min of norepinephrine) at arginine vasopressin initiation had a lower 28-day mortality rate compared with norepinephrine-only infusion (26.5 vs. 35.7%; $P = 0.05$).

Terlipressin (TP) is a synthetic analogue of AVP characterized by greater selectivity for the V_1 receptor than AVP [66]. The elimination half-life of TP is longer than that of AVP (50 vs. 6 min). Bolus administration of TP has been associated with several adverse effects in both preclinical and clinical studies such as reduction in cardiac index or coronary vasoconstriction [58]. The adverse effects after intermittent TP bolus injections are probably due to excessive systemic and regional vasoconstriction. Consequently, it has been suggested that administration of lower TP boluses at shorter intervals or continuous infusion of TP may be equally effective in restoring systemic blood pressure, thereby avoiding the risk of uncontrolled vasoconstriction [67]. TP use has been demonstrated to be efficient in cases of catecholamine-resistant septic shock [68]. Nevertheless, based on current knowledge, it remains unclear whether AVP or TP should be preferred in the treatment of vasodilatory shock states unresponsive to conventional vasopressor agents.

Activated protein C

Recombinant human activated protein C (APC) has been demonstrated to reduce the mortality rate of adult patients with septic shock [69]. Initially, this effect was thought to be related to a reduction in coagulation and, to a lesser extent, to a reduction in inflammatory response to sepsis. Indeed, data from the PROWESS study demonstrated that the use of APC was associated with a quicker reduction in cardiovascular failure. Post-PROWESS investigative areas have been associated with a myriad of cellular studies [70] demonstrating that APC, through reactions mediated by the endothelial protein C receptor (EPCR) [71] and the effector receptor (protease activated receptor-1), acts directly on cells to exert multiple cytoprotective effects including: (a) downregulation of proinflammatory gene expression [72]; (b) anti-apoptotic activity [73]; (c) antioxidant properties; and (d) protection of endothelial barrier function [74]. Recent animal [75] and human [76] data have suggested that APC may improve both vascular and myocardial dysfunction and vascular reactivity to catecholamines during endotoxin and/or septic challenges. Nevertheless, despite a high recommendation level [52], the use of APC remains controversial. A multicenter study is currently investigating the effects of APC in a more severe (catecholamine dependent) and homogeneous group of septic shock patients.

Hydrocortisone

Hydrocortisone is widely used in patients with septic shock. Annane et al. [77] found a survival benefit only in patients who remained hypotensive after fluid and vasopressor resuscitation and whose plasma cortisol levels did not rise appropriately after the administration of corticotropin. On the other hand, Sprung et al. [39] found that hydrocortisone did not improve survival or reversal of shock in patients with septic shock, either overall or in patients who did not respond to corticotropin, although hydrocortisone hastened the reversal of shock in patients in whom shock was ultimately reversed. Clearly, hydrocortisone [5] treatment allows for a more rapid weaning of catecholamines in patients with severe septic shock treated with high doses of catecholamine, by reducing among others the production of interleukin-6 [77]. Furthermore, by decreasing the expression of NF-κB, corticoids also decrease the production of NO via iNOS. The detailed mechanisms of action of corticosteroids involve genomic as well as non-genomic effects after activation of their nuclear receptor [78]. Beneficial effects of glucocorticoids have also been found in non-infectious shock states such as vascular failure in post-cardiac surgical patients [79]. Currently, both the Surviving Sepsis Campaign [52] and the American College of Critical Care Medicine International Consensus [37] recommend giving stress-dose steroid therapy only in septic shock after blood pressure is identified to be poorly responsive to fluid and vasopressor therapy (grade 2C).

Conclusions

As previously described, the pathophysiology of shock-induced vascular hyporeactivity to vasopressor agents involves many mechanisms and a number of cellular pathways. Indeed, despite this vast amount of scientific knowledge, there is currently no "vascular-directed therapy" that has proven its efficiency in human septic shock. Indeed, many of the therapeutic approaches that have proved their efficiency in animal models and especially therapies directed against a particular compound have failed when used in human shock.

The most obvious conclusion is that preventing or decreasing the global cellular consequences of septic shock may prevent the overproduction of the involved mediators. For example, manipulating innate immunity with a peptide derived from the triggering receptor expressed on myeloid cells-1 (TREM-1) has been shown to improve hemodynamics and mortality in various forms of shock [80].

Another example stems from the Rivers study [81], in which patients who benefited from a goal-directed therapeutic approach required less vasopressor therapy after 24 h of treatment, hence demonstrating that early treatment of vascular failure accompanied by sound commonsense practices (antibiotic therapy, monitoring) enables one to reduce the impact of sepsis on vascular failure, likely by reducing the consequences of tissue hypoperfusion.

References

1. Angus DC, Linde-Zwirble WT, Lidicker J, Clermont G, Carcillo J, Pinsky MR (2001) Epidemiology of severe sepsis in the United States: analysis of incidence, outcome, and associated costs of care. Crit Care Med 29:1303–1310
2. Merx MW, Weber C (2007) Sepsis and the heart. Circulation 116:793–802
3. Matsuda N, Hattori Y (2007) Vascular biology in sepsis: pathophysiological and therapeutic significance of vascular dysfunction. J Smooth Muscle Res 43:117–137
4. Umans JG, Wylam ME, Samsel RW, Edwards J, Schumacker PT (1993) Effects of endotoxin in vivo on endothelial and smooth-muscle function in rabbit and rat aorta. Am Rev Respir Dis 148:1638–1645
5. Annane D, Bellissant E, Cavaillon JM (2005) Septic shock. Lancet 365:63–78
6. Bernardin G, Pradier C, Tiger F, Deloffre P, Mattei M (1996) Blood pressure and arterial lactate level are early indicators of short-term survival in human septic shock. Intensive Care Med 22:17–25
7. Abid O, Akca S, Haji-Michael P, Vincent JL (2000) Strong vasopressor support may be futile in the intensive care unit patient with multiple organ failure. Crit Care Med 28:947–949
8. Lamia B, Chemla D, Richard C, Teboul JL (2005) Clinical review: interpretation of arterial pressure wave in shock states. Crit Care 9:601–606
9. Benchekroune S, Karpati PC, Berton C, Nathan C, Mateo J, Chaara M, Riche F, Laisne MJ, Payen D, Mebazaa A (2008) Diastolic arterial blood pressure: a reliable early predictor of survival in human septic shock. J Trauma 64:1188–1195
10. Benedict CR, Rose JA (1992) Arterial norepinephrine changes in patients with septic shock. Circ Shock 38:165–172
11. Landry DW, Oliver JA (2001) The pathogenesis of vasodilatory shock. N Engl J Med 345:588–595
12. Alvarez S, Boveris A (2004) Mitochondrial nitric oxide metabolism in rat muscle during endotoxemia. Free Radic Biol Med 37:1472–1478
13. Lundberg JO, Weitzberg E (2005) NO generation from nitrite and its role in vascular control. Arterioscler Thromb Vasc Biol 25:915–922
14. Rees DD, Monkhouse JE, Cambridge D, Moncada S (1998) Nitric oxide and the haemodynamic profile of endotoxin shock in the conscious mouse. Br J Pharmacol 124:540–546
15. Julou-Schaeffer G, Gray GA, Fleming I, Schott C, Parratt JR, Stoclet JC (1990) Loss of vascular responsiveness induced by endotoxin involves L-arginine pathway. Am J Physiol 259:H1038–H1043
16. Boyle WA 3rd, Parvathaneni LS, Bourlier V, Sauter C, Laubach VE, Cobb JP (2000) iNOS gene expression modulates microvascular responsiveness in endotoxin-challenged mice. Circ Res 87:E18–E24
17. Walker TA, Curtis SE, King-VanVlack CE, Chapler CK, Vallet B, Cain SM (1995) Effects of nitric oxide synthase inhibition on regional hemodynamics and oxygen transport in endotoxic dogs. Shock 4:415–420
18. Vincent JL, Zhang H, Szabo C, Preiser JC (2000) Effects of nitric oxide in septic shock. Am J Respir Crit Care Med 161:1781–1785
19. Lopez A, Lorente JA, Steingrub J, Bakker J, McLuckie A, Willatts S, Brockway M, Anzueto A, Holzapfel L, Breen D, Silverman MS, Takala J, Donaldson J, Arneson C, Grove G, Grossman S, Grover R (2004) Multiple-center, randomized, placebo-controlled, double-blind study of the nitric oxide synthase inhibitor 546C88: effect on survival in patients with septic shock. Crit Care Med 32:21–30
20. Levy B, Valtier M, de Chillou C, Bollaert PE, Cane D, Mallie JP (1999) Beneficial effects of L-canavanine, a selective inhibitor of inducible nitric oxide synthase, on lactate metabolism and muscle high energy phosphates during endotoxic shock in rats. Shock 11:98–103
21. Cauwels A (2007) Nitric oxide in shock. Kidney Int 72:557–565
22. Cauwels A, Buys ES, Thoonen R, Geary L, Delanghe J, Shiva S, Brouckaert P (2009) Nitrite protects against morbidity and mortality associated with TNF- or LPS-induced shock in a soluble guanylate cyclase-dependent manner. J Exp Med 206:2915–2924

23. Wang P, Zhou M, Cioffi WG, Bland KI, Ba ZF, Chaudry IH (2000) Is prostacyclin responsible for producing the hyperdynamic response during early sepsis? Crit Care Med 28:1534–1539
24. Schildknecht S, Bachschmid M, Baumann A, Ullrich V (2004) COX-2 inhibitors selectively block prostacyclin synthesis in endotoxin-exposed vascular smooth muscle cells. FASEB J 18:757–759
25. Höcherl K, Schmidt C, Kurt B, Bucher M (2008) Activation of the PGI(2)/IP system contributes to the development of circulatory failure in a rat model of endotoxic shock. Hypertension 52:330–335
26. Bernard GR, Wheeler AP, Russell JA, Schein R, Summer WR, Steinberg KP, Fulkerson WJ, Wright PE, Christman BW, Dupont WD, Higgins SB, Swindell BB (1997) The effects of ibuprofen on the physiology and survival of patients with sepsis. The Ibuprofen in Sepsis Study Group. N Engl J Med 336:912–918
27. Pacher P, Beckman JS, Liaudet L (2007) Nitric oxide and peroxynitrite in health and disease. Physiol Rev 87:315–424
28. Szabo C, Salzman AL, Ischiropoulos H (1995) Endotoxin triggers the expression of an inducible isoform of nitric oxide synthase and the formation of peroxynitrite in the rat aorta in vivo. FEBS Lett 363:235–238
29. Macarthur H, Westfall TC, Riley DP, Misko TP, Salvemini D (2000) Inactivation of catecholamines by superoxide gives new insights on the pathogenesis of septic shock. Proc Natl Acad Sci U S A 97:9753–9758
30. Salvemini D, Wang ZQ, Zweier JL, Samouilov A, Macarthur H, Misko TP, Currie MG, Cuzzocrea S, Sikorski JA, Riley DP (1999) A nonpeptidyl mimic of superoxide dismutase with therapeutic activity in rats. Science 286:304–306
31. Landry DW, Oliver JA (1992) The ATP-sensitive K^+ channel mediates hypotension in endotoxemia and hypoxic lactic acidosis in dog. J Clin Invest 89:2071–2074
32. Buckley JF, Singer M, Clapp LH (2006) Role of KATP channels in sepsis. Cardiovasc Res 72:220–230
33. Warrillow S, Egi M, Bellomo R (2006) Randomized, double-blind, placebo-controlled crossover pilot study of a potassium channel blocker in patients with septic shock. Crit Care Med 34:980–985
34. Morelli A, Lange M, Ertmer C, Broeking K, Van Aken H, Orecchioni A, Rocco M, Bachetoni A, Traber DL, Landoni G, Pietropaoli P, Westphal M (2007) Glibenclamide dose response in patients with septic shock: effects on norepinephrine requirements, cardiopulmonary performance, and global oxygen transport. Shock 28:530–535
35. Cauwels A, Brouckaert P (2008) Critical role for small and large conductance calcium-dependent potassium channels in endotoxemia and TNF toxicity. Shock 29:577–582
36. Pickkers P, Dorresteijn MJ, Bouw MP, van der Hoeven JG, Smits P (2006) In vivo evidence for nitric oxide-mediated calcium-activated potassium-channel activation during human endotoxemia. Circulation 114:414–421
37. Marik PE, Pastores SM, Annane D, Meduri GU, Sprung CL, Arlt W, Keh D, Briegel J, Beishuizen A, Dimopoulou I, Tsagarakis S, Singer M, Chrousos GP, Zaloga G, Bokhari F, Vogeser M (2008) Recommendations for the diagnosis and management of corticosteroid insufficiency in critically ill adult patients: consensus statements from an international task force by the American College of Critical Care Medicine. Crit Care Med 36:1937–1949
38. Annane D, Maxime V, Ibrahim F, Alvarez JC, Abe E, Boudou P (2006) Diagnosis of adrenal insufficiency in severe sepsis and septic shock. Am J Respir Crit Care Med 174:1319–1326
39. Sprung CL, Annane D, Keh D, Moreno R, Singer M, Freivogel K, Weiss YG, Benbenishty J, Kalenka A, Forst H, Laterre PF, Reinhart K, Cuthbertson BH, Payen D, Briegel J (2008) Hydrocortisone therapy for patients with septic shock. N Engl J Med 358:111–124
40. Briegel J, Sprung CL, Annane D, Singer M, Keh D, Moreno R, Mohnle P, Weiss Y, Avidan A, Brunkhorst FM, Fiedler F, Vogeser M (2009) Multicenter comparison of cortisol as measured by different methods in samples of patients with septic shock. Intensive Care Med 35:2151–2156
41. Wu LL, Tang C, Liu MS (1997) Hyper- and hypocardiodynamic states are associated with externalization and internalization, respectively, of alpha-adrenergic receptors in rat heart during sepsis. Shock 7:318–323
42. McMillan M, Chernow B, Roth BL (1986) Hepatic alpha 1-adrenergic receptor alteration in a rat model of chronic sepsis. Circ Shock 19:185–193
43. Hwang TL, Lau YT, Huang SF, Chen MF, Liu MS (1994) Changes of alpha 1-adrenergic receptors in human liver during intraabdominal sepsis. Hepatology 20:638–642
44. de Montmollin E, Aboab J, Mansart A, Annane D (2009) Bench-to-bedside review: β-adrenergic modulation in sepsis. Crit Care 13:230
45. Pacheco ME, Beltran A, Redondo J, Manso AM, Alonso MJ, Salaices M (2006) High glucose enhances inducible nitric oxide synthase expression. Role of protein kinase C-betaII. Eur J Pharmacol 538:115–123
46. Ellger B, Richir MC, van Leeuwen PA, Debaveye Y, Langouche L, Vanhorebeek I, Teerlink T, Van den Berghe G (2008) Glycemic control modulates arginine and asymmetrical-dimethylarginine levels during critical illness by preserving dimethylarginine-dimethylaminohydrolase activity. Endocrinology 149:3148–3157
47. Holger JS, Dries DJ, Barringer KW, Peake BJ, Flottemesch TJ, Marini JJ (2010) Cardiovascular and metabolic effects of high-dose insulin in a porcine septic shock model. Acad Emerg Med 17:429–435
48. Annane D, Cariou A, Maxime V, Azoulay E, D'Honneur G, Timsit JF, Cohen Y, Wolf M, Fartoukh M, Adrie C, Santre C, Bollaert PE, Mathonet A, Amathieu R, Tabah A, Clec'h C, Mayaux J, Lejeune J, Chevret S (2010) Corticosteroid treatment and intensive insulin therapy for septic shock in adults: a randomized controlled trial. JAMA 303:341–348
49. Mitchell JA, Kohlhaas KL, Sorrentino R, Warner TD, Murad F, Vane JR (1993) Induction by endotoxin of nitric oxide synthase in the rat mesentery: lack of effect on action of vasoconstrictors. Br J Pharmacol 109:265–270
50. Stoclet JC, Martinez MC, Ohlmann P, Chasserot S, Schott C, Kleschyov AL, Schneider F, Andriantsitohaina R (1999) Induction of nitric oxide synthase and dual effects of nitric oxide and cyclooxygenase products in regulation of arterial contraction in human septic shock. Circulation 100:107–112
51. Spronk PE, Ince C, Gardien MJ, Mathura KR, Oudemans-van Straaten HM, Zandstra DF (2002) Nitroglycerin in septic shock after intravascular volume resuscitation. Lancet 360:1395–1396

52. Dellinger RP, Levy MM, Carlet JM, Bion J, Parker MM, Jaeschke R, Reinhart K, Angus DC, Brun-Buisson C, Beale R, Calandra T, Dhainaut JF, Gerlach H, Harvey M, Marini JJ, Marshall J, Ranieri M, Ramsay G, Sevransky J, Thompson BT, Townsend S, Vender JS, Zimmerman JL, Vincent JL (2008) Surviving Sepsis Campaign: international guidelines for management of severe sepsis and septic shock: 2008. Intensive Care Med 34:17–60
53. De Backer D, Biston P, Devriendt J, Madl C, Chochrad D, Aldecoa C, Brasseur A, Defrance P, Gottignies P, Vincent JL (2010) Comparison of dopamine and norepinephrine in the treatment of shock. N Engl J Med 362:779–789
54. LeDoux D, Astiz ME, Carpati CM, Rackow EC (2000) Effects of perfusion pressure on tissue perfusion in septic shock. Crit Care Med 28:2729–2732
55. Breslow MJ, Ligier B (1991) Hyperadrenergic states. Crit Care Med 19:1566–1579
56. Insel PA (1996) Seminars in medicine of the Beth Israel Hospital, Boston. Adrenergic receptors—evolving concepts and clinical implications. N Engl J Med 334:580–585
57. Katsaragakis S, Kapralou A, Theodorou D, Markogiannakis H, Larentzakis A, Stamou KM, Drimousis P, Bramis I (2006) Refractory septic shock: efficacy and safety of very high doses of norepinephrine. Methods Find Exp Clin Pharmacol 28:307–313
58. Lange M, Ertmer C, Westphal M (2008) Vasopressin vs. terlipressin in the treatment of cardiovascular failure in sepsis. Intensive Care Med 34:821–832
59. Kirov MY, Evgenov OV, Evgenov NV, Egorina EM, Sovershaev MA, Sveinbjornsson B, Nedashkovsky EV, Bjertnaes LJ (2001) Infusion of methylene blue in human septic shock: a pilot, randomized, controlled study. Crit Care Med 29:1860–1867
60. Honore PM, Matson JR (2002) Short-term high-volume hemofiltration in sepsis: perhaps the right way is to start with. Crit Care Med 30:1673–1674
61. Ataman K, Jehmlich M, Kock S, Neumann S, Leischik M, Filipovic Z, Hopf HB (2002) Short-term cardiovascular effects of plasmapheresis in norepinephrine-refractory septic shock. Intensive Care Med 28:1164–1167
62. Landry DW, Levin HR, Gallant EM, Ashton RC Jr, Seo S, D'Alessandro D, Oz MC, Oliver JA (1997) Vasopressin deficiency contributes to the vasodilation of septic shock. Circulation 95:1122–1125
63. Sharshar T, Carlier R, Blanchard A, Feydy A, Gray F, Paillard M, Raphael JC, Gajdos P, Annane D (2002) Depletion of neurohypophyseal content of vasopressin in septic shock. Crit Care Med 30:497–500
64. Leone M, Boyle WA (2006) Decreased vasopressin responsiveness in vasodilatory septic shock-like conditions. Crit Care Med 34:1126–1130
65. Russell JA, Walley KR, Singer J, Gordon AC, Hebert PC, Cooper DJ, Holmes CL, Mehta S, Granton JT, Storms MM, Cook DJ, Presneill JJ, Ayers D (2008) Vasopressin versus norepinephrine infusion in patients with septic shock. N Engl J Med 358:877–887
66. Westphal M, Traber DL (2005) Low-dose terlipressin for hemodynamic support in sepsis and systemic inflammatory response syndrome: art for (he)art's sake or state of the art? Crit Care Med 33:455–457
67. Broking K, Lange M, Morelli A, Ertmer C, Aken HV, Luecke M, Rehberg S, Bowering N, Bone HG, Traber DL, Westphal M (2008) Employing dobutamine as a useful agent to reverse the terlipressin-linked impairments in cardiopulmonary hemodynamics and global oxygen transport in healthy and endotoxemic sheep. Shock 29:71–77
68. Lange M, Morelli A, Ertmer C, Broking K, Rehberg S, Van Aken H, Traber DL, Westphal M (2007) Role of adenosine triphosphate-sensitive potassium channel inhibition in shock states: physiology and clinical implications. Shock 28:394–400
69. Bernard GR, Vincent JL, Laterre PF, LaRosa SP, Dhainaut JF, Lopez-Rodriguez A, Steingrub JS, Garber GE, Helterbrand JD, Ely EW, Fisher CJ Jr (2001) Efficacy and safety of recombinant human activated protein C for severe sepsis. N Engl J Med 344:699–709
70. Mosnier LO, Zlokovic BV, Griffin JH (2007) The cytoprotective protein C pathway. Blood 109:3161–3172
71. Esmon CT (2006) The endothelial protein C receptor. Curr Opin Hematol 13:382–385
72. Joyce DE, Gelbert L, Ciaccia A, DeHoff B, Grinnell BW (2001) Gene expression profile of antithrombotic protein C defines new mechanisms modulating inflammation and apoptosis. J Biol Chem 276:11199–11203
73. Bilbault P, Lavaux T, Launoy A, Gaub MP, Meyer N, Oudet P, Pottecher T, Jaeger A, Schneider F (2007) Influence of drotrecogin alpha (activated) infusion on the variation of Bax/Bcl-2 and Bax/Bcl-xl ratios in circulating mononuclear cells: a cohort study in septic shock patients. Crit Care Med 35:69–75
74. Nacira S, Meziani F, Dessebe O, Cattan V, Collin S, Montemont C, Gibot S, Asfar P, Ramaroson A, Regnault V, Slama M, Lecompte T, Lacolley P, Levy B (2009) Activated protein C improves lipopolysaccharide-induced cardiovascular dysfunction by decreasing tissular inflammation and oxidative stress. Crit Care Med 37:246–255
75. Favory R, Lancel S, Marechal X, Tissier S, Neviere R (2006) Cardiovascular protective role for activated protein C during endotoxemia in rats. Intensive Care Med 32:899–905
76. Monnet X, Lamia B, Anguel N, Richard C, Bonmarchand G, Teboul JL (2005) Rapid and beneficial hemodynamic effects of activated protein C in septic shock patients. Intensive Care Med 31:1573–1576
77. Annane D, Sebille V, Charpentier C, Bollaert PE, Francois B, Korach JM, Capellier G, Cohen Y, Azoulay E, Troche G, Chaumet-Riffaut P, Bellissant E (2002) Effect of treatment with low doses of hydrocortisone and fludrocortisone on mortality in patients with septic shock. JAMA 288:862–871
78. Prigent H, Maxime V, Annane D (2004) Clinical review: corticotherapy in sepsis. Crit Care 8:122–129
79. Kilger E, Weis F, Briegel J, Frey L, Goetz AE, Reuter D, Nagy A, Schuetz A, Lamm P, Knoll A, Peter K (2003) Stress doses of hydrocortisone reduce severe systemic inflammatory response syndrome and improve early outcome in a risk group of patients after cardiac surgery. Crit Care Med 31:1068–1074
80. Gibot S, Massin F, Alauzet C, Montemont C, Lozniewski A, Bollaert PE, Levy B (2008) Effects of the TREM-1 pathway modulation during mesenteric ischemia-reperfusion in rats. Crit Care Med 36:504–510
81. Rivers E, Nguyen B, Havstad S, Ressler J, Muzzin A, Knoblich B, Peterson E, Tomlanovich M (2001) Early goal-directed therapy in the treatment of severe sepsis and septic shock. N Engl J Med 345:1368–1377

Daniel De Backer
Gustavo Ospina-Tascon
Diamantino Salgado
Raphaël Favory
Jacques Creteur
Jean-Louis Vincent

Monitoring the microcirculation in the critically ill patient: current methods and future approaches

Abstract *Purpose:* To discuss the techniques currently available to evaluate the microcirculation in critically ill patients. In addition, the most clinically relevant microcirculatory alterations will be discussed. *Methods:* Review of the literature on methods used to evaluate the microcirculation in humans and on microcirculatory alterations in critically ill patients. *Results:* In experimental conditions, shock states have been shown to be associated with a decrease in perfused capillary density and an increase in the heterogeneity of microcirculatory perfusion, with non-perfused capillaries in close vicinity to perfused capillaries. Techniques used to evaluate the microcirculation in humans should take into account the heterogeneity of microvascular perfusion. Microvideoscopic techniques, such as orthogonal polarization spectral (OPS) and sidestream dark field (SDF) imaging, directly evaluate microvascular networks covered by a thin epithelium, such as the sublingual microcirculation. Laser Doppler and tissue O_2 measurements satisfactorily detect global decreases in tissue perfusion but not heterogeneity of microvascular perfusion. These techniques, and in particular laser Doppler and near-infrared spectroscopy, may help to evaluate the dynamic response of the microcirculation to a stress test. In patients with severe sepsis and septic shock, the microcirculation is characterized by a decrease in capillary density and in the proportion of perfused capillaries, together with a blunted response to a vascular occlusion test. *Conclusions:* The microcirculation in humans can be evaluated directly by videomicroscopy (OPS/SDF) or indirectly by vascular occlusion tests. Of note, direct videomicroscopic visualization evaluates the actual state of the microcirculation, whereas the vascular occlusion test evaluates microvascular reserve.

Keywords Microcirculation · Cardiac output · Hemodynamic monitoring · Capillaries · Oxygen delivery · Outcome

Introduction

The microcirculation plays a fundamental role in gas and nutrient exchange; it must constantly adapt by controlling vascular tone. In disease states, increased permeability may be necessary to provide the inflammatory response, including leukocyte diapedesis. It is difficult to simultaneously evaluate these different aspects of the microcirculation. In this review, we will focus on the role of the microcirculation in oxygenation, dealing with the evaluation of blood flow and its implication for cellular oxygenation.

M.R. Pinsky et al. (eds.), *Applied Physiology in Intensive Care Medicine 2: Physiological Reviews and Editorials*,
DOI 10.1007/978-3-642-28233-1_26,

In experimental conditions, intravital microscopy is considered as a gold standard, allowing measurement of blood flow in individual vessels and could be coupled with measurements of oxygenation, endothelial activation (including generation of reactive oxygen species), and permeability measurements. Unfortunately, this technique is not applicable as such in humans, as it can only be applied on organs that can be submitted to transillumination, with light coming from the opposite side to the microscope objective, such as cremaster muscle, liver edge, intestine, and dorsal skinfold. It also uses specific dyes that are often not registered for human use.

In humans, and especially in critically ill patients, the evaluation of the microcirculation has long been difficult. Recent years have witnessed the development of new techniques that can either directly visualize or indirectly evaluate microvascular perfusion. In order to appreciate the information provided by the various techniques, it is important to understand the architecture of the microcirculation and its behavior in health and disease.

Characteristics of the normal and the diseased microcirculation

The microcirculation comprises vessels smaller than 100 microns, i.e., arterioles, capillaries, and venules. Arterioles divide into small branches, and the terminology of A1, A2-An is used to define each vessel before bifurcation (1st bifurcation for A1, 2nd for A2,...). Arterioles are mostly responsible for vascular tone, with a considerable decrease in blood pressure from proximal to terminal arterioles. Local modulation of arteriolar tone in first-order arterioles is responsible for adapting microvascular perfusion to local O_2 demand [1]. Capillaries originate from the terminal arterioles, are covered by a thin endothelial surface, and are mostly responsible for O_2 and nutrient exchange, as well as elimination of cellular waste products. Capillary networks vary in density and architecture. Capillary architecture differs somewhat among organs, with arborescence being the most common form, but the gut, liver, and kidney have different architecture. In general, arterioles divide into smaller and smaller vessels until the capillaries, and these never merge. The length and orientation of the capillaries may vary from one organ to another. Capillaries flow into small venules which merge into larger ones, and contact between venules and arterioles/capillaries is limited. In some organs, the specific architecture may favor countercurrent exchange mechanisms [2]. Leukocyte adhesion, rolling, and migration, as well as permeability changes take place mostly in venules, although again there may be some variability among organs [3]. Although arterioles are responsible for fine tuning microcirculatory perfusion, events occurring at capillary and even venular sites may affect capillary perfusion as cross-talk occurs within endothelial cells [1, 4].

Typical microcirculatory alterations in disease states

Numerous experimental studies have reported that microvascular blood flow is altered in sepsis. Shortly after endotoxin administration, functional capillary density (FCD) is decreased, and this effect is directly dose-dependent [5]. This decrease in FCD is associated with an increase in the diffusion distance for O_2 [6]. As the shutdown of capillaries is heterogeneous, some areas become deprived of capillaries while others are not, so that perfused capillaries are in close vicinity to non-perfused capillaries [7, 8].

Low-flow conditions such as hemorrhage or cardiogenic shock are associated with a progressive decrease in arteriolar diameter [9], associated with a substantial decrease in FCD [10] as a result of shutting down some capillaries while others remain perfused with reduced flow. The severity of the decrease in FCD is directly related to a poor outcome [10]. When global flow returns, the microcirculation becomes more heterogeneous as a result of the inflammatory response associated with reperfusion [10].

What are the consequences of the heterogeneity of microvascular perfusion?

In normal circumstances, heterogeneity is minimal [11], and matching of perfusion to metabolism improves in hypoxic or low-flow conditions [7, 12]. In sepsis, heterogeneity cannot be improved in response to changes in O_2 demand or to decreases in O_2 delivery [7], and tissue perfusion and oxygenation are, therefore, compromised [13]. Similar findings can be observed in reperfusion injury [11, 14].

Heterogeneity of the microvascular perfusion is associated with heterogeneity in O_2 diffusion distance, with a shift to higher median values [6]. As a result, an O_2 extraction defect is observed, with an increased mixed venous O_2 saturation (SvO_2) [7, 8], even though O_2 extraction in a single perfused capillary may be increased [15]. Importantly, tissues tolerate better a homogeneous decrease in blood flow better than a heterogeneous one [16]. As shown in a theoretical example in Fig. 1, a 50% decrease in flow in a homogeneously perfused tissue is accompanied by preserved tissue O_2 consumption, as a result of increased O_2 extraction. A 50% reduction in capillary density, resulting in heterogeneous perfusion, is associated with a reduction in tissue O_2 consumption (and hence tissue hypoxia) as a result of increased diffusion distance. In these conditions, venous PO_2/SO_2 will

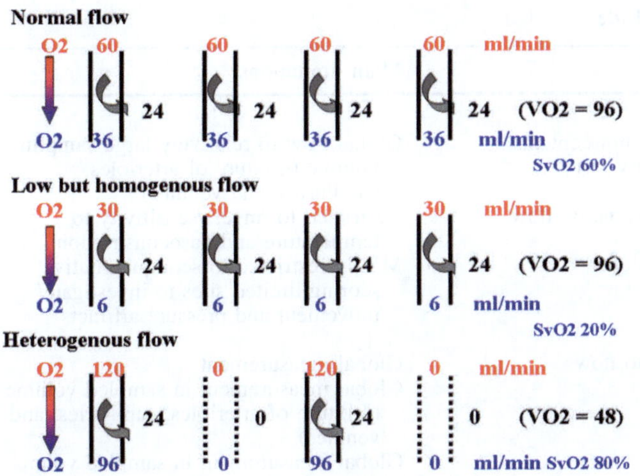

Fig. 1 Impact of heterogenous perfusion on tissue metabolism and venous oxygen saturation. Normal situation (*top panel*): O_2 is delivered at 240 ml/min in four perfused capillaries. The tissues extract oxygen to meet cellular oxygen consumption. Low flow but homogeneous perfusion (*middle panel*): half the oxygen is delivered to the tissue but all the capillaries are perfused. The amount of oxygen is sufficient to meet oxygen requirement of the cells. Hence, VO_2 is preserved even though venous oxygen saturation is severely decreased. Heterogeneous flow (*bottom panel*): even though total oxygen delivery is preserved (240 ml/min) only 50% of the capillaries are perfused. Cells close to the perfused capillaries consume the normal amount of oxygen. Cell too far away from perfused capillaries do not receive enough oxygen to meet their oxygen requirements and become hypoxic. As a consequence, hypoxic zones can be encountered in the presence of an elevated venous oxygen saturation. Note: this schematic presentation is simplified. In normal conditions, recruitment of microcirculation is not maximal and a mild degree of heterogeneity can be observed. In response to systemic low flow, such as illustrated in *middle panel*, the microcirculation tends to adapt by recruiting previously unfilled capillaries and decreasing perfusion heterogeneity [13, 118]. When endothelial dysfunction occurs and heterogeneity develops, such as in *bottom panel*, these adaptive mechanisms are lost. In addition to these, tissues try to limit the impact of decreases in perfusion by decreasing metabolism, which leads to a decrease in O_2 consumption (concept of oxygen conformance [119])

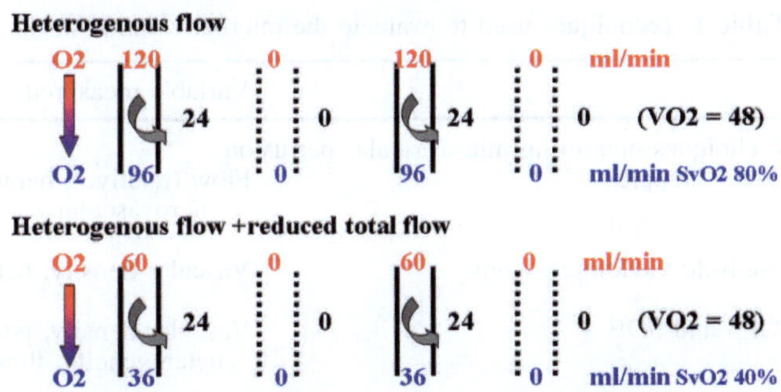

Fig. 2 Venous O_2 saturation can be low in conditions associated with microvascular shunting. When perfusion is heterogeneous, a low venous oxygen saturation can also be encountered. If total flow to the tissue is decreased (*bottom panel*), venous oxygen saturation decreases but this fails to reflect an improvement in perfusion heterogeneity

increase; this explains the typically high SvO_2 in sepsis. Nevertheless, SvO_2 can still decrease in sepsis [17]: as illustrated in Fig. 2, if blood flow decreases by 50% without further altering heterogeneity, SvO_2 will decrease as a result of the increase in extraction in perfused capillaries.

The heterogeneity of tissue perfusion may not be revealed by all methods used to evaluate the microcirculation: these techniques should have a sufficient spatial resolution to detect heterogeneity in blood flow or in PO_2.

Techniques used to evaluate the microcirculation

The evaluation of the microcirculation can include assessment of its transport and exchange functions, permeability, and regulation of inflammation and coagulation. In this manuscript we will focus on the transport and exchange functions. The latter can be assessed by using markers of microvascular perfusion and indirectly by indices of tissue oxygenation (Table 1).

By definition, any device looking at the microcirculation can only evaluate the microcirculation in the microvascular bed in which it is implemented. The ability of that specific window to represent other beds depends on the mechanisms implicated in microvascular disease (generalized, diffuse but somewhat heterogeneous or localized), on organ microvascular architecture, and on local factors (local vasoconstriction/pressure). Some areas may be more relevant than others, as illustrated by a relationship with microcirculatory alterations in that area with outcome. Nevertheless one should, at best, consider that the area being investigated is a window that reflects the minimal alterations that are likely to be observed in other areas, provided that local factors do not exacerbate the lesion in the investigated area.

Evaluation of microvascular perfusion

Clinical evaluation and biomarkers

An impaired microcirculation may be suspected in the presence of mottled skin, acrocyanosis, slow recoloration time, or increased central to toe temperature gradient [18, 19]. These signs of impaired cutaneous perfusion lack specificity (and even sensitivity) for disclosing more central microcirculatory alterations, including the sublingual microcirculation [19]. Skin vasoconstriction is a physiological response to low cardiac output, in an attempt to redistribute blood flow to more central compartments. Accordingly, it is fair to say that these clinical signs indicate the severity of cardiovascular impairment [18] and are, therefore, associated with a poor outcome

Table 1 Techniques used to evaluate the microcirculation at the bedside

	Variable measured	Main limitations
Techniques measuring microvascular perfusion		
Laser Doppler	Flow (relative), hemoglobin content/ microvascular reactivity test	Global flow to relatively large sampling volume (mixture of arterioles, capillaries, and venules)
Nailfold videomicroscopy	Vascular density, heterogeneity, flow	Restricted to fingers/sensitivity to temperature and vasoconstriction
OPS and SDF	Vascular density, perfusion heterogeneity, flow	Mostly restricted to semiquantitative scoring/limited sites to investigate/ movement and pressure artifacts
Techniques measuring tissue oxygenation		
SvO_2	Adequacy of perfusion to flow	Global measurement
O_2 electrodes	Tissue PO_2	Global measurement in sampled volume (mixture of arterioles, capillaries, and venules)
NIRS	Tissue O_2 saturation	Global measurement in sampled volume (mixture of arterioles, capillaries, and venules)
Reflectance spectroscopy	O_2 saturation/microvascular reactivity test	Global measurement in sampled volume (mixture of arterioles, capillaries, and venules) unless SO_2 histograms are provided
Gastric tonometry	Tissue CO_2 (reflects inadequate perfusion and/or anaerobic metabolism)	Interference (feeding/reflux)/difficult discrimination between low flow and anaerobic metabolism
Sublingual capnometry	Tissue CO_2 (reflects inadequate perfusion and/or anaerobic metabolism)	Availability limited/difficult discrimination between low flow and anaerobic metabolism
Microdialysis and equilibrium dialysis	Lactate/pyruvate	Time lag/limited sites to investigate

OPS orthogonal polarization spectral imaging technique; *SDF* sidestream dark field imaging technique; *SvO_2* mixed-venous oxygen saturation; *NIRS* near-infrared spectroscopy; *EMPHO* Erlangen MicroPHOtometer

[20], but they do not provide relevant information on the central microcirculation [19].

Biological markers can also be used. Blood lactate levels may be considered, but they lack sensitivity and specificity. Nevertheless, several trials have shown that therapeutic interventions inducing improvement in microvascular perfusion are associated with an inverse and proportional decrease in lactate levels [21, 22].

In experimental conditions, increased plasma hyaluronan levels were associated with impaired microcirculation in sepsis and therapies that improved the microcirculation also caused a decrease in hyaluronan levels [23]. Whether these levels can be used to detect microvascular alterations in critically ill patients remains to be determined.

Laser Doppler flowmetry

Laser Doppler techniques are frequently used to measure microvascular blood flow. They can be applied on various tissues and probes can even be inserted in the upper digestive tract through a nasogastric tube [24]. As laser Doppler techniques provide measurements of blood flow in relative units (mV), one can only assess relative changes from baseline. The main limitation of this technique is that it measures flow in a variable volume of tissue and it is unable to detect it in individual vessels. The sampling volume of current laser Doppler devices is between 0.5 and 1 mm^3, so that the flow that is measured represents the average flow in at least 50 vessels, including arterioles, capillaries, and venules of variable size, direction, and perfusion. Given the heterogeneous aspect of microvascular alterations, these will be missed by these devices that measure only total blood flow to a piece of tissue.

Scanning laser Doppler and reflected-mode confocal laser scanning microscopy are two attractive developments as they can both visualize the field of interest, allowing semiquantitative evaluation of heterogeneity of perfusion [25, 26]. As with traditional laser Doppler techniques, the resolution of the beam is crucial, the confocal aspect allowing narrowing of the laser beam. With a confocal technique, measurements of vascular density, diameters, and blood flow can be obtained [26, 27]. As a result of the size of the device, it can currently only be applied in humans to study skin perfusion.

Laser Doppler devices allow a vasoreactivity test, based on the fact that after transient ischemia obtained by arterial occlusion with a cuff placed around the arm the speed of flow recovery will mostly be determined by the capacity of the microvasculature to recruit arterioles and capillaries. The ascending slope after transient occlusion is a marker of endothelial reactivity and blood rheology, and can thus be used as a surrogate for the functional integrity of the microvasculature [28]. Although it may not reflect the actual state of the microcirculation, this test provides quantitative information on microvascular reserve within a couple of minutes.

Microvideoscopic techniques

Intravital microvideoscopy is used as a "classical" technique in experimental conditions, but in humans fixed tissue preparations and dyes cannot be used. Microvideoscopy techniques apply light on superficial organs and need technical devices to discard light reflected by the superficial layers of the tissues. Their application in humans requires that either the organ is thin enough to be illuminated from behind (e.g., fingers) or that organs can be made translucent by reflected light.

Nailfold videocapillaroscopy

Nailfold microvideoscopy was the first method used at the bedside [29]. The junction between cuticle and nail is coated with transparent oil and placed on the stage of an ordinary microscope. In addition to morphological abnormalities, mostly encountered in chronic diseases of the microcirculation, capillary density and microvascular blood flow can be measured [30]. This technique is particularly suitable for investigating the microvascular effects of chronic diseases, such as diabetes, vasculitis, and arteritis. Unfortunately, the nailfold area is very sensitive to changes in temperature: one can control ambient but not body temperature. Peripheral vasoconstriction can also occur during chills and acute circulatory failure with or without vasopressor agents. Hence, this area is of limited use in critically ill patients.

Orthogonal polarization spectral and sidestream darkfield imaging techniques

Orthogonal polarization spectral (OPS) and sidestream darkfield (SDF) are two videomicroscopic imaging techniques that can be applied at the bedside. Both are based on the same general principles developed more than 20 years ago [31, 32], but were only recently implemented in handheld devices. If one applies a light source on a tissue, the light is reflected by the deeper layers of the tissue providing transillumination of the superficial layers of the tissue [32]. With both techniques, the selected wavelength (530 nm) is absorbed by the hemoglobin contained in the red blood cells, independently of its oxygenation state, so that these can be seen as black/gray bodies. In OPS (Fig. 3), the applied light is polarized

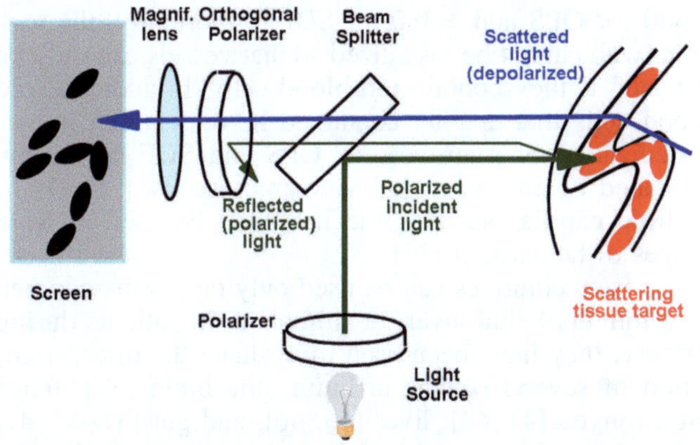

Fig. 3 Orthogonal polarization spectral (OPS) imaging technique. Polarized light is directed to the tissue. Light reflected by the superficial layers is still polarized and discarded by the orthogonal filter. Light reflected from the depth of the tissues has encountered many scattering events and has lost its polarized characteristics so is not discarded by the orthogonal filter; this light is absorbed by hemoglobin contained in red blood cells so that these will be seen as gray/black bodies on the screen

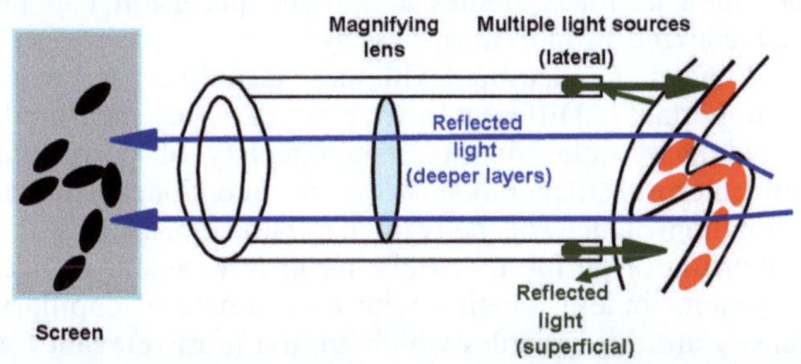

Fig. 4 Sidestream dark field (SDF) imaging technique. Green light is provided by the lateral sides of the device. Light reflected by superficial layers fails to reach the center of the device where the optics are located. Light reflected from the depth of the tissues reaches the center of the device; this light is absorbed by hemoglobin contained in red blood cells so that these will be seen as gray/black bodies on the screen

and the reflected light is depolarized, due to multiple hits on cells in the deep layers of the tissue [33]. The light reflected by the surface of the tissue is still polarized and can easily be discarded by a polarizer filter [33]. The SDF technique (Fig. 4) uses pulsed green light which is provided to the tissue by multiple peripheral emitting diodes while the optics are located centrally [34]. As a result of the isolation of the light source from the inner lenses, the light reflected by the superficial layers is perpendicular to the light source and does not reach the optics. Both devices provide good quality images of microvascular vessels filled with red blood cells. As a result of the peripheral location of multiple stroboscopic diodes and synchronization of light emission and camera frame rate, SDF provides more detailed visualization of capillaries, with sharper and less granular images than OPS [34]. Using the ×5 objective, the on-screen magnification is

×340 for OPS and ×380 for SDF. Importantly, the vascular wall cannot be visualized so that vessels can only be detected if they contain red blood cells. In addition, red blood cells that are not contained in vessels can impair visualization of microvessels. OPS and SDF have been validated against intravital videomicroscopy [35–37] or nailfold capillaroscopy [38]. They can be used at wide ranges of hematocrit [35].

These techniques can be used only on organs covered by a thin epithelial layer. In animals or in patients during surgery, they have been used to evaluate the microcirculation of several organs including the brain [39], lungs [40], tongue [41–44], liver [45, 46], and gut [41–44, 47, 48]. In intact humans, this technique can be applied to the skin [38, 49–51], conjunctiva [52], gingiva [53], sublingual area [54–57], ileostomies or colostomies [58], and rectal mucosa [59]. In the sublingual area, which is the area that has been investigated most, capillaries and venules of variable size (resolution is 2–3 μm) can be visualized; arterioles are usually not visualized because they are located in deeper layers. Red blood cells are identified as black bodies and tissue perfusion can be characterized in individual vessels.

What can be measured with these techniques and what is important? Different variables can be measured, including vascular density, heterogeneity of perfusion, and microvascular blood flow. As mentioned above, estimation of heterogeneity of perfusion (measuring the proportion of perfused vessels, mean flow index, or heterogeneity index) together with an estimate of capillary density are the variables which are the most relevant for tissue perfusion [60]. These are usually measured using a semiquantitative analysis, which can easily be performed by experienced investigators, with excellent reliability (intra- and interobserver variabilities within 5–10% [54, 61, 62] and excellent agreement between investigators [63]). Semiquantitative analysis can even be obtained as a point of care measurement [64], but this kind of analysis has been validated only for a single score and cannot be used to assess capillary density; it should, therefore, only be used for rapid evaluation of the microcirculation. Of note, measurement of blood flow cannot be obtained with these semiquantitative scores. These techniques can be used to quantify flow in various organs. In animals, measurements of gut microvascular perfusion can be made in a similar way to measurements of the sublingual microcirculation, and it has been shown that the evolution over time during sepsis is similar in both sites [43]. However, semiquantitative measurements of gut microcirculation may be more difficult to obtain and less reproducible than measurement of sublingual microcirculation [44], probably because of the specific gut architecture.

New software for computer-assisted microcirculation assessment is currently being developed. With this software, it is usually feasible to measure vessel density and blood flow in microvessels. Unfortunately, manual intervention is still needed for vessel identification as well as for blood flow measurement [65].

Is it relevant to measure blood flow in microvessels? Measuring blood flow in selected microvessels is probably irrelevant, as an increase in flow in a single vessel may reflect improved tissue perfusion as well as an increase in shunt flow. Measuring blood flow in all visible vessels and comparing histograms of blood flow distribution is probably more relevant, but this is not yet feasible as it would take hours to obtain such measurements.

Several limitations should be acknowledged. Secretions and movement artifacts may impair image quality. In addition, movement artifacts can spuriously interrupt flow in some microvessels. Special care should be taken to prevent this. To limit movement artifacts and to decrease the risk of pressure artifacts, use of stabilization devices has been proposed [43, 66]. These are especially convenient in experimental conditions but their application in humans is still anecdotal. Sterile cover caps need to be used, but these do not impair image quality. Finally, the investigation of the sublingual area is only feasible in sedated or cooperative patients. It is also impossible to evaluate the sublingual microcirculation in hypoxemic patients who are being treated with non-invasive mechanical ventilation.

Evaluation of tissue oxygenation (SvO_2/NIRS/PO_2 electrodes/reflectance spectroscopy)

Measurements of O_2 tension or saturation in a piece of tissue reflect the balance between O_2 transport and O_2 consumption in that tissue. These measurements are, therefore, influenced by flow but also by hemoglobin content, arterial PO_2, and O_2 consumption.

Venous oxygen saturation

Venous O_2 saturation is often considered as a gauge for the circulation [17, 67], but this measurement can be misleading. As illustrated in Figs. 1 and 2, venous O_2 saturation is a poor indicator of microvascular dysfunction: venous O_2 saturation can be high or low for the same degree of microvascular shunting. Several studies have shown that measuring SvO_2 does not provide much information about microvascular alterations [54, 68, 69].

PO_2 electrodes

PO_2 can be measured in tissues with Clark-type electrodes, which are made of multiple platinum wires that measure PO_2 in the surrounding tissue. These electrodes accurately measure tissue PO_2 when PO_2 is homogenously decreased but they are not suitable in conditions of PO_2 heterogeneity, as they are sensitive to the highest PO_2 in the sampling volume. The most modern tissue PO_2 electrodes measure PO_2 on a tissue surface of 8 mm^2 over a depth of a few microns [70]. This represents a sampling volume of at least 0.5 mm^3. Such a volume includes at least 100 microvessels, including arterioles, capillaries, and venules, as well as interstitium and other cells, which all contribute to the PO_2 value.

Some investigators have used PO_2 electrodes [62, 70–73], but they are not useful to assess microvascular perfusion. They can be used to assess adequacy of perfusion and/or oxygenation in a piece of tissue, especially in low-flow conditions [72].

Reflectance spectroscopy

Reflectance spectroscopy measures tissue SO_2. Light generated with a rapidly rotating filter disk at 64 different wavelengths of 2-nm increments in the range 502–628 nm is directed through a microlight guide to the tissues. The use of different wavelengths allows SO_2 measurement due to light absorption by oxy- and deoxyhemoglobin. The resolution of the probe is very sharp (1 nm) allowing SO_2 measurements in a very small area. Nevertheless, the depth of the tissue sampled is quite large [74], so that the sampling volume is not so small. A histogram of tissue SO_2 is generated, which provides information on the heterogeneity in tissue oxygenation. Reporting only the mean value of tissue SO_2 is misleading [75, 76], and no conclusions can be drawn on the presence or absence of hypoxic areas. Initially, this technique, known under the name of Erlangen MicroPHOtometer (EMPHO), was mostly used in experimental conditions and heterogeneity of tissue oxygenation was reported in several conditions [74, 77]. Some investigators have been able to embed this technique on an endoscope, enabling measurement of human gastric SO_2 [78]. Recent developments have allowed miniaturization of the technique, making it suitable for measurement of skin and sublingual SO_2 [76], but unfortunately these new devices only provide mean SO_2.

Near-infrared spectroscopy

Near-infrared spectroscopy (NIRS) is a technique that utilizes near-infrared light to measure chromophores (oxy- and deoxyhemoglobin, myoglobin, and cytochrome aa3) in tissues [79]. The fractions of oxy- and deoxyhemoglobin are used to calculate tissue O_2 saturation (StO_2). In addition, total light absorption is used to compute total tissue hemoglobin (HbT) and the absolute tissue hemoglobin index (THI), two indicators of blood volume in the region of microvasculature sensed by the probe [80]. According to Beer's law, the NIRS signal is limited to vessels that have a diameter less than 1 mm (arterioles, capillaries, and venules), but, as 75% of the blood in a skeletal muscle is venous, NIRS StO_2 measurements mostly represent local venous hemoglobin O_2 saturation. This represents the aggregate of O_2 saturations in the sampling volume and this technique is not suitable in conditions of heterogeneous blood flow. Indeed, even though StO_2 is slightly lower in septic patients compared to healthy volunteers, there is a huge overlap between the groups [81, 82]. StO_2 also differs from $ScvO_2$ saturation in sepsis [68].

The analysis of changes in StO_2 during a brief episode of forearm ischemia enables quantification of microvascular dysfunction [83–85]. This technique, which can easily be repeated [83], is particularly promising as it provides quantitative information on microvascular function within a few minutes. One should bear in mind that NIRS does not measure microcirculatory blood flow, making interpretation of the absolute StO_2 value in terms of tissue oxygenation difficult. As StO_2 represents the balance between O_2 delivery and O_2 consumption, any change in StO_2 can reflect a change in flow in the same direction and/or a change in metabolism in the opposite direction. More importantly, proportional changes in flow and metabolism may be associated with unchanged StO_2. In addition, the vasoreactivity test evaluates a different aspect of microvascular function than flow: it evaluates microvascular reserve more than actual microvascular perfusion.

NIRS-derived measurements are influenced by adipose tissue thickness as well as the presence of edema; hence, in the majority of studies, the thenar eminence has been used because the thickness of skin and adipose tissue covering this muscle is less influenced by any increase in fluid content or body mass index. The influence of temperature and vasoactive substances on NIRS-derived variables obtained in the thenar eminence need to be evaluated. Likewise, the relationship between peripheral and more central microvascular beds need to be further studied in critically ill patients.

Finally, NIRS devices vary in terms of wavelength and number of wavelengths, optode spacing, and algorithms [86]. Accordingly, the data reported with the different devices may vary somewhat and this absence of standardization may limit comparisons of results from different trials.

PCO_2-derived measurements

Tissue CO_2 represents the balance between CO_2 production and flow to the tissue. It is influenced by arterial CO_2, so that the tissue to arterial gradient, or PCO_2 gap, is usually calculated. The PCO_2 gap reflects more the adequacy of flow than the presence of tissue hypoxia, unless very high PCO_2 gap values are reached [87, 88]. Tissue PCO_2 can be measured by electrodes inserted in tissues, probes in contact with the tissue, or tonometry. Even though the sampling volume is large, the measured value reflects the most abnormal (highest) value in the sampled volume. Hence, this measurement can detect zones of impaired perfusion and/or tissue hypoxia even when total perfusion is preserved but heterogeneous.

Gastric tonometry raised a lot of interest. A gastric PCO_2 gap above 20 mmHg discriminated survivors from non-survivors [87]. More importantly, these variables had a stronger prognostic value when systemic variables were already corrected [89]. But what does PCO_2 gap really measure? Does it reflect splanchnic, serosal, or mucosal blood flow? Even though it was initially proposed as a surrogate of splanchnic perfusion, several studies suggest that it mostly reflects gut mucosal microcirculation. In experimental conditions, there was a close relationship between mucosal PCO_2 and mucosal perfusion [41, 42, 48]. In patients with sepsis, there was no correlation between the gastric PCO_2 gap and total splanchnic perfusion [90], although changes in mucosal PCO_2 correlated with changes in mucosal perfusion [91]. The technique has now been abandoned, mostly because of technical problems. In particular, duodeno-gastric reflux and feeding can interfere with PCO_2 measurements. Sublingual and buccal PCO_2 monitoring have been developed [92, 93]. Sublingual PCO_2 is often increased in sepsis, especially in non-survivors [94–96]. Using this technique, we demonstrated that sublingual PCO_2 tracks microvascular blood flow, as the sublingual PCO_2 gap is inversely related to the proportion of perfused capillaries [97]. This technique, although attractive, is unfortunately not easily available at the present time (available for research purposes only).

Microdialysis and equilibrium dialysis

Microdialysis allows measurements of different molecules in the extracellular space. Soluble substances equilibrate through a semipermeable membrane of hollow fiber perfused at a constant rate with saline, and are recovered in the dialysate. In the equilibrium dialysis technique, a probe covered by a semipermeable membrane is used without infusing fluids, solutes slowly equilibrate through the membrane, and the content of the probe is sampled intermittently for analysis (and replaced by saline). Lactate and pyruvate can be measured; measurements of the lactate/pyruvate ratio are particularly appealing, as this variable is less sensitive to dialysate perfusion rate and problems of incomplete recovery (absence of full equilibration).

Although the sampling volume of this device is large, measurements are influenced by the most abnormal values so that it should be able to detect the consequence of tissue heterogeneity. Using this technique, several studies have shown that the lactate/pyruvate ratio may be increased in septic shock [98–100].

Importantly, measurements of the lactate/pyruvate ratio may be useful to detect the occurrence of tissue hypoxia but cannot identify whether it is because of insufficient flow or other causes of tissue hypoxia. In addition, it cannot detect alterations in microvascular perfusion before they are associated with cellular hypoxia.

Microcirculatory alterations in critically ill patients

In the following sections, we will illustrate some of the main disease states with involvement of the microcirculation. The list is far from exhaustive and microcirculatory alterations have been found in many other circumstances.

Severe sepsis and septic shock

Using the OPS technique, we [54] evaluated the sublingual microcirculation in 50 patients with severe sepsis and in a cohort of healthy volunteers and non-infected intensive care unit (ICU) controls. We observed a significant decrease in vessels density and, more importantly, a decreased proportion of perfused small vessels (<20 μm), mostly capillaries, from 90% in controls to 48% in septic patients. This decrease in the proportion of well-perfused small vessels was due to a combined increase in non-perfused and intermittently perfused vessels. In addition, the heterogeneity between areas distant by a few microns was also increased. These results are in line with experimental findings and were later confirmed by other groups of investigators [57, 101]. These alterations can be observed very early in the course of sepsis, even within a few hours of hospital admission [57, 101]. Similar alterations, of lower magnitude, can be induced by low-dose endotoxin administration in healthy volunteers [102].

Interestingly, microcirculatory alterations were more severe in non-survivors than in survivors [54, 101, 103]. More importantly these microcirculatory changes rapidly resolved in response to therapy in survivors but persisted in patients dying in acute circulatory failure or later from organ failure after recovery from shock [103]. Changes in microvascular perfusion during the first day of ICU admission are more strongly associated with outcome than changes in cardiac output, arterial pressure, or SvO_2 [103]. Trzeciak et al. [104] showed that early improvement in microvascular perfusion in response to goal-directed therapy was associated with an improvement in organ function. Even though these data strongly suggest that microcirculatory alterations are implicated in the development of organ failure, interventional studies guiding therapy at the microcirculation should be conducted to evaluate whether improving microcirculatory alterations may be associated with an improvement in organ dysfunction.

Using a vascular occlusion test combined with NIRS measurements, several studies have shown that patients with severe sepsis frequently have profound alterations in microvascular reactivity [81, 84, 85, 105, 106] and that these alterations are associated with a high risk of organ dysfunction [105] and death [81].

Cardiogenic shock

We observed that, compared to patients with coronary artery or valvular disease who were scheduled for cardiac surgery, patients admitted to the ICU for acute decompensation of severe heart failure or cardiogenic shock had microvascular alterations, consisting of a decrease in vessel density and in the proportion of perfused capillaries [55]. These findings were later confirmed by other groups of investigators [107–110]. More severe alterations were observed in patients with higher lactate levels [110] and poor outcome [55]. These alterations could be improved by nitroglycerin [107, 108] or mechanical support such as aortic counterpulsation [109, 111] or ventricular assist devices [112].

High-risk surgery

High-risk surgery is a new area in which microcirculatory alterations have been observed. In patients submitted to high-risk non-cardiac surgery, Jhanji et al. [62] observed that the density and proportion of perfused capillaries was lower in the 14 patients who subsequently developed postoperative complications than in the 11 patients with an uneventful postoperative course. Subcutaneous tissue PO_2 and laser Doppler cutaneous blood flow did not differ between the groups, further highlighting the lack of sensitivity of these methods to detect heterogeneous perfusion. Interestingly, there was no significant difference in global O_2 delivery between the groups; it would be interesting to evaluate the impact of hemodynamic optimization on these microvascular alterations, as this approach has been shown to improve outcome in high-risk surgical patients [113]. Although the link between global hemodynamics and microvascular perfusion is quite loose, interventions aimed at improving global hemodynamics also have microvascular effects [21, 22, 114], which may be mediated by effects independent of changes in global hemodynamics. Further studies should address this issue.

Microcirculatory alterations may also occur in patients undergoing cardiac surgery. Bauer et al. [115] first reported that microcirculatory perfusion was transiently altered in humans after cardiopulmonary bypass. Similar findings were reported more recently by other groups [116, 117]. More importantly, these alterations can also be observed in patients who undergo surgery without cardiopulmonary bypass [117]; of note, the sublingual microcirculation was still slightly abnormal up to 24 h after surgery in these patients [117]. As in non-cardiac surgery, the severity of perioperative microvascular alterations correlated with peak lactate levels and severity of organ dysfunction after surgery [117].

Conclusions

Microcirculatory alterations are frequently observed in critically ill patients, and especially in patients with severe sepsis. These alterations are characterized by a decrease in capillary density and an increase in heterogeneity of perfusion with non-perfused in close vicinity to well-perfused capillaries. As a heterogeneous decrease in perfusion is less well tolerated than a homogenously decreased perfusion, the diagnostic tool used to assess the microcirculation should be able to detect heterogeneity of perfusion. This is best achieved with handheld microvideoscopic techniques, such as OPS and SDF. The use of vascular occlusion tests with laser Doppler or NIRS investigates microvascular reactivity, another important, but different, aspect of microvascular function. Combining techniques may be of interest in the future.

Guiding resuscitation with the use of these tools may allow more complete resuscitation and improve outcomes.

References

1. Beach JM, McGahren ED, Duling BR (1998) Capillaries and arterioles are electrically coupled in hamster cheek pouch. Am J Physiol 275:H1489–H1496
2. Haglund U, Rasmussen I (1993) Oxygenation of the gut mucosa. Br J Surg 80:955–956
3. Aird WC (2007) Phenotypic heterogeneity of the endothelium: II. Representative vascular beds. Circ Res 100:174–190
4. Collins DM, McCullough WT, Ellsworth ML (1998) Conducted vascular responses: communication across the capillary bed. Microvasc Res 56:43–53
5. Hangai-Hoger N, Nacharaju P, Manjula BN, Cabrales P, Tsai AG, Acharya SA, Intaglietta M (2006) Microvascular effects following treatment with polyethylene glycol-albumin in lipopolysaccharide-induced endotoxemia. Crit Care Med 34:108–117

6. Bateman RM, Tokunaga C, Kareco T, Dorscheid DR, Walley KR (2007) Myocardial hypoxia-inducible HIF-1α, VEGF and GLUT1 gene expression is associated with microvascular and ICAM-1 heterogeneity during endotoxemia. Am J Physiol Heart Circ Physiol 293:H448–H456
7. Farquhar I, Martin CM, Lam C, Potter R, Ellis CG, Sibbald WJ (1996) Decreased capillary density in vivo in bowel mucosa of rats with normotensive sepsis. J Surg Res 61:190–196
8. Goldman D, Bateman RM, Ellis CG (2006) Effect of decreased O_2 supply on skeletal muscle oxygenation and O_2 consumption during sepsis: role of heterogeneous capillary spacing and blood flow. Am J Physiol Heart Circ Physiol 290:H2277–H2285
9. Borgstrom P, Bruttig SP, Lindbom L, Intaglietta M, Arfors KE (1990) Microvascular responses in rabbit skeletal muscle after fixed volume hemorrhage. Am J Physiol 259:H190–H196
10. Kerger H, Waschke KF, Ackern KV, Tsai AG, Intaglietta M (1999) Systemic and microcirculatory effects of autologous whole blood resuscitation in severe hemorrhagic shock. Am J Physiol 276:H2035–H2043
11. Zuurbier CJ, van Iterson M, Ince C (1999) Functional heterogeneity of oxygen supply-consumption ratio in the heart. Cardiovasc Res 44:488–497
12. Stein JC, Ellis CG, Ellsworth ML (1993) Relationship between capillary and systemic venous PO2 during nonhypoxic and hypoxic ventilation. Am J Physiol 265:H537–H542
13. Humer MF, Phang PT, Friesen BP, Allards MF, Goddard CM, Walley KR (1996) Heterogeneity of gut capillary transit times and impaired gut oxygen extraction in endotoxemic pigs. J Appl Physiol 81:895–904
14. Ince C, Vink H, Wieringa PA, Giezeman M, Spaan JA (1990) Heterogeneous NADH fluorescence during post-anoxic reactive hyperemia in saline perfused rat heart. Adv Exp Med Biol 277:477–482
15. Ellis CG, Bateman RM, Sharpe MD, Sibbald WJ, Gill R (2002) Effect of a maldistribution of microvascular blood flow on capillary O_2 extraction in sepsis. Am J Physiol 282:H156–H164
16. Goldman D, Bateman RM, Ellis CG (2004) Effect of sepsis on skeletal muscle oxygen consumption and tissue oxygenation: interpreting capillary oxygen transport data using a mathematical model. Am J Physiol Heart Circ Physiol 287:H2535–H2544
17. Rivers E, Nguyen B, Havstadt S, Ressler J, Muzzin A, Knoblich B, Peterson E, Tomlanovich M (2001) Early goal-directed therapy in the treatment of severe sepsis and septic shock. N Engl J Med 345:1368–1377
18. Joly HR, Weil MH (1969) Temperature of the great toe as an indication of the severity of shock. Circulation 39:131–138
19. Boerma EC, Kuiper MA, Kingma WP, Egbers PH, Gerritsen RT, Ince C (2008) Disparity between skin perfusion and sublingual microcirculatory alterations in severe sepsis and septic shock: a prospective observational study. Intensive Care Med 34:1294–1298
20. Lima A, Jansen TC, van Bommel J, Ince C, Bakker J (2009) The prognostic value of the subjective assessment of peripheral perfusion in critically ill patients. Crit Care Med 37:934–938
21. De Backer D, Creteur J, Dubois MJ, Sakr Y, koch M, Verdant C, Vincent JL (2006) The effects of dobutamine on microcirculatory alterations in patients with septic shock are independent of its systemic effects. Crit Care Med 34:403–408
22. Ospina-Tascon G, Neves AP, Occhipinti G, Donadello K, Buchele G, Simion D, Chierego M, Oliveira Silva T, Fonseca A, Vincent JL, De Backer D (2010) Effects of fluids on microvascular perfusion in patients with severe sepsis. Intensive Care Med 36:949–955
23. Marechal X, Favory R, Joulin O, Montaigne D, Hassoun S, Decoster B, Zerimech F, Neviere R (2008) Endothelial glycocalyx damage during endotoxemia coincides with microcirculatory dysfunction and vascular oxidative stress. Shock 29:572–576
24. Duranteau J, Sitbon P, Teboul JL, Vicaut E, Anguel N, Richard C, Samii K (1999) Effects of epinephrine, norepinephrine, or the combination of norepinephrine and dobutamine on gastric mucosa in septic shock. Crit Care Med 27:893–900
25. Boyle NH, Roberts PC, Ng B, Berkenstadt H, McLuckie A, Beale RJ, Mason RC (1999) Scanning laser Doppler is a useful technique to assess foot cutaneous perfusion during femoral artery cannulation. Crit Care 3:95–100
26. Altintas MA, Altintas AA, Guggenheim M, Aust MC, Niederbichler AD, Knobloch K, Vogt PM (2010) Insight in microcirculation and histomorphology during burn shock treatment using in vivo confocal-laser-scanning microscopy. J Crit Care 25:1–7
27. Altintas MA, Altintas AA, Guggenheim M, Steiert AE, Aust MC, Niederbichler AD, Herold C, Vogt PM (2009) Insight in human skin microcirculation using in vivo reflectance-mode confocal laser scanning microscopy. J Digit Imaging. doi:10.1007/s10278-009-9219-3
28. Lamblin V, Favory R, Boulo M, Mathieu D (2006) Microcirculatory alterations induced by sedation in intensive care patients. Effects of midazolam alone and in association with sufentanil. Crit Care 10:R176
29. Fagrell B, Fronek A, Intaglietta M (1977) A microscope-television system for studying flow velocity in human skin capillaries. Am J Physiol 233:H318–H321
30. Awan ZA, Wester T, Kvernebo K (2010) Human microvascular imaging: a review of skin and tongue videomicroscopy techniques and analysing variables. Clin Physiol Funct Imaging 30:79–88
31. Sherman H, Klausner S, Cook WA (1971) Incident dark-field illumination: a new method for microcirculatory study. Angiology 22:295–303
32. Slaaf DW, Tangelder GJ, Reneman RS, Jager K, Bollinger A (1987) A versatile incident illuminator for intravital microscopy. Int J Microcirc Clin Exp 6:391–397
33. Groner W, Winkelman JW, Harris AG, Ince C, Bouma GJ, Messmer K, Nadeau RG (1999) Orthogonal polarization spectral imaging: a new method for study of the microcirculation. Nat Med 5:1209–1212
34. Goedhart P, Khalilzada M, Bezemer R, Merza J, Ince C (2007) Sidestream dark field (SDF) imaging: a novel stroboscopic LED ring-based imaging modality for clinical assessment of the microcirculation. Optics Express 15:15101–15114
35. Harris AG, Sinitsina I, Messmer K (2001) Validation of OPS imaging for microvascular measurements during isovolumic hemodilution and low hematocrits. Am J Physiol Heart Circ Physiol 282:H1502–H1509
36. Laemmel E, Tadayoni R, Sinitsina I, Boczkowski J, and Vicaut E (2000) Using orthogonal polarization spectral imaging for the experimental study of microcirculation: comparison with intravital microscopy. In: Messmer K (ed) Orthogonal polarization spectral imaging—Progress in applied microcirculation, vol 26, pp 50–60. Basel, Karger

37. Harris AG, Sinitsina I, Messmer K (2000) The Cytoscan™ Model E-II, a new reflectance microscope for intravital microscopy: comparison with the standard fluorescence method. J Vasc Res 37:469–476
38. Mathura KR, Vollebregt KC, Boer K, De Graaff JC, Ubbink DT, Ince C (2001) Comparison of OPS imaging and conventional capillary microscopy to study the human microcirculation. J Appl Physiol 91:74–78
39. Pennings FA, Ince C, Bouma GJ (2006) Continuous real-time visualization of the human cerebral microcirculation during arteriovenous malformation surgery using orthogonal polarization spectral imaging. Neurosurgery 59:167–171
40. den Uil CA, Bezemer R, Miranda DR, Ince C, Lagrand WK, Hartman M, Bogers AJ, Spronk PE, Simoons ML (2009) Intra-operative assessment of human pulmonary alveoli in vivo using sidestream dark field imaging: a feasibility study. Med Sci Monit 15:137–141
41. Dubin A, Edul VS, Pozo MO, Murias G, Canullan CM, Martins EF, Ferrara G, Canales HS, Laporte M, Estenssoro E, Ince C (2008) Persistent villi hypoperfusion explains intramucosal acidosis in sheep endotoxemia. Crit Care Med 36:535–542
42. Dubin A, Pozo MO, Ferrara G, Murias G, Martins E, Canullan C, Canales HS, Kanoore Edul V, Estenssoro E, Ince C (2009) Systemic and microcirculatory responses to progressive hemorrhage. Intensive Care Med 35:556–564
43. Verdant CL, De Backer D, Bruhn A, Clausi C, Su F, Wang Z, Rodriguez H, Pries AR, Vincent JL (2009) Evaluation of sublingual and gut mucosal microcirculation in sepsis: a quantitative analysis. Crit Care Med 37:2875–2881
44. Bracht H, Krejci V, Hiltebrand L, Brandt S, Sigurdsson G, Ali SZ, Takala J, Jakob SM (2008) Orthogonal polarization spectroscopy to detect mesenteric hypoperfusion. Intensive Care Med 34:1883–1890
45. Langer S, von Dobschuetz E, Harris AG, Krombach F, Messmer K (2000) Validation of the orthogonal polarization spectral imaging technique on solid organs. In: Messmer K (ed) Orthogonal polarization spectral imaging—Progress in applied microcirculation, vol 24, pp 32–46. Basel, Karger
46. Puhl G, Schaser KD, Vollmar B, Menger MD, Settmacher U (2003) Noninvasive in vivo analysis of the human hepatic microcirculation using orthogonal polorization spectral imaging. Transplantation 75:756–761
47. Biberthaler P, Langer S, Luchting B, Khandoga A, Messmer K (2001) In vivo assessment of colon microcirculation: comparison of the new OPS imaging technique with intravital microscopy. Eur J Med Res 6:525–534
48. Tugtekin I, Radermacher P, Theisen M, Matejovic M, Stehr A, Ploner F, Matura K, Ince C, Georgieff M, Trager K (2001) Increased ileal-mucosal-arterial PCO2 gap is associated with impaired villus microcirculation in endotoxic pigs. Intensive Care Med 27:757–766
49. Lupi O, Semenovitch I, Treu C, Bouskela E (2008) Orthogonal polarization technique in the assessment of human skin microcirculation. Int J Dermatol 47:425–431
50. Genzel-Boroviczeny O, Strotgen J, Harris AG, Messmer K, Christ F (2002) Orthogonal polarization spectral imaging (OPS): a novel method to measure the microcirculation in term and preterm infants transcutaneously. Pediatr Res 51:386–391
51. Kroth J, Weidlich K, Hiedl S, Nussbaum C, Christ F, Genzel-Boroviczeny O (2008) Functional vessel density in the first month of life in preterm neonates. Pediatr Res 64:567–571
52. Schaser KD, Settmacher U, Puhl G, Zhang L, Mittlmeier T, Stover JF, Vollmar B, Menger MD, Neuhaus P, Haas NP (2003) Noninvasive analysis of conjunctival microcirculation during carotid artery surgery reveals microvascular evidence of collateral compensation and stenosis-dependent adaptation. J Vasc Surg 37:789–797
53. Lindeboom JA, Mathura KR, Harkisoen S, van den Akker HP, Ince C (2005) Effect of smoking on the gingival capillary density: assessment of gingival capillary density with orthogonal polarization spectral imaging. J Clin Periodontol 32:1208–1212
54. De Backer D, Creteur J, Preiser JC, Dubois MJ, Vincent JL (2002) Microvascular blood flow is altered in patients with sepsis. Am J Respir Crit Care Med 166:98–104
55. De Backer D, Creteur J, Dubois MJ, Sakr Y, Vincent JL (2004) Microvascular alterations in patients with acute severe heart failure and cardiogenic shock. Am Heart J 147:91–99
56. Spronk PE, Ince C, Gardien MJ, Mathura KR, Oudemans-van Straaten HM, Zandstra DF (2002) Nitroglycerin in septic shock after intravascular volume resuscitation. Lancet 360:1395–1396
57. Trzeciak S, Dellinger RP, Parrillo JE, Guglielmi M, Bajaj J, Abate NL, Arnold RC, Colilla S, Zanotti S, Hollenberg SM (2007) Early microcirculatory perfusion derangements in patients with severe sepsis and septic shock: relationship to hemodynamics, oxygen transport, and survival. Ann Emerg Med 49:88–98
58. Boerma EC, van der Voort PH, Spronk PE, Ince C (2007) Relationship between sublingual and intestinal microcirculatory perfusion in patients with abdominal sepsis. Crit Care Med 35:1055–1060
59. Dondorp AM, Ince C, Charunwatthana P, Hanson J, van Kuijen A, Faiz MA, Rahman MR, Hasan M, Bin YE, Ghose A, Ruangveerayut R, Limmathurotsakul D, Mathura K, White NJ, Day NP (2008) Direct in vivo assessment of microcirculatory dysfunction in severe falciparum malaria. J Infect Dis 197:79–84
60. De Backer D, Hollenberg S, Boerma C, Goedhart P, Buchele G, Ospina-Tascon G, Dobbe I, Ince C (2007) How to evaluate the microcirculation: report of a round table conference. Crit Care 11:R101
61. Buchele GL, Silva E, Ospina-Tascon G, Vincent JL, De Backer D (2009) Effects of hydrocortisone on microcirculatory alterations in patients with septic shock. Crit Care Med 37:1341–1347
62. Jhanji S, Lee C, Watson D, Hinds C, Pearse RM (2009) Microvascular flow and tissue oxygenation after major abdominal surgery: association with post-operative complications. Intensive Care Med 35:671–677
63. Boerma EC, Mathura KR, van der Voort PH, Spronk PE, Ince C (2005) Quantifying bedside-derived imaging of microcirculatory abnormalities in septic patients: a prospective validation study. Crit Care 9:R601–R606
64. Arnold RC, Parrillo JE, Phillip DR, Chansky ME, Shapiro NI, Lundy DJ, Trzeciak S, Hollenberg SM (2009) Point-of-care assessment of microvascular blood flow in critically ill patients. Intensive Care Med 35:1761–1766
65. Salgado DR, Favory R, Creteur J, Vincent JL, De Backer D (2009) Automate microcirculation analysis still requires a human intervention. Intensive Care Med 35:S27 (abstract)
66. Lindert J, Werner J, Redlin M, Kuppe H, Habazettl H, Pries AR (2002) OPS imaging of human microcirculation: a short technical report. J Vasc Res 39:368–372

67. Pinsky MR, Vincent JL (2005) Let us use the pulmonary artery catheter correctly and only when we need it. Crit Care Med 33:1119–1122
68. Podbregar M, Mozina H (2007) Skeletal muscle oxygen saturation does not estimate mixed venous oxygen saturation in patients with severe left heart failure and additional severe sepsis or septic shock. Crit Care 11:R6
69. Marik PE, Bankov A (2003) Sublingual capnometry versus traditional markers of tissue oxygenation in critically ill patients. Crit Care Med 31:818–822
70. Dyson A, Stidwill R, Taylor V, Singer M (2009) The impact of inspired oxygen concentration on tissue oxygenation during progressive haemorrhage. Intensive Care Med 35:1783–1791
71. VanderMeer TJ, Wang H, Fink MP (1995) Endotoxemia causes ileal mucosal acidosis in the absence of mucosal hypoxia in a normodynamic porcine model of septic shock. Crit Care Med 23:1217–1225
72. Dyson A, Stidwill R, Taylor V, Singer M (2007) Tissue oxygen monitoring in rodent models of shock. Am J Physiol Heart Circ Physiol 293:H526–H533
73. Jhanji S, Stirling S, Patel N, Hinds CJ, Pearse RM (2009) The effect of increasing doses of norepinephrine on tissue oxygenation and microvascular flow in patients with septic shock. Crit Care Med 37:1961–1966
74. Schwarz B, Hofstotter H, Salak N, Pajk W, Knotzer H, Mayr A, Labeck B, Kafka R, Ulmer H, Hasibeder W (2001) Effects of norepinephrine and phenylephrine on intestinal oxygen supply and mucosal tissue oxygen tension. Intensive Care Med 27:593–601
75. Albuszies G, Radermacher P, Vogt J, Wachter U, Weber S, Schoaff M, Georgieff M, Barth E (2005) Effect of increased cardiac output on hepatic and intestinal microcirculatory blood flow, oxygenation, and metabolism in hyperdynamic murine septic shock. Crit Care Med 33:2332–2338
76. Sakr Y, Gath V, Oishi J, Klinzing S, Simon TP, Reinhart K, Marx G (2010) Characterization of buccal microvascular response in patients with septic shock. Eur J Anaesthesiol 27:388–394
77. Vollmar B, Rüttinger D, Menger MD (1997) Monitoring of microvascular hemoglobin oxygenation in liver and skeletal muscle tissue of endotoxin-exposed rats using reflection spectrophotometry. Adv Exp Med Biol 428:397–402
78. Temmesfeld-Wollbrück B, Szalay A, Mayer K, Olschewski H, Seeger W, Grimminger F (1998) Abnormalities of gastric mucosal oxygenation in septic shock. Am J Respir Crit Care Med 157:1586–1592
79. Jobsis FF (1977) Noninvasive, infrared monitoring of cerebral and myocardial oxygen sufficiency and circulatory parameters. Science 198:1264–1267
80. Myers DE, Anderson LD, Seifert RP, Ortner JP, Cooper CE, Beilman GJ, Mowlem JD (2005) Noninvasive method for measuring local hemoglobin oxygen saturation in tissue using wide gap second derivative near-infrared spectroscopy. J Biomed Opt 10:034017
81. Creteur J, Carollo T, Soldati G, Buchele G, De Backer D, Vincent JL (2007) The prognostic value of muscle StO_2 in septic patients. Intensive Care Med 33:1549–1556
82. Mulier KE, Skarda DE, Taylor JH, Myers DE, McGraw MK, Gallea BL, Beilman GJ (2008) Near-infrared spectroscopy in patients with severe sepsis: correlation with invasive hemodynamic measurements. Surg Infect (Larchmt) 9:515–519
83. Gomez H, Torres A, Polanco P, Kim HK, Zenker S, Puyana JC, Pinsky MR (2008) Use of non-invasive NIRS during a vascular occlusion test to assess dynamic tissue O_2 saturation response. Intensive Care Med 34:1600–1607
84. Pareznik R, Knezevic R, Voga G, Podbregar M (2006) Changes in muscle tissue oxygenation during stagnant ischemia in septic patients. Intensive Care Med 32:87–92
85. De Blasi RA, Palmisani S, Alampi D, Mercieri M, Romano R, Collini S, Pinto G (2005) Microvascular dysfunction and skeletal muscle oxygenation assessed by phase-modulation near-infrared spectroscopy in patients with septic shock. Intensive Care Med 31:1661–1668
86. Boushel R, Piantadosi CA (2000) Near-infrared spectroscopy for monitoring muscle oxygenation. Acta Physiol Scand 168:615–622
87. Levy B, Gawalkiewicz P, Vallet B, Briancon S, Nace L, Bollaert PE (2003) Gastric capnometry with air-automated tonometry predicts outcome in critically ill patients. Crit Care Med 31:474–480
88. Schlichtig R, Bowles SA (1994) Distinguishing between aerobic and anaerobic appearance of dissolved CO2 in intestine during low flow. J Appl Physiol 76:2443–2451
89. Poeze M, Solberg BC, Greve JW, Ramsay G (2005) Monitoring global volume-related hemodynamic or regional variables after initial resuscitation: what is a better predictor of outcome in critically ill septic patients? Crit Care Med 33:2494–2500
90. Creteur J, De Backer D, Vincent JL (1999) Does gastric tonometry monitor splanchnic perfusion? Crit Care Med 27:2480–2484
91. Nevière R, Mathieu D, Chagnon JL, Lebleu N, Wattel F (1996) The contrasting effects of dobutamine and dopamine on gastric mucosal perfusion in septic patients. Am J Respir Crit Care Med 154:1684–1688
92. Weil MH, Nakagawa Y, Tang W, Sato Y, Ercoli F, Finegan R, Grayman G, Bisera J (1999) Sublingual capnometry: a new noninvasive measurement for diagnosis and quantitation of severity of circulatory shock. Crit Care Med 27:1225–1229
93. Cammarata GA, Weil MH, Castillo CJ, Fries M, Wang H, Sun S, Tang W (2009) Buccal capnometry for quantitating the severity of hemorrhagic shock. Shock 31:207–211
94. Marik PE (2001) Sublingual capnography: a clinical validation study. Chest 120:923–927
95. Baron BJ, Dutton RP, Zehtabchi S, Spanfelner J, Stavile KL, Khodorkovsky B, Nagdev A, Hahn B, Scalea TM (2007) Sublingual capnometry for rapid determination of the severity of hemorrhagic shock. J Trauma 62:120–124
96. Rackow EC, O'Neil P, Astiz ME, Carpati CM (2001) Sublingual capnometry and indexes of tissue perfusion in patients with circulatory failure. Chest 120:1633–1638
97. Creteur J, De Backer D, Sakr Y, koch M, Vincent JL (2006) Sublingual capnometry tracks microcirculatory changes in septic patients. Intensive Care Med 32:516–523
98. de Boer J, Potthoff H, Mulder PO, Dofferhoff AS, van Thiel RJ, Plijter-Groendijk H, Korf J (1994) Lactate monitoring with subcutaneous microdialysis in patients with shock: a pilot study. Circ Shock 43:57–63
99. Jorgensen VL, Nielsen SL, Espersen K, Perner A (2006) Increased colorectal permeability in patients with severe sepsis and septic shock. Intensive Care Med 32:1790–1796
100. Jorgensen VL, Reiter N, Perner A (2006) Luminal concentrations of L- and D-lactate in the rectum may relate to severity of disease and outcome in septic patients. Crit Care 10:R163

101. Spanos A, Jhanji S, Vivian-Smith A, Harris T, Pearse RM (2010) Early microvascular changes in sepsis and severe sepsis. Shock 33:387–391
102. Draisma A, Bemelmans R, van der Hoeven JG, Spronk P, Pickkers P (2009) Microcirculation and vascular reactivity during endotoxemia and endotoxin tolerance in humans. Shock 31:581–585
103. Sakr Y, Dubois MJ, De Backer D, Creteur J, Vincent JL (2004) Persistant microvasculatory alterations are associated with organ failure and death in patients with septic shock. Crit Care Med 32:1825–1831
104. Trzeciak S, McCoy JV, Phillip DR, Arnold RC, Rizzuto M, Abate NL, Shapiro NI, Parrillo JE, Hollenberg SM (2008) Early increases in microcirculatory perfusion during protocol-directed resuscitation are associated with reduced multi-organ failure at 24 h in patients with sepsis. Intensive Care Med 34:2210–2217
105. Doerschug KC, Delsing AS, Schmidt GA, Haynes WG (2007) Impairments in microvascular reactivity are related to organ failure in human sepsis. Am J Physiol Heart Circ Physiol 293:H1065–H1071
106. Skarda DE, Mulier KE, Myers DE, Taylor JH, Beilman GJ (2007) Dynamic near-infrared spectroscopy measurements in patients with severe sepsis. Shock 27:348–353
107. den Uil CA, Caliskan K, Lagrand WK, van der Ent M, Jewbali LS, van Kuijk JP, Spronk PE, Simoons ML (2009) Dose-dependent benefit of nitroglycerin on microcirculation of patients with severe heart failure. Intensive Care Med 35:1893–1899
108. den Uil CA, Lagrand WK, Spronk PE, van der Ent M, Jewbali LS, Brugts JJ, Ince C, Simoons ML (2009) Low-dose nitroglycerin improves microcirculation in hospitalized patients with acute heart failure. Eur J Heart Fail 11:386–390
109. den Uil CA, Lagrand WK, van der Ent M, Jewbali LS, Brugts JJ, Spronk PE, Simoons ML (2009) The effects of intra-aortic balloon pump support on macrocirculation and tissue microcirculation in patients with cardiogenic shock. Cardiology 114:42–46
110. Jung C, Ferrari M, Rodiger C, Fritzenwanger M, Goebel B, Lauten A, Pfeifer R, Figulla HR (2009) Evaluation of the sublingual microcirculation in cardiogenic shock. Clin Hemorheol Microcirc 42:141–148
111. Jung C, Rodiger C, Fritzenwanger M, Schumm J, Lauten A, Figulla HR, Ferrari M (2009) Acute microflow changes after stop and restart of intra-aortic balloon pump in cardiogenic shock. Clin Res Cardiol 98:469–475
112. Jung C, Ferrari M, Gradinger R, Fritzenwanger M, Pfeifer R, Schlosser M, Poerner TC, Brehm BR, Figulla HR (2008) Evaluation of the microcirculation during extracorporeal membrane-oxygenation. Clin Hemorheol Microcirc 40:311–314
113. Pearse R, Dawson D, Fawcett J, Rhodes A, Grounds M, Bennett D (2005) Early goal directed therapy following major surgery reduces complications and duration of hospital stay. A randomized, controlled trial. Crit Care 9:R687–R693
114. Pottecher J, Deruddre S, Teboul JL, Georger J, Laplace C, Benhamou D, Vicaut E, Duranteau J (2010) Both passive leg raising and intravascular volume expansion improve sublingual microcirculatory perfusion in severe sepsis and septic shock. Intensive Care Med. doi:10.1007/s00134-010-1966-6
115. Bauer A, Kofler S, Thiel M, Eifert S, Christ F (2007) Monitoring of the sublingual microcirculation in cardiac surgery using orthogonal polarization spectral imaging: preliminary results. Anesthesiology 107:939–945
116. den Uil CA, Lagrand WK, Spronk PE, van Domburg RT, Hofland J, Luthen C, Brugts JJ, van der Ent M, Simoons ML (2008) Impaired sublingual microvascular perfusion during surgery with cardiopulmonary bypass: a pilot study. J Thorac Cardiovasc Surg 136:129–134
117. De Backer D, Dubois MJ, Schmartz D, koch M, Ducart A, Barvais L, Vincent JL (2009) Microcirculatory alterations in cardiac surgery: effects of cardiopulmonary bypass and anesthesia. Ann Thorac Surg 88:1396–1403
118. Parthasarathi K, Lipowsky HH (1999) Capillary recruitment in response to tissue hypoxia and its dependence on red blood cell deformability. Am J Physiol 277:H2145–H2157
119. Schumacker PT, Chandel N, Agusti AGN (1993) Oxygen conformance of cellular respiration in hepatocytes. Am J Physiol 265:L395–L402

E. Christiaan Boerma
Can Ince

The role of vasoactive agents in the resuscitation of microvascular perfusion and tissue oxygenation in critically ill patients

Abstract *Purpose:* The clinical use of vasoactive drugs is not only intended to improve systemic hemodynamic variables, but ultimately to attenuate derangements in organ perfusion and oxygenation during shock. This review aims (1) to discuss basic physiology with respect to manipulating vascular tone and its effect on the microcirculation, and (2) to provide an overview of available clinical data on the relation between vasoactive drugs and organ perfusion, with specific attention paid to recent developments that have enabled direct in vivo observation of the microcirculation and concepts that have originated from it. *Methods:* A MedLine search was conducted for clinical articles in the English language over the last 15 years pertainig to shock, sepsis, organ failure, or critically ill patients in combination with vasoactive drugs and specific variables of organ perfusion/oxygenation (e.g., tonometry, indocyanine clearance, laser Doppler, and sidestream dark field imaging). *Results:* Eighty original papers evaluating the specific relationship between organ perfusion/oxygenation and the use of vasoactive drugs were identified and are discussed in light of physiological theory of vasomotor tone. *Conclusions:* Solid clinical data in support of the idea that increasing blood pressure in shock improves microcirculatory perfusion/oxygenation seem to be lacking, and such a concept might not be in line with physiological theory of microcirculation as a low-pressure vascular compartment. In septic shock no beneficial effect on microcirculatory perfusion above a mean arterial pressure of 65 mmHg has been reported, but a wide range in interindividual effect seems to exist. Whether improvement of microcirculatory perfusion is associated with better patient outcome remains to be elucidated.

Keywords Organ perfusion · Oxygenation · Microcirculation · Vasoactive · Shock · Vasomotor tone

Introduction

Although shock is defined in terms of a critically low blood pressure, a more generally accepted and physiology-based definition of shock is: the inability of the circulation to sustain the cellular respiration needed to maintain normal organ function [1]. This controversy in definition reflects an underlying dilemma with profound effects at bedside. Although intensivists are aware of the physiology-based mechanisms of shock, they have to rely on surrogate global upstream (e.g., blood pressure) and/or downstream (e.g., SvO_2) hemodynamic variables to

M.R. Pinsky et al. (eds.), *Applied Physiology in Intensive Care Medicine 2: Physiological Reviews and Editorials*,
DOI 10.1007/978-3-642-28233-1_27, © Springer-Verlag Berlin Heidelberg 2012

diagnose 'inadequate' organ perfusion and guide therapy. Attempts to integrate regional indicators such as intestinal CO_2, lactate and indocyanine green (ICG) clearance, which have all been associated with prognosis, have had limited success.

Apart from these general limitations, it becomes clear that in distributive shock shunting in the microcirculation is an intrinsic complexity. Although theoretically the concept of shunting has been well known for many decades [2], new technologies have elucidated the role of 'microcirculatory weak units.' In a model of ischemia reperfusion, a speckled pattern of NADH fluorescence and pO_2 emerged after re-oxygenation, indicating an inhomogeneous distribution of cells more vulnerable to ischemic insults than others. Microsphere embolization determined these so-called 'weak units' at the capillary level [3]. Provided upstream oxygen delivery is adequate, shunted parts of the microcirculation remain hypoxic in the presence of well-maintained venous pO_2, explaining the persistence of elevated lactate and regional pCO_2 levels [4] not sensed by the downstream variables such as SvO_2 [5]. The net systemic result is an inability to increase tissue oxygen uptake, despite efforts to '(supra)normalize' oxygen delivery, but whether this reflects a true extraction deficit as result of a preceded cellular metabolic shutdown or a potentially correctable state of inhomogeneous hypo perfusion remains to be established [6]. Because of the introduction of direct in vivo observation of the microcirculation [7], heterogeneity of blood flow has now become a key feature of distributive shock. It has not only been reported within the microcirculation [8], but also between different organs, within different regions of one organ, in response to therapeutic interventions and in a time-dependent way [4, 9], all challenging the simplicity of systemic hemodynamic monitoring under such conditions.

At first evaluation, these observations seem to add more data to the already dazzling complexity of treatment modalities in the critically ill. However, these new insights have established two main findings: (1) the independent perfusion behavior of the microcirculation in relation to classically measured systemic hemodynamic variables, albeit within certain absolute limits of minimal perfusion pressure [8], and (2) persistence of microcirculatory alterations are associated with morbidity and mortality under various conditions, irrespective of correction of systemic hemodynamics [10, 11]. The issue to be resolved is whether correction of microcirculatory distributive alterations will improve organ function and morbidity. In order to explore this exiting concept, it is not sufficient to 'simply' find novel therapeutic approaches that specifically aim to reopen the microcirculation directly. We also have to be prepared to (re)evaluate our current strategies at the bedside in the light of its potential effects from the perspective of the microcirculation and relate it to organ function and outcome.

Administration of vasoactive compounds and fluid therapy are the cornerstone of hemodynamic management of critically ill patients. In this paper we will review reported effects of vasoactive substances on microcirculatory perfusion and tissue oxygenation in shock. These compounds have been advocated to improve systemic perfusion pressure and oxygen delivery, with subsequent improvement of tissue perfusion and oxygen uptake [12]. But do they behave the way we expect them to do? Since shock is a syndrome rather than a well-defined pathophysiologic entity, disease itself as well as treatment might contribute to the clinical picture [13]. An appreciation of basic physiology with respect to manipulating vascular tone and its effect on the microcirculation is followed by a systematic review of the literature. We will focus our review on recent clinical research that includes microcirculatory effects of three classes of vasoactive substances: vasopressors, inotropes and vasodilators, and follow the suggested classification of shock etiology [2]. Preclinical studies will only be discussed in so far as they pertain to the clinical studies.

Materials and methods

In MedLine the following search strategy was performed. Article titles containing shock or sepsis or septic or organ failure or critically ill in combination with vasopressor or vasoactive or inotrope or inotropic or vasodilator or several specific vasoactive drugs [e.g., (nor)adrenaline/(nor)epinephrine, vasopressin, dopamine, dobutamine, nitroglycerin] were selected. The search was restricted to clinical studies in the English language, published over the last 15 years, where indicators of microcirculatory or regional perfusion were specifically mentioned, or in case the effect was evaluated with aid of specific microcirculatory or regional techniques [e.g., tonometry/capnography, ICG, orthogonal polarization spectral (OPS)/side-stream dark field (SDF) imaging, spectrophotometry (Table 1)].

Results

Physiology

Microcirculatory perfusion pressure is the net result of precapillary inflow pressure minus venular outflow pressure. Most of the pressure drop occurs upstream in small arterioles (resistance vessels) as the principal site of active diameter changes to achieve regulation of blood flow. Mean capillary pressure is therefore much closer to venous pressure than to arterial pressure, which is relevant for the maintenance of tissue fluid balance [14].

Table 1 Summary of techniques for the quantification of (microvascular) organ perfusion and oxygenation

Technique	Principle	Data expressed as	Area of interest	Remarks
Tonometry	Balloon content (saline: tonometry, air: capnography) equilibrates with mucosal cellular fluid/gas. Content is quantified with classical bloodgas technology (pH, pCO_2, HCO_3^-)	Intestinal pH or difference between intestinal and arterial ($pCO_{2\ g\text{-}a}$)	Mucosal capillary blood flow	Detects mucosal dysoxia (imbalance between oxygen demand and supply) as a result of inadequate microvascular perfusion. Hypoxic hypoxia is not detected, serosal perfusion can influence measurements.
Indocyanine green clearance	Dye dilution method. The flow is related to the quantity of the injected indicator dye divided by the area under the curve of the downstream dye concentration, according to the Stewart-Hamilton equation	l/min	Hepatosplanchnic vascular compartment	Indocyanine green clearance is dependent on overall hepatosplanchnic blood flow and hepatic cellular clearance function (altered in liver failure)
Laser-Doppler flowmetry	Shift in frequency between emitted and received signal related to (red) blood cell velocity (Doppler principle); flow = velocity × probe catchment area	m/s (velocity) or l/min (flow)	Catchment volume incorporates arteriolar, capillary and venular blood flow	
Spectrophotometry	Light with a specific wavelength is emitted by a spectrometer. Given a specific distance, the solute concentration or color between the spectrometer and the receiving photometer determines the (change in) received light intensity, according to Beer's law	Optical density units from which hemoglobin saturation (%) is calculated	Catchment area incorporates capillary and venular hemoglobin saturation	Hemoglobin saturation may be normal or elevated under conditions of microvascular heterogeneity in capillary blood flow due to shunting
Orthogonal polarization spectral imaging	Direct in vivo video microscopy. Absorbance of green light (540 nm) by hemoglobin projects red blood cells as black dots. Polarization prevents scattering of light	Semi-quantitative: microvascular blood flow index (convective transport) and perfused capillary density (diffusion distance) quantative: functional capillary density (software analysis needed)	Images less than 1 mm^2 discriminates between capillaries and venules	Visualization of vessels depends on presence of red blood cells. Enables to visualize distributive changes in blood flow between individual capillaries
Sidestream dark field imaging	Direct in vivo video microscopy. Absorbance of green light (540 nm) by hemoglobin projects red blood cells as black dots. Ring of stroboscopic light emitting diodes around the camera prevents scattering of light	Semi-quantitative: microvascular blood flow index (convective transport) and perfused capillary density (diffusion distance). Quantative: functional capillary density (software analysis needed)	Images less than 1 mm^2 discriminates between capillaries and venules	Visualization of vessels depends on presence of red blood cells. Enables to visualize distributive changes in blood flow between individual capillaries

Under normal conditions sympathic vasoconstriction is reduced in case of venular hypoxia. This signal is forwarded upstream electrophysiologically via endothelial cells connected by gap junctions proximal to arterioles causing upstream dilatation. This process is regulated per microcirculatory unit arising from the respective arteriole feed vessels [15]. It is proposed that the 'sensor' for detecting changes in ambient pO_2 is located downstream and acts by release of nitric oxide (NO) in the venules [16]. In this respect additional exogenous precapillary and postcapillary vasoconstriction by means of a vasopressive drug results in a reduced net perfusion pressure over the microcirculation [17], despite increment of systemic blood pressure (Fig. 1). At the same time shunting may disrupt the normal venular signaling process for vasodilatation to prevent local hypoxia. Indeed, in ischemia/reperfusion local hypoxia persists in 'microcirculatory weak units' after restoration of oxygen delivery in a speckled pattern that appears to be determined at the capillary level, but not at the arteriolar level [3].

Apart from interference in the complex regulation of tissue perfusion, vasoactive drugs may also influence the homeostasis of tissue oxygenation. Tissue oxygenation is not only dependent on convective properties of red blood cells (flow), but is also determined by diffusion. Given the gas-specific characteristics, oxygen diffusion is related to the pressure gradient and inversely related to the distance between the capillary and the cell (Fig. 2). Closing

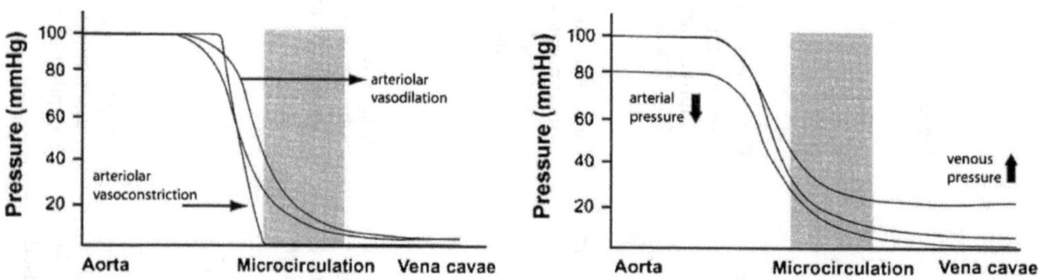

Fig. 1 *Left panel* arteriolar vasodilation increases the opening pressure of the microcirculation as result of a decrease in pressure drop prior to the microvascular compartment. *Right panel* combined arteriolar and venular increment of vascular tone reduces the net driving pressure over the microvascular compartment (from [17] by permission)

Fig. 2 Convective transport of oxygen through the capillaries depends on red blood cell velocity, capillary hematocrit and oxygen saturation. Oxygen transport from the capillary to the cell via diffusion is inversely related to the diffusion distance (D_1 and D_2) according to Fick's law

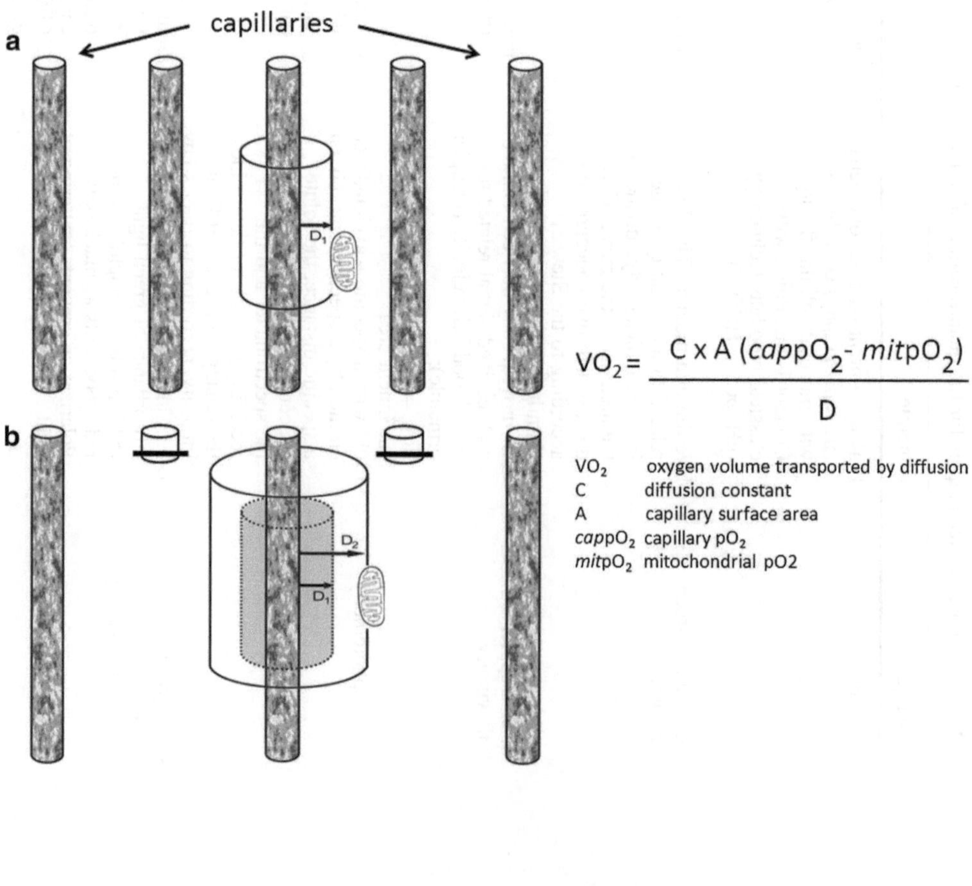

capillaries in order to maintain perfusion pressure increases diffusion distance and vice versa. Under resting conditions capillaries constantly perform changes in caliber in order to serve both purposes [15].

A third factor that influences microcirculatory oxygen delivery is capillary hematocrit. Mechanical interaction between red blood cells and vessel walls induces the formation of a plasma layer adjacent to the wall and increases hematocrit in the center. Since blood flow-velocity distribution has a parabolic shape, from zero next to the wall to a maximum at the center, the average red cell velocity is higher than overall blood velocity. As a consequence, red cell transit time is reduced. This results in dynamic lowering of the capillary hematocrit in comparison to the entering and discharge hematocrit, and is known as the Fahraeus effect [18]. Additional to this effect, capillary hematocrit is also determined by a phenomenon, originally described by Krogh as 'plasma skimming' [19]. At the diverging branches of the capillary network, distribution of red cells is related to the diameter of the daughter vessels (Fig. 3). During in vitro experiments at a systemic hematocrit of 50%, capillary hematocrit ranged from 6.8% during vasoconstriction to 38% under vasodilatation [20], with profound implications on capillary oxygen transport. From the perspective of microcirculation, the dilemma of the use of vasopressors to enhance organ perfusion and oxygenation cannot be better expressed than in the original observations by Krogh: 'This plasma skimming is usually very pronounced when adrenaline is applied in small drops to muscle arteries of which all branches, even the smallest, react and show a contraction, which in a short time may become complete. The portion of the muscle supplied by the contracting artery becomes blanched and the capillaries often disappear completely from view, while application of adrenaline to capillaries and venules alone shows that these vessels do not react visibly to the substance' [19].

Despite abundant experimental data, little is known about human in vivo alterations of vasomotor tone during shock. Direct in vivo observations of the microcirculation in animal endotoxemia demonstrated loss of arterial vasomotion. Interestingly, not all vessels were affected at once, but areas with stagnant blood flow were observed next to areas with brisk flow [21]. In humans, topical endotoxin exposure produced acute venous hyporesponsiveness to NE or sympathic nervous system activation. This was inhibited by glucocorticoids, but not mitigated by NO synthase- or cyclo-oxygenase inhibitors, suggesting other mediators than NO or prostanoids contribute to the overall vascular response to endotoxin [22]. Systemic LPS injection in healthy volunteers blunted the vascular baroreflex response against nitroprusside-induced hypotension and caused complete uncoupling of the cardiac baroreflex from prevailing blood pressure [23]. At present, no direct observations of the microcirculation, other than in tongue or skin, are available from human endotoxemia models.

Human studies

Vasopressors

Norepinephrine (α and β-adrenergic, Table 2) is the most commonly advocated vasopressive drug in septic shock to maintain mean arterial pressure (MAP) at a minimum level of 65 mmHg [12]. Although suggested, improvement of outcome as a result of the use of NE has never been established [24]. Recent studies, which included direct in vivo observation of the microcirculation with Sidestream Dark Field (SDF) imaging, have established that in human sepsis further increment of MAP above 65 mmHg by means of NE does not improve sublingual microcirculatory perfusion, intestinal pCO_2 concentrations or arterial lactate levels [25, 26]. This confirmed previous reports in which stepwise increases of MAP with

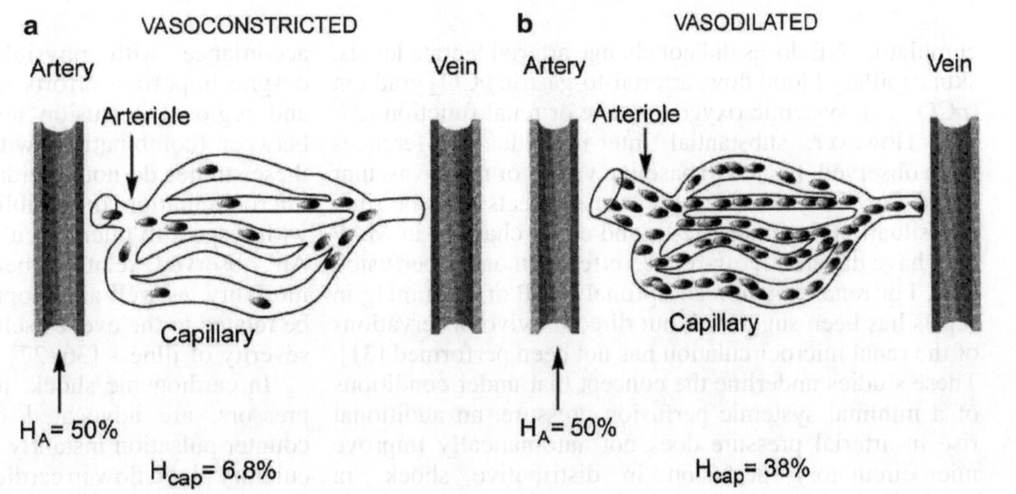

Fig. 3 Under experimental conditions with a systemic hematocrit (H_A) of 50%, capillary hematocrit (H_{cap}) ranges from 6.8% under vasoconstriction to 38% under vasodilation. (From [20] by permission)

Table 2 Adrenergic vasopressors (summary of effects in human studies on microvascular perfusion, oxygenation and organ function)

Study [ref]	Vasopressor	Setting	Technique(s)	Effects	Remarks
[11, 25]	Norepinephrine	Septic shock, $n = 20$, $n = 20$	SDF-imaging, tonometry, laser-Doppler	No change in sublingual microvascular blood flow, lactate or $pCO_{2\ g\text{-}a}$	Stepwise increase MAP from 65 to 85 mmHg, individual effect baseline-dependent
[27]	Norepinephrine	Septic shock, $n = 10$	Laser-Doppler, tonometry	No difference in skin capillary blood flow, $pCO_{2\ g\text{-}a}$, lactate or urine output	Stepwise increase MAP from 65 to 85 mmHg
[28]	Norepinephrine	Septic shock, $n = 28$	Creatinine clearance	No difference in lactate, urine output or creatinine clearance	Comparison between MAP 65 and 85 mmHg
[31]	Norepinephrine	Septic shock, $n = 11$	Doppler ultrasonography, creatinine clearance	Decrease in renal resistive index, increase in urine output, no change in creatinine clearance	Effect between MAP 65 and 75, no further change at 85 mmHg
[42]	Epinephrine	Septic shock, $n = 8$	Tonometry, hepatic vein lactate, ICG clearance	Decrease in mucosal pH and splanchnic blood flow, increase in hepatic vein lactate	Cross-over, in addition to norepinephrine plus dobutamine
[34]	Phenylephrine	Septic shock, $n = 32$	Tonometry, ICG clearance	No change in splancnic blood flow, $pCO_{2\ g\text{-}a}$, lactate, urine output or creatinine clearance	Increment MAP from 65 to 75 mmHg, comparison between norepinephrine and phenylephrine
[44]	Phenylephrine	Septic shock, $n = 15$	Tonometry, ICG clearance	Decrease in splanchnic blood flow, $pCO_{2\ g\text{-}a}$, lactate or creatinine clearance	Switching from norepinephrine to phenylephrine under steady state MAP at 70 mmHg
[45]	Phenylephrine	Cardiopulmonary bypass, $n = 15$	SDF-imaging, laser-Doppler flowmetry, spectrophotometry	Decrease in sublingual capillary blood flow together with an increase in microcirculatory hemoglobin oxygen saturation and overall sublingual blood flow, suggesting shunt	Increment MAP from 47 to 68 mmHg under steady state cardiac output
[74]	Dopamine (high dose)	Septic shock, $n = 20$	Tonometry	Decrease in gastric mucosal pH	Increment MAP from $\leq$60 to $\geq$75 mmHg, under norepinephrine intestinal pH decreased

SDF Sidestream dark field, $pCO_{2\ g\text{-}a}$ arterial-to-gastric pCO_2 gradient, *MAP* mean arterial pressure, *ICG* indocyanine green

cumulating NE doses did not change arterial lactate levels, skin capillary blood flow, arterial-to-gastric pCO_2 gradient ($pCO_{2\ g\text{-}a}$), systemic oxygen uptake or renal function [27, 28]. However, substantial inter-individual differences were observed, related to baseline values of microvascular blood flow [25]. Furthermore, these effects may be time and situation dependent [29], and equal changes in MAP may have different drug-related effects on organ perfusion [30]. For renal function an optimal MAP of 75 mmHg in sepsis has been suggested, but direct in vivo observations of the renal microcirculation has not been performed [31]. These studies underline the concept that under conditions of a minimal systemic perfusion pressure, an additional rise in arterial pressure does not automatically improve microcirculatory perfusion in distributive shock, in accordance with physiological theory [17]. Clearly, despite important efforts to compare mortality, systemic and regional perfusion and cardiovascular side effects between (combinations with) NE and other vasopressors, these studies do not elucidate its individual effects on the microcirculation or establish a critical minimum MAP with respect to microcirculatory organ perfusion [32–35]. An observed relation between both hypotension and mortality, as well as vasopressor load and mortality, may be related to the event itself, but may also be a marker for severity of illness [36, 37].

In cardiogenic shock, inotropic agents, but not vasopressors, are advocated [38, 39]. Intra-aortic balloon counter pulsation instantly improved sublingual microcirculatory blood flow in cardiogenic shock, but additional NE dosage was inversely correlated with microcirculatory blood flow [40].

Epinephrine (α and β-adrenergic, Table 2) in the treatment of septic shock has been subject to controversy. Hyperlactatemia during use of epinephrine in sepsis treatment may be caused by tissue hypoxia, but may also be explained by direct metabolic effects [32, 41]. Human data about direct effects of epinephrine on microcirculatory perfusion in sepsis are not available, but only in comparison to NE. In a crossover design, in comparison to NE plus dobutamine, epinephrine was associated with lower intestinal pH (pH_i) and higher hepatic venous lactate levels under equal systemic hemodynamic conditions [42], but again interpretation of these data with respect to splanchnic perfusion is complicated by the intrinsic effect of epinephrine to cause hyperlactatemia and systemic acidosis [41, 43].

Phenylephrine (α-adrenergic, Table 2) has been used to increase MAP in human sepsis from 65 to 75 mmHg over a 12-h period [34]. Gastric-to-arterial pCO_2 difference, indocyanine clearance, arterial lactate levels and urine output/creatinine clearance were found to be unaltered over time and in comparison to NE, indicating that intestinal microcirculatory organ perfusion neither improved nor deteriorated as a result of a phenylephrine-induced rise in MAP. However, switching from NE to phenylephrine in patients with septic shock while maintaining MAP at 70 mmHg at steady-state systemic hemodynamic variables revealed a rise in $pCO_{2\ g\text{-}a}$ and a decrease in ICG clearance and urine output/creatinine clearance [44]. These indicators of impaired splanchnic and renal perfusion during phenylephrine infusion disappeared after switch-back to NE again.

In cardiopulmonary bypass (CPB)-induced hypotension, phenylephrine was used to increase MAP from 47 to 68 mmHg [45]. During hypotension, SDF-measured microcirculatory blood flow of sublingual capillaries was unchanged in comparison to pre-CPB hypotension, but after correction with phenylephrine microcirculatory blood flow was significantly reduced. At the same time, global tissue blood flow (laser Doppler) and spectophotometric microvascular hemoglobin oxygen saturation (Hbi_{O2}) of the tongue increased, underlining the distributive changes that take place as a result of phenylephrine administration, not sensed in the absence of direct observation of the microcirculation. Interestingly, in an animal model of CPB-induced hypotension, administration of phenylephrine also reduced tissue perfusion to all visceral organs despite correction of MAP from 40 to 65 mmHg [46]. However, correction of hypotension by increasing pump flow improved perfusion of the pancreas, colon and kidneys.

Vasopressin (Table 3) depletion is believed to play a causative role in sepsis-induced vasodilatory shock [47]. In a mixed population with catecholamine-resistant vasodilatory shock, additional low-dose arginine vasopressin (AVP) was associated with an increment of $pCO_{2\ g\text{-}a}$ over time, but lower than NE alone [48]. Direct in vivo observation of the sublingual microcirculation with OPS imaging in a patient with non-septic distributive shock revealed marked microcirculatory alterations, which did not change after AVP injection [49]. In a randomized controlled open-label trial in patients with septic shock, additional use of AVP disclosed no changes in $pCO_{2\ g\text{-}a}$ and a higher creatinine clearance in comparison to NE alone [50]. This was in contrast to other reports of patients with septic shock; both additional continuous infusion of low dose AVP as well as replacement of NE by high dose AVP resulted in a significant increase of $pCO_{2\ g\text{-}a}$ [51, 52]. Equally conflicting data in animal studies are suggested to be related to volume status and cardiac performance [53]. AVP administration in sepsis has been associated with ischemic skin and tongue lesions in up to 30% [54], although in a recent trial the reported incidence was considerably lower and not different from norepinephrine [55].

In post-CPB cardiac surgery patients with high output failure, replacement of NE by AVP during steady-state MAP at 75 mmHg resulted in augmentation of $pCO_{2\ g\text{-}a}$ and diminished laser Doppler-measured jejunal mucosal perfusion, but this was in conjunction with a significantly lower cardiac index [56]. In hemodynamically stable post-CPB patients, incremental doses of AVP were associated with a decline in renal blood flow and impairment of the renal oxygen demand/supply relationship, in the absence of changes in MAP [57].

Terlipressin (Table 3) not only acts as a long-lasting prodrug for AVP with a high V1a receptor affinity, but is also a fast-acting vasopressor peptide per se that evokes coronary vasoconstriction with reduction in cardiac output [58]. It was originally described as rescue therapy in catecholamine-resistant septic shock [59]. The dilemma of its use in septic shock is outlined in a case report in which a bolus of terlipressin produced significantly higher MAP and urine output while tapering NE doses, but was also associated with a complete shutdown of sublingual microcirculatory perfusion and progressive acidosis [60]. More human data of direct effects of terlipressin on microcirculatory perfusion are not available, but only in comparison to other (combinations of) vasopressors. In septic shock after volume resuscitation, there was no difference between a bolus terlipressin or NE with respect to lactate levels and creatinine clearance [61]. Additional terlipressin to NE in septic shock was accompanied by a rise in bilirubin and aminotransferases [62], but not in $pCO_{2\ g\text{-}a}$ [63]. As with AVP, ischemic skin lesions are reported frequently [64].

With respect to splanchnic perfusion in relation to terlipressin, it is of note that it has become an established treatment modality in hepatorenal syndrome and gastrointestinal bleeding in liver cirrhosis. This condition is characterized by a marked vasoconstrictive state in the liver in combination with systemic vasoplegia. As

Table 3 Vasopressin and analogues (summary of effects in human studies on microvascular perfusion, oxygenation and organ function)

Study [ref]	Vasopressor	Setting	Technique(s)	Effects	Remarks
[48]	AVP	Vasodilatory shock, $n = 48$	Tonometry	Increase in $pCO_{2\ g\text{-}a}$ and bilirubin concentrations over time	Additional to 0.5 mcg/kg/min norepinephrine, MAP ≥70 mmHg; increase in $pCO_{2\ g\text{-}a}$ lower in comparison to norepinephrine alone
[49]	AVP	Vasodilatory shock, $n = 1$	OPS-imaging	No difference in capillary perfusion	Baseline capillary perfusion markedly impaired
[50]	AVP	Vasodilatory shock, $n = 23$	Tonometry	No change in $pCO_{2\ g\text{-}a}$ over time and in comparison to norepinephrine, no change in lactate, increase in creatinine clearance	In comparison to norepinephrine lower SOFA score, despite higher bilirubin
[51, 52]	AVP	Septic shock, $n = 11$, $n = 12$	Tonometry	Increase in $pCO_{2\ g\text{-}a}$	In addition to norepinephrine or replacement of norepinephrine respectively
[56]	AVP	Vasodilatory shock, post cardiac surgery, $n = 8$	Tonometry, laser-Doppler flowmetry	Decrease in jejuna mucosal blood flow, increase in $pCO_{2\ g\text{-}a}$	No change in MAP, decrease in cardiac output
[57]	AVP	Vasodilatory shock, post cardiac surgery, $n = 8$	Renal vein thermodilution, ^{51}Cr-EDTA	Decrease in renal blood flow, increase in glomerular filtration rate, impairment of renal oxygen supply/demand relationship	No change in MAP
[60]	Terlipressin	Septic shock, $n = 1$	OPS-imaging	Complete shutdown sublingual microcirculatory blood flow, increase in urine output	Rise in MAP from 58 to 105 mmHg
[62, 63]	Terlipressin	Septic shock, $n = 17$, $n = 15$	Tonometry, laser-Doppler flowmetry	Increase of urine output and creatinine clearance, rise in bilirubin, no significant change in $pCO_{2\ g\text{-}a}$	

AVP Argenine vasopressin, *OPS* orthogonal polarization spectral, $pCO_{2\ g\text{-}a}$ arterial-to-gastric pCO_2 gradient, *MAP* mean arterial pressure, *EDTA* ethylenediaminetetraacetic acid

opposed to septic shock, its potent ability to reduce splanchnic blood flow has become beneficial under these conditions, either to increase risk of bleeding or to redirect flow to the kidney [65].

Inotropes

Dobutamine (predominantly β_2-adrenergic, Table 4) has both inotropic and mild vasodilatory effects. In an open-label setting addition of dobutamine in septic patients was associated with improved OPS-measured sublingual microcirculatory perfusion over time, irrespective of changes in systemic hemodynamic variables [66]. Interestingly, topical application of acetylcholine further improved microcirculatory perfusion, challenging the widespread concept of an irresponsive endothelium in sepsis-induced hypotension. In a crossover setting, dobutamine attenuated intramucosal acidosis during sepsis, whereas dopamine did not change $pCO_{2\ g\text{-}a}$ under equal effects in systemic hemodynamics [67]. Addition of dobutamine to NE in septic patients revealed a lower $pCO_{2\ g\text{-}a}$, but no change in ICG plasma clearance [68, 69]; this could either be due to a direct effect on the microcirculation or a result of an increase in cardiac output. Whether an increase in general splanchnic perfusion indeed is followed by improved organ function is still a matter of debate [70].

Dopamine (β_2-adrenergic and dopaminergic, Table 4; in high-dose also α-adrenergic, Table 2) was used in sepsis for many years in low concentrations for its potential beneficial effects on renal function as a result of afferent renal vessel dilatation. However, results of multiple studies have made such an effect of clinical relevance very unlikely [71]. Low-dose dopamine in addition to NE did not alter pH_i despite increased overall splanchnic oxygen consumption [72, 73]. High-dose dopamine decreased pH_i despite a rise in cardiac output, whereas NE increased pH_i at the same MAP [74].

Dopexamine (predominantly dopaminergic, also β_2-adrenergic, Table 4) initially was introduced as an inotropic agent with specific pro splanchnic perfusion abilities [75]. However, though dopexamine infusion was associated with a partial correction of spectrophotometric gastric Hbi_{O2}, $pCO_{2\ g\text{-}a}$ remained unaltered [76]. This might be compatible with persistence of microcirculatory weak units

Table 4 Inotropic agents (summary of effects in human studies on microvascular perfusion, oxygenation and organ function)

Study [ref]	Inotrope	Setting	Technique(s)	Effects	Remarks
[66]	Dobutamine	Septic shock, $n = 22$	OPS-imaging	Increase in sublingual capillary perfusion over time	Microcirculatory effects irrespective of systemic hemodynamics
[67–69]	Dobutamine	Septic shock, $n = 10$, $n = 14$, $n = 12$	Tonometry, laser-Doppler flowmetry, ICG clearance	Decrease in $pCO_{2\ g\text{-}a}$, increase in gastric mucosal perfusion, no change in overall hepatosplachnic perfusion	Substantial rise in cardiac output
[72, 73]	Dopamine (low dose)	Septic shock, $n = 11$, $n = 16$	Tonometry, ICG clearance	No change in intestinal pH despite increase in overall splanchnic blood flow	Effect on splanchnic blood flow baseline-dependent
[76]	Dopexamine	Septic shock, $n = 15$	Tonometry, spectrophotometry	Increase in microvascular hemoglobin saturation, no change in intestinal pH	These combined observations suggest distributive failure
[77]	Dopexamine	Septic shock, $n = 22$	Laser-Doppler flowmetry	Increase in gastric mucosal blood flow	In addition to norepinephrine and in comparison to epinephrine
[79, 80]	Dopexamine	Cardiac surgery, $n = 19$, $n = 14$	Tonometry, ICG clearance	Increase in splanchnic blood flow and oxygen consumption, no change in intestinal pH	Significant rise in cardiac output
[83]	Levosimendan	Septic shock, $n = 28$	Tonometry, laser-Doppler flowmetry	Decrease in $pCO_{2\ g\text{-}a}$ and lactate, increase in gastric mucosal perfusion and urine output	In comparison to dobutamine
[84]	Levosimendan	Abdominal aneurysm repair, $n = 20$	Tonometry, ICG clearance	Overall splanchnic blood flow remained unaltered, $pCO_{2\ g\text{-}a}$ decreased	In comparison to placebo during aortic clamping, significantly higher cardiac output

OPS Orthogonal polarization spectral, $pCO_{2\ g\text{-}a}$ arterial-to-gastric pCO_2 gradient, *ICG* indocyanine green

in combination with shunting, not sensed by spectrophotometry due to incorporation of arteriolar and venular hemoglobin. The same dilemma was illustrated in another study. Dopexamine, in addition to volume loading and dobutamine, increased ICG-derived splanchnic blood flow, but with a concomitant decrease in pH_i [77]. Apart from this heterogeneity in blood flow between regional circulation and microcirculation, experimental data also suggested regional heterogeneity in blood flow between the gastric and colon region during the use of dopexamine in sepsis [78].

In postoperative cardiac surgery no difference in $pCO_{2\ g\text{-}a}$ between low-dose dopexamine and placebo could be detected [79]. In another study pH_i did not rise despite an increment in ICG-measured splanchnic blood flow and cardiac output [80]. Apart from thermogenetic effects of dopexamine, this might also be explained by a distributive effect. To date, in postoperative non-cardiac surgery, the use of dopexamine remains a matter of debate [81, 82].

Levosimendan (calcium sensitizer, Table 4) improves cardiac contractility and has slight vasodilatory effects. In patients with sepsis-induced myocardial depression levosimendan in addition to NE plus dobutamine was superior to an incremental dose of dobutamine, with respect to $pCO_{2\ g\text{-}a}$, laser Doppler-measured gastric mucosal perfusion, arterial lactate levels and creatinine clearance, either as a direct effect or as result of improved cardiac output [83]. After abdominal aortic aneurysm surgery $pCO_{2\ g\text{-}a}$ was lower in the levosimendan group in comparison to placebo, but despite a higher cardiac output this was not a result of better regional splanchnic perfusion [84]. In an experimental setting attenuation of sepsis-induced cellular hypoxia was observed, but simultaneous SDF-imaging failed to detect changes in microvascular blood flow [85].

Vasodilators

Nitroglycerin (NTG, Table 5) as well as other organic nitrates undergo intracellular metabolism in order to produce nitric oxide (NO)-mediated vasodilatation [86].

Table 5 Vasodilators (summary of effects in human studies on microvascular perfusion, oxygenation and organ function)

Study [ref]	Inotrope	Setting	Technique(s)	Effects	Remarks
[91]	Nitroglycerin	Septic shock, $n = 8$	OPS-imaging	Instantaneous increase in sublingual microcirculatory blood flow after a 0.5 mg iv bolus	Open label, after fulfilment of static pressure resuscitation endpoint
[92]	Nitroglycerin	Septic shock, $n = 70$	SDF-imaging	No difference in sublingual microcirculatory blood flow after 24 h	Placebo controlled double-blind, after fulfilment of dynamic resuscitation endpoints.
[94]	Nitroglycerin	Cardiogenic shock, $n = 20$	SDF-imaging	Increase in sublingual perfused capillary density	Effect ceased after stop medication
[99]	Ketanserin	Cardiac surgery, $n = 6$	SDF-imaging	No change in sublingual perfused capillary density and microvascular blood flow	MAP dropped from 86 to 68 mmHg
[102]	Prostacyclin	Septic shock, $n = 16$	Tonometry	Increase in gastric mucosal pH	Intravenous prostacyclin
[103]	Prostacyclin	Septic shock, $n = 16$	Tonometry, ICG clearance	Decrease in $pCO_{2\ g\text{-}a}$, no change in overall splanchnic perfusion	Patients with septic shock and pulmonary hypertension, aerosolized prostacyclin; effects in comparison to baseline and inhaled nitric oxyde

OPS Orthogonal polarization spectral, *SDF* sidestream dark field, $pCO_{2\ g\text{-}a}$ arterial-to-gastric pCO_2 gradient, *ICG* indocyanine green, *MAP* mean arterial pressure

Despite the fact that overwhelming NO production is believed to play an important role in sepsis-induced hypotension, it has also been suggested as therapeutic strategy to overcome heterogeneity in microcirculatory blood flow [5, 87]. This dilemma is illustrated by the fact that unselective blocking of NO-synthase indeed was associated with a substantial increase in blood pressure, but also with a higher mortality [88, 89]. The general idea that increasing MAP results in a higher net microcirculatory perfusion pressure is not in line with physiological theory of the microcirculation as a low-pressure vascular compartment [17]. For example, in the brain of healthy volunteers (with intact autoregulation), NE was unable to increase estimated cerebral perfusion pressure despite a rise in MAP, whereas glyceryl trinitrate increased estimated cerebral perfusion pressure as a result of a lower zero flow pressure, even at a lower MAP [90].

In an uncontrolled setting, NTG was administered to septic patients who fulfilled static systemic hemodynamic resuscitation endpoints [91]. Despite fulfilment of these endpoints sublingual microcirculatory flow remained severely impaired. After a single bolus of NTG, instant improvement of microcirculatory blood flow was observed, indicating an NO-mediated endothelial ability for vasodilatation, which based on the analogy of topical acetylcholine challenged the general idea of endothelial hyporesponsiveness in sepsis-induced hypotension [66]. However, in a double-blind placebo-controlled setting, after fulfillment of dynamic systemic hemodynamic resuscitation endpoints, sublingual microcrocirculatory perfusion improved significantly over time, but no effect of NTG in comparison to placebo could be demonstrated [92]. In the uncontrolled setting, baseline values for microvascular blood flow in large vessels was considerably lower in comparison to the controlled setting, suggesting marked differences in systemic volume status.

In cardiogenic shock, impairment of sublingual microcirculation has also been observed and associated with morbidity and mortality [93]. Application of low-dose NTG in addition to standard care for cardiogenic shock was associated with a rise in sublingual perfused capillary density [94]. This was not accompanied by a change in cardiac output or MAP and disappeared after cessation of NTG administration. Interestingly, non-pulsatile systemic circulatory flow support by means of a percutaneous left ventricular assist device after acute myocardial infarction was also reflected in a better sublingual microcirculatory flow score [95].

In the specific setting of gastric tube reconstruction, topical application of NTG improved laser Doppler blood in the fundus without changes in local Hbi_{O2} [96]. However, no effect was observed during intravenous NTG in the same setting, suggesting potential interference with bioactivation [97].

Ketanserin (serotonin 5-HT_2 antagonist and weak α_1-adrenergic blocker, Table 5) has been used in the treatment of hypertension with a reported beneficial effect on microhemodynamics and hemorheology due vasodilatation and inhibition of platelet aggregation [98]. Administration of ketanserin in hypertensive post-CPB cardiac surgery patients effectively lowered MAP, while sublingual capillary blood flow was preserved [99].

Prostacyclin (cyclic adenosine monophosphate activator, Table 5) was initially propagated as a drug for improvement of oxygen extraction deficits, suspected to cause tissue dysoxia [100]. Since then it has been studied extensively, especially in experimental settings, for its potential beneficial effect on organ perfusion, as it plays a crucial role in the physiological endothelial vasodilatory response to ischemia/reperfusion [101]. Administration of intravenous prostacyclin after conventional resuscitation was associated with higher pH_i and indicative for outcome [102]. Similar effects on pH_i were reported during aerosolized prostacyclin despite unaltered ICG clearance in patients with pulmonary hypertension [103].

During CPB, infusion of prostacyclin blunted jejunal vasomotion, resulting in a reduced ability to maintain laser Doppler-measured jejunal perfusion constant under variation of blood pressure (autoregulation) [104]. On the other hand, jejunal perfusion increased significantly in parallel to a drop in MAP, but unfortunately $pCO_{2\ g\text{-}a}$ was not measured to establish the overall effect on jejunal microcirculatory perfusion.

Conclusions

Regardless of practical limitations, there is a growing perception that shock should be defined at the level of the microcirculation. Previous clinical research was limited to surrogate markers of organ microcirculatory blood perfusion such as tonometry, laser Doppler flowmetry and ICG clearance. Recent developments have brought direct in vivo observation of the microcirculation in critically ill patients within reach, albeit limited to accessible organs. To date there are no data available in support of the idea that increasing MAP is beneficial from the perspective of microcirculatory perfusion and/or oxygenation, and such an idea is not in line with the physiological theory of the microcirculation as a low-pressure vascular compartment. In septic shock several reports have demonstrated an absence of effect on microcirculatory perfusion above a MAP of 65 mmHg, but a lower threshold has not been established. The role of vasodilators in sepsis as a therapeutic strategy to recruit 'microcirculatory weak units' is yet to be elucidated. In cardiogenic shock neither vasopressors nor inotropic agents have been proven beneficial in terms of organ perfusion, but increasing systemic flow by means of several assist devices are now associated with better microcirculatory flow.

Acknowledgments We thank M. Koopmans and C. Kesting for their assistance in the design of Fig. 2

Conflict of interest ECB has no conflict of interest. CI holds a patent on SDF imaging, has stock in Microvision Medical and has received educational grants from Hutchinison Technology, Baxter, Novartis and Eli Lilly.

References

1. Vincent JL, International Sepsis Forum (2001) Hemodynamic support in septic shock. Intensive Care Med 27(Suppl 1):S80–S92
2. Weil MH, Shubin H (1971) Proposed reclassification of shock states with special reference to distributive defects. Adv Exp Med Biol 23:13–23
3. Ince C, Ashruf JF, Avontuur JA, Wieringa PA, Spaan JA, Bruining HA (1993) Heterogeneity of the hypoxic state in rat heart is determined at capillary level. Am J Physiol 264:H294–H301
4. Dubin A, Edul VSK, Pozo MO et al (2008) Persistent villi hypoperfusion explains intramucosal acidosis in sheep endotoxemia. Crit Care Med 36:535–542. doi:10.1097/01.CCM.0000300083.74726.43
5. Buwalda M, Ince C (2002) Opening the microcirculation: can vasodilators be useful in sepsis? Intensive Care Med 28:1208–1217. doi:10.1007/s00134-002-1407-2
6. Mongardon N, Dyson A, Singer M (2009) Is MOF an outcome parameter or a transient, adaptive state in critical illness? Curr Opin Crit Care 15:431–436. doi:10.1097/MCC.0b013e3283307a3b
7. Groner W, Winkelman JW, Harris AG, Ince C, Bouma GJ, Messmer K, Nadeau RG (1999) Orthogonal polarization spectral imaging: a new method for study of the microcirculation. Nat Med 5:1209–1212. doi:10.1038/13529
8. Trzeciak S, Dellinger RP, Parrillo JE et al (2007) Early microcirculatory perfusion derangements in patients with severe sepsis and septic shock: relationship to hemodynamics, oxygen transport, and survival. Ann Emerg Med 49:88–98, 98.e1–2. doi:10.1016/j.annemergmed.2006.08.021
9. Boerma EC, van der Voort PHJ, Spronk PE, Ince C (2007) Relationship between sublingual and intestinal microcirculatory perfusion in patients with abdominal sepsis. Crit Care Med 35:1055–1060. doi:10.1097/01.CCM.0000259527.89927.F9
10. Sakr Y, Dubois MJ, De Backer D, Creteur J, Vincent JL (2004) Persistent microcirculatory alterations are associated with organ failure and death in patients with septic shock. Crit Care Med 32:1825–1831
11. Jhanji S, Lee C, Watson D, Hinds C, Pearse RM (2009) Microvascular flow and tissue oxygenation after major abdominal surgery: association with post-operative complications. Intensive Care Med 35:671–677. doi:10.1007/s00134-008-1325-z

12. Dellinger RP, Levy MM, Carlet JM et al (2008) Surviving Sepsis Campaign: international guidelines for management of severe sepsis and septic shock: 2008. Intensive Care Med 34:17–60. doi:10.1007/s00134-007-0934-2
13. Ince C (2005) The microcirculation is the motor of sepsis. Crit Care 9(Suppl 4): S13–S19. doi:10.1186/cc3753
14. Pries AR, Secomb TW, Gaehtgens P (1996) Biophysical aspects of blood flow in the microvasculature. Cardiovasc Res 32:654–667
15. Segal SS (2005) Regulation of blood flow in the microcirculation. Microcirculation 12:33–45. doi: 10.1080/10739680590895028
16. Stamler JS, Jia L, Eu JP, McMahon TJ, Demchenko IT, Bonaventura J, Gernert K, Piantadosi CA (1997) Blood flow regulation by *S*-nitrosohemoglobin in the physiological oxygen gradient. Science 276:2034–2037
17. Taylor AE, Moore TM (1999) Capillary fluid exchange. Am J Physiol 277:S203–S210
18. Fahraeus R (1929) The suspension stability of the blood. Physiol Rev 1929:241–271
19. Krogh A (1921) Studies on the physiology of capillaries: II. The reactions to local stimuli of the blood-vessels in the skin and web of the frog. J Physiol 55:412–422
20. Duling BR, Desjardins C (1987) Capillary hematocrit–what does it mean. News Physiol Sci 1987:66–69
21. Delaunay A, Lebrun J, Delaunay M (1948) Le mode d'action des endotoxines bactériennes IV.Les troubles vase-moteurs chez les animaux intoxiqués et leurs conséquences. J Physiol Paris 40:89–110
22. Bhagat K, Collier J, Vallance P (1996) Local venous responses to endotoxin in humans. Circulation 94:490–497
23. Sayk F, Vietheer A, Schaaf B, Wellhoener P, Weitz G, Lehnert H, Dodt C (2008) Endotoxemia causes central downregulation of sympathetic vasomotor tone in healthy humans. Am J Physiol Regul Integr Comp Physiol 295:R891–R898. doi: 10.1152/ajpregu.90444.2008
24. Martin C, Viviand X, Leone M, Thirion X (2000) Effect of norepinephrine on the outcome of septic shock. Crit Care Med 28:2758–2765
25. Dubin A, Pozo MO, Casabella CA, Palizas F, Murias G, Moseinco MC, Kanoore Edul VS, Estenssoro E, Ince C (2009) Increasing arterial blood pressure with norepinephrine does not improve microcirculatory blood flow: a prospective study. Crit Care 13:R92. doi:10.1186/cc7922
26. Jhanji S, Stirling S, Patel N, Hinds CJ, Pearse RM (2009) The effect of increasing doses of norepinephrine on tissue oxygenation and microvascular flow in patients with septic shock*. Crit Care Med 37:1961–1966. doi: 10.1097/CCM.0b013e3181a00a1c
27. LeDoux D, Astiz ME, Carpati CM, Rackow EC (2000) Effects of perfusion pressure on tissue perfusion in septic shock. Crit Care Med 28:2729–2732
28. Bourgoin A, Leone M, Delmas A, Garnier F, Albanèse J, Martin C (2005) Increasing mean arterial pressure in patients with septic shock: effects on oxygen variables and renal function. Crit Care Med 33:780–786
29. Albanèse J, Leone M, Garnier F, Bourgoin A, Antonini F, Martin C (2004) Renal effects of norepinephrine in septic and nonseptic patients. Chest 126:534–539. doi: 10.1378/chest.126.2.534
30. Nakajima Y, Baudry N, Duranteau J, Vicaut E (2006) Effects of vasopressin, norepinephrine, and L-arginine on intestinal microcirculation in endotoxemia. Crit Care Med 34:1752–1757. doi: 10.1097/01.CCM.0000218812.73741.6C
31. Deruddre S, Cheisson G, Mazoit JX, Vicaut E, Benhamou D, Duranteau J (2007) Renal arterial resistance in septic shock: effects of increasing mean arterial pressure with norepinephrine on the renal resistive index assessed with Doppler ultrasonography. Intensive Care Med 33:1557–1562. doi:10.1007/s00134-007-0665-4
32. Myburgh JA, Higgins A, Jovanovska A, Lipman J, Ramakrishnan N, Santamaria J, CAT Study investigators (2008) A comparison of epinephrine and norepinephrine in critically ill patients. Intensive Care Med 34:2226–2234. doi:10.1007/s00134-008-1219-0
33. Annane D, Vignon P, Renault A et al (2007) Norepinephrine plus dobutamine versus epinephrine alone for management of septic shock: a randomised trial. Lancet 370:676–684. doi:10.1016/S0140-6736(07)61344-0
34. Morelli A, Ertmer C, Rehberg S et al (2008) Phenylephrine versus norepinephrine for initial hemodynamic support of patients with septic shock: a randomized, controlled trial. Crit Care 12:R143. doi:10.1186/cc7121
35. De Backer D, Biston P, Devriendt J et al (2010) Comparison of dopamine and norepinephrine in the treatment of shock. N Engl J Med 362:779–789. doi:10.1056/NEJMoa0907118
36. Dünser MW, Takala J, Ulmer H et al (2009) Arterial blood pressure during early sepsis and outcome. Intensive Care Med 35:1225–1233. doi:10.1007/s00134-009-1427-2
37. Dünser MW, Ruokonen E, Pettilä V, Ulmer H, Torgersen C, Schmittinger CA, Jakob S, Takala J (2009) Association of arterial blood pressure and vasopressor load with septic shock mortality: a post hoc analysis of a multicenter trial. Crit Care 13:R181. doi:10.1186/cc8167
38. Spahn DR, Cerny V, Coats TJ et al (2007) Management of bleeding following major trauma: a European guideline. Crit Care 11:R17. doi:10.1186/cc5686
39. Gowda RM, Fox JT, Khan IA (2008) Cardiogenic shock: basics and clinical considerations. Int J Cardiol 123:221–228. doi: 10.1016/j.ijcard.2006.03.099
40. Jung C, Rödiger C, Fritzenwanger M, Schumm J, Lauten A, Figulla HR, Ferrari M (2009) Acute microflow changes after stop and restart of intra-aortic balloon pump in cardiogenic shock. Clin Res Cardiol 98:469–475. doi:10.1007/s00392-009-0018-0
41. Levy B, Gibot S, Franck P, Cravoisy A, Bollaert PE (2005) Relation between muscle Na+K+ ATPase activity and raised lactate concentrations in septic shock: a prospective study. Lancet 365:871–875. doi:10.1016/S0140-6736(05)71045-X
42. Meier-Hellmann A, Reinhart K, Bredle DL, Specht M, Spies CD, Hannemann L (1997) Epinephrine impairs splanchnic perfusion in septic shock. Crit Care Med 25:399–404
43. Uusaro A, Takala J (1998) Vasoactive drugs and splanchnic perfusion in septic shock. Crit Care Med 26:1458–1460
44. Morelli A, Lange M, Ertmer C et al (2008) Short-term effects of phenylephrine on systemic and regional hemodynamics in patients with septic shock: a crossover pilot study. Shock 29:446–451. doi: 10.1097/shk.0b013e31815810ff
45. Maier S, Hasibeder WR, Hengl C, Pajk W, Schwarz B, Margreiter J, Ulmer H, Engl J, Knotzer H (2009) Effects of phenylephrine on the sublingual microcirculation during cardiopulmonary bypass. Br J Anaesth 102:485–491. doi:10.1093/bja/aep018

46. O'Dwyer C, Woodson LC, Conroy BP, Lin CY, Deyo DJ, Uchida T, Johnston WE (1997) Regional perfusion abnormalities with phenylephrine during normothermic bypass. Ann Thorac Surg 63:728–735
47. Landry DW, Oliver JA (2001) The pathogenesis of vasodilatory shock. N Engl J Med 345:588–595
48. Dünser MW, Mayr AJ, Ulmer H, Knotzer H, Sumann G, Pajk W, Friesenecker B, Hasibeder WR (2003) Arginine vasopressin in advanced vasodilatory shock: a prospective, randomized, controlled study. Circulation 107:2313–2319. doi: 10.1161/01.CIR.0000066692.71008.BB
49. Dubois MJ, De Backer D, Creteur J, Anane S, Vincent JL (2003) Effect of vasopressin on sublingual microcirculation in a patient with distributive shock. Intensive Care Med 29:1020–1023. doi: 10.1007/s00134-003-1742-y
50. Lauzier F, Lévy B, Lamarre P, Lesur O (2006) Vasopressin or norepinephrine in early hyperdynamic septic shock: a randomized clinical trial. Intensive Care Med 32:1782–1789. doi: 10.1007/s00134-006-0378-0
51. van Haren FMP, Rozendaal FW, van der Hoeven JG (2003) The effect of vasopressin on gastric perfusion in catecholamine-dependent patients in septic shock. Chest 124:2256–2260
52. Klinzing S, Simon M, Reinhart K, Bredle DL, Meier-Hellmann A (2003) High-dose vasopressin is not superior to norepinephrine in septic shock. Crit Care Med 31:2646–2650. doi: 10.1097/01.CCM.0000094260.05266.F4
53. Asfar P, Bracht H, Radermacher P (2008) Impact of vasopressin analogues on the gut mucosal microcirculation. Best Pract Res Clin Anaesthesiol 22:351–358
54. Dünser MW, Mayr AJ, Tür A, Pajk W, Barbara F, Knotzer H, Ulmer H, Hasibeder WR (2003) Ischemic skin lesions as a complication of continuous vasopressin infusion in catecholamine-resistant vasodilatory shock: incidence and risk factors. Crit Care Med 31:1394–1398. doi:10.1097/01.CCM.0000059722.94182.79
55. Russell JA, Walley KR, Singer J et al (2008) Vasopressin versus norepinephrine infusion in patients with septic shock. N Engl J Med 358:877–887. doi:10.1056/NEJMoa067373
56. Nygren A, Thorén A, Ricksten SE (2009) Vasopressin decreases intestinal mucosal perfusion: a clinical study on cardiac surgery patients in vasodilatory shock. Acta Anaesthesiol Scand 53:581–588. doi:10.1111/j.1399-6576.2008.01900.x
57. Bragadottir G, Redfors B, Nygren A, Sellgren J, Ricksten SE (2009) Low-dose vasopressin increases glomerular filtration rate, but impairs renal oxygenation in post-cardiac surgery patients. Acta Anaesthesiol Scand 53:1052–1059. doi: 10.1111/j.1399-6576.2009.02037.x
58. Ryckwaert F, Virsolvy A, Fort A, Murat B, Richard S, Guillon G, Colson PH (2009) Terlipressin, a provasopressin drug exhibits direct vasoconstrictor properties: consequences on heart perfusion and performance. Crit Care Med 37:876–881. doi: 10.1097/CCM.0b013e31819b8199
59. O'Brien A, Clapp L, Singer M (2002) Terlipressin for norepinephrine-resistant septic shock. Lancet 359:1209–1210. doi: 10.1016/S0140-6736(02)08225-9
60. Boerma EC, van der Voort PHJ, Ince C (2005) Sublingual microcirculatory flow is impaired by the vasopressin-analogue terlipressin in a patient with catecholamine-resistant septic shock. Acta Anaesthesiol Scand 49:1387–1390. doi: 10.1111/j.1399-6576.2005.00752.x
61. Albanèse J, Leone M, Delmas A, Martin C (2005) Terlipressin or norepinephrine in hyperdynamic septic shock: a prospective, randomized study. Crit Care Med 33:1897–1902
62. Leone M, Albanèse J, Delmas A, Chaabane W, Garnier F, Martin C (2004) Terlipressin in catecholamine-resistant septic shock patients. Shock 22:314–319
63. Morelli A, Rocco M, Conti G et al (2004) Effects of terlipressin on systemic and regional haemodynamics in catecholamine-treated hyperkinetic septic shock. Intensive Care Med 30:597–604. doi:10.1007/s00134-003-2094-3
64. Mégarbané H, Barete S, Khosrotehrani K, Izzedine H, Moguelet P, Chosidow O, Frances C, Aractingi S (2009) Two observations raising questions about risk factors of cutaneous necrosis induced by terlipressin (Glypressin). Dermatology 218:334–337. doi:10.1159/000195676
65. Döhler KD, Meyer M (2008) Vasopressin analogues in the treatment of hepatorenal syndrome and gastrointestinal haemorrhage. Best Pract Res Clin Anaesthesiol 22:335–350
66. De Backer D, Creteur J, Dubois MJ, Sakr Y, Koch M, Verdant C, Vincent JL (2006) The effects of dobutamine on microcirculatory alterations in patients with septic shock are independent of its systemic effects. Crit Care Med 34:403–408
67. Nevière R, Mathieu D, Chagnon JL, Lebleu N, Wattel F (1996) The contrasting effects of dobutamine and dopamine on gastric mucosal perfusion in septic patients. Am J Respir Crit Care Med 154:1684–1688
68. Joly LM, Monchi M, Cariou A, Chiche JD, Bellenfant F, Brunet F, Dhainaut JF (1999) Effects of dobutamine on gastric mucosal perfusion and hepatic metabolism in patients with septic shock. Am J Respir Crit Care Med 160:1983–1986
69. Duranteau J, Sitbon P, Teboul JL, Vicaut E, Anguel N, Richard C, Samii K (1999) Effects of epinephrine, norepinephrine, or the combination of norepinephrine and dobutamine on gastric mucosa in septic shock. Crit Care Med 27:893–900
70. Reinelt H, Radermacher P, Fischer G, Geisser W, Wachter U, Wiedeck H, Georgieff M, Vogt J (1997) Effects of a dobutamine-induced increase in splanchnic blood flow on hepatic metabolic activity in patients with septic shock. Anesthesiology 86:818–824
71. Debaveye YA, Van den Berghe GH (2004) Is there still a place for dopamine in the modern intensive care unit? Anesth Analg 98:461–468
72. Meier-Hellmann A, Bredle DL, Specht M, Spies C, Hannemann L, Reinhart K (1997) The effects of low-dose dopamine on splanchnic blood flow and oxygen uptake in patients with septic shock. Intensive Care Med 23:31–37
73. Olson D, Pohlman A, Hall JB (1996) Administration of low-dose dopamine to nonoliguric patients with sepsis syndrome does not raise intramucosal gastric pH nor improve creatinine clearance. Am J Respir Crit Care Med 154:1664–1670
74. Marik PE, Mohedin M (1994) The contrasting effects of dopamine and norepinephrine on systemic and splanchnic oxygen utilization in hyperdynamic sepsis. JAMA 272:1354–1357

75. Smithies M, Yee TH, Jackson L, Beale R, Bihari D (1994) Protecting the gut and the liver in the critically ill: effects of dopexamine. Crit Care Med 22:789–795
76. Temmesfeld-Wollbrück B, Szalay A, Mayer K, Olschewski H, Seeger W, Grimminger F (1998) Abnormalities of gastric mucosal oxygenation in septic shock: partial responsiveness to dopexamine. Am J Respir Crit Care Med 157:1586–1592
77. Seguin P, Laviolle B, Guinet P, Morel I, Mallédant Y, Bellissant E (2006) Dopexamine and norepinephrine versus epinephrine on gastric perfusion in patients with septic shock: a randomized study [NCT00134212]. Crit Care 10:R32. doi:10.1186/cc4827
78. Tenhunen JJ, Martikainen TJ, Uusaro A, Ruokonen E (2003) Dopexamine reverses colonic but not gastric mucosal perfusion defects in lethal endotoxin shock. Br J Anaesth 91:878–885
79. Gårdebäck M, Settergren G, Ohquist G, Tirén C (1995) Effect of dopexamine on calculated low gastric intramucosal pH following valve replacement. Acta Anaesthesiol Scand 39:599–604
80. Uusaro A, Ruokonen E, Takala J (1995) Gastric mucosal pH does not reflect changes in splanchnic blood flow after cardiac surgery. Br J Anaesth 74:149–154
81. Pearse RM, Belsey JD, Cole JN, Bennett ED (2008) Effect of dopexamine infusion on mortality following major surgery: individual patient data meta-regression analysis of published clinical trials. Crit Care Med 36:1323–1329. doi: 10.1097/CCM.0b013e31816a091b
82. Gopal S, Jayakumar D, Nelson PN (2009) Meta-analysis on the effect of dopexamine on in-hospital mortality. Anaesthesia 64:589–594. doi: 10.1111/j.1365-2044.2009.05896.x
83. Morelli A, De Castro S, Teboul JL et al (2005) Effects of levosimendan on systemic and regional hemodynamics in septic myocardial depression. Intensive Care Med 31:638–644. doi: 10.1007/s00134-005-2619-z
84. Leppikangas H, Tenhunen JJ, Lindgren L, Salenius JP, Ruokonen E (2008) Effects of levosimendan on indocyanine green plasma disappearance rate and the gastric mucosal-arterial pCO_2 gradient in abdominal aortic aneurysm surgery. Acta Anaesthesiol Scand 52:785–792. doi:10.1111/j.1399-6576.2008.01659.x
85. Fries M, Ince C, Rossaint R, Bleilevens C, Bickenbach J, Rex S, Mik EG (2008) Levosimendan but not norepinephrine improves microvascular oxygenation during experimental septic shock. Crit Care Med 36:1886–1891. doi: 10.1097/CCM.0b013e31817cede9
86. Münzel T, Wenzel P, Daiber A (2007) Do we still need organic nitrates? J Am Coll Cardiol 49:1296–1298. doi: 10.1016/j.jacc.2007.01.007
87. Trzeciak S, Cinel I, Phillip Dellinger R, Shapiro NI, Arnold RC, Parrillo JE, Hollenberg SM, Microcirculatory Alterations in Resuscitation, Shock (MARS) Investigators (2008) Resuscitating the microcirculation in sepsis: the central role of nitric oxide, emerging concepts for novel therapies, and challenges for clinical trials. Acad Emerg Med 15:399–413. doi: 10.1111/j.1553-2712.2008.00109.x
88. Bakker J, Grover R, McLuckie A et al (2004) Administration of the nitric oxide synthase inhibitor NG-methyl-L-arginine hydrochloride (546C88) by intravenous infusion for up to 72 hours can promote the resolution of shock in patients with severe sepsis: results of a randomized, double-blind, placebo-controlled multicenter study (study no. 144-002). Crit Care Med 32:1–12. doi:10.1097/01.CCM.0000105118.66983.19
89. López A, Lorente JA, Steingrub J et al (2004) Multiple-center, randomized, placebo-controlled, double-blind study of the nitric oxide synthase inhibitor 546C88: effect on survival in patients with septic shock. Crit Care Med 32:21–30. doi:10.1097/01.CCM.0000105581.01815.C6
90. Moppett IK, Sherman RW, Wild MJ, Latter JA, Mahajan RP (2008) Effects of norepinephrine and glyceryl trinitrate on cerebral haemodynamics: transcranial Doppler study in healthy volunteers. Br J Anaesth 100:240–244. doi:10.1093/bja/aem374
91. Spronk PE, Ince C, Gardien MJ, Mathura KR, Oudemans-van Straaten HM, Zandstra DF (2002) Nitroglycerin in septic shock after intravascular volume resuscitation. Lancet 360:1395–1396
92. Boerma EC, Koopmans M, Konijn A et al (2010) Effects of nitroglycerin on sublingual microcirculatory blood flow in patients with severe sepsis/septic shock after a strict resuscitation protocol: a double-blind randomized placebo controlled trial. Crit Care Med 38:93–100. doi:10.1097/CCM.0b013e3181b02fc1
93. De Backer D, Creteur J, Dubois MJ, Sakr Y, Vincent JL (2004) Microvascular alterations in patients with acute severe heart failure and cardiogenic shock. Am Heart J 147:91–99
94. den Uil CA, Lagrand WK, Spronk PE, van der Ent M, Jewbali LSD, Brugts JJ, Ince C, Simoons ML (2009) Low-dose nitroglycerin improves microcirculation in hospitalized patients with acute heart failure. Eur J Heart Fail 11:386–390. doi: 10.1093/eurjhf/hfp021
95. Lam K, Sjauw KD, Henriques JPS, Ince C, de Mol BA (2009) Improved microcirculation in patients with an acute ST-elevation myocardial infarction treated with the Impella LP2.5 percutaneous left ventricular assist device. Clin Res Cardiol 98:311–318. doi: 10.1007/s00392-009-0006-4
96. Buise MP, Ince C, Tilanus HW, Klein J, Gommers D, van Bommel J (2005) The effect of nitroglycerin on microvascular perfusion and oxygenation during gastric tube reconstruction. Anesth Analg 100:1107–1111. doi:10.1213/01.ANE.0000147665.60613.CA
97. Buise M, van Bommel J, Jahn A, Tran K, Tilanus H, Gommers D (2006) Intravenous nitroglycerin does not preserve gastric microcirculation during gastric tube reconstruction: a randomized controlled trial. Crit Care 10:R131. doi:10.1186/cc5043
98. Konishi M, Sakakura M, Tsushima N (1990) Effects of ketanserin on microhemodynamics and hemorheology in patients with essential hypertension. Cardiovasc Drugs Ther 4 Suppl 1:101–104
99. Elbers PWG, Ozdemir A, van Iterson M, van Dongen EPA, Ince C (2009) Microcirculatory imaging in cardiac anesthesia: ketanserin reduces blood pressure but not perfused capillary density. J Cardiothorac Vasc Anesth 23:95–101. doi: 10.1053/j.jvca.2008.09.013
100. Bihari D, Smithies M, Gimson A, Tinker J (1987) The effects of vasodilation with prostacyclin on oxygen delivery and uptake in critically ill patients. N Engl J Med 317:397–403
101. Scheeren T, Radermacher P (1997) Prostacyclin (PGI2): new aspects of an old substance in the treatment of critically ill patients. Intensive Care Med 23:146–158

102. Radermacher P, Buhl R, Santak B, Klein M, Kniemeyer HW, Becker H, Tarnow J (1995) The effects of prostacyclin on gastric intramucosal pH in patients with septic shock. Intensive Care Med 21:414–421

103. Eichelbrönner O, Reinelt H, Wiedeck H, Mezödy M, Rossaint R, Georgieff M, Radermacher P (1996) Aerosolized prostacyclin and inhaled nitric oxide in septic shock–different effects on splanchnic oxygenation? Intensive Care Med 22:880–887

104. Nygren A, Thorén A, Houltz E, Ricksten SE (2006) Autoregulation of human jejunal mucosal perfusion during cardiopulmonary bypass. Anesth Analg 102:1617–1622. doi: 10.1213/01.ANE.0000219596.34753.72

J.-F. Augusto
J.-L. Teboul
P. Radermacher
P. Asfar

Interpretation of blood pressure signal: physiological bases, clinical relevance, and objectives during shock states

Abstract Achievement of a mean blood pressure (MBP) target is one of the hemodynamic goals to ensure an adequate blood perfusion pressure in critically ill patients. Arterial catheter allows for a continuous and precise monitoring of arterial pressure signal. In addition to giving a precise MBP monitoring, analysis of the blood pressure wave provides information that may help the clinician to interpret hemodynamic status. The interpretation of BP wave requires the understanding of simple principles. In this review, we first discuss the physiological mechanism responsible for arterial pressure generation. We then emphasize the interpretation of the static indexes and the dynamic indexes generated by heart–lung interactions derived from arterial pressure wave. Finally, we focus on MBP value as a therapeutic target in critically ill patients. We discuss the recommended target MBP value by reviewing available data from experimental and clinical studies.

Keywords Mean blood pressure · Arterial pressure · Hemodynamics · Septic shock

Abbreviations

ARDS	Acute respiratory distress syndrome
BP	Blood pressure
C	Compliance
CO	Cardiac output
DBP	Diastolic blood pressure
HR	Heart rate
LV	Left ventricle
MBP	Mean blood pressure
PEEP	Positive end-expiratory pressure
PP	Pulse pressure
RV	Right ventricle
SBP	Systolic blood pressure
SV	Stroke volume
SVR	Systemic vascular resistance
RAP	Right atrial pressure

Introduction

The blood pressure (BP) signal provides information, which aids the physician in assessing the patient's hemodynamic status, and guides treatment. Interpreting the BP wave requires the understanding of simple principles. In this review, we summarize these physiological principles; we then detail the information provided by the indexes obtained from BP curve analysis and their clinical contribution. Lastly, we focus on mean blood pressure (MBP) as a therapeutic objective in critically ill patients, and the MBP target to be reached during septic shock.

M.R. Pinsky et al. (eds.), *Applied Physiology in Intensive Care Medicine 2: Physiological Reviews and Editorials*,
DOI 10.1007/978-3-642-28233-1_28, © Springer-Verlag Berlin Heidelberg 2012

Fundamental bases and hemodynamic principles

The BP signal fluctuates around a mean value according to a complex mechanism. From this value, BP reaches systolic blood pressure (SBP), and diastolic blood pressure (DBP). The difference between both values is the arterial pulse pressure (PP; PP = SBP − DBP). The BP signal undergoes changes along its course from the proximal aorta (aortic pressure) to the peripheral arteries (peripheral blood pressure) that may be modeled by wave reflection and pulse wave amplification phenomena.

The arterial system may be considered as a functional unit interposed between the left ventricle (LV) and the capillary exchange and is divided into two subunits, namely the large arteries (characterized by their capacitive function) and the distal arterioles (characterized by high resistance). These features enable the transformation of the pulsatile flow into a continuous flow.

The major hemodynamic principles are derived from the dynamics of a Newtonian fluid (water) circulating continuously in rigid tubes. Neither conditions are met in physiology where the assumptions are that the flow is described by linear equations and that the pressure/flow relationship obeys Ohm's law.

Continuous flow hemodynamics

In this model, cardiac output (CO) is considered continuous rather than pulsatile. MBP would be the pressure required to obtain an identical CO in the absence of pulsatility.

Hydrostatic and hydrodynamic pressures

Pascal's first principle of fluid pressure establishes that below the fluid surface there is a hydrostatic pressure. Similarly, blood exerts hydrostatic pressure on vascular wall, called mean systemic filling pressure, which would be observed under no-flow conditions. Blood is a moving fluid which exerts additional pressure (hydrodynamic pressure). This moving pressure, called MBP, is generated by cardiac activity.

Resistance

Resistance is the frictional force opposing blood flow. If blood is assimilated to a Newtonian fluid under of a laminar regimen, Hagen and Poiseuille's law may be applied to blood circulation:

$$R(\text{SVR}) = \frac{8L\mu}{\pi r^4}$$

Systemic vascular resistances (SVR) are directly proportional to blood vessel length (L) and blood viscosity, and varies inversely with mean blood vessel radius (r). As shown by this relationship, the radius plays a predominant role in vascular resistance. Therefore, because of their large diameter, the large capacitance vessels (aorta and peripheral arteries) provide little flow resistance. Conversely, a minor change in arteriolar radius leads to a significant variation in resistance.

Darcy's law

Darcy's law establishes the relationship between flow (Q), pressure gradient ($P_1 - P_2$), and resistance (R):

$$Q = C \times (P_1 - P_2) = \frac{1}{R} \times (P_1 - P_2)$$

Flow is linearly proportional to the pressure difference. C is the hydraulic conductance of fluid, and hydraulic resistance ($C = 1/R$) is its opposite. Poiseuille's law can be expressed as follows:

$$Q = \frac{\pi r^4}{8L\mu} \times \Delta P$$

Application to hemodynamics

Applying Darcy's law to blood circulation leads to the key relationship governing hemodynamics:

$$\text{CO} = \frac{(\text{MBP} - \text{RAP})}{\text{SVR}}$$

MBP may be expressed by the following equation:

$$\begin{aligned}\text{MBP} &= \text{CO} \times \text{SVR} + \text{RAP}\\ &= (\text{HR} \times \text{SV}) \times \text{SVR} + \text{RAP}\end{aligned}$$

in which HR represents the heart rate; SV, the stroke volume; and RAP, the right atrial pressure. Based on the hypothesis that the RAP is negligible, the relationship is simplified as follows:

$$\text{MBP} = \text{CO} \times \text{SVR} = (\text{HR} \times \text{SV}) \times \text{SVR}$$

MBP's determinants are CO and SVR. This relationship shows that for a given MBP value, CO depends largely on SVR, regardless of how it is generated (high HR/low SV or low HR/high SV). SVR is the "reactive variable": whereas in low SVR states (i.e., septic shock) SVR drives the equation with CO limiting, this contrasts with cardiogenic shock where elevated SVR is a reaction to the low CO. Furthermore, this equation provides a good illustration of the impact of the treatments used in patients presenting shock. Such treatments are aimed at increasing MBP, either by enhancing CO (volume administration and positive inotropic agents), or increasing SVR (vasopressor amines). Hemodynamic principles are based on the study of a Newtonian fluid circulation in rigid tubes under laminar conditions. As blood is not a perfect fluid, and as CO is generated in a pulsatile mode, some of these laws must be adapted to the cardiovascular system's specific features, and lead us to consider pulsatile flow hemodynamics.

Pulsatile flow hemodynamics

As cardiac activity is biphasic, blood flow and hydrodynamic pressure vary when the LV is in systole (increased velocity and pressure) or diastole (decreased velocity and pressure). Thus, BP fluctuates between a maximum (SBP) and a minimum (DBP). The degree of these fluctuations, reflected by the pulse pressure (PP), depends on ventricular ejection volume and rate, peripheral resistances, and arterial walls' viscoelastic properties.

Compliance

The aorta is capable of absorbing part of the SV during ventricular systole, releasing it during diastole. This property is linked to its elasticity, known as compliance, and allows for the offset of systolic ejection, thereby limiting BP elevation and converting pulsatile flow into continuous peripheral flow. The Windkessel simplified model may be applied to the aorta [1] and the overall compliance (C) may be estimated by using the following formula:

$$C = \frac{\text{SV}}{\text{aorticPP}}$$

Reflected waves and amplification of the pulse wave

Aortic pressure may be modeled as the summation of incident BP and reflected waves. The incident BP wave propagates distally from the proximal aorta at high velocity (8–10 m s^{-1}). On its path, it encounters arterial bifurcations and arteriolar blocks, resulting in reflected waves, which are added to the incident wave at the aortic root during diastole. This phenomenon is responsible for coronary perfusion, which mainly occurs during diastole. In specific pathological conditions with decreased vascular compliance (hypertension and the elderly), the velocity of the incident and reflected wave is greater and instead of adding to the diastolic part of the aortic BP wave, it adds to its systolic part, resulting in aortic SBP increase [2]. The same phenomenon may be observed in subjects of short height because of a shortened return of the reflected wave. The addition occurs at the systolic time instead of the diastolic time, increasing the aortic SBP with its deleterious consequences (increased risk of stroke, increased left ventricular afterload) and decreasing the coronary perfusion pressure.

Pulse wave amplification reflects the BP increase measured peripherally, as compared to the aortic level. SBP and PP mainly increase peripherally, leading to a central SBP and PP overestimation of approximately 15 mmHg. This phenomenon is primarily accounted for by increasing differences in arterial caliber and compliance, from the center towards the periphery [3]. Although this amplification is more pronounced in young male subjects and in cases of vasodilation (high compliance), it tends to fade in elderly subjects, hypertensive patients, and in cases of vasoconstriction [4, 5].

Pulse wave amplification has little effect on MBP and DBP, which both tend to remain constant from the aorta to the periphery [3].

Data obtained from blood pressure signal analysis in intensive care units

BP curve analysis provides three types of data on the patient's hemodynamic status. The first approach relies on the interpretation of BP static indices (MBP, SBP, DBP, and PP). The second approach relies on the analysis of BP variations induced by applying positive inspiratory pressure which is aimed at predicting hemodynamic effects of volume loading. The third approach is the mathematical analysis of the pulse wave shape.

Static indexes

Mean blood pressure

Measurement methods for MBP. Intensive care monitors measure MBP by calculating the integral of the BP wave (area under the curve). MBP may also be estimated from SBP and DBP by using the following formula:

$$\begin{aligned} \text{MBP} &= \frac{2}{3}\text{DBP} + \frac{1}{3}\text{SBP} = \text{DBP} + \frac{1}{3}(\text{SBP} - \text{DBP}) \\ &= \text{DBP} + \frac{1}{3}\text{PP} \end{aligned}$$

DBP contributes twice as much to MBP as SBP. This formula was shown to provide an accurate MBP assessment in critically ill patients [6].

MBP determinants and informative value. The determinants of MBP are CO, SVR, and mean systemic filling pressure, which is assumed to be equal to RAP in clinical practice. In intensive care patients, isolated or combined failure of one of these factors may result in an MBP decrease when physiological compensation mechanisms are overwhelmed. Thus, an MBP decrease may be accounted for by either a decrease in CO, insufficiently compensated by increased vascular peripheral resistances, or by inadequate vasodilation along with insufficient cardiac compensation. Analysis of MBP separately does not allow for determining the mechanisms responsible for shock.

Two pathological situations may lead to an erroneous MBP interpretation. The first condition is related to high extravascular pressure, responsible for decreased perfusion pressure of the peripheral organ. This is observed in cases of intracranial hypertension, intra-abdominal hypertension, and compartment syndrome. The second is seen in right heart diseases, which are associated with significant RAP elevation, which can no longer be ignored in the MBP equation (MBP = (CO × SVR) + RAP). In such cases, observed MBP underestimates the true perfusion pressure.

Diastolic, pulsed, and systolic blood pressures

In healthy subjects, DBP remains nearly constant from the aorta to the peripheral arteries. Its main determinant is vascular tone. Thus, a low vascular tone (sepsis, vasodilators) is responsible for a drop in DBP. The DBP also depends on the duration of the diastole and BP decay time constant. A short diastole (tachycardia) is associated with high DBP, whereas a prolonged diastole (bradycardia) is associated with low DBP. If we assume that BP decreases monoexponentially during diastole, it has a time constant (Tau) which is equal to the product of SVR multiplied by compliance. Tau shortening is associated with a decrease in DBP, which is related to either decreased resistances (vasomotor tone decrease), or decreased arterial compliance. In summary, low DBP is observed in cases of vasodilatation, bradycardia, or decreased arterial compliance.

The PP is determined by SV and compliance of large arteries (PP = SV/*C*). A decrease in SV is associated with decreased PP, whereas a decrease in compliance is associated with increased PP. The decrease in vascular compliance with age causes a decrease in DBP along with an increase in PP and SBP [7]. Thus, detecting a lowered PP in the elderly is indicative of a decrease in stroke volume. The main determinants for SBP are SV, arterial compliance, and SVR. SBP is physiologically an essential determinant of LV afterload. In some cases, the combined analysis of various BP indexes (MBP, PP, SBP, and DBP) and patient characteristics (age and cardiovascular disease) may allow for a precise assessment of hemodynamic status. For instance, an elderly patient presenting a DBP of 60 mmHg and SBP of 80 mmHg (MBP 66 mmHg) is likely to experience a decreased SV, as PP is lowered to 20 mmHg. If SV was normal, PP would have been close to 60 or 70 mmHg, i.e., enlarged, because of age-related decreased arterial compliance. In such a patient with low PP, hypovolemia or cardiac failure must be considered, potentially requiring volume administration or positive inotropic agents, depending on the clinical context.

Dynamic indexes of preload-dependence, derived from the blood pressure curve

The analysis of short-term variations in BP related to positive pressure ventilation allows for the assessment of existing preload-dependence. This dynamic approach is aimed at selecting those patients who would respond to volume expansion.

Physiological bases

The Frank–Starling relationship describes SV variation depending on ventricular preload [8]. In healthy subjects, this relationship is curvilinear, and the ventricles function on the ascending part of the curve to such a degree that a preload increase is associated with significantly increased SV and thus increased CO (preload reserve). In acute cases, a preload increase may not lead to increased SV, either because the ventricles function on the flat part of the Franck–Starling curve, or because the preload/SV relationship is modified (heart failure), which is referred to as preload-independence, and in which fluid challenge might be deleterious.

Cyclic variations in alveolar pressures induced by mechanical ventilation are responsible for modifications in ventricular preload and afterload. Upon insufflations, the increase in intrathoracic and transpulmonary pressures (alveolar pressure–pleural pressure) causes a decrease in right ventricular (RV) preload, an increase in RV afterload, and increased LV preload. The SV of the right ventricle is thus decreased during insufflations, which is responsible for a decrease in left ventricular (LV) preload and in its SV, two to four systoles later. The more the LV is on the initial part of the Frank–Starling relationship (preload-dependence), the more the decrease in SV is pronounced. As SV is a determinant of BP, its variations induce modifications of the BP wave.

Respiratory variation in systolic blood pressure: delta SBP and delta down

ΔSBP is the difference between maximum and minimal SBP during a respiratory cycle. ΔSBP was broken down into two other indexes: delta up (Δup) and delta down (Δdown). The measurement of these two indexes is performed with reference to the SBP measured during an

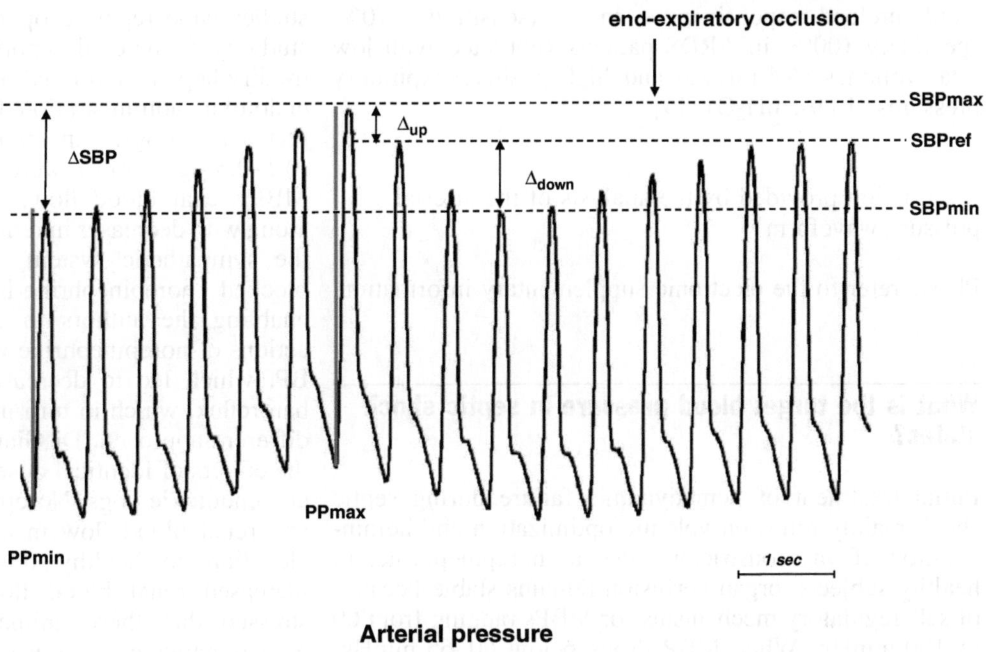

Fig. 1 Dynamic indexes of preload-dependence derived from the blood pressure curve. *SBP* systolic blood pressure, *SBPmax* maximal systolic blood pressure, *SBPmin* minimal systolic blood pressure, *SBPref* reference systolic blood pressure, *PPmax* maximal pulse pressure, *PPmin* minimal pulse pressure

end-expiratory pause (SBPref). Δdown is the difference between SBPref and the lowest value obtained during the respiratory cycle. Δdown illustrates the decrease in LV preload and SV during expiration as an out-of-phase response to the RV decrease in SV occurring during insufflation (Fig. 1).

The clinical relevance of ΔSBP and Δdown as predictors of preload-dependence was validated in a study by Tavernier et al. involving septic shock patients [9]. In that study ΔSBP ≥ 10 mmHg and Δdown ≥ 5 mmHg were predictors of an SV increase of at least 15% in response to fluid administration, with excellent positive and negative predictive values (>90%).

Respiratory variation in pulse pressure: delta PP

The PP is determined by SV and arterial compliance. Considering the absence of significant changes in arterial compliance over the respiratory cycle, it has been assumed that the respiratory variability of PP should accurately predict fluid responsiveness [10]. In the study by Michard et al. [11], conducted on 40 mechanically ventilated septic shock patients, a high delta PP (ΔPP > 13%) enabled the differentiation between responders and non-responders to volume expansion (increase in cardiac index of >15%), with a 94% sensitivity and a 96% specificity. Subsequently, these results were confirmed by numerous other studies [12, 13]. Similarly to Δdown, baseline ΔPP correlates with the degree of response to volume administration. Furthermore, ΔPP analysis would allow the prediction of the hemodynamic effects secondary to an increase in positive end-expiratory pressure (PEEP). It was shown that the higher ΔPP at the zero PEEP, the higher the decrease in cardiac output induced by application of PEEP in patients with acute respiratory distress syndrome (ARDS) [14].

Limits of dynamic indexes

Dynamic indexes have been validated in mechanically ventilated and sedated patients, without spontaneous breathing, presenting regular cardiac rhythm. These indexes cannot be used in patients with arrhythmia. In patients with spontaneous respiration, the specificity of ΔPP is low [15]. A recent study [16] suggests that, in mechanically ventilated patients with spontaneous breathing, the elevation of PP by more than 5 mmHg at the end of a 15-s end-expiratory pause could be useful (sensitivity 87%, specificity 100%) to predict a beneficial effect of fluid infusion.

The relevance of respiratory BP variations also depends on the tidal volume. In the studies that have validated these indexes, tidal volumes were greater than 8 mL/kg of predicted weight. The use of low tidal volumes during ARDS diminishes their sensitivity [17]. However, as a result of decreased pulmonary compliance, marked cyclic variations in alveolar pressure are likely to occur during ARDS, generating marked cyclic variations in transpulmonary pressure and intrathoracic pressure, even in the case of low tidal volume [18]. In this regard, the study by Huang et al. suggests that ΔPP remains a valid preload-responsiveness index (sensitivity 70%, specificity 100%) in ARDS patients ventilated with low tidal volumes (6.4 mL/kg) and high positive expiratory pressures (13.9 cmH_2O) [19].

Information provided by the analysis of the arterial pressure waveform

Please refer to the electronic supplementary information.

What is the target blood pressure in septic shock states?

Initial treatment of hemodynamic failure during septic shock mainly relies on volemic optimization and administration of vasoconstrictors such as norepinephrine. In healthy subjects, organ perfusion remains stable because of self-regulatory mechanisms for MBPs ranging from 60 to 100 mmHg. When MBP drops below 60–65 mmHg, perfusion becomes dependent on the MBP level ("critical MBP"), decreasing linearly with MBP [20].

According to the Surviving Sepsis Campaign guidelines, MBP should be elevated to at least 65 mmHg in order to avoid organ hypoperfusion in patients with septic shock [21]. Nevertheless, these recommendations neither define a target MBP level, nor propose a precise MBP objective to be reached in function of patient's characteristics (age and cardiovascular diseases). During septic shock, vasomotor and microcirculation disorders might upregulate self-regulatory thresholds towards higher MBP values [22], which would require MBP levels greater than 65 mmHg to ensure sufficient tissue perfusion pressure.

Following volume status optimization, norepinephrine is the most commonly used vasopressor to increase MBP, which relies on strong experimental and clinical arguments. Optimal dosage and treatment objectives in terms of target MBP levels are, however, poorly assessed, and remain controversial.

Scientific literature is scarce and contradictory with regard to the dose-dependent effects of catecholamines and the optimal MBP level to be reached. Published data refer mainly to experimental models using incremental doses of norepinephrine, with only few clinical studies.

Experimental data

Norepinephrine causes vasoconstriction (via alpha-agonist receptors) with the potential to result in decreased blood flow to the organs. Accordingly, following norepinephrine administration, decreased splanchnic [23] and renal [24] blood flows were observed under various conditions (hypotension, normotension, and hypertension). Other studies have reported opposite results. For instance, the study by Zhang et al. reported that norepinephrine did not modify hepatic and renal blood flow in dogs submitted to endotoxin administration [25]. Anderson et al. showed that, in dogs, incremental norepinephrine doses (0.1–0.4 μg/kg/min) were associated with increases in MBP, renal blood flow, and glomerular filtration rate, along with decreases in renal resistances [26]. Inhibition of the sympathetic system using pentolinium completely blocked norepinephrine-induced renal vasodilatation, enabling the authors to conclude that the vasodilator actions of norepinephrine were due to increased systemic BP, which led to decreased sympathetic tonus via the baroreflex, which in turn induced vasodilatation. Using a different approach, Di Giantomasso et al. [27] compared the effects of identical doses of norepinephrine in healthy and endotoxic dogs. Norepinephrine increased both MBP and renal blood flow in endotoxic dogs, whereas MBP elevation in healthy dogs was not associated with increased renal blood flow. Nevertheless, it must be stressed that these animal studies do not reflect the hemodynamic conditions observed in septic shock, which is generally characterized by a hyperdynamic state combining high CO and low peripheral vascular resistances.

Clinical data

As the aim of the present review was to focus on the target blood pressure and not to discuss the differential effects of vasoactive drugs both on systemic and regional blood flows (please see [28, 29]), we selected the few clinical studies that have addressed the dose–response effects of vasopressor amines (Table 1). In two studies [30, 31] in septic shock patients, elevation of MBP from 65 to 85 mmHg with norepinephrine did not result in any improvement in metabolic parameters and regional perfusion at the high MBP level. Deruddre et al. [32], however, reported increases in cardiac index and diuresis and a decrease in renal arterial resistance index (measured using Doppler) when MBP increased from 65 to 75 mmHg with norepinephrine in 11 septic shock patients. However, when norepinephrine doses were increased further in order to achieve an MBP of 85 mmHg, no additional benefits were observed. More recently, two prospective studies assessed macrocirculation and microcirculation with a similar design (increment of MBP by 10 mmHg). In the study by Jhanji et al. [33], the increase in MBP from 60 to 90 mmHg increased cardiac index, cutaneous tissue PtO_2 (measured using a Clark electrode), and cutaneous red blood cell flux (assessed using laser Doppler flowmetry), whereas sublingual microvascular flow (assessed using sidestream darkfield imaging) did not change. In the study by Dubin et al. the incremental doses of norepinephrine led to a progressive increase in MBP (from 65 to 75 mmHg and

Table 1 Summary of relevant prospective studies

Study patients (n)	Incremental increases in the MBP (mmHg) (time for each step of MBP)	Measures	Results
Bourgoin et al. [30] (2 × 14)	MBP 65 versus 85 (4 h)	Hemodynamics, renal function	↑CI
Ledoux et al. [31] (10)	65, 75, 85 (105′)	Hemodynamics, tonometry, laser Doppler, renal function	↑CI
Deruddre et al. [32] (11)	65, 75, 85 (120′)	Hemodynamics, renal function, renal resistance index	For 65–75 mmHg step, ↑urine output, ↓renal resistance index
Jhanji et al. [33] (16) CCM 2009	60, 70, 80, 90 (45′)	Hemodynamics, PtO_2, LD, SDI	↑DO_2, ↑PtO_2↑LD. SDI ns
Dubin et el. [34] (20)	65, 75, 85 (30′)	Hemodynamics, tonometry, SDI	↑CI, DO_2 ns, tonometry ns, SDI ns

MBP mean blood pressure, *CI* cardiac index, *PtO_2* cutaneous tissue PtO_2, *LD* laser Doppler. *SDI* sidestream darkfield imaging, *DO_2* oxygen delivery, *ns* result not significant

then to 85 mmHg) and in oxygen delivery. Overall, these systemic changes did not influence the sublingual microcirculatory blood flow assessed by using sidestream darkfield imaging [34]. However, the sublingual perfusion response was different among individuals. The sublingual perfusion was better for an MBP of 65 mmHg in some patients, for an MBP of 75 or of 85 mmHg in others [34]. Finally, it should be added that in these prospective studies, very few patients were included and the time of equilibrium between the incremental increases in MBP was rather short with a range of 30 min [34] for the shorter time to 4 h for the longer time [30].

Finally, using another approach, Varpula et al. retrospectively assessed the hemodynamic values that were likely to be associated with the patient's outcome [35]. In their 111-patient cohort, only MBP and venous blood oxygen saturation values were independently associated with mortality. The best predictor of death was the cumulative time spent below the 65 mmHg MBP threshold. Although this threshold must be considered as the minimum MBP target, the value does not represent a fixed and definitive objective during the resuscitation of critically ill patients. The aforementioned studies have several limitations. First, sample sizes were small. Second, the norepinephrine dose increases were tested far after the onset of septic shock. In contrast, clinical studies that revealed the benefits of an aggressive hemodynamic strategy generally included patients straight upon septic shock diagnosis [36]. In their study comparing standard versus aggressive strategy guided by precise hemodynamic objectives (central venous pressure >8 mmHg, MBP > 65 mmHg, diuresis >0.5 mL/kg/h, and $ScvO_2 > 70\%$), Rivers et al. observed statistically significant benefits in terms of mortality and morbidity in the aggressive strategy arm. Interestingly, the MBP of patients of the aggressive strategy arm was significantly higher, at hour 6 of resuscitation, than that measured in patients of the standard strategy arm (95 ± 19 vs. 81 ± 18 mmHg), far beyond the objectives set by the protocol or the current recommendations.

Other prospective studies, which were not aimed at assessing the effects of various MBP levels, reported mean MBP values ranging from 75 to 90 mmHg, without any notable deleterious effects [37–39]. Only one single study evaluating a non-specific NO synthase inhibitor revealed an abnormally high mortality rate in the patient arm receiving this treatment [40]. This abnormally high mortality rate was ascribed to cardiovascular failure and excessive vasoconstriction induced by this agent as suggested by very high MBP (>95 mmHg) levels in 25% of patients receiving the NO synthase inhibitor.

Published data did not reveal whether increasing MBP target above 65 mmHg can actually improve the patient's survival. Furthermore, target MBP is likely to differ from patient to patient, depending on the underlying condition (preexisting hypertension or cardiovascular disease). Currently, there is no study comparing the effects of two different MBP targets at an early stage of septic shock. The SEPSISPAM study (funded by Programme Hospitalier de Recherche Clinique National, 2009, clinicaltrials.gov identifier NCT01149278) has been designed to provide some answers. The study was aimed at comparing two early resuscitation strategies based on two different MBP targets: a control arm ("standard MBP") with an MBP target between 65 and 70 mmHg, in conformity with the current recommendations, and an interventional arm ("high MBP") with an MBP target between 80 and 85 mmHg to be reached by using incremental doses of norepinephrine. The main evaluation criterion will be mortality rate, irrespective of the cause, at day 28. The secondary end points of the SEPSISPAM trial are related to the potential side effects of increase in MBP during septic shock resuscitation (i.e., life-threatening arrhythmias, acute myocardial infarction, mesenteric ischemia, and digital necrosis). This study, scheduled to include 800 patients, will allow for subgroup analyses, depending on patient's characteristics such as preexisting hypertension.

Conclusion

Invasive BP monitoring seems indispensable for guiding resuscitation of patients with circulatory shock, as it provides reliable and continuous MBP values. The optimal MBP target remains a matter of debate and justifies being pursued in both clinical and fundamental research.

In addition to MBP levels, the BP curve provides valuable information. Its correct interpretation may help to identify the mechanisms responsible for the hemodynamic failure, thereby guiding fluid therapy and vasoactive drugs administration.

References

1. Chemla D, Hebert JL, Coirault C, Zamani K, Suard I, Colin P, Lecarpentier Y (1998) Total arterial compliance estimated by stroke volume-to-aortic pulse pressure ratio in humans. Am J Physiol 274:H500–H505
2. O'Rourke MF, Nichols WW (2005) Aortic diameter, aortic stiffness, and wave reflection increase with age and isolated systolic hypertension. Hypertension 45:652–658
3. Kroeker EJ, Wood EH (1955) Comparison of simultaneously recorded central and peripheral arterial pressure pulses during rest, exercise and tilted position in man. Circ Res 3:623–632
4. O'Rourke MF, Pauca AL (2004) Augmentation of the aortic and central arterial pressure waveform. Blood Press Monit 9:179–185
5. O'Rourke MF (2009) Time domain analysis of the arterial pulse in clinical medicine. Med Biol Eng Comput 47:119–129
6. Michard F, Teboul JL, Richard C, Lecarpentier Y, Chemla D (2003) Arterial pressure monitoring in septic shock. Intensive Care Med 29:659
7. Nichols WW, O'Rourke MF (1998) McDonald's blood flow in arteries: theoretical, experimental and clinical principles. Arnold, London
8. Braunwald E, Sonnenblick E, Ross J (1988) Mechanisms of cardiac contraction and relaxation. In: Braunwald E (ed) Heart disease. Saunders, Philadelphia, pp 383–425
9. Tavernier B, Makhotine O, Lebuffe G, Dupont J, Scherpereel P (1998) Systolic pressure variation as a guide to fluid therapy in patients with sepsis-induced hypotension. Anesthesiology 89:1313–1321
10. Michard F, Teboul JL (2000) Using heart–lung interactions to assess fluid responsiveness during mechanical ventilation. Crit Care 4:282–289
11. Michard F, Boussat S, Chemla D, Anguel N, Mercat A, Lecarpentier Y, Richard C, Pinsky MR, Teboul JL (2000) Relation between respiratory changes in arterial pulse pressure and fluid responsiveness in septic patients with acute circulatory failure. Am J Respir Crit Care Med 162:134–138
12. Marik PE, Cavallazzi R, Vasu T, Hirani A (2009) Dynamic changes in arterial waveform derived variables and fluid responsiveness in mechanically ventilated patients: a systematic review of the literature. Crit Care Med 37:2642–2647
13. Monnet X, Teboul JL (2007) Volume responsiveness. Curr Opin Crit Care 13:549–553
14. Michard F, Chemla D, Richard C, Wysocki M, Pinsky MR, Lecarpentier Y, Teboul JL (1999) Clinical use of respiratory changes in arterial pulse pressure to monitor the hemodynamic effects of PEEP. Am J Respir Crit Care Med 159:935–939
15. Soubrier S, Saulnier F, Hubert H, Delour P, Lenci H, Onimus T, Nseir S, Durocher A (2007) Can dynamic indicators help the prediction of fluid responsiveness in spontaneously breathing critically ill patients? Intensive Care Med 33:1117–1124
16. Monnet X, Osman D, Ridel C, Lamia B, Richard C, Teboul JL (2009) Predicting volume responsiveness by using the end-expiratory occlusion in mechanically ventilated intensive care unit patients. Crit Care Med 37:951–956
17. De Backer D, Heenen S, Piagnerelli M, Koch M, Vincent JL (2005) Pulse pressure variations to predict fluid responsiveness: influence of tidal volume. Intensive Care Med 31:517–523
18. Teboul JL, Vieillard-Baron A (2005) Clinical value of pulse pressure variations in ARDS. Still an unresolved issue? Intensive Care Med 31:499–500
19. Huang CC, Fu JY, Hu HC, Kao KC, Chen NH, Hsieh MJ, Tsai YH (2008) Prediction of fluid responsiveness in acute respiratory distress syndrome patients ventilated with low tidal volume and high positive end-expiratory pressure. Crit Care Med 36:2810–2816
20. Johnson PC (1986) Autoregulation of blood flow. Circ Res 59:483–495
21. Dellinger RP, Levy MM, Carlet JM, Bion J, Parker MM, Jaeschke R, Reinhart K, Angus DC, Brun-Buisson C, Beale R, Calandra T, Dhainaut JF, Gerlach H, Harvey M, Marini JJ, Marshall J, Ranieri M, Ramsay G, Sevransky J, Thompson BT, Townsend S, Vender JS, Zimmerman JL, Vincent JL (2008) Surviving sepsis campaign: international guidelines for management of severe sepsis and septic shock: 2008. Crit Care Med 36:296–327
22. Terborg C, Schummer W, Albrecht M, Reinhart K, Weiller C, Rother J (2001) Dysfunction of vasomotor reactivity in severe sepsis and septic shock. Intensive Care Med 27:1231–1234
23. Shepherd AP, Pawlik W, Mailman D, Burks TF, Jacobson ED (1976) Effects of vasoconstrictors on intestinal vascular resistance and oxygen extraction. Am J Physiol 230:298–305
24. Gombos EA, Hulet WH, Bopp P, Goldringw, Baldwin DS, Chasis H (1962) Reactivity of renal and systemic circulations to vasoconstrictor agents in normotensive and hypertensive subjects. J Clin Invest 41:203–217
25. Zhang H, Smail N, Cabral A, Rogiers P, Vincent JL (1997) Effects of norepinephrine on regional blood flow and oxygen extraction capabilities during endotoxic shock. Am J Respir Crit Care Med 155:1965–1971
26. Anderson WP, Korner PI, Selig SE (1981) Mechanisms involved in the renal responses to intravenous and renal artery infusions of noradrenaline in conscious dogs. J Physiol 321:21–30

27. Di Giantomasso D, Morimatsu H, May CN, Bellomo R (2003) Intrarenal blood flow distribution in hyperdynamic septic shock: effect of norepinephrine. Crit Care Med 31:2509–2513
28. Asfar P, De Backer D, Meier-Hellmann A, Radermacher P, Sakka SG (2004) Clinical review: influence of vasoactive and other therapies on intestinal and hepatic circulations in patients with septic shock. Crit Care 8:170–179
29. Hollenberg SM (2009) Inotrope and vasopressor therapy of septic shock. Crit Care Clin 25:781–802
30. Bourgoin A, Leone M, Delmas A, Garnier F, Albanese J, Martin C (2005) Increasing mean arterial pressure in patients with septic shock: effects on oxygen variables and renal function. Crit Care Med 33:780–786
31. LeDoux D, Astiz ME, Carpati CM, Rackow EC (2000) Effects of perfusion pressure on tissue perfusion in septic shock. Crit Care Med 28:2729–2732
32. Deruddre S, Cheisson G, Mazoit JX, Vicaut E, Benhamou D, Duranteau J (2007) Renal arterial resistance in septic shock: effects of increasing mean arterial pressure with norepinephrine on the renal resistive index assessed with Doppler ultrasonography. Intensive Care Med 33:1557–1562
33. Jhanji S, Stirling S, Patel N, Hinds CJ, Pearse RM (2009) The effect of increasing doses of norepinephrine on tissue oxygenation and microvascular flow in patients with septic shock. Crit Care Med 37:1961–1966
34. Dubin A, Pozo MO, Casabella CA, Palizas F Jr, Murias G, Moseinco MC, Kanoore Edul VS, Palizas F, Estenssoro E, Ince C (2009) Increasing arterial blood pressure with norepinephrine does not improve microcirculatory blood flow: a prospective study. Crit Care 13:R92
35. Varpula M, Tallgren M, Saukkonen K, Voipio-Pulkki LM, Pettila V (2005) Hemodynamic variables related to outcome in septic shock. Intensive Care Med 31:1066–1071
36. Rivers E, Nguyen B, Havstad S, Ressler J, Muzzin A, Knoblich B, Peterson E, Tomlanovich M (2001) Early goal-directed therapy in the treatment of severe sepsis and septic shock. N Engl J Med 345:1368–1377
37. Russell JA, Walley KR, Singer J, Gordon AC, Hebert PC, Cooper DJ, Holmes CL, Mehta S, Granton JT, Storms MM, Cook DJ, Presneill JJ, Ayers D (2008) Vasopressin versus norepinephrine infusion in patients with septic shock. N Engl J Med 358:877–887
38. Annane D, Vignon P, Renault A, Bollaert PE, Charpentier C, Martin C, Troche G, Ricard JD, Nitenberg G, Papazian L, Azoulay E, Bellissant E (2007) Norepinephrine plus dobutamine versus epinephrine alone for management of septic shock: a randomised trial. Lancet 370:676–684
39. Gattinoni L, Brazzi L, Pelosi P, Latini R, Tognoni G, Pesenti A, Fumagalli R (1995) A trial of goal-oriented hemodynamic therapy in critically ill patients. SvO2 Collaborative Group. N Engl J Med 333:1025–1032
40. Lopez A, Lorente JA, Steingrub J, Bakker J, McLuckie A, Willatts S, Brockway M, Anzueto A, Holzapfel L, Breen D, Silverman MS, Takala J, Donaldson J, Arneson C, Grove G, Grossman S, Grover R (2004) Multiple-center, randomized, placebo-controlled, double-blind study of the nitric oxide synthase inhibitor 546C88: effect on survival in patients with septic shock. Crit Care Med 32:21–30

Pratik Sinha
Oliver Flower
Neil Soni

Deadspace ventilation: a waste of breath!

Abstract Problems with ventilatory efficiency results in abnormal CO_2 clearance. Measuring deadspace ventilation should be the most reliable method of monitoring ventilatory efficiency in mechanically ventilated patients. Since its first description by Bohr in the late 19th century to the current use of single-breath test for volumetric CO_2, our understanding of the physiological deadspace has vastly improved. Yet indices of oxygenation seem to be the mainstay when instigating or fine-tuning ventilatory strategies. Deadspace and with it ventilatory efficiency has been largely forgotten. Recently though there has been a resurgence of interest in ventilatory efficiency. Several indices have been described that either predict deadspace or track ventilatory efficiency at the bedside. Thus making it more accessible and easy to monitor and study in large groups of patients, factors which have perhaps resulted in its under-utilisation in critical care. This review revisits the physiological concepts and methods of measuring deadspace. Described are the various clinical applications of deadspace measurements in the critically unwell. The potential reasons that have led to the variable being under-used are also examined. Finally we describe the indices currently available to track ventilatory efficiency at the bedside.

Keywords Deadspace · Dead space · Ventilatory efficiency · ALI · ARDS

Introduction

Alveolar ventilation is the amount of air per unit time that is involved in gas exchange. Ventilatory efficiency describes this volume as a proportion of the tidal volume. The remainder of the tidal volume is not involved in gas exchange and is conceptually known as the physiological deadspace. Whilst deadspace ventilation is probably of minimal consequence in normal conditions, its inherent clinical importance is that pathophysiological states of the lung result in its increase and hence a reduction in ventilatory efficiency. At the bedside this will manifest as altered carbon dioxide clearance. Such pathological processes are common in the critically ill and measurement of physiological deadspace should be a most valuable and intuitive tool to manage ventilation, yet it is seldom used.

The importance of carbon dioxide clearance was first appreciated in the Danish polio epidemic when clinicians rapidly realised that existing methods such as negative pressure ventilation resulted in deaths despite adequate oxygenation. The turning point was the realization that most deaths were due to inadequate ventilation [1, 2]. This led to the birth of positive pressure ventilation, respiratory physiological monitoring and with it intensive care medicine. The initial primacy of carbon dioxide clearance in monitoring during mechanical ventilation was key. Since then emphasis in practice has slowly changed and adequacy of oxygenation has replaced carbon dioxide as the principle focus for managing such

M.R. Pinsky et al. (eds.), *Applied Physiology in Intensive Care Medicine 2: Physiological Reviews and Editorials*,
DOI 10.1007/978-3-642-28233-1_29,

patients. Yet the indirect role of ventilation in oxygenation is illustrated by the ability to oxygenate by insufflation. Carbon dioxide and its clearance has been considered of still lesser importance especially with the advent of permissive hypercapnia. This correctly identifies the relatively innocuous nature of mild hypercapnia but in doing so obscures the obvious fact that hypercapnia with adequate ventilation implies a significant increase in physiological deadspace with or without alterations in shunt. The pathophysiology underlying permissive hypercapnia is directly related to the underlying disease processes yet it is considered of secondary importance. It is a clinical paradox that while the concept of physiological deadspace has been known since the late 19th century, in the critical care setting it remains an underused and poorly understood variable.

It is time to revisit this neglected subject and the aims of this review are to examine current physiological concepts of deadspace, describe methods of measurement, and describe its common uses as a clinical tool in the critical care setting. Also examined are the current available methods to assess ventilatory efficiency at the bedside.

Terminology

Deadspace is the portion of tidal volume that does not participate in gas exchange i.e. 'wasted'. Physiological deadspace (VD^{phys}) is a composed of airway deadspace (VD^{aw}) and alveolar deadspace (VD^{alv}):

$$VD^{phys} = VD^{aw} + VD^{alv} \tag{1}$$

In mechanically ventilated patients airway deadspace (VD^{aw}) is the sum of anatomical deadspace (conducting airways) and apparatus deadspace. Alveolar deadspace is a construct that accounts for the remainder of the tidal volume that does not participate in gas exchange. In normal healthy subjects the alveolar deadspace is expected to be negligible.

The history of physiological deadspace

Bohr equation

Tidal volume (V_T) is the sum of alveolar ventilation (V_A) and physiological deadspace (V_D):

$$V_T = V_A + V_D \tag{2}$$

In 1891 Bohr made two basic assumption when considering his approach to calculating deadspace [3]. Firstly a two-lung model was assumed whereby there was either gas exchange (alveolar ventilation) or deadspace. The 'deadspace' in this instance was assumed to be a fixed entity derived from previous cadaveric measurements (airway deadspace). Bohr proposed using Eq. 2 to calculate the alveolar volume. He also assumed that there was no carbon dioxide in inspired air. Therefore all carbon dioxide measured in mixed expired gas came from alveolar ventilation. The latter assumption is used in most current methods used to calculate deadspace.

Inserting the appropriate fractioned CO_2 concentration (F) into each of the three volumes in Eq. 2 and given that the concentration of CO_2 in deadspace gas ($F_{D_{CO_2}}$) is 0, using the conservation of mass principle Eq. 2 can be restated as:

$$V_T \cdot F_{E_{CO_2}} = V_A \cdot F_{A_{CO_2}} \tag{3}$$

From Eq. 2 we also know that $V_A = V_T - V_D$ therefore:

$$V_T \cdot F_{E_{CO_2}} = (V_T - V_D) \cdot F_{A_{CO_2}} \tag{4}$$

Solving for V_D/V_T we get:

$$\frac{V_D}{V_T} = \frac{F_{A_{CO_2}} - F_{E_{CO_2}}}{F_{A_{CO_2}}} \tag{5}$$

where $F_{A_{CO_2}}$ is the alveolar fractional concentration of CO_2 and $F_{E_{CO_2}}$ is the mixed expired fractional concentration of CO_2. This equation was originally used by Bohr to obtain $F_{A_{CO_2}}$ and the associated alveolar volume. Equation 5 is commonly known as Bohr's equation.

Since then Eq. 5 is frequently restated substituting fractioned CO_2 concentration with partial pressures of CO_2 (PCO_2):

$$\frac{V_D}{V_T} = \frac{P_{A_{CO_2}} - P_{E_{CO_2}}}{P_{A_{CO_2}}} \tag{6}$$

where $P_{A_{CO_2}}$ is the alveolar P_{CO_2} and $P_{E_{CO_2}}$ is the mixed expired P_{CO_2}. Subsequent to the work of Bohr it was recognized that deadspace was a varying entity. The introduction of gas analysis allowed the use of expired CO_2 as a surrogate for alveolar CO_2 [4]. Mixed expired CO_2 was collected in a reservoir bag and thereby enabling the calculation of deadspace using Eq. 6 [5].

Enghoff modification of Bohr's equation

One of the limitations of Bohr's method of calculating deadspace has been accurately measuring alveolar PCO_2 ($P_{A_{CO_2}}$). Given the inter-alveoli heterogeneity of ventilation-perfusion ratio and the uneven emptying of lung units due to varied time constants, end-tidal CO_2 is an inaccurate representation of $P_{A_{CO_2}}$ [6]. This is especially true in the case of diseased lungs where there is increased disparity in the homogeneity of the $\dot{V}/\dot{Q}$ matching and alveolar emptying. By assuming that there was no difference in the values of alveolar P_{CO_2} and arterial P_{CO_2} ($P_{a_{CO_2}}$), in 1938

Enghoff modified the Bohr deadspace equation by substituting P_{ACO_2} with P_{aco_2} [7]. Accounting for this substitution we can restate Eq. 6:

$$\frac{V_D}{V_T} = \frac{P_{aco_2} - P_{ECO_2}}{P_{aco_2}} \qquad (7)$$

Equation 7 is known as the Bohr–Enghoff equation and to this day remains the most commonly used method to calculate deadspace using mixed-expired CO_2.

Fowler's airway deadspace

Fowler's novel method was to use continuous nitrogen gas analysis to calculate deadspace [8]. His subjects inhaled 99.6% oxygen and the expired volume and concentration of nitrogen were continuously measured. Fowler defined 'physiological deadspace' as the volume representing the conducting airways. He described it as the point where a large change in the gas composition occurred. Effectively this is the volume represented by what we now know as the airway deadspace. Fowler proposed analyzing the graphform of the nitrogen volume-concentration of expired gas to calculate the deadspace (Fig. 1).

Since then Bartels and colleagues demonstrated that the deadspace for carbon dioxide was the same as that of nitrogen and Fowler's methods could be applied to calculate deadspace using single breath analysis of expired CO_2 [9].

More recently Langley and colleagues plotted the expired CO_2 volume against the expired total volume and described an alternative method of calculating airway deadspace [10]. This curvilinear graph is shown in Fig. 2. A straight best-fit line is extrapolated from the linear portion of the graph and the intercept of this line on the volume axis (x axis) is representative of the deadspace (Fig. 2). This method correlates with Fowler's method for calculating VD^{aw} but with the added advantage that it does not rely on the visual interpretation for determining equal areas [11, 12].

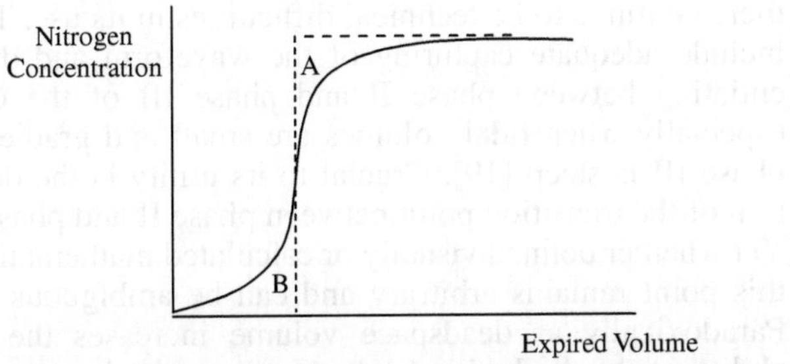

Fig. 1 Fowler's method of calculating deadspace. The *vertical dashed line* is drawn such that the areas marked *A* and *B* are equal. The deadspace volume is represented by the volume where the line intercepts the *x* axis. A similar waveform can be drawn for expired CO_2 concentration

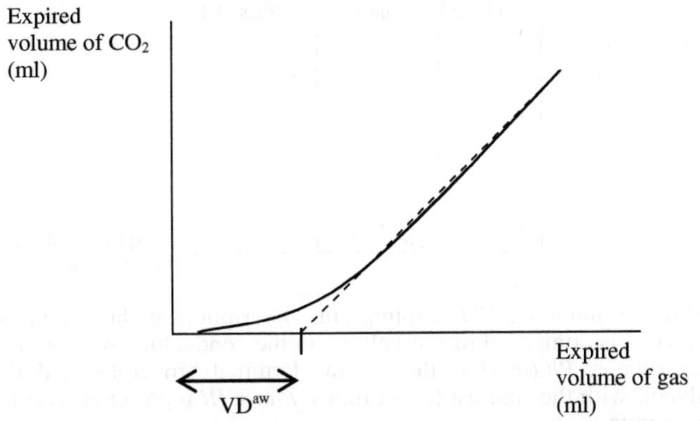

Fig. 2 Langley's method for calculating anatomical deadspace. Plotted is the volume of expired CO_2 against the volume of expired gas. The *dotted line* represents the best-fit line of the linear segment of the graph. The point of interception of the *dotted line* on the *x* axis represents the airway deadspace volume

While several factors can influence airway deadspace, in the critical care setting this volume remains relatively unchanged. Large stepwise changes in airway deadspace in mechanically ventilated patients are usually as a result of equipment deadspace and hence easily quantifiable. Any changes in measured physiological deadspace, without added equipment deadspace, are mostly a result of changes in alveolar deadspace. It is alveolar deadspace and its inherent interaction with physiological deadspace that is clearly most important clinically.

Measuring physiological deadspace and ventilatory efficiency

Single breath test for carbon dioxide

The CO_2 single breath test (SBT-CO_2) of volumetric capnography can be used to extract useful information about ventilatory efficiency. Breath-by-breath analysis of expired CO_2 concentrations plotted against the total expired volume allows for meaningful calculations of the area under the graph. The volumetric SBT-CO_2 expirogram can be divided into three phases (Fig. 3). Phase I is the volume of gas that is in the airway (and the apparatus volume in ventilated patients). Phase II is composed of gas from the terminal airways and from the alveoli with the shortest transit times. Phase III is also known as the alveolar plateau and represents majority of the alveolar emptying.

The slopes of phase II and III can impart useful information on visual analysis. A flat alveolar plateau (phase III) would be indicative of homogenous lung emptying. Conversely an expirogram with an alveolar plateau with a steep continuous gradient represents heterogeneity in alveolar emptying. This is frequently encountered in diseased lung states. Inhomogeneity in

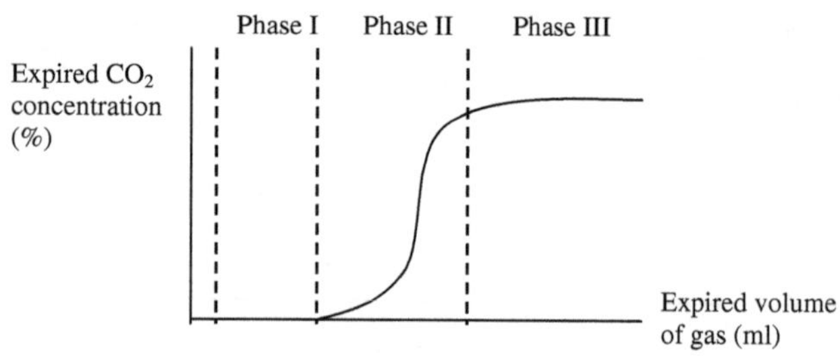

Fig. 3 Volumetric CO_2 expirogram. Description of the 3 phases. *Phase I* is composed of the volume in the conducting airways and equipment. *Phase II* is the volume terminal broncioles and the alveoli with the shortest transit times. *Phase III* represents alveolar emptying

alveolar emptying could either result from within the alveolar units where in the more distal alveoli there is likely to be lower $\dot{V}/\dot{Q}$ ratio or due to inter-unit heterogeneity [6].

Fletcher further analyzed the SBT-CO_2 and gave a detailed proposal of measuring the various parts that contribute to physiological deadspace [13, 14]. Figure 4 shows that the area under the graph (x) is the volume of CO_2 eliminated in a breath. The area ABCDA describes the maximum (hypothetical) volume of gas that could be excreted in the breath. 'Efficiency' which is the portion of volume participating in gas exchange is described as:

$$\text{Efficiency} = \frac{X}{\text{ABCDA}} \tag{8}$$

1 − efficiency represents the same fraction as deadspace. Therefore 'E' or efficiency can be restated as a product of more familiar terms:

$$E = \frac{V_A}{V_E} = 1 - \frac{V_D}{V_T} = \text{Efficiency}_{\text{Fletcher}} \tag{9}$$

where V_A represents the alveolar volume (ml) and V_E represents the expired tidal volume (ml).

In diseased lungs where there is significant $\dot{V}/\dot{Q}$ mismatch the peak P_{CO_2} of the alveolar plateau seldom equals alveolar P_{CO_2} or arterial P_{CO_2}. Fletcher proposed using this discrepancy to calculate the alveolar deadspace. As shown in Fig. 5A a horizontal line is drawn from the point on the y axis that represents the arterial P_{CO_2}. As per Fowler's method a vertical line is drawn to elicit equal areas p and q. Area X once again represents the volume of CO_2 eliminated, area Y represents the VD^{alv} and area Z represents VD^{aw}.

Therefore from the analysis we can deduce that anatomical deadspace fraction is:

$$\frac{V_D^{aw}}{V_T} = \frac{Z}{X + Y + Z} \tag{10}$$

alveolar deadspace fraction is:

$$\frac{V_D^{alv}}{V_T} = \frac{Y}{X + Y + Z} \tag{11}$$

and physiological deadspace can be defined as:

$$\frac{V_D^{phys}}{V_T} = \frac{Y + Z}{X + Y + Z} \tag{12}$$

SBT-CO_2 deadspace calculations have been validated against the V_D^{bohr} in both animal models and humans [15, 16]. There are several advantages to using volumetric capnography (SBT-CO_2) over the Douglas Bag method for measuring deadspace in mechanically ventilated patients. Collecting mixed expired gas in a Douglas bag is subject to inherent accuracies due to gas compression predominantly within the ventilator circuit [17, 18]. On expiration this compressed gas will dilute the mixed expired CO_2 concentration in the bag, and therefore lower the measured $PeCO_2$, resulting in falsely elevated physiological deadspace. Volumetric capnography measures the expired CO_2 closer to the endotracheal tube and therefore the measurements do not require a correction factor accounting for the gas compression in the ventilator circuit. Additionally volumetric capnography provides breath to breath analysis of the CO_2 capnograph and enables frequent assessment of deadspace changes.

Although recent developments in both software and capnography have made this method more accessible there continue to be technical difficulties in its use. These include adequate capturing of the waveform and differentiating between phase II and phase III of the curve especially when tidal volumes are small and gradient of phase III is steep [19]. Crucial to its utility is the definition of the transition point between phase II and phase III. Yet whether defined visually or calculated mathematically this point remains arbitrary and can be ambiguous [16]. Paradoxically as deadspace volume increases the reliability of the method is further compromised.

To overcome these shortcomings Romero et al. used the SBT-CO_2 to propose an alternative method to analyse ventilatory efficiency. This moves away from the visual description of the transition from phase II to phase III.

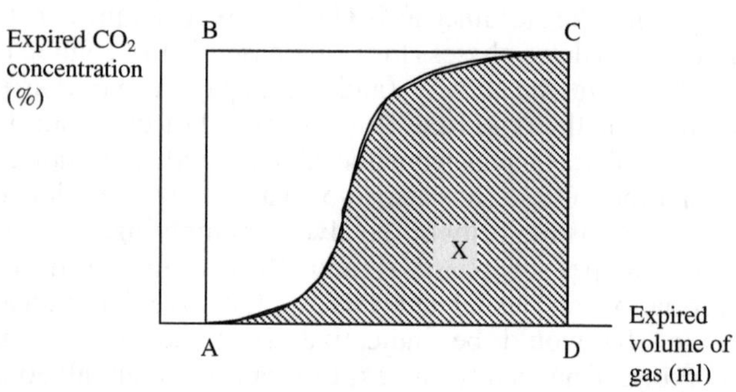

Fig. 4 SBT-CO_2 demonstrating the fraction of 'efficiency'. The *shaded area X* represents the volume of CO_2 eliminated. The area *ABCDA* represents the potential maximum volume of elimination

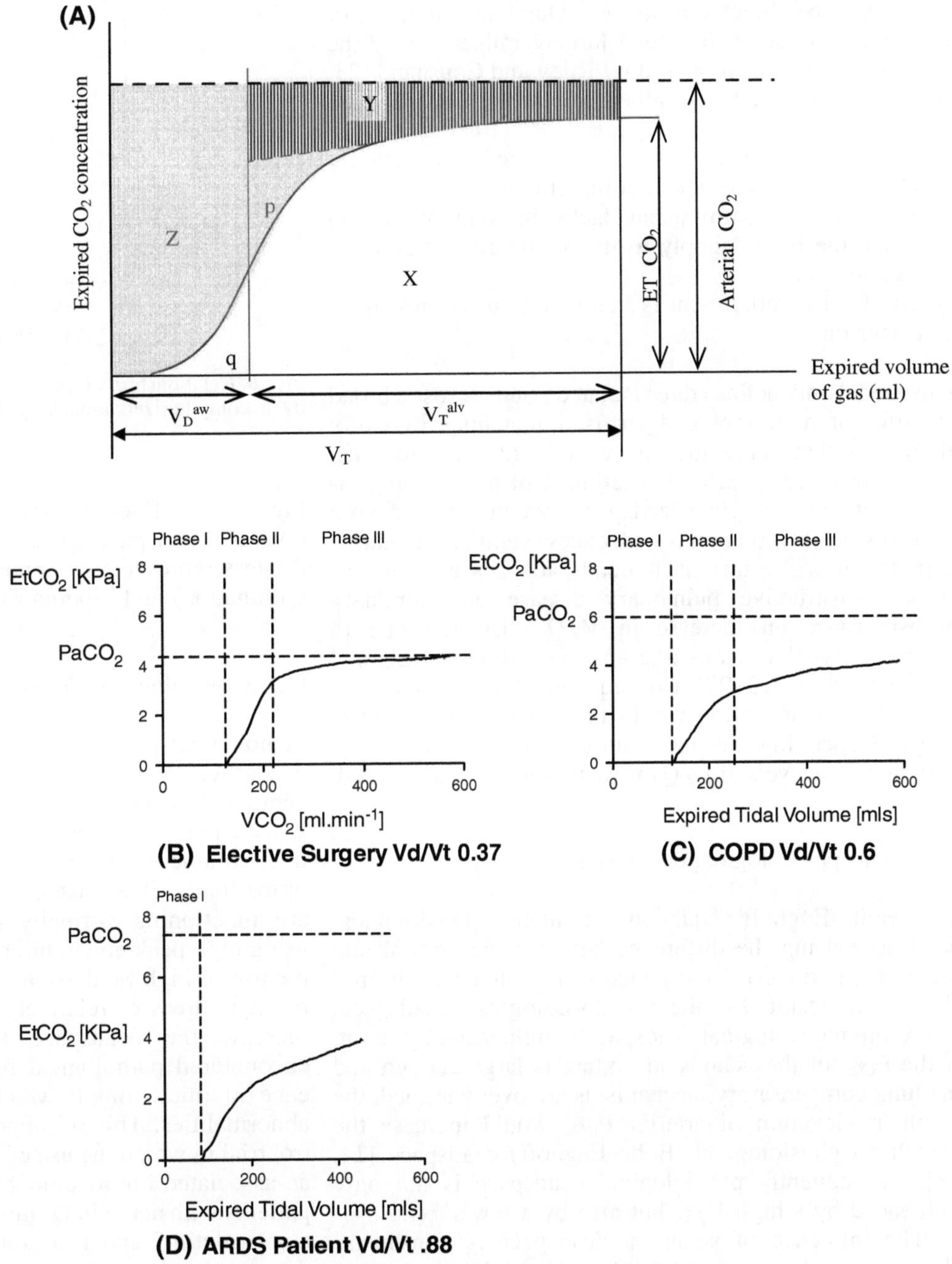

Fig. 5 **a** Components of SBT-CO_2 expirogram as described by Fletcher. Area *X* represents the CO_2 elimination volume, area *Y* is the alveolar deadspace volume, and area *Z* is the airway deadspace volume, where areas *p* and *q* are equal. **b** Shows the SBT-CO_2 expirogram for a mechanically ventilated patient undergoing elective surgery. **c** Shows the SBT-CO_2 expirogram for a mechanically ventilated patient with COPD admitted to intensive care, the slope of phase III is steeper. **d** shows SBT-CO_2 expirogram of a mechanically ventilated patient with ARDS, the transition between *phase II* and *phase III* is harder to define

Instead, as in Fig. 2 they plot the expired volume of CO_2 against the expired tidal volume to describe the term alveolar ejection volume (V_{AE}) as the predicted point on the VCO_2 curve where alveolar emptying begins. This volume attempts quantification of the phase III of the slope. The alveolar ejection volume versus tidal volume ratio (V_{AE}/V_t) [20] is an index that monitors alveolar heterogeneity and has been shown to correlate with severity of lung diseases as well as being a useful predictor of outcome [21, 22]. Limitations of this index as a clinical tool include the requirement of relatively simple software to calculate [22] the values and that it is not a previously described physiological term.

Current concepts in deadspace

Ventilation-perfusion mismatch

Physiological deadspace is a marriage of a tangible anatomical entity and an intangible physiological function that cannot be directly measured. Our understanding of deadspace and shunt has been largely influenced by the three lung model as proposed by Riley and Cournand [23, 24]. In this proposed model there are three compartments:

a) The first compartment is both ventilated and perfused. This is the most efficient compartment.
b) The second compartment lacks in ventilation and hence the blood supply to this compartment contributes to shunt.
c) The final compartment is ventilated but is lacking in perfusion.

This model only defines three isolated points across a broad spectrum of ventilation and perfusion matching. In reality all factors that cause inequality of $\dot{V}/\dot{Q}$ mismatch will contribute to deadspace ventilation. Not all alveoli contributing to physiological deadspace are completely devoid of perfusion. Alveolar units with excess ventilation relative to perfusion will contribute to deadspace. Diseases such as chronic obstructive pulmonary disease or pulmonary fibrosis cause an increase in $\dot{V}/\dot{Q}$ mismatch due to defective alveolar gas mixing and inequalities in regional gas distribution [25–27]. Consequently there is heterogeneous $\dot{V}/\dot{Q}$ distribution within lung units and the entire lungs. Depending on the nature and severity of the pathology the levels of $\dot{V}/\dot{Q}$ mismatch can be vastly varied.

Shunt and physiological deadspace

The Bohr–Enghoff equation calculates physiological deadspace using the difference between the arterial and mixed-expired CO_2, so any factor that influences arterial P_{CO_2} will result in altered physiological deadspace. Therefore physiological deadspace is influenced by shunt. If the P_{CO_2} of the venous admixture is large enough and the lung compensatory mechanisms are overwhelmed, the resultant elevation of arterial P_{CO_2} would increase the calculated physiological (Bohr–Enghoff) deadspace [14, 28]. Consequently physiological deadspace is not only influenced by a high $\dot{V}/\dot{Q}$ but also by a low $\dot{V}/\dot{Q}$.

The influence of shunt on deadspace is non-linear. P_{aco_2} and consequently physiological deadspace is only affected in disease processes that result in large shunt. At shunt fractions (Q_s/Q_t) of 0.2 the influence of shunt on P_{aco_2} is negligible [29]. Due to the nature of the variables involved it is very difficult to directly measure the influence of shunt on physiological deadspace. Figure 6 shows the effects of shunt on P_{aco_2} and hence Bohr–Enghoff deadspace in a high-fidelity computer model [30]. Shunt fractions of greater than 0.5 shows a rapid increase in physiological deadspace [28, 31].

Although shunt plays a role in increasing physiological deadspace, alveolar deadspace has a much more profound impact on CO_2 elimination as illustrated by

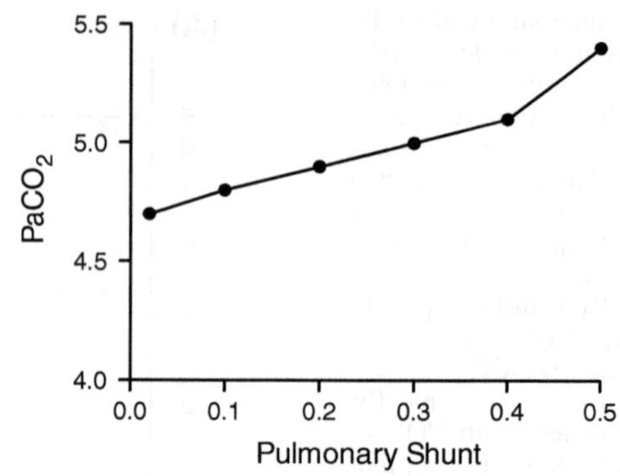

Fig. 6 Relationship of pulmonary shunt and P_{aco_2} as proposed by a computerized model by Tang and colleagues [30]

Fig. 7 [32]. Even though the contributions of shunt to alveolar deadspace are not strictly "deadspace", it none-the-less represents an abnormality in gas exchange (CO_2 elimination) and a pointer to abnormal pathology.

Pathophysiology of deadspace in ALI/ARDS

Pathological processes can alter measured physiological deadspace in many ways. For example in mechanically ventilated patients with severe ARDS, increased deadspace can result from increased alveolar deadspace as the tidal volume is distributed to poorly or non-perfused parts of the lungs. Over-distension of segments of the lung that are functioning normally either as a manifestation of using high peak end expiratory pressure (PEEP) or due to the use of high tidal volumes/ventilatory pressures would result in areas of relatively high $\dot{V}/\dot{Q}$ which would also increase the deadspace fraction. Another frequently encountered pathological features in ARDS is the presence of microemboli which can further result in $\dot{V}/\dot{Q}$ abnormalities. This is supported by the randomized control trial in which the use of activated protein C resulted in an associated improvement in physiological deadspace in patients with acute lung injury [33]. Elsewhere the ratio of angiopoietin 2 and 1, a proposed indicator of endothelial damage, has been shown to have a prognostic interaction with deadspace fraction in such patients. This suggests that endothelial damage and the resultant disruption in pulmonary microcirculation may also lead to increases in ventilation-perfusion mismatching in ALI [34]. Additionally, as the severity of illness increases the level of intra-pulmonary shunt increases, which would further contribute to the deadspace fraction. Theoretically a drop in cardiac output and a resultant drop in the pulmonary perfusion pressures could also contribute to raising the $\dot{V}/\dot{Q}$ ratio. In these situations positive pressure ventilation itself may actively redistribute ventilation according to local compliance and radically alter $\dot{V}/\dot{Q}$ ratio.

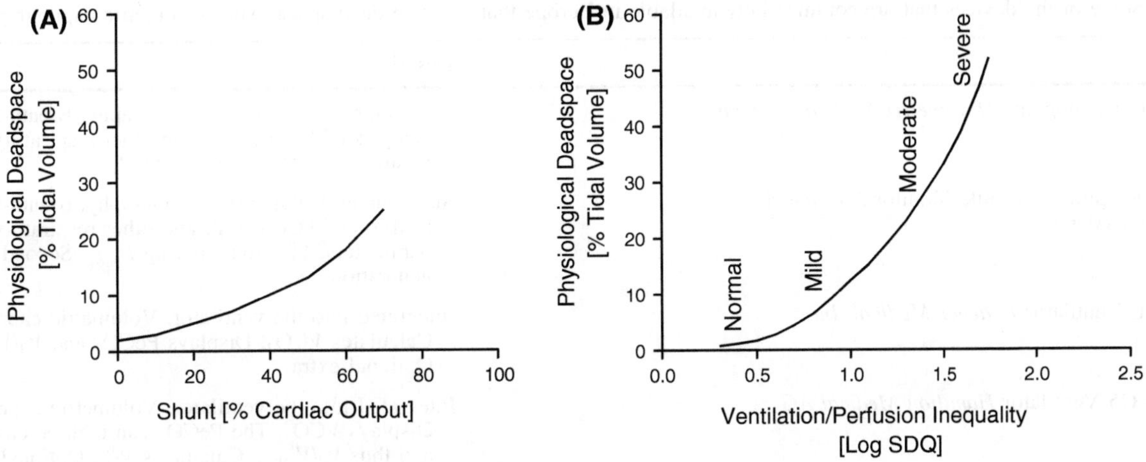

Fig. 7 Comparison of the relative effects of shunt (**a**) and $\dot{V}/\dot{Q}$ (**b**) mismatch on calculated physiological deadspace. Log SDQ, second moment (dispersion) of the ventilation/perfusion distribution on a log scale. Figure recreated with permission from Wagner [32]

The current position of deadspace measurement in critical care practice

In the critical care setting carbon dioxide clearance or ventilatory efficiency is influenced by a limited number of factors which include ventilation, perfusion and to a lesser extent CO_2 production. This contrasts with indices of oxygenation which are determined by numerous factors that are both intrinsic (pathological) and extrinsic (physics) to the body. These factors are frequently independent of ventilation. Studies on Mount Everest with impressively low oxygen indices in exercising climbers [35, 36] clearly demonstrate that the relationship of oxygenation to clinical well-being is relatively indirect. Nevertheless oxygenation continues to be used as the primary tool for the initiation and structuring of ventilatory strategies [37]. This may partly be due to the key but weak association between commonly used indices of oxygenation and survival [38]. Equally important is that it is not conventional practice to be guided by deadspace either whilst describing or monitoring the severity of pulmonary failure. It may be argued that whilst describing conditions such as such as ALI/ARDS it would be more relevant to also incorporate ventilatory efficiency for categorizing disease severity. As this is in effect unexplored, there is a reasonable reluctance amongst clinicians to use this most relevant of parameters.

Recently there has been a resurgence in interest in using deadspace measurements and in particular using SBT-CO_2 in the clinical setting. Yet given the potential usefulness of ventilatory efficiency/deadspace the reasons for its absence deserve explanation:

1. The methods to calculate deadspace as described above are either time-honoured but cumbersome (Douglas bag) or expensive and ancillary (volumetric capnography) [39]. There are only a few reliable automated commercially available methods of measuring deadspace and they are not yet fully integrated into standard monitoring systems (see Table 1).
2. As it is seldom measured there is a lack of clinical familiarity with the measurement and a therefore natural tendency to continue with a standard approach based on oxygenation.
3. Similarly there is a paucity of information regarding interventions that directly manipulate deadspace and hence an assumption that it is of limited value.
4. As it is rarely measured there are very few large studies describing its behaviour in critically unwell patients and its true value as a clinical tool has yet to be evaluated.

Indices of ventilatory efficiency

Recently there has been increasing interest in developing more simple 'user-friendly' indices to monitor changes in ventilatory efficiency at the bedside. These are summarized in Table 2. All the indices use variables measured at the bedside and broadly fall into 2 main categories. The first use complex calculations to predict numerical values for V_d/V_t. Unfortunately some of the assumed values inherent to either the method of derivation or the proposed calculations will inevitably lead to inaccuracies. The second do not offer explicit quantification of deadspace but rather look at tracking ventilatory efficiency using bedside variables. The latter whilst easier to reproduce and calculate would be subject to similar inaccuracies.

Most of these methods have yet to be adequately validated. The bedside method proposed by Saddiki et al.

Table 1 Some of the devices that are commercially available in Europe that measure dead space using volumetric capnography

Device	Description
CO_2SMO® Capnograph *Novametrix Medical Systems*	Stand alone. Volumetric capnography. Breath-by-breath analysis of VCO_2, V_D^{aw}, and other respiratory parameters. V_D^{phys} on entering P_{aco_2}
NICO®2 Respiratory Profile Monitor *Novametrix Medical Systems*	Stand alone. Volumetric capnography. Breath-by-breath analysis of VCO_2, V_D^{aw}, and other respiratory parameters. V_D^{phys} on entering P_{aco_2}. Second generation
Evita® XL Ventilator *Draeger Medical, Inc*	Integrated into the ventilator. Volumetric capnography. Calculates VCO_2. Displays $PeCO_2$ and V_d/V_{tphys}. Optional extra
Hamilton G5 Ventilator *Hamilton Medical AG*	Integrated into the ventilator. Volumetric capnography. Displays VCO_2. The $PeCO_2$ can then be calculated and thus V_d/V_{tphys}. Calculates V_D^{aw}. Optional extra

[40] uses the alveolar gas equation to estimate V_d/V_t. In order to obtain quantitative values of V_d/V_t they have used the Harris–Benedict equation to estimate values of VCO_2 for a given patient. The Harris–Benedict equation is not only complex to calculate but also has been shown to be unreliable in the critical care setting [41, 42]. This brings into question the validity of the V_d/V_t values extracted from the equation.

An alternative approach from Frankenfield et al. uses regression analysis to derive a predictive equation to estimate V_d/V_t. The equation has been validated for patients in steady state with an $FiO_2 < 0.6$. Although there is good correlation between measured and calculated values of V_d/V_t, this remains validated in a very small select group of patients. The difference between arterial and end-tidal ($PaCO_2$-$EtCO_2$) has been proposed to be used to either predict V_d^{alv}/V_t^{alv} using [43] or to track changes in V_d^{alv}/V_t^{alv} [44]. Once again neither methods have been validated in patients. Conceptually using $EtCO_2$ as a tool to monitor deadspace is likely to lead to inaccuracies due to its dependence on the ventilatory patterns and tidal volumes.

Lastly ventilatory ratio (VR) uses similar principles as those applied in respiratory medicine to stipulate a predicted standard of ventilation to obtain an ideal $PaCO_2$. Measured values are then compared to these values. Whilst this is a simple method that has been physiologically defined it remains to be validated as a clinical tool.

Clinical utility

In the critical care setting there are diverse but isolated examples of deadspace measurements being used as a clinical tool. In pulmonary embolism deadspace-tidal volume fraction in conjunction with D-Dimer assays, has been shown to be of diagnostic value [48–50]. Deadspace fraction has also been used to predict likelihood of successful extubation in paediatric patients [51]. It would seem likely that from first principles monitoring ventilatory efficiency could play a vital role in weaning and prediction of extubation. The negative impact of rising deadspace on weaning has been demonstrated in the neonatal population [52]. Although these population groups are distinct from adults, the pathophysiologcial principles that result in difficult weaning stand true in all populations. Currently the most widely used index to predict successful weaning is the frequency-tidal volume ratio and it focuses on the endurance of breathing [53]. This index is simple to calculate and shows high sensitivity but has low specificity. It does not incorporate the corresponding efficiency of CO_2 elimination. A combination of the work of breathing and ventilatory efficiency would in theory provide a more refined index to predict successful weaning. Studies have demonstrated the superiority of such combined indices in small groups of patients resulting in increased specificity as compared to f/V_T [54, 55]. Larger studies are needed to explore the advantages of using a combined index that intuitively appears to offer a more comprehensive evaluation of the pathophysiology of weaning failure.

Deadspace measurements have been used to assess the impact of varying PEEP on carbon dioxide elimination and to determine the optimum levels of PEEP during lung recruitment [56, 57]. The SBT-CO_2 has been used to study the effects of PEEP on the 2 individual components of deadspace (VD^{aw} and VD^{alv}) in patients with acute lung injury [58]. This showed that there was no uniform response to PEEP.

In animal studies it has been shown that deadspace is highly specific and sensitive in monitoring lung collapse [59]. In these studies the lungs use a surfactant-depleted model and show large changes with recruitment techniques. This contrasts with the findings in adults with acute lung injury where recruitment is far less effective

Table 2 Description of bedside indices to monitor ventilatory efficiency

Authors	Index	Derivation/Validation	Advantages	Disadvantages
Hardman and Aitkenhead [44]	$P_{a\text{-}\acute{E}}CO_2/P_aCO_2$ Arterial-end-tidal CO_2 gradient is divided by arterial PCO_2 as a measurement to track $(VD_{alv}/VT_{alv})_{Bohr\text{–}Enghoff}$ at the bedside	Nunn and Hill first described the relationship of $P_{a\text{-}\acute{E}}CO_2$ and alveolar deadspace [45]. Authors calculated $(VD_{alv}/VT_{alv})_{Bohr\text{–}Enghoff}$ and $P_{a\text{-}\acute{E}}CO_2/P_aCO_2$ whilst altering variables in a computational physiological model. Linear relationship between the 2 fractions is demonstrated	Easy to calculate at the bedside Negates the influence of airway deadspace Stable under various conditions	Untested in clinical/animal setting No evident physiological derivation No clinical data available Not quantitative
Sinha et al. [46]	$VR = \frac{\dot{V}_{E_{measured}} \times P_{aCO_{2measured}}}{\dot{V}_{E_{predicted}} \times P_{aCO_{2predicted}}}$ Ventilatory Ratio (VR) Predicted V_E = 100 ml kg^{-1}.min of ideal body weight. Predicted $PaCO_2$ is 5 kPa	Compares measured values against predicted values derived from population normograms Physiological analysis shows VR is influenced by physiological deadspace and CO_2 production.	Easy to calculate at the bedside Physiological analysis shows the ratio is intuitive	Not clinically validated Reflects changes in 2 variables
Frankfield et al. [47]	$V_d/V_t = 0.32 + 0.0106\ (PaCO_2 - ETCO_2) + 0.003\ (RR) + 0.0015\ (age)$	Regression analysis used to derive a predictive equation for V_d/V_t. Measurements of ventilatory and clinical variables were made in 135 patients. Respiratory rate, $PaCO_2$–$ETCO_2$, and age were factors that significantly influenced V_d/V_t. Measured V_d/V_t was validated against estimated V_d/V_t for that population.	Quantitative value for V_d/V_t Calculated using values at the bedside	Derived from measured values Not intuitive Not tested in varying clinical conditions Not tested in patient with $FiO_2 > 0.6$
Siddiki et al. [40]	$V_d/V_t = 1 - [(0.86 \times VCO_2^{est})/(V_E \times PaCO_2)]$ VCO_2est is the estimated CO_2 Production calculated from the Harris Benedict equation and *0.863* is a correction constant	Uses the alveolar gas equation Uses the Harris–Benedict equation to estimate VCO_2	Quantitative value for V_d/V_t Can be calculated at the bedside Equation in physiologically intuitive	Not validated against measured V_d/V_t Harris–Benedict equation is unreliable Equation unreliable in unsteady state Complicated to calculate

and excessive PEEP may exert a negative influence on $\dot{V}/\dot{Q}$ matching secondary to overdistension [60]. Nevertheless lung recruitment manoeuvres have been evaluated using deadspace fraction or ventilatory efficiency [61–63]. It appears to be a more useful means of assessing the efficacy of recruitment than using indices of oxygenation [64].

Deadspace and acute lung injury

Perhaps of greatest interest and relevance in the critical care setting is the utility of deadspace measurements in the context of ALI, ARDS, and modes of ventilation. In patients with ARDS a range of pathophysiological mechanisms increase ventilatory inefficiency. Hence as one might anticipate deadspace measurements have been shown to be a useful prognostic marker for patients with ARDS. This has been clearly demonstrated in several studies where non-survivors have been shown to have a significantly higher deadspace ratio than survivors [40, 65–67]. Similarly using a measurement of ventilatory efficiency, V_{AE}/V_t, has been shown to be a useful predictor of outcome in patients with lung injury [22]. The timing and the magnitude of the deadspace abnormality has also been shown to predict the clinical outcome in patients with lung injury. While prognostic indicators have their place, measurements that allow both monitoring and manipulation of ventilatory management have more immediate clinical usefulness. Kallet and colleagues demonstrated that serial measurements of deadspace could be used to monitor disease progression in ARDS [68, 69]. Others have demonstrated its use in monitoring manoeuvres such as prone positioning that are designed to improve gas exchange [70, 71]. Patients with ALI/ARDS that demonstrate a decrease in arterial P_{CO_2} i.e. increased ventilatory efficiency on prone-positioning have shown improved survival compared to those patients that show no improvement in arterial P_{CO_2} [72]. Clearly measurement of ventilatory efficiency has a potential role in the management of ventilation.

There is more recently, linkage between prognosis and potential pathophysiological mechanisms underlying deadspace changes. Ong and colleagues have demonstrated a prognostic association between dead space fraction and the ratio of angiopoietin 2 and 1 which are proposed markers of endothelial damage. The interaction between deadspace and pulmonary capillary perfusion is clearly important and this may prove an exciting and fruitful new direction for clinical study [34].

In the rapidly evolving field of ventilatory management where modalities such as extracorporeal membrane CO_2 removal and high frequency oscillatory ventilation are becoming increasing prevalent, a fresh look at our methods of monitoring gas exchange in ventilated patients is essential. CO_2 clearance is a crucial part of these strategies and needs to be monitored. Routine monitoring of ventilatory efficiency could lead to more appropriate diagnostic categorization of respiratory failure in terms of CO_2 clearance rather than just oxygenation. This may in turn be helpful in earlier instigation of these novel therapies. Additionally monitoring efficiency of CO_2 clearance during treatment could aide in the management of the finer aspects of extracorporeal membrane CO_2 removal such as assessing device efficacy and deciding the timeliness of return to more conventional ventilation.

The two common themes in these reports across a spectrum of clinical activity are that potential usefulness of measuring ventilatory efficiency has been demonstrated but to date investigation and application of these measurements are very limited. That should in itself be enough to stimulate interest across other areas of clinical practice.

Conclusion

Recently there has been a growing trend in the literature pointing to the use of deadspace measurement as a monitoring tool in mechanically ventilated patients. Whilst the introduction of more sophisticated and advanced measurement devices and software have increased our understanding of deadspace ventilation, it has not increased its use in intensive care medicine. Clearly if there were more affordable, simpler and integrated methods to track ventilatory efficiency our use of this measurement would increase and thereby enhance our understanding of it as a clinical tool. Early and repeated measurements in lung disease could provide clinicians with valuable information for prognostication and disease monitoring. Although several relatively easy to use bedside tools to monitor deadspace have been described in the literature they need to be validated in real-time against established methods of deadspace measurement but interest in these techniques is growing.

With the advent of extracorporeal gas exchange management of respiratory failure is rapidly changing and carbon dioxide clearance will return to the fore. Early detection of deadspace abnormalities may be useful for monitoring and optimizing ventilatory modes. This may lead to managing ventilation through assessment of ventilatory efficiency and potentially developing methods of influencing and manipulating deadspace. More importantly it may lead to new avenues in our understanding of the pathophysiology and progression of respiratory failure. Even if a fraction of these ideas come to fruition it would justify a resurgence in clinical interest in ventilatory efficiency. It is the authors' contention that in the next decade critical care will rediscover the importance of carbon dioxide clearance.

References

1. Andersen EW, Ibsen B (1954) The anaesthetic management of patients with poliomyelitis and respiratory paralysis. Br Med J 1:786–788
2. Ibsen B (1954) The anaesthetist's viewpoint on the treatment of respiratory complications in poliomyelitis during the epidemic in Copenhagen, 1952. Proc R Soc Med 47:72–74
3. Bohr C (1891) Ueber die Lungenathmung. Skand Arch Physiol 2:236–238
4. Haldane JS, Priestley JG (1905) The regulation of the lung-ventilation. J Physiol 32:225–266
5. Douglas CG, Haldane JS (1912) The capacity of the air passages under varying physiological conditions. J Physiol 45:235–238
6. Drummond GB, Fletcher R (2006) Deadspace: invasive or not? Br J Anaesth 96:4–7
7. Englhoff H (1938) Volumen inefecax. Bemerkungen zur Frage des schaedlichen Raumes. Uppsala Lä k Fö r Fö rh 44:191–218
8. Fowler WS (1948) Lung function studies; the respiratory dead space. Am J Physiol 154:405–416
9. Bartels J, Severinghaus JW, Forster RE, Briscoe WA, Bates DV (1954) The respiratory dead space measured by single breath analysis of oxygen, carbon dioxide, nitrogen or helium. J Clin Invest 33:41–48
10. Langley FE, Duroux P, Nicolas RL, Cumming G (1975) Ventilatory consequences of unilateral pulmonary artery occlusion. Les Colloques de l'Institut National de la Santeet de la Recherche Medicale 51:209–212
11. Fletcher R (1984) Airway deadspace, end-tidal CO2, and Christian Bohr. Acta Anaesthesiol Scand 28:408–411
12. Blanch L, Romero PV, Lucangelo U (2006) Volumetric capnography in the mechanically ventilated patient. Minerva Anestesiol 72:577–585
13. Fletcher R, Jonson B (1984) Deadspace and the single breath test for carbon dioxide during anaesthesia and artificial ventilation. Effects of tidal volume and frequency of respiration. Br J Anaesth 56:109–119
14. Fletcher R, Jonson B, Cumming G, Brew J (1981) The concept of deadspace with special reference to the single breath test for carbon dioxide. Br J Anaesth 53:77–88
15. Riou Y, Leclerc F, Neve V, Dupuy L, Noizet O, Leteurtre S, Sadik A (2004) Reproducibility of the respiratory dead space measurements in mechanically ventilated children using the CO2SMO monitor. Intensive Care Med 30:1461–1467
16. Arnold JH, Thompson JE, Arnold LW (1996) Single breath CO2 analysis: description and validation of a method. Crit Care Med 24:96–102
17. Forbat AF, Her C (1980) Correction for gas compression in mechanical ventilators. Anesth Analg 59:488–493
18. Crossman PF, Bushnell LS, Hedley-Whyte J (1970) Dead space during artificial ventilation: gas compression and mechanical dead space. J Appl Physiol 28:94–97
19. Wenzel U, Wauer RR, Schmalisch G (1999) Comparison of different methods for dead space measurements in ventilated newborns using CO2-volume plot. Intensive Care Med 25:705–713
20. Romero PV, Lucangelo U, Lopez Aguilar J, Fernandez R, Blanch L (1997) Physiologically based indices of volumetric capnography in patients receiving mechanical ventilation. Eur Respir J 10:1309–1315
21. Blanch L, Lucangelo U, Lopez-Aguilar J, Fernandez R, Romero PV (1999) Volumetric capnography in patients with acute lung injury: effects of positive end-expiratory pressure. Eur Respir J 13:1048–1054
22. Lucangelo U, Bernabe F, Vatua S, Degrassi G, Villagra A, Fernandez R, Romero PV, Saura P, Borelli M, Blanch L (2008) Prognostic value of different dead space indices in mechanically ventilated patients with acute lung injury and ARDS. Chest 133:62–71
23. Riley RL, Cournand A (1949) Ideal alveolar air and the analysis of ventilation-perfusion relationships in the lungs. J Appl Physiol 1:825–847
24. Riley RL, Cournand A, Donald KW (1951) Analysis of factors affecting partial pressures of oxygen and carbon dioxide in gas and blood of lungs; methods. J Appl Physiol 4:102–120
25. Wagner PD, Naumann PF, Laravuso RB (1974) Simultaneous measurement of eight foreign gases in blood by gas chromatography. J Appl Physiol 36:600–605
26. Wagner PD, Dantzker DR, Dueck R, Clausen JL, West JB (1977) Ventilation-perfusion inequality in chronic obstructive pulmonary disease. J Clin Invest 59:203–216
27. Yamaguchi K, Mori M, Kawai A, Takasugi T, Oyamada Y, Koda E (1997) Inhomogeneities of ventilation and the diffusing capacity to perfusion in various chronic lung diseases. Am J Respir Crit Care Med 156:86–93
28. Niklason L, Eckerstrom J, Jonson B (2008) The influence of venous admixture on alveolar dead space and carbon dioxide exchange in acute respiratory distress syndrome: computer modelling. Crit Care 12:R53
29. Kuwabara S, Duncalf D (1969) Effect of anatomic shunt on physiologic deadspace-to-tidal volume ratio—a new equation. Anesthesiology 31:575–577
30. Tang Y, Turner MJ, Baker AB (2005) Effects of alveolar dead-space, shunt and *V*/*Q* distribution on respiratory dead-space measurements. Br J Anaesth 95:538–548
31. Mecikalski MB, Cutillo AG, Renzetti AD Jr (1984) Effect of right-to-left shunting on alveolar dead space. Bull Eur Physiopathol Respir 20:513–519
32. Wagner PD (2008) Causes of a high physiological dead space in critically ill patients. Crit Care 12:148
33. Liu KD, Levitt J, Zhuo H, Kallet RH, Brady S, Steingrub J, Tidswell M, Siegel MD, Soto G, Peterson MW, Chesnutt MS, Phillips C, Weinacker A, Thompson BT, Eisner MD, Matthay MA (2008) Randomized clinical trial of activated protein C for the treatment of acute lung injury. Am J Respir Crit Care Med 178:618–623
34. Ong T, McClintock DE, Kallet RH, Ware LB, Matthay MA, Liu KD (2010) Ratio of angiopoietin-2 to angiopoietin-1 as a predictor of mortality in acute lung injury patients. Crit Care Med 38:1845–1851
35. West JB, Hackett PH, Maret KH, Milledge JS, Peters RM Jr, Pizzo CJ, Winslow RM (1983) Pulmonary gas exchange on the summit of Mount Everest. J Appl Physiol 55:678–687
36. Grocott MP, Martin DS, Levett DZ, McMorrow R, Windsor J, Montgomery HE (2009) Arterial blood gases and oxygen content in climbers on Mount Everest. N Engl J Med 360:140–149
37. Gowda MS, Klocke RA (1997) Variability of indices of hypoxemia in adult respiratory distress syndrome. Crit Care Med 25:41–45
38. Ware LB (2005) Prognostic determinants of acute respiratory distress syndrome in adults: impact on clinical trial design. Crit Care Med 33:S217–S222

39. Badal JJ, Chen KJ, Loeb RG (2011) Measurement of Dead Space in Subjects Under General Anesthesia Using Standard Anesthesia Equipment. Anesth Analg 112(2):375–377
40. Siddiki H, Kojicic M, Li G, Yilmaz M, Thompson TB, Hubmayr RD, Gajic O (2010) Bedside quantification of dead-space fraction using routine clinical data in patients with acute lung injury: secondary analysis of two prospective trials. Crit Care 14:R141
41. Flancbaum L, Choban PS, Sambucco S, Verducci J, Burge JC (1999) Comparison of indirect calorimetry, the Fick method, and prediction equations in estimating the energy requirements of critically ill patients. Am J Clin Nutr 69:461–466
42. Frankenfield D, Hise M, Malone A, Russell M, Gradwell E, Compher C (2007) Prediction of resting metabolic rate in critically ill adult patients: results of a systematic review of the evidence. J Am Diet Assoc 107:1552–1561
43. Hardman JG, Aitkenhead AR (1999) Estimation of alveolar deadspace fraction using arterial and end-tidal CO2: a factor analysis using a physiological simulation. Anaesth Intensive Care 27:452–458
44. Hardman JG, Aitkenhead AR (2003) Estimating alveolar dead space from the arterial to end-tidal CO(2) gradient: a modeling analysis. Anesth Analg 97:1846–1851
45. Nunn JF, Hill DW (1960) Respiratory dead space and arterial to end-tidal carbon dioxide tension difference in anesthetized man. J Appl Physiol 15:383–389
46. Sinha P, Fauvel NJ, Singh S, Soni N (2009) Ventilatory ratio: a simple bedside measure of ventilation. Br J Anaesth 102:692–697
47. Frankenfield DC, Alam S, Bekteshi E, Vender RL (2010) Predicting dead space ventilation in critically ill patients using clinically available data. Crit Care Med 38:288–291
48. Kline JA, Israel EG, Michelson EA, O'Neil BJ, Plewa MC, Portelli DC (2001) Diagnostic accuracy of a bedside D-dimer assay and alveolar dead-space measurement for rapid exclusion of pulmonary embolism: a multicenter study. JAMA 285:761–768
49. Kline JA, Kubin AK, Patel MM, Easton EJ, Seupal RA (2000) Alveolar dead space as a predictor of severity of pulmonary embolism. Acad Emerg Med 7:611–617
50. Verschuren F, Liistro G, Coffeng R, Thys F, Roeseler J, Zech F, Reynaert M (2004) Volumetric capnography as a screening test for pulmonary embolism in the emergency department. Chest 125:841–850
51. Hubble CL, Gentile MA, Tripp DS, Craig DM, Meliones JN, Cheifetz IM (2000) Deadspace to tidal volume ratio predicts successful extubation in infants and children. Crit Care Med 28:2034–2040
52. Estay A, Claure N, D'Ugard C, Organero R, Bancalari E (2010) Effects of instrumental dead space reduction during weaning from synchronized ventilation in preterm infants. J Perinatol 30:479–483
53. Yang KL, Tobin MJ (1991) A prospective study of indexes predicting the outcome of trials of weaning from mechanical ventilation. N Engl J Med 324:1445–1450
54. Jabour ER, Rabil DM, Truwit JD, Rochester DF (1991) Evaluation of a new weaning index based on ventilatory endurance and the efficiency of gas exchange. Am Rev Respir Dis 144:531–537
55. Gluck EH (1996) Predicting eventual success or failure to wean in patients receiving long-term mechanical ventilation. Chest 110:1018–1024
56. Maisch S, Reissmann H, Fuellekrug B, Weismann D, Rutkowski T, Tusman G, Bohm SH (2008) Compliance and dead space fraction indicate an optimal level of positive end-expiratory pressure after recruitment in anesthetized patients. Anesth Analg 106:175–181 table of contents
57. Suter PM, Fairley B, Isenberg MD (1975) Optimum end-expiratory airway pressure in patients with acute pulmonary failure. N Engl J Med 292:284–289
58. Beydon L, Uttman L, Rawal R, Jonson B (2002) Effects of positive end-expiratory pressure on dead space and its partitions in acute lung injury. Intensive Care Med 28:1239–1245
59. Tusman G, Suarez-Sipmann F, Bohm SH, Pech T, Reissmann H, Meschino G, Scandurra A, Hedenstierna G (2006) Monitoring dead space during recruitment and PEEP titration in an experimental model. Intensive Care Med 32:1863–1871
60. Lucangelo U, Blanch L (2004) Dead space. Intensive Care Med 30:576–579
61. Tusman G, Bohm SH, Sipmann FS, Maisch S (2004) Lung recruitment improves the efficiency of ventilation and gas exchange during one-lung ventilation anesthesia. Anesth Analg 98:1604–1609 table of contents
62. Tusman G, Bohm SH, Suarez-Sipmann F, Turchetto E (2004) Alveolar recruitment improves ventilatory efficiency of the lungs during anesthesia. Can J Anaesth 51:723–727
63. Gattinoni L, Caironi P, Cressoni M, Chiumello D, Ranieri VM, Quintel M, Russo S, Patroniti N, Cornejo R, Bugedo G (2006) Lung recruitment in patients with the acute respiratory distress syndrome. N Engl J Med 354:1775–1786
64. Calzia E, Radermacher P, Bein T (2006) Unveiling alveolar recruitment: the fascinating trail between theory and practice. Intensive Care Med 32:1686–1688
65. Nuckton TJ, Alonso JA, Kallet RH, Daniel BM, Pittet JF, Eisner MD, Matthay MA (2002) Pulmonary dead-space fraction as a risk factor for death in the acute respiratory distress syndrome. N Engl J Med 346:1281–1286
66. Shimada Y, Yoshiya I, Tanaka K, Sone S, Sakurai M (1979) Evaluation of the progress and prognosis of adult respiratory distress syndrome. Simple respiratory physiologic measurement. Chest 76:180–186
67. Raurich JM, Vilar M, Colomar A, Ibanez J, Ayestaran I, Perez-Barcena J, Llompart-Pou JA (2010) Prognostic value of the pulmonary dead-space fraction during the early and intermediate phases of acute respiratory distress syndrome. Respir Care 55:282–287
68. Valta P, Uusaro A, Nunes S, Ruokonen E, Takala J (1999) Acute respiratory distress syndrome: frequency, clinical course, and costs of care. Crit Care Med 27:2367–2374
69. Kallet RH, Alonso JA, Pittet JF, Matthay MA (2004) Prognostic value of the pulmonary dead-space fraction during the first 6 days of acute respiratory distress syndrome. Respir Care 49:1008–1014
70. Johannigman JA, Davis K Jr, Miller SL, Campbell RS, Luchette FA, Frame SB, Branson RD (2000) Prone positioning for acute respiratory distress syndrome in the surgical intensive care unit: who, when, and how long? Surgery 128:708–716
71. Davis K Jr, Johannigman JA, Campbell RS, Marraccini A, Luchette FA, Frame SB, Branson RD (2001) The acute effects of body position strategies and respiratory therapy in paralyzed patients with acute lung injury. Crit Care 5:81–87
72. Gattinoni L, Vagginelli F, Carlesso E, Taccone P, Conte V, Chiumello D, Valenza F, Caironi P, Pesenti A (2003) Decrease in PaCO2 with prone position is predictive of improved outcome in acute respiratory distress syndrome. Crit Care Med 31:2727–2733

Editorials 2

The role of the right ventricle in determining cardiac output in the critically ill

M. R. Pinsky
University of Pittsburgh, Pennsylvania, USA

Assessment and management of cardiovascular homeostasis represent a cornerstone in the teaching and practice of critical care medicine. Indeed, most invasive hemodynamic monitoring is done in an attempt to understand cardiovascular status and its response to specific therapies. Bedside insertion of a flow-directed balloon-tipped pulmonary arterial chatheter to measure pulmonary artery occlusion pressure (Ppao) (as an estimate of left ventricular filling pressure) and cardiac output (by the thermodilution technique) in the hemodynamically unstable patient is now routine [1]. Using these data and derived parameters of left ventricular (LV) function [2] has allowed the clinician to diagnose common causes of cardiovascular instability, such as acute myocardial infarction, tamponade, and other causes of LV failure versus hypovolemia [3]. From the time of its introduction onward, the flow-directed balloon-tipped pulmonary artery catheter has been within the domain of the intensivist.

Since a reasonable goal in the management of the hemodynamically unstable patient is the preservation of blood flow to the tissues, determinations of whether the observed hemodynamic instability is due primarily to cardiac or peripheral vascular causes has refocused attention on the broader issues of assessment of global oxygen transport (DO_2) and peripheral vascular resistance as well [4]. This new focus has identified an important peripheral vascular component to the clinical picture of septic shock and underscored the importance of examining the entire cardiovascular system when assessing cardiovascular status and of using these parameters as therapeutic end points rather than as simple monitors of mean arterial pressure and Ppao [5].

Thus, the stage was set recently for the "*rediscovery of the right ventricle*" as a potential cause of cardiovascular dysfunction in the critically ill [6]. It has long been appreciated that acute and chronic right ventricular (RV) dysfunction occurs in the setting of increased pulmonary vascular resistance as may occur during acute pulmonary embolism [7], end-stage acute lung injury with vascular obliteration [8], and chronic obstructive lung disease [9]. All these diseases share an associated increase in pulmonary vascular resistance, a condition known to be poorly tolerated by the right ventricle. However, recently it has been suggested that RV dysfunction may occur in conditions other than those associated with pulmonary hypertension. In such conditions RV contractility is presumed to be primarily reduced. Examples of this include selective RV infarction [10], a "relative" decrease in systemic arterial pressure in the face of pulmonary hypertension [11], and possibly sepsis-related impairment in myocardial contractility [12].

In this regard, the study by Redl et al. [13] in this volume is most interesting. These authors examined the hemodynamic data of 27 patients in the early stages of hypotensive septic shock prior to resuscitation using invasive hemodynamic monitoring, which allowed them to estimate RV volumes using a rapid response thermistor-type pulmonary arterial catheter (RVef-1, Baxter-Edwards, Santa Ana, CA). They saw that those patients who could be adequately resuscitated using volume resuscitation alone (as defined by restoration of a mean arterial pressure >60 mmHg and an increase in DO_2) had a pre-resuscitation RV ejection fraction (EFrv) of >45%. By contrast, those in whom resuscitative efforts required the addition of an inotrope or vasoactive support to the fluid resuscitation therapy had a pre-resuscitation EFrv of <45%. Furthermore, these workers could not find a significant relation between pooled Ppao and DO_2 data in the patients with an EFrv <45%. They conclude that RV function may be an important isolated determinant of clinical response to fluid resuscitation in septic patients.

Aside from important issues as to whether or not the rapid response thermistor-pulmonary arterial catheter system can accurately measure Efrv [14] and how one can define RV function [15], this study raises several questions which need to be addressed before its results can be applied clinically and before the logic expressed above can be accepted. First, it is not clear if the septic patients described by Redl et al. [13] also had concomitant reductions in LV function as well. As Parker et al. have demonstrated [16] LV function is impaired early in sepsis. Thus, these data may just demonstrate that RV function, like

M.R. Pinsky et al. (eds.), *Applied Physiology in Intensive Care Medicine 2: Physiological Reviews and Editorials*,
DOI 10.1007/978-3-642-28233-1_30, © Springer-Verlag Berlin Heidelberg 2012

LV function, is impaired in sepsis. The correlation between RV and LV function has been clearly demonstrated in post-cardiopulmonary bypass patients [17]. Second, although pooled data may show population characteristics, they do not model the clinical scenario nor the physiologic assessment usually done in critically ill patients. Most clinicians measure caridovascular function serially to ascertain if changes in measures of cardiac function (such as LV stroke work) increase as estimates of preload (such as Ppao) are varied by therapy. The study by Redl et al. [13] does not allow us that comparison. Thus, it is not clear if septic individuals would behave uniformly as defined solely by pretreatment EFrv. Third, the determinants of RV function are poorly understood [18], but include RV coronary perfusion pressure, end-diastolic wall stress, pulmonary artery input impedance, RV wall inotropy. None of these factors was assessed in the present study. Thus, the differences seen between patient subgroups described above may reflect factors not analyzed but which are both known to be relevant to RV function and can be manipulated clinically.

The right ventricle may fail in an isolated fashion, but this probably occurs rarely if processes such as RV infarction, RV valvulopathy, acute pulmonary hypertension, and selective RV hypoperfusion (ischemia) are excluded. However, if global myocardial dysfunction is present and increased cardiac output increases pulmonary arterial pressure more than systemic arterial pressure, a condition often met in septic patients owing to loss of peripheral vasomotor tone and increased pulmonary vascular resistance [19], then the stage is set for selective RV dysfunction (cor pulmonale), which on its own could limit DO_2 and further impair LV function in the critically ill. Accordingly, sepsis-related cardiovascular dysfunction may reflect a unique constellation of cardiovascular derangements which will manifest selective RV dysfunction in the resuscitated patient. Sitting, as it were, at the gate between systemic venous return and LV filling, the right ventricle could and does limit cardiac output under a variety of conditions [20].

Thus, this study and others like it which attempt to define the limits of resuscitability imposed by the right ventricle in sepsis are important, if validated by prospective clinical trials, because they suggest different options of therapy. The rationale for such studies would be: *Since both excessive fluid resuscitation alone and the use of vasoactive drug therapy in the face of inadequate fluid resuscitation are potentially detrimental to organ-system function, it would be useful to define a cardiovascular parameter that could reliably predict when further fluid resuscitation is no longer expected to improve organ perfusion pressure, owing to limitations of cardiac output responsiveness, so that inotropic and vasoactive support can be instituted in a timely fashion.* Serial measures of RV function in the critically ill may provide such a parameter in selected patients. The question remains unanswered, however, if such knowledge will direct specific therapies which will ultimately alter the clinical course of septic shock.

References

1. Swan HCJ, Ganz W, Forrester JS et al (1970) Catheterization of the heart in man with use of a flow-directed balloon-tipped catheter. N Engl J Med 283:447–451
2. Elzinga G, Westerhof N (1973) How to quantify pump function of the heart. The value of variables derived from measurement on isolated muscle. Circ Res 32:178–186
3. Forrester JS, Diamond G, McHugh et al (1971) Filling pressure in the right and left sides of the heart in acute myocardial infarction: a reappraisal of central venous pressure monitoring. N Engl J Med 285:190–192
4. Reinhart K, Hannermann L, Kuss B (1990) Optimal oxygen delivery in the critically ill patient. Intensive Care Med 16:149–155
5. Shoemaker WC, Apple M, Kram HB et al (1988) Prospective trial of supranormal values of survivors as therapeutic goals in high-risk surgical patients. Chest 94:1176–1186
6. Pinsky MR (1989) The rediscovery of the right ventricle. Reanim Soins Intensifs Méd Urgence 5:89–90
7. MacIntyre KN, Sasahara AA (1974) Determinations of the right ventricular function and hemodynamics after pulmonary embolism. Chest 65:534–543
8. Calvin JE, Quinn B (1989) Right ventricular pressure overload during acute lung injury: cardiac mechanics and the pathophysiology of right systolic dysfunction. J Crit Care 4:251–265
9. Bergofsky EH (1983) Tissue oxygenation and cor pulmonale in chronic obstructive pulmonary disease. N Engl J Med 308: 1092–1094
10. Cohn JN, Gwha NH, Broder ML et al (1974) Right ventricular infarction. Clinical and hemodynamic features. Am J Cardiol 33:209–214
11. Fixler DE, Archie JP, Ullyot DJ (1973) Effects of acute right ventricular hypertension on regional myocardial blood flow in anesthetized dogs. Am Heart J 85:491–499
12. Parker MP, Shelhammer JH, Bararach SL et al (1984) Profound but reversible myocardial depression in patients with septic shock. Ann Intern Med 100:483–490
13. Redl G, Germann P, Plattner H et al (1993) Right ventricular function in early septic shock states. Intensive Care Med 19:3–7
14. Dhainaut JF, Brunet F, Monsallier JF et al (1987) Bedside evaluation of right ventricular performance using a rapid computerized thermodilution method. Crit Care Med 15:148–152
15. Pinsky MR (1989) Asssessment of right ventricular function in the critically ill: fact, fancy, perspective. In: Vincent JL (ed) Update in intensive care and emergency medicine, vol 8. Springer, Berlin Heidelberg New York, pp 518–523
16. Parker MP, McCarthy, Ognibene FP et al (1990) Right ventricular dysfunction and dilation, similar to left ventricular changes, characterize the cardiac depression seen in septic shock. Chest 97:126–131
17. Brisblatt WM, Stein KL, Wolfe CJ et al (1990) Acute myocardial dysfunction and recovery: a common occurrence after coronary bypass surgery. J Am Coll Cardiol 15:1261–1269
18. Wiedermann HP, Matthay MA (1985) Acute right heart failure. Crit Care Clin 1:631–661
19. Sibbald WJ, Paterson NA, Holliday RL et al (1978) Pulmonary hypertension in sepsis. Measurement by the pulmonary artery diastolic-wedge pressure gradient and the influence of passive and active factors. Chest 73:583–591
20. Guyton AC, Lindsey AW, Abernathy B et al (1957) Venous return at various right atrial pressures and the normal venous return curve. Am J Physiol 189:609–615

M. R. Pinsky, MD
604 Scaife Hall
3550 Terrace Street
Pittsburgh, PA 15261
USA

Beyond global oxygen supply-demand relations: in search of measures of dysoxia

M. R. Pinsky

Division of Critical Care Medicine, Department of Anesthesiology and Critical Care Medicine, University of Pittsburgh, Pittsburgh, Pennsylvania, USA

Central to the management of the hemodynamically unstable patient are resuscitative therapies for circulatory shock and the hemodynamic monitoring used to guide such therapies. In this context, shock can be considered to reflect inadequate O_2 utilization by the tissues, due to either inadequate O_2 delivery or inadequate O_2 uptake. Inadequate O_2 delivery usually reflects either hypoperfusion or arterial desaturation, whereas impaired O_2 utilization by the tissues reflects an abnormal O_2 metabolism or dysoxia [1]. In the last 10 years increased attention has been directed at the assessment of O_2 consumption and delivery in the critically ill patient using data derived from pulmonary arterial and systemic arterial catheterization. Initial clinical studies suggested that as O_2 delivery was varied, O_2 uptake co-varied in a similar fashion [2–4]. Since this phenomenon in critically ill patients was contrary to previously proposed mechanisms in the normal relation between O_2 delivery and uptake, it was referred to as "pathological O_2 supply dependency" [5]. Much confusion and controversy has arisen in the published reports of further attempts to assess O_2 metabolism in critically ill. In two papers in this volume, Hanique and coworkers address primary issues in this controversy [6, 7]. Although not the first to examine these concepts, these investigators did an excellent job of evaluating many of the relevant issues and reached conclusions now held by an enlarging majority of this field. One hopes that their results and conclusions will lay to rest some of these issues, so that future clinical studies on O_2 metabolism will go beyond the analysis of global O_2 supply-demand relations. Nevertheless, it is instructive to consider the process by which our thinking has arrived at this juncture.

Some previous studies of critically ill patients being resuscitated from shock have demonstrated a co-variance of O_2 uptake and delivery. Covariance has usually been defined from two or more data pairs per subject collected over time, demonstrating that O_2 uptake increases as O_2 delivery increases [3, 4, 8, 9]. The determinants of this perceived covariance were an additional source of controversy and have given rise to three principles that should be addressed in any study of O_2 delivery and consumption [10]. First, because measures of O_2 delivery and consumption derived from common data of cardiac output and arterial and venous O_2 contents share two of their three variables, the resultant shared errors lead naturally to the coupling of these variables. Second, because, under most conditions, the "independent variable" is O_2 consumption, not delivery, and varying O_2 demand induces proportional changes in O_2 delivery, it is reasonable to assume that O_2 uptake and delivery should covary in patients with varying metabolic demand. To avoid these problems O_2 uptake and delivery should be measured by independent means, and the testing environment should ensure that changes in O_2 uptake due to changes in metabolic rate are kept minimal. The important methodological problem can be resolved by minimizing muscular and sympathetic activity by sedating, paralyzing, and ventilating the subject [11, 12]. Furthermore, by actively varying O_2 delivery rather than observing the relation between oxygen delivery and consumption as both are allowed to vary will further minimize the potential documentation of normal covariance of the two as metabolic rate varies [13]. Third, to ascertain the degree to which O_2 delivery and consumption co-vary, multiple data pairs should be collected for each subject over a wide range of O_2 delivery values.

No evidence of covariance between O_2 delivery and consumption has been demonstrated when all three of the criteria listed above have been met [14–16]. Thus, it seems unlikely that co-variance of O_2 delivery and consumption occurs as a function of deranged O_2 metabolism in most critically ill patients. How, then, did the issue of supply-dependence of O_2 consumption first arise? It appears that clinicians applied sound physiological principles at the bedside, but with the wrong set of assumptions.

Correspondence to: M. R. Pinsky, MD, 604 Scaife Hall, 3550 Terrace Street, Pittsburgh, PA 15261, USA

M.R. Pinsky et al. (eds.), *Applied Physiology in Intensive Care Medicine 2: Physiological Reviews and Editorials*,
DOI 10.1007/978-3-642-28233-1_31, © Springer-Verlag Berlin Heidelberg 2012

Using the model of acute hemorrhagic shock and principles derived from exercise physiology, it can be argued that tissue hypoperfusion reduces tissue O_2 delivery below levels at which extraction can maintain adequate cellular O_2 flux to support oxidative phosphorylation at a level sufficient to maintain function. Short-term adaptations include almost complete reliance on inefficient anaerobic metabolism to produce high-energy phosphate. This cellular strategy is limited in its ability to maintain energy production, because of residual acidosis induced by unopposed hydrolysis of ATP and lactic acid accumulation, coupled with the relatively low rates at which new ATP can be regenerated [17]. The end results are organ dysfunction, decreased metabolism, and lactic acidosis. Some degree of "oxygen debt" occurs because of the excessive but limited production of lactic acid, which in the absence of molecular oxygen is a metabolic end product. If O_2 delivery to the tissues can be reinstituted before irreversible tissue death, then O_2 uptake will increase transiently to supranormal levels as the "oxygen debt" is repaid, organ system function will improve, and lactic acidosis will resolve [18]. Oxygen consumption will then decrease again toward baseline preshock levels after a finite and relatively short interval as the "oxygen debt" is paid off. This process will be manifest as a transient O_2 delivery-dependent O_2 uptake [18]. It may signal pre-existent oxygen debt and may suggest that therapies preventing a decrease in O_2 to pre-resuscitation levels would aid survival [19]. Continuing this logic, if a little increase in O_2 is good, then a lot may be better, because one can never know if pockets of ischemic tissue exist at the borders of perfused regions in the critically ill. This logic forms the basis for the use of hyper-resuscitated values for oxygen delivery in critically ill patients to prevent tissue dysoxia and organ system dysfunction [20]. Although a reasonable first approximation, since pockets of ischemic tissue may exist despite otherwise normal values for global blood flow in critically ill patients, a recently published prospective study addressing this issue failed to demonstrate a survival benefit from hyper-resuscitation [21].

Several investigators have studied the effects of varying O_2 delivery and examining its effect on O_2 uptake using the three principles stated above. The results of these studies demonstrate that under most conditions and with most organs O_2 uptake remains relatively constant as O_2 delivery falls, because O_2 extraction increases until some threshold value, below which extraction mechanisms can not compensate for the reduction in O_2 delivery, and O_2 uptake becomes coupled to delivery, leading to tissue hypoxia [1, 5, 23, 24]. The level of O_2 delivery at which O_2 consumption becomes limited has been referred to as the critical O_2 delivery (DO_2crit). DO_2crit is not the same for all organs or for the whole body as sepsis or endotoxemia develops [1, 5, 22–24]. Thus, in the hemodynamically unstable patient, some areas of the body may become ischemic at higher levels of global O_2 delivery than do others. The gut mucosa appears to be one such tissue bed at risk for early ischemia [25]. However, even in well-controlled animal studies assessing O_2 supply/uptake relations, O_2 uptake data derived at levels of O_2 deliveries below the DO_2crit reflected very unstable preparations, or those with limited capacity to be resuscitated quickly back to the baseline states. Thus, it is not clear what clinically relevant information can be derived from O_2 data taken below DO_2crit in these preparations.

Furthermore, since metabolically active organs, such as the heart, brain, kidney, gut, and liver cannot survive long when perfused below their DO_2crit, the issue of whether sustained O_2 supply-dependency is present in critically ill patients seems mute. Though an O_2 debt must occur before a metabolic shut-down develops in shock, it cannot be excessive, because of the lack of substrate and associated cellular toxicity of the metabolic end product. Is there, then, no place in our monitoring of critically ill patients for an assessment of O_2 uptake and delivery? Perhaps not if used in a global and blinded fashion. However, when analysis of O_2 supply-uptake relations is used in conjunction with analyses of individual organ-system function or as threshold values to prevent further hypoperfusion and organ ischemia, it seems warranted. The constraint, however, rests in our limited ability to identify and follow specific markers that reflect organ-specific tissue wellness and that will improve as dysoxia subsides. For the heart and brain, these limits are less of a problem, because in the absence of vascular disease powerful protective autonomic mechanisms maintain cardiac and cerebral perfusion pressure. Below this perfusion pressure threshold the patient rapidly dies. However, visceral organs including the liver, gut, and kidney have little autonomic protection and may become severely dysfunctional or fail because of hyperfusion despite apparently adequate levels of arterial pressure [5, 23, 26]. This problem is of great clinical importance because patient survival after acute renal, hepatic, or gut failure induced by hypoperfusion is poor despite the most heroic therapies. Thus, if we are to use information on global O_2 supply-uptake effectively to prevent tissue dysoxia, organ failure, and death, we must define organ-specific markers of function for the gut, liver, and kidney that vary with dysoxia.

At present, only one clinical study using gastric intraluminal pH to identify gut ischemia and to define adequacy of resuscitative efforts has been published [27]. The results appear very promising, and have been initially duplicated in a smaller study [28]. We await, however, the results of further, better defined, and larger clinical studies before we can accept this measure of gut perfusion as a clinically valid guide to resuscitation.

We have come a long way from initial thinking that adequate global O_2 delivery was synonymous with adequate organ blood flow, through the era of comparison of O_2 delivery with uptake relations, to our present state. We now aim at specific organs to assess whether tissue dysoxia is present, to judge whether our therapies can reverse it, and to decide what measures of tissue function can be used to assess our resuscitative efforts. When these markers of tissue function are validated and become available clinically, we finally will be able to address whether any form of resuscitation in critically ill patients actually improves organ system function, and ultimately improves survival.

References

1. Schlichtig R, Kramer D, Pinsky MR (1991) Flow redistribution during progressive hemorrhage is a determinant of critical O_2 delivery. J Appl Physiol 70:169–178
2. Danek SJ, Lynch JP, Weg JG, Dantzker DR (1980) The dependence of oxygen uptake on oxygen delivery in the adult respiratory distress syndrome. Am Rev Respir Dis 122:387–395
3. Haupt MT, Gilbert EM, Carlson RW (1985) Fluid loading increases oxygen consumption in septic patients with lactic acidosis. Am Rev Respir Dis 131:912–916
4. Kaufman BS, Rackow EC, Falk JL (1984) The relationship between oxygen delivery and consumption during fluid resuscitation of hypovolemic and septic shock. Chest 85:336–340
5. Nelson DP, Beyer C, Samsel RW, Wood LDH, Schumacker PT (1987) Pathological supply dependence of O_2 uptake during bacteremia in dogs. J Appl Physiol 63:1487–1492
6. Hanique G, Dugernier T, Laterre PF et al (1994) Evaluation of oxygen uptake and delivery in critically ill patients: A statistical reappraisal. Intensive Care Med 20:19–26
7. Hanique G, Dugernier T, Laterre PF et al (1994) Significance of pathologic oxygen supply dependency in the critically ill: Comparison between measured and calculated methods. Intensive Care Med 20:12–18
8. Astiz ME, Rackow EC, Kaufman B, Falk JL, Weil MH (1988) Relationship of oxygen delivery and mixed venous oxygenation to lactic acidosis in patients with sepsis and acute myocardial infarction. Crit Care Med 16:655–658
9. Gilbert EM, Haupt MT, Mandanas RY, Huaringa AJ, Carlson RW (1986) The effect of fluid loading, blood transfusion, and catecholamine infusion on oxygen delivery and consumption in patients with sepsis. Am Rev Respir Dis 134:873–878
10. Bartlett RH, Dechert RE (1990) Oxygen kinetics: pitfalls in clinical research [editorial]. J Crit Care 5:77–80
11. Chiolero R, Flatt J-P, Revelly J-P, Jequier E (1991) Effects of catecholamines on oxygen consumption and oxygen delivery in critically ill patients. Chest 100:1676–1684
12. Ruokonen E, Takala J, Uusaro A (1991) Effect of vasoactive treatment on the relationship between mixed venous and regional oxygen saturation. Crit Care Med 19:1365–1369
13. Palazzo MG, Suter PM (1991) Delivery dependent oxygen consumption in patients with septic shock: daily variations, relationships with outcome and the sick-euthyroid syndrome. Intensive Care Med 17:325–332
14. Annat G, Viale J-P, Percival C, Froment M, Motin J (1986) Oxygen delivery and uptake in the adult respiratory distress syndrome. Am Rev Respir Dis 133:999–1001
15. Ronco JJ, Phang PT, Walley KR, Wiggs B, Fenwick JC, Russell JA (1991) Oxygen consumption is independent of changes in oxygen delivery in severe adult respiratory distress syndrome. Am Rev Respir Dis 143:1267–1273
16. Vermeij CG, Feenstra BWA, Adrichem WJ, Bruning HA (1991) Independent oxygen uptake and oxygen delivery in septic and postoperative patients. Chest 99:1438–1443
17. Hotchkiss RS, Karl IE (1992) Reevaluation of the role of cellular hypoxia and bioenergetic failure in sepsis. JAMA 267:1503–1510
18. Fahey JT, Lister G (1987) Oxygen transport in low cardiac output states. J Crit Care 2:288–305
19. Shoemaker WC, Appel PL, Kram HR (1988) Tissue oxygen debt as a determinant of lethal and non-lethal postoperative organ failure. Crit Care Med 16:1117–1120
20. Shoemaker WC, Appel PL, Kram HR, Waxman K, Lee T-S (1988) Prospective trial of supranormal values of survivors as therapeutic goals in high-risk surgical patients. Chest 94:1176–1186
21. Tuchschmidt J, Fired J, Astiz M, Rackow E (1992) Elevation of cardiac output and oxygen delivery improves outcome in septic shock. Chest 102:216–220
22. Pinsky MR, Matuschak GM (1986) Cardiovascular determinants of the hemodynamic response to acute endotoxemia in the dog. J Crit Care 1:18–31
23. Rasmussen I, Arvidsson D, Zak A, Haglund U (1992) Splanchnic and total body oxygen consumption in experimental fecal peritonitis in pigs: effects of dextran and Iloprost. Circ Shock 36:299–306
24. Schlichtig R, Klions HA, Kramer DJ, Nemoto EM (1992) Hepatic dysoxia commences during O_2 supply dependence. J Appl Physiol 72:1499–1505
25. Fink MP, Kaups KL, Wang H, Rotschild HR (1991) Maintenance of superior mesenteric arterial perfusion prevents increased intestinal mucosal permeability in endotoxic pigs. Surgery 110:154–161
26. Kobayashi S, Clemens MG (1992) Kupffer cell exacerbation of hepatocyte hypoxia/reoxygenation injury. Circ Shock 37:245–252
27. Gutierrez G, Palizas F, Doglio G, Wainsztein N, Gallesio A, Pacin J, Dubin A, Schaivi E, Jorge M, Pusajo J (1992) Gastric intramucosal pH as a therapeutic index of tissue oxygenation in critically ill patients. Lancet 339:195–199
28. Gutierrez G, Bismar H, Dantzker DR, Silva N (1992) Comparison of gastric intramucosal pH with measures of oxygen transport and consumption in critically ill patients. Crit Care Med 20:451–457

Michael R. Pinsky

Breathing as exercise:

The cardiovascular response to weaning from mechanical ventilation

It is axiomatic that exercise increases oxygen (O_2) demand if within the bounds of cardiovascular reserve, results in a proportional increase in whole body oxygen consumption (VO_2). Exercise physiologists have long known that it does not really matter what form of exercise is performed, VO_2 will increase in response to all forms of exercise, although the degree to which the increased VO_2 demand is met by increasing cardiac output and O_2 extraction varies with conditioning and underlying disease [1]. Interestingly, the type of exercise also influences the efficiency of the performance, defined as the ratio of external work performed to VO_2.[2]. The reasons for this discrepancy probably reflect motor efficiency and vascular conditioning as much as cardiac reserve. Thus, some subjects with prior training in a specific event will increase their cardiac outputs more during that stress than less conditioned subjects. These other less conditioned subjects may not increase cardiac output as much and will support the increased O_2 demand by increasing O_2 extraction across the capillary beds.

Using this paradigm, DeBacker and colleagues demonstrated that all ventilator-dependent patients following cardiovascular surgery who were challenged by weaning to spontaneous ventilation and in whom weaning was successful demonstrated markedly different cardiac output and O_2 extraction responses, depending on their underlying pathology [3]. Those subjects with primarily peripheral vascular disease (vascular surgery patients) responded to this challenge with an increase in cardiac output, whereas those subjects with progressively lesser levels of cardiac responsiveness increased their O_2 extract more. Importantly, it did not matter why cardiac output responsiveness was limited, the overall response was predictable. Thus, subjects with normal autonomic tone and cardiovascular responsiveness (status – post coronary artery surgery) increased their cardiac output more than subjects with denervated hearts (cardiac transplant recipients) whose chronotropic response is usually blunted. These data are interesting to the practicing clinician for several reasons.

First, they underscore the obvious fact that spontaneous breathing is exercise. This statement alone needs to be heard. Numerous studies before this present one have documented that the transition from mechanical ventilation to spontaneous ventilation induces increased cardiac stress that can induce myocardial ischemia in subjects with coronary artery disease [4, 5, 6, 7]. Similarly, the act of spontaneous inspiratory efforts can precipitate left ventricular (LV) dilation [8] and cardiogenic shock [9] in subjects without coronary artery disease. Importantly, clinically relevant cardiovascular improvements during weaning often occur in these patients only if inotropic agents are given [10] or aggressive diuresis reverses cor pulmonale [9]. Thus, clinicians need to appreciate that spontaneous ventilation can place an excessive cardiovascular burden on the heart, induce myocardial ischemia and promote cardiogenic shock. Simple clinical observation and a review of the large clinical literature on this subject adequately document this point.

Second, how cardiovascular stress is manifest in a given patient during weaning is as much a function of their cardiovascular reserves and conditioning as it is the level of metabolic load imposed by the weaning tri-

M.R. Pinsky et al. (eds.), *Applied Physiology in Intensive Care Medicine 2: Physiological Reviews and Editorials*,
DOI 10.1007/978-3-642-28233-1_32, © Springer-Verlag Berlin Heidelberg 2012

al. Jabran et al. [11] demonstrated recently that although all patients with chronic obstructive lung disease increased their cardiac outputs during weaning trials, those who failed to wean also increased their arterio-venous O_2 saturation difference, demonstrating that patients who fail to wean do so as part of cardiovascular decompensation. Thus, occult cardiovascular insufficiency occurs during weaning failure in critically ill patients and may be the primary cause of weaning failures in many patients.

Given that these statements are true and relevant to clinical practice, where should we go from here? For starters, it is incumbent on the bedside clinician to be able to identify the etiology of cardiovascular failure. Dynamic hyperinflation-induced cor pulmonale or tamponade can cause weaning failure [12]. Acute LV failure associated with LV enlargement and pulmonary edema also occurs during weaning trials [13]. Though both these scenarios will present with an increasing arterio-venous O_2 gradient, the management of each is quite different. Hyperinflation is usually treated with maneuvers tending to prolong expiratory time and match extrinsic positive end-expiratory pressure (PEEP) to the dynamic hyperinflation-induced intrinsic PEEP [14]. Whereas, acute LV failure is best treated with inotropic agents and therapies aimed at minimizing the negative swings in intrathoracic pressure during spontaneous inspiration [15]. Thus, accurate diagnosis and management of cardiovascular insufficiency during weaning trials requires careful attention to both the underlying pulmonary dysfunction and the overall cardiovascular response, not just the change in VO_2.

Furthermore, since cardiovascular insufficiency is commonplace in subjects who fail to wean from mechanical ventilation, reliable bedside monitoring tools and tests need to be developed to aid the clinician in titrating cardiovascular therapies during weaning trials. One recent technique described by Mechard et al. [16] uses arterial pulse pressure variation during positive-pressure breath as a cardiovascular forcing function to identify preload-responsive states. Since arterial pulse pressure variation approximates LV stroke volume variation from beat to beat, these authors reasoned that increasing arterial pulse pressure variation would reflect positive-pressure ventilation-induced phasic decreases in venous return. Thus, the greater the pulse pressure variation, the more preload-dependent would be the subject. They demonstrated that arterial pulse pressure variation predicted the subsequent decrease in cardiac output as PEEP was increased by 10 cmH_2O. Similarly, the decreases in pulmonary artery diastolic pressure, and presumably arterial diastolic pressure, can be used to monitor the spontaneous ventilation-induced decreases in intrathoracic pressure [17]. This measure would allow the bedside clinician to estimate the work-cost of breathing, an important determinant of the increased VO_2 during weaning.

Thus, although some bedside tools are presently available to monitor cardiac vascular status, the list of such tools is short and the validity of each technique in different situations is unknown. This is an area where new investigation is necessary and where real progress can be expected, primarily because of the excellent basic physiological foundations present for their interpretation. Finally, the exact mechanisms by which LV failure can occur, as manifest by an increasing arterio-venous O_2 difference, remains to be defined. Non-invasive bedside tests that can accurately identify and differentiate different pathophysiological processes need to be developed. This is an important issue because process-specific therapies are often very effective at improving cardiovascular support, whereas non-specific therapies are often of marginal benefit and can be harmful.

At the end of the day we are left with the satisfaction of knowing that cardiovascular dysfunction may be the missing piece in predicting weaning success, and that cardiovascular monitoring can be useful in the diagnosis and management of ventilator-dependent patients, especially when weaning trials are being considered. The fact that increasing arterio-venous O_2 content monitoring identifies patients at risk to fail wean trials can aid clinicians in identifying the etiology of the cardiovascular dysfunction and, hopefully, improve outcome in this high-cost, high-mortality patient population.

References

1. Adams WC, McHenry MN, Bernauer EN (1974) Long-term physiologic adaptations to exercise with special reference to performance and cardiorespiratory function in health and disease. Am J Cardiol 33: 765–775
2. Chester EH, Belman MJ, Bahler RC, Baum GL, Schey G, Buch P (1977) Multidisciplinary treatment of chronic pulmonary insufficiency 3. The effect of physical training on cardiopulmonary performance in patients with chronic obstructive pulmonary disease. Chest 72: 695–702
3. DeBacker D, El Haddad P, Preiser J-C, Vincent J-L (2000) Haemodynamic responses to successful weaning from mechanical ventilation after cardiovascular surgery. Intensive Care Med (this issue)
4. Richard C, Teboul J-L, Archambaud F, Hebert J-L, Michaut P, Auzepy P (1994) Left ventricular function during weaning of patients with chronic obstructive pulmonary disease. Intensive Care Med 20: 181–186

5. Hurford WE, Lynch KE, Strauss HW (1991) Myocardial perfusion as assessed by Thallium-201 scintigraphy during discontinuation of mechanical ventilation in ventilated patients. Anesthesiology 74: 1007–1016
6. Chatila W, Ani S, Guaglianone D, Jacob B, Amoateng-Adjepong Y, Manthous CA (1995) Cardiac ischemia during weaning from MV. Chest 109: 1421–1422
7. Hurford WE, Favorito F (1995) Association of myocardial ischemia with failure to wean. Crit Care Med 23: 1475–1480
8. Buda AJ, Pinsky MR, Ingles NB, Daughters GT, Alderman EL (1979) Effect of intrathoracic pressure on left ventricular performance. N Engl J Med 301: 453–459
9. Lemaire F, JL Teboul, L Cinoti, G Giotto, F Abrouk, G Steg, I Macquin-Mavier, WM Zapol (1988) Acute left ventricular dysfunction during unsuccessful weaning from mechanical ventilation. Anesthesiology 69: 171–179
10. Beach T, Millen E, Grenvik (1973) Hemodynamic response to discontinuance of mechanical ventilation. Crit Care Med 1: 85–90
11. Jubran A. Mathru M. Dries D. Tobin MJ (1998) Continuous recordings of mixed venous oxygen saturation during weaning from mechanical ventilation and the ramifications thereof. Am J Respir Crit Care Med 158: 1763–1769
12. Pinsky MR (1994) Though the past darkly: ventilatory management of patients with chronic obstructive pulmonary disease. Crit Care Med 22: 1714–1717
13. Rasanen J, Nikki P, Heikkila J (1984) Acute myocardial infarction complicated by respiratory failure. The effects of mechanical ventilation. Chest 85: 21–28
14. Ranieri VM, Giuliani R, Cinnella G, et al. (1993) Physiologic effects of positive end-expiratory pressure in patients with chronic obstructive lung disease during acute ventilatory failure and controlled mechanical ventilation. Am Rev Respir Dis 147: 5–13
15. Rasanen J, Vaisanen IT, Heikkila J, et al. (1985) Acute myocardial infarction complicated by left ventricular dysfunction and respiratory failure. The effects of continuous positive airway pressure. Chest 87: 158–162
16. Michard F, Chemla D, Richard C, Wysocki M, Pinsky MR, Lecarpentier Y, Teboul JL (1999) Clinical use of respiratory changes in arterial pulse pressure to monitor the hemodynamic effects of PEEP. Am J Respir Crit Care Med 159 (3): 935–939
17. Teboul J-L, Besbes M, Andrivet P, Axler O, Douguet D, Zelter M, Lemaire F, Brun-Bussian C (1992) A bedside index assessing the reliability of pulmonary artery occlusion pressure measurements during mechanical ventilation with positive end-expiratory pressure. J Crit Care 7: 22–29

S. M. Jakob
J. Takala

Variability of splanchnic blood flow measurements in patients with sepsis – physiology, pathophysiology or measurement errors?

Splanchnic blood flow and sepsis

Impaired tissue oxygenation, especially in the splanchnic region, may play a central role both in the pathogenesis of multiple organ dysfunction and in the development of complications in various groups of intensive care patients [1, 2]. In severe inflammation such as SIRS, septic infection, and septic shock, the metabolic demand for oxygen in the splanchnic region is increased [3, 4, 5]. This is explained in part by an increased hepatic metabolism [6, 7]. In patients with normal or hyperdynamic hemodynamics, hepato-splanchnic blood flow is higher than normal, but the increase in oxygen consumption is disproportionate to the increase in blood flow. Hence, splanchnic oxygen extraction has to be increased. It is therefore evident that splanchnic tissue perfusion is at risk, should any deterioration of systemic oxygen transport occur. This is clinically relevant especially in septic shock, where early myocardial depression is common [8, 9]. During experimental cardiac tamponade, endotoxin infusion appears to impair the hepatic microcirculatory blood flow: while mesenteric and liver blood flow increased similarly, the liver capillary blood flow increased less than the intestinal mucosal blood flow [10]. In addition, the critical oxygen delivery required to maintain oxygen uptake constant is higher in the liver as compared to the intestine.

Assessment of splanchnic blood flow

The aim of monitoring hepato-splanchnic perfusion is to detect, prevent, and reverse tissue hypoperfusion. This may help to improve the outcome of these patients. The available methods to evaluate splanchnic perfusion include among others dye-extraction methods, ultrasound and laser Doppler flowmetry, tonometry, and spectrophotometry. Both the appropriate use of each method and the correct interpretation of the measurements are of fundamental importance.

In critically ill patients estimation of splanchnic blood flow is usually based on hepatic uptake of substances, which are metabolized by the liver and distributed in the plasma [11, 12, 13]. Indocyanine green dye has become the most often used substance. However, estimated hepatic blood flow calculated from systemic indocyanine green clearance correlates poorly with blood flow obtained using hepatic vein catheterization and the Fick principle [12]. In case of normal liver function, pharmacokinetic modeling improves the accuracy substantially. Because vasoactive drugs change acutely the hepatic extraction of indocyanine green, the use of methods without hepatic venous catheterization is not valid.

M.R. Pinsky et al. (eds.), *Applied Physiology in Intensive Care Medicine 2: Physiological Reviews and Editorials*,
DOI 10.1007/978-3-642-28233-1_33, © Springer-Verlag Berlin Heidelberg 2012

Variability of physiological signals in critically ill patients

When effects of drugs or other interactions on the splanchnic perfusion are assessed, it is important to measure the respective blood flows under steady state conditions. In addition, when constant dye infusion methods are used, stable blood concentrations during the measurements are mandatory. Most investigators measure the blood dye concentrations three times per measurement period in intervals of 5 min to prove stable conditions. In the August issue of this journal, Dr. Sakka and coworkers assessed the variability of splanchnic blood flow in eight sedated, mechanically ventilated patients during a stable 4-h period [14]. By using the continuous indocyanine green method they found a standard error of 31 % for repeated measurements with 5-min distances and of 26 % for average values with 2-h distances. In contrast, coefficients of variation for triplicate cardiac output measurements using the thermodilution method were low (between 3 % and 4 %). The high variability of the splanchnic blood flow measurements could neither be explained by unstable indocyanine green concentrations (coefficients of variation between 4 % and 6 %), nor by inaccuracies in hematocrit (coefficient of variation 2 %). The pumps for the infusion of the indocyanine green solution were calibrated. The authors conclude that splanchnic blood flow may exhibit significant variability in patients with sepsis, even when systemic haemodynamic parameters are stable. They suggest that this spontaneous variability could explain the non-uniform behavior of changes in splanchnic blood flow in response to therapeutic interventions such as vasoactive drugs: for instance, treatment of hyperdynamic septic shock with norepinephrine and dopamine had little effect on systemic oxygen transport but was associated with major changes in splanchnic blood flow and oxygen transport [15]. Regional changes were unpredictable from systemic changes. In patients with pancreatitis, dobutamine had inconsistent effects on splanchnic blood flow: in individual patients, splanchnic blood flow even decreased [16]. In patients with septic shock, low-dose dopamine increased splanchnic perfusion in patients with low fractional splanchnic blood flow but not in patients with high fractional splanchnic blood flow [17]. Therefore, if the variability of splanchnic blood flow is high, small effects of drugs may not become apparent, and effects attributed to the infusion of drugs may have occurred just by chance.

The physiologic variability of hemodynamic and respiratory variables is well known in healthy subjects [18, 19]. Heart rate and blood pressure variability are signs of an intact autonomic nervous system. In patients with cardiovascular disease a strong association has been found between impaired heart rate variability and both all-cause and cardiovascular mortality rates [20, 21, 22]. Age and heart rate are the major determinants of the selected heart rate variability measures [23, 24]. Heritable factors have also been proposed [25]. In diabetic patients, heart rate variability is reduced and inversely associated with plasma glucose levels [26]. In septic patients, cardiac variability and sympathovagal balance are impaired [27].

Splanchnic blood flow demonstrates circadian variation [28]. By using magnetic resonance velocity mapping, Lycklama a Nijeholt and co-workers found an intra-individual variability for portal vein flow measurements of approximately 7 % [29]. The variability did not increase after a meal and was independent of the technique used (Echo-Doppler measurements vs magnetic resonance velocity mapping). Some of the variability in regional (and potentially systemic) blood flow measurements can be explained by movement of the diaphragm during the respiratory cycle: in a recent study venous return from the legs was monitored using an ultrasonic flow recorder placed over the femoral veins in ten subjects [30]. Quiet inspiration was associated with a fall in femoral venous blood flow of 65 % of the end-expiratory value. Between-subjects variability could be largely explained by differences in abdominal pressure swings. The amount of fall in femoral blood flow during inspiration varied in proportion to the diaphragmatic contribution to tidal volume. Isovolume belly-in maneuvers and external compression of the abdomen also caused cessation of femoral blood flow. In line with the findings of Dr. Sakka and co-workers, there is some evidence from animals studies that splanchnic hemodynamic parameters could exhibit a more pronounced variability as compared to systemic hemodynamics [31]: in conscious rats a major oscillation at around 160 mHz was present in the mesenteric, but not in hindquarter circulation. Cross-spectral analysis performed between mean arterial pressure and mesenteric blood flow indicated that fractional changes in flow were twice as much as those in mean arterial pressure. We have measured the variability of gastric mucosal $PrCO_2$ in 40 patients and systemic hemodynamic parameters in 100 patients with acute respiratory or circulatory failure during the first 24 h after admission to the intensive care unit [32]. We found at the most a slightly higher coefficient of variation for gastric mucosal $PrCO_2$ (15 %) as compared to heart rate (6 %), mean arterial pressure (9 %), and thermodilution cardiac output (10 %). Using the same technique as Dr. Sakka and colleagues, Uusaro reported a coefficient of variation of 7 % for splanchnic blood flow in 136 critically ill patients. In the subgroup of patients with septic shock the coefficient of variation was 9 %. This is well below the variability of splanchnic blood flow reported in the study by Dr. Sakka and co-workers. In septic patients and in healthy volunteers challenged with endotoxin, heart rate variability is decreased rather than increased [27, 33]. What could explain these differences? Different patient populations and undetected methodological errors may play a role. The authors explain that the high standard error of 31 % for repeated measurements with 5-min distances in their septic patients was due to a few (less than 10 %) outliers. One may wonder whether there were also outliers in their measurements of the systemic hemodynamic parameters of the patients. Unfortunately, the authors do not indicate intra-patient variability measures for any of these variables, except cardiac output. The statement that the global haemodynamic parameters were more stable than the splanchnic blood flow is therefore not convincingly demonstrated. Nevertheless, their study reminds us that spontaneous changes in hemodynamic parameters including splanchnic blood flow do occur and have to be taken into account when effects of therapeutic interventions are assessed. Inclusion of an appropriate control group and the graphical display of individual data always enhance the possibility to distinguish between spontaneous variability and true intervention-induced changes.

References

1. Kirton OC, Windsor J, Wedderburn R, Hudson-Civetta J, Shatz DV, Mataragas NR, Civetta JM (1998) Failure of splanchnic resuscitation in the acutely injured trauma patient correlates with multiple organ system failure and length of stay in the ICU. Chest 113: 1064–1069
2. Swank GM, Deitch EA (1996) Role of the gut in multiple organ failure: bacterial translocation and permeability changes. World J Surg 20: 411–417
3. Dahn MS, Lange P, Lobdell K, Hans B, Jacobs LA, Mitchell RA (1987) Splanchnic and total body oxygen consumption differences in septic and injured patients. Surgery 101: 69–80
4. Dahn MS, Lange MP, Wilson RF, Jacobs LA, Mitchell RA (1990) Hepatic blood flow and splanchnic oxygen consumption measurements in clinical sepsis. Surgery 107: 295–301
5. Ruokonen E, Takala J, Kari A, Saxen H, Mertsola J, Hansen EJ (1993) Regional blood flow and oxygen transport in septic shock. Crit Care Med 21: 1296–1303
6. Dahn MS, Mitchell RA, Lange MP, Smith S, Jacobs LA (1995) Hepatic metabolic response to injury and sepsis. Surgery 117: 520–530
7. Reinelt H, Radermacher P, Fischer G, Geisser W, Wachter U, Wiedeck H, Georgieff M, Vogt J (1997) Effects of a dobutamine-induced increase in splanchnic blood flow on hepatic metabolic activity in patients with septic shock. Anesthesiology 86: 818–824
8. Parker MM, Shelhamer JH, Bacharach SL, Green MV, Natanson C, Frederick TM, Damske BA, Parrillo JE (1984) Profound but reversible myocardial depression in patients with septic shock. Ann Intern Med 100: 483–490
9. Giroir BP, Stromberg D (2000) Myocardial depression versus myocardial destruction: integrating the multiple mechanisms of myocardial dysfunction during sepsis. Crit Care Med 28: 3111–3112
10. Zhang H, Smail N, Cabral A, Cherkaoui S, Peny MO, Vincent JL (1999) Hepato-splanchnic blood flow and oxygen extraction capabilities during experimental tamponade: effects of endotoxin. J Surg Res 81: 129–138
11. Bradley SE, Ingelfinger FJ, Bradley GP, Curry JJ (1945) The estimation of hepatic blood flow in man. J Clin Invest 24: 890–897
12. Leevy CV, Mendehall CL, Lesko W, Howard MK (1962) Estimation of hepatic blood flow with indocyanine green. J Clin Invest 41: 1169–1179
13. Uusaro A, Ruokonen E, Takala J (1995) Estimation of splanchnic blood flow by the Fick principle in man and problems in the use of indocyanine green. Cardiovasc Research 30: 106–112
14. Sakka SG, Reinhart K, Wegscheider K, Meier-Hellmann A (2001) Variability of splanchnic blood flow in patients with sepsis. Intensive Care Med 8: 1281–1287
15. Ruokonen E, Takala J, Kari A, Saxen H, Mertsola J, Hansen EJ (1993) Regional blood flow and oxygen transport in septic shock. Crit Care Med 21: 1296–1303
16. Ruokonen E, Uusaro A, Alhava E, Takala J (1997) The effect of dobutamine infusion on splanchnic blood flow and oxygen transport in patients with acute pancreatitis. Intensive Care Med 23: 732–737
17. Meier-Hellmann A, Bredle DL, Specht M, Spies C, Hannemann L, Reinhart K (1997) The effects of low-dose dopamine on splanchnic blood flow and oxygen uptake in patients with septic shock. Intensive Care Med 23: 31–37
18. Nobrega AC, dos Reis AF, Moraes RS, Bastos BG, Ferlin EL, Ribeiro JP (2001) Enhancement of heart rate variability by cholinergic stimulation with pyridostigmine in healthy subjects. Clin Auton Res 11: 11–17
19. Jauregui-Renaud K, Hermosillo AG, Marquez MF, Ramos-Aguilar F, Hernandez-Goribar M, Cardenas M (2001) Repeatability of heart rate variability during simple cardiovascular reflex tests on healthy subjects. Arch Med Res 32: 21–26
20. Gillman MW, Kannel WB, Belanger A, D'Agostino RB (1993) Influence of heart rate on mortality among persons with hypertension: the Framingham Heart Study. Am Heart J 125: 1148–1154
21. Kannel WB, Kannel C, Paffenbarger RSJ, Cupples LA (1987) Heart rate and cardiovascular mortality: the Framingham Study. Am Heart J 113: 1489–1494
22. Dyer AR, Persky V, Stamler J, Paul O, Shekelle RB, Berkson DM, Lepper M, Schoenberger JA, Lindberg HA (1980) Heart rate as a prognostic factor for coronary heart disease and mortality: findings in three Chicago epidemiologic studies. Am J Epidemiol 112: 736–749
23. Tsuji H, Venditti FJ Jr, Manders ES, Evans JC, Larson MG, Feldman CL, Levy D (1996) Determinants of heart rate variability. J Am Coll Cardiol 28: 1539–1546
24. Kuch B, Hense HW, Sinnreich R, Kark JD, von Eckardstein A, Sapoznikov D, Bolte HD (2001) Determinants of short-period heart rate variability in the general population. Cardiology 95: 131–138
25. Singh JP, Larson MG, O'Donnell CJ, Tsuji H, Evans JC, Levy D (1999) Heritability of heart rate variability (The Framingham Heart Study). Circulation 99: 2251–2254

26. Singh JP, Larson MG, O'Donnell CJ, Wilson PF, Tsuji H, Lloyd-Jones DM, Levy D (2000) Association of hyperglycemia with reduced heart rate variability (The Framingham Heart Study). Am J Cardiol 86: 309–312
27. Korach M, Sharshar T, Jarrin I, Fouillot JP, Raphael JC, Gajdos P, Annane D (2001) Cardiac variability in critically ill adults: influence of sepsis. Crit Care Med 29: 1380–1385
28. Lemmer B, Nold G (1991) Circadian changes in estimated hepatic blood flow in healthy subjects. Br J Clin Pharmacol 32: 627–629
29. Lycklama a Nijeholt GJ, Burggraaf K, Wasser MN, Schultze Kool LJ, Schoemaker RC, Cohen AF, de Roos A (1997) Variability of splanchnic blood flow measurements using MR velocity mapping under fasting and post-prandial conditions-comparison with echo-Doppler. J Hepatol 26: 298–304
30. Willeput R, Rondeux C, De Troyer A (1984) Breathing affects venous return from legs in humans. J Appl Physiol 57: 971–976
31. Letienne R, Julien C, Zhang ZQ, Barres C (1998) Characterization of a major slow oscillation in the mesenteric circulation of conscious rats. Clin Exp Pharmacol Physiol 25: 820–824
32. Jakob SM, Parviainen I, Ruokonen E, Takala J (2000) Variability of continually measured gastric-mucosal PCO_2 in critically ill patients and effect of ranitidine. Intensive Care Med 26:S429
33. Godin PJ, Fleisher LA, Eidsath A, Vandivier RW, Preas HL, Banks SM, Buchman TG, Suffredini AF (1996) Experimental human endotoxemia increases cardiac regularity: results from a prospective, randomized, crossover trial. Crit Care Med 1996 24: 1117–1124

Michael R. Pinsky

Functional hemodynamic monitoring

The management of the critically ill patient often requires continual monitoring of cardiovascular status. Numerous invasive and noninvasive technologies have been used to monitor cardiovascular status. Presently, highly invasive hemodynamic monitoring appears to be needed to define and treat the specific causes of cardiovascular instability. However, these complex monitoring systems often require pulmonary arterial catheterization and have not been shown to provide critically ill patients with a survival advantage [1]. In fact, the utility of hemodynamic monitoring itself has never been documented to improve survival. In part, this lack of benefit from hemodynamic monitoring may reflect the use of poorly validated systems of hemodynamic profile analysis and unproven treatments.

In the assessment and management of critically ill patients, the actual hemodynamic monitoring questions are physiological in their language but need to be practical and concrete in their application. Perhaps the most pertinent function hemodynamic question is: Will cardiac output increase with volume loading? Documenting that an unstable patient is preload-responsive defines the initial treatment as fluid resuscitation. Since a majority of the patients presenting with cardiovascular insufficiency are preload-responsive and often show dramatic improvement in their cardiac output and organ perfusion with fluid resuscitation alone, this is an important initial therapeutic question. However, in those unstable patients who are not preload-responsive, fluid resuscitation may induce acute heart failure or pulmonary edema, if cor pulmonale or acute left ventricular (LV) failure, respectively, are the causes of cardiovascular insufficiency. Thus, being able to identify preload responsiveness quickly, accurately, and with a minimum of invasive risk prior to actually performing a fluid challenge is highly desirable.

Data from numerous clinical trials have documented repeatedly that neither right atrial pressure (P_{ra}) or pulmonary artery occlusion pressure (P_{pao}) predict well the subsequent response of the subject to an intravascular fluid challenge [2]. Furthermore, measures of absolute LV volumes are only slightly better at predicting preload responsiveness. Clearly, subjects with small LV end-diastolic volumes can have a limited response to a volume challenge if their filling is limited either by tamponade, cor pulmonale, or diastolic stiffening. Furthermore, ventilation and ventilatory therapies, such as the use of positive end-expiratory pressure often complicates this analysis by dissociating filling pressures from measured intrathoracic vascular pressure because of both increasing intrathoracic pressure and cardiac compression by lung expansion [3]. However, ventilation, by phasically altering P_{ra} also serves as a sine wave forcing function on venous return and can be used to define cardiovascular performance. Several groups have applied this concept to assess preload responsiveness. The importance of these applications to bedside monitoring is finally being understood.

Since P_{ra} is the backpressure to venous return, if P_{ra} should decrease during spontaneous inspiration, venous return will transiently increase, increasing cardiac output. If, however, the right ventricle is unable to dilate further, P_{ra} will not decrease during inspiration even though intrathoracic pressure decreases. At the extreme, spontaneous inspiration-associated increases in P_{ra} reflect severe right ventricular failure and are referred to as Kussmaul's sign. Madger et al. [4] used the fall in P_{ra} to predict which patients would increase their cardiac outputs in response to a defined fluid challenge. They found

M.R. Pinsky et al. (eds.), *Applied Physiology in Intensive Care Medicine 2: Physiological Reviews and Editorials*,
DOI 10.1007/978-3-642-28233-1_34, © Springer-Verlag Berlin Heidelberg 2012

that if P_{ra} decreased by more than 2 mmHg during a spontaneous breath, cardiac output increased in 16 or 19 patients in response to 250–500 ml saline bolus infusion. If P_{ra} did not decrease, cardiac output increased in only one of 14 patients. These data are important because they focus on both right ventricular function and spontaneous ventilation, two areas of study with markedly few clinical trials.

More studies focus on the effects of positive-pressure ventilation on LV output. Positive-pressure ventilation induces phasic changes in LV stroke volume although similar cyclic changes in venous return. The magnitude of these changes in stroke volume are a function of the size of the tidal breath, the subsequent increase in intrathoracic pressure, and the extent that changes in LV output are determined by changes in LV filling pressure. Beat-to-beat changes in LV stroke volume can be easily monitored as beat-to-beat changes in arterial pulse pressure variation (PVV), since the only other determinants of pulse pressure, arterial resistance, and compliance cannot change enough to alter pulse pressure during a single breath. Based on this logic, Perel et al. [5] and Szold et al. [6] examined the systolic pressure variation (SPV) induced by a defined positive-pressure breath both in animals made hypovolemic and in humans with heart failure, demonstrating that the SPV, as specifically the decrease in systolic pressure from an apneic baseline, referred to a Δdown, identified hemorrhage and was minimized by fluid resuscitation. Tavernier et al. [7] subsequently validated these findings. The concept of SPV assumes that all the changes in systolic pressure can be explained by parallel changes in LV stroke volume.

Unfortunately, Denault et al. [8] could not demonstrate any relationship between LV stroke volume, estimated by transesophageal echocardiographic analysis, and SPV, suggesting that factors other than LV stroke volume contribute to SPV. Michard et al. [9, 10] reasoned that arterial PVV rather than SPV would more accurately reflect changes in LV stroke volume because arterial PVV is not influenced by the intrathoracic pressure-induced changes in both systolic and diastolic arterial pressure. They compared SPV with PPV as predictors of the subsequent increase in cardiac output in response to fluid loading in septic ventilator-dependent patients. Their data convincingly demonstrated that both PPV and SPV greater than 15% were far superior to measures of either P_{ra} or P_{pao} in predicting an increase in cardiac output response to volume loading. Furthermore, the greater the PPV or SPV was, the greater the subsequent increase in cardiac output. However, PPV claimed a slight although significant advantage over SPV in terms of greater precision and less bias. Since PPV attempts to monitor LV stroke volume changes, it was not surprising that Feissel et al. [11] demonstrated that aortic flow variation, as measured by transesophageal two-dimensional echocardiography pulsed Doppler of the aortic outflow tract, followed a similar response to PPV in response to fluid loading. The flow variation data are very important because flow it is the primary variable from which SPV and APP derive their validity. Although less invasive than arterial pressure monitoring, echocardiographic analysis is far from ideal as a hemodynamic monitoring tool. It requires the continuous presence of an experienced operator. Echocardiography requires using expensive and often scare equipment. Finally, measures of aortic root flow variation cannot be made on-line or continuously over prolonged periods of time.

Thus, Reuter et al. [12] attempted to apply the same stroke volume variation (SVV) logic using an alternative method that by-passes these limitations. They used a relatively old technology [13] referred to as the arterial pulse contour technique. The technique calculates LV stroke volume from the impedance characteristics of the pulse pressure waveform using a complex and proprietary algorithm [14]. The technique has enjoyed limited success in the critical care arena [15]. The measure of SVV then comes from the beat-to-beat analysis of these measures over a breath. Reuter et al. measured a vast variety of independent measures of cardiovascular status, namely echocardiographic measures of cross-sectional LV area, intrathoracic blood volume index, and both central venous pressure and P_{pao}. They demonstrated that their pulse contour SVV measures behaves in a fashion predicted from previous studies of SVP, arterial PPV, and aortic flow wherein actual measures were made. If these data are correct, this study marks a major step forward in the use of functional measures of hemodynamic status. The greater the SVV, the more cardiac output can be expected to increase in response to volume loading. Furthermore, if the SVV is less than 10%, cardiac output does not increase in response to volume loading and may be avoided as a therapeutic challenge.

The study by Reuter et al. [12] has some limitations, however, that make the application of these data in the management of patients today unadvisable. First, the arterial PPV data of Michard et al. [10] used a tidal volume of only 6 ml/kg, whereas the present study used a much larger tidal volume of 13–15 ml/kg. It is not clear whether similar SVV would be seen by this technique if the tidal volumes used were in the range of clinically relevant breaths. This is important because the measure of SVV by the pulse contour method has not been validated under positive-pressure ventilation conditions. The pulse contour method accurately tracks mean cardiac output [15]. However, it has never been validated for its accuracy to assess beat-to-beat variations in LV stroke volume. This is not a minor point. Denault et al. [8] demonstrated that much of the power signal of the arterial pulse is altered by ventilation, making the measure of SVV variation by the pulse contour technique questionable at best since it uses the power spectral analysis to estimate volume. That the authors saw a variation in their derived "stroke volume" variable and that it changed as expected in response to volume loading is encouraging but not definitive in allowing us to embrace this monitoring technique as a simpler method of measuring preload responsiveness. Second, and perhaps more concerning, the study design did not test the hypothesis that the cardiac output response to volume loading in critically ill patients could be predicted by SVV. The authors merely showed that a post hoc analysis of changes in SVV were correlated with subsequent stroke index changes in hemodynamically stable patients. Clearly, over time in postoperative patients arterial tone and rheology change, and these variables can alter pulse contour characteristics in unforeseen ways. Thus, this technique needs to be validated.

Hemodynamic monitoring has many roles in medicine. One is to diagnose disease and define cardiac performance. In the cardiac catheterization laboratory where all these techniques had their birth, that goal was clear. However, as we evolved into a treatment-oriented clinical practice, the paradigm of physiological status evolved as well into functional performance, a much different measure. The trend in hemodynamic monitoring toward more performance-based measures, such as preload responsiveness, is encouraging and marks the pathway toward more effective patient management, which at the end of the day is the reason why we use invasive monitoring at all.

References

1. Connors AF Jr, Speroff T, Dawson NV, Thomas C, Harrell FE Jr, Wagner D, Desbiens N, Goldman L, Wu AW, Califf RM, Fulkerson WJ Jr, Vidaillet H, Broste S, Bellamy P, Lynn J, Knaus WA (1996) The effectiveness of right heart catheterization in the initial care of critically ill patients. SUPPORT Investigators. JAMA 276:889–8897
2. Lichtwarck-Aschoff M, Zeravik J, Pfeiffer UJ (1992) Intrathoracic blood volume accurately reflects circulatory volume status in critically ill patients with mechanical ventilation. Intensive Care Med 18:137–138
3. Pinsky MR, Vincent JL, DeSmet JM (1991) Estimating left ventricular filling pressure during positive end-expiratory pressure in humans. Am Rev Respir Dis 143:25–31
4. Magder S, Georgiadis G, Cheong T (1992) Respiratory variations in right atrial pressure predict the response to fluid challenge. J Crit Care 7:76–85
5. Perel A, Pizov R, Cotev S (1987) Systolic blood pressure variation is a sensitive indicator of hypovolemia in ventilated dogs subjected to graded hemorrhage. Anesthesiology 67:498–502
6. Szold A, Pizov R, Segal E, Perel A (1989) The effect of tidal volume and intravascular volume state on systolic pressure variation in ventilated dogs. Intensive Care Med 15:368–371
7. Tavernier B, Makhotine O, Lebuffe G, Dupont J, Scherpereel P (1998) Systolic pressure variation as a guide to fluid therapy in patients with sepsis-induced hypotension. Anesthesiology 89:1313–1321
8. Denault AY, Gasior TA, Gorcsan J, Mandarino WA, Deneault LG, Pinsky MR (2000) Determinants of aortic pressure variation during positive-pressure ventilation in man. Chest 116:176–86
9. Michard F, Chemla D, Richard C, Wysocki M, Pinsky MR, Lecarpentier Y, Teboul JL (1999) Clinical use of respiratory changes in arterial pulse pressure to monitor the hemodynamic effects of PEEP. Am J Respir Crit Care Med 159:935–939
10. Michard F, Boussat S, Chemla D, Anguel N, Mercat A, Lecarpentier Y, Richard C, Pinsky MR, Teboul JL (2000) Relation between respiratory changes in arterial pulse pressure and fluid responsiveness in septic patients with acute circulatory failure. Am J Respir Crit Care Med 162:134–138
11. Feissel M, Michard F, Mangin I, Ruyer O, Faller JP, Teboul JL (2001) Respiratory changes in aortic blood velocity as an indicator of fluid responsiveness in ventilated patients with septic shock. Chest 119:867–873
12. Reuter DA, Felbinger TW, Schmidt C, Kilger E, Goedje O, Lamm P, Goetz AE (2002) Stroek volume variations for assessment of cardiac responsiveness to volume loading in mechanically ventilated patients after cardiac surgery. Intensive Care Med http://dx.doi.org/10.1007/s00134-002-1211-z
13. Frank O (1899) Die Grundform des arteriellen Pulses. Z Biol 37:483–526
14. Wesseling K, Wit BD, Weber J, Smith NT (1983) A simple device for the continuous measurement of cardiac output. Adv Cardiovasc Physiol 5:16–52
15. Bock J, Barker B, Mackersie R, Tranbaugh R, Lewis F (1989) Cardiac output measurement using femoral artery dilution in patients. J Crit Care 4:106–111

M.W. Elliott

Non-invasive ventilation in acute exacerbations of chronic obstructive pulmonary disease: a new gold standard?

Non-invasive ventilation (NIV) has been shown to be an effective treatment for ventilatory failure resulting from acute exacerbations of chronic obstructive pulmonary disease in a number of randomised controlled trials (RCTs) and in a recent meta-analysis [1]. It has been used in a variety of countries and settings, with different ventilator modes and interfaces and in differing degrees of severity.

In the studies in which NIV was applied in the ICU [2, 3, 4, 5] the most striking finding was a reduction in the need for endotracheal intubation (ETI) and mechanical ventilation (MV), which in the largest study translated into improved survival, reduced complication rates and length of both intensive care unit (ICU) and hospital stay [2]. These studies showed that NIV is feasible in acute exacerbations of COPD, and that the prevention of ETI is advantageous. Because paralysis and sedation are not needed with NIV, ventilation outside the ICU is an option; given the considerable pressure on ICU beds in most countries, the high costs and the fact that for some patients admission to ICU is a distressing experience [6], this is an attractive option. NIV can be instituted at an earlier stage in the natural history of the condition before mechanical ventilation would normally be considered necessary. There have been a number of prospective randomised controlled studies of NIV outside the ICU either on general wards or in accident and emergency departments [7, 8, 9, 10, 11, 12, 13]. NIV was instituted at a higher pH than that reported in the ICU studies and most failed to show any significant advantage to NIV when analysed on an intention to treat basis, but in one study [7] when those unable to tolerate NIV were excluded a significant survival benefit was seen (9/30 vs. 1/26, $p=0.014$). These studies were all relatively small and may have lacked sufficient statistical power to show a difference in the need for intubation and mortality given that most patients with a mild exacerbation of COPD (defined by the degree of acidosis) would not be expected to need ETI and MV anyway [14]. In a large ($n=236$) multicentre RCT of NIV in acute exacerbations of COPD on general respiratory wards in 13 centres [12] 'treatment failure', a surrogate for the need for intubation, defined by a priori criteria, was reduced from 27% to 15% by NIV ($p<0.05$). In-hospital mortality was also reduced from 20% to 10% ($P<0.05$). Sub-group analysis suggested that the outcome in patients with pH lower than 7.30 after initial treatment was inferior to that in the studies performed in the ICU. NIV was applied by the usual ward staff, most of whom had had little or no previous experience of NIV, using a bilevel device in spontaneous mode, according to a simple protocol. This study suggests that with adequate staff training NIV can be applied with benefit outside the ICU and that the early (pH <7.35 on admission to the ward) introduction of NIV on a general ward results in a better outcome than providing no ventilatory support for acidotic patients outside the ICU. The results in the more severely affected patients (pH<7.30 after initial management) were not as good as those seen in the ICU studies suggesting that this simple approach is not appropriate in these patients, and that they are best managed in a higher dependency setting with a more sophisticated ventilator individually adjusted to their requirements.

None of these studies involved the use of a placebo arm because of concern that this was impractical and might make the patients worse; it is therefore possible that the results may have been influenced by bias. However, a recent study [15] of patients with acute cardiogenic pulmonary oedema or an acute exacerbation of

M.R. Pinsky et al. (eds.), *Applied Physiology in Intensive Care Medicine 2: Physiological Reviews and Editorials*,
DOI 10.1007/978-3-642-28233-1_35, © Springer-Verlag Berlin Heidelberg 2012

COPD presenting to the emergency department found that placebo NIV had no effect upon physiological measures, such as arterial blood gas tensions and respiratory rate, and in all cases rescue therapy with active NIV or intubation was required. In seven of the ten patients the institution of active NIV resulted in a prompt improvement. By contrast there was a rapid improvement in physiological variables in all patients in the group treated with active NIV from the outset and none required intubation.

A number of studies have suggested that NIV is less likely to be successful in more severely affected patients [2, 16, 17], and all the studies reported to date have excluded patients who required immediate ETI and MV. The study of Wood et al. [9] suggested that failure to move to ETI in a timely fashion may have explained a trend towards a worse survival in the NIV group. The concern has been voiced therefore that, particularly in the more severely ill, NIV may be harmful by delaying the institution of the "gold" standard therapy, namely ETI and MV.

Conti et al. [18] report in this journal a prospective RCT of NIV vs. immediate ETI and MV in patients with an exacerbation of COPD. Not surprisingly their patients were sicker than those reported in previous studies, as evidenced by the mean pH of 7.2, compared with 7.27 in the study of Brochard et al. [2] and 7.32 in the study of Plant et al. [12]. In these sicker patients they showed that NIV was no worse than ETI and MV. In those who could be managed successfully with NIV there was an advantage both in the short term but also in the year after hospital discharge. This confirms the findings of two previous studies comparing NIV patients with historical controls who had been invasively ventilated [19, 20]. Imperfect matching is one possible explanation in these studies [21], but patients who are intubated and mechanically ventilated may lose a considerable amount of muscle bulk rendering them susceptible to further episodes of ventilatory failure [22, 23, 24, 25]. Longer term follow-up from the study of Plant et al. [17] failed to show any statistically significant benefit from NIV compared with conventional therapy, although, importantly, the study showed a median survival in both groups of over 1 year, indicating that the patients salvaged by NIV were not just those who had a very poor prognosis. It may be significant that few patients in either group were intubated and ventilated and this is an important difference when compared with the studies mentioned above. The intubation rate of 52% in the NIV group in the study by Conti et al. [18] was higher than in other RCTs, which is not surprising given that these were a sicker group of patients. It does, however, reinforce the view that NIV is best instituted early [26].

In common with other studies some patients were still excluded, in particular those intubated prior to transfer to the ICU or those with respiratory arrest or pauses, psychomotor agitation requiring sedation, heart rate below 60 or systolic blood pressure below 80 mmHg. NIV remains a complimentary technique to invasive ventilation but for patients intubated, either from the outset or after a failed trial of NIV, non-invasive ventilation may have a role in weaning [27, 28] or in the management of respiratory failure following extubation [29]. Further studies are needed but NIV is likely to be useful in selected patients.

There are no absolute contraindications to NIV, although a number have been suggested [16, 30]. These include coma or confusion, inability to protect the airway, severe acidosis at presentation, significant co-morbidity, vomiting, obstructed bowel, haemodynamic instability (two studies have shown only small changes in cardiac output when NIV is initiated [31, 32], but haemodynamic collapse comparable to that often seen when patients are intubated is very rare), radiological evidence of consolidation, and orofacial abnormalities which interfere with the mask/face interface. In part, these "contraindications" have been determined by the fact that they were exclusion criteria for the controlled trials. It is therefore more correct to state that NIV is not proven in these circumstances rather than that it is contraindicated. In a recent epidemiological study of 42 ICUs over a 3-week period NIV was never used in coma [33]. Although mask positive pressure ventilation is far away the most widely used non-invasive modality, negative pressure ventilation using an iron lung still has its advocates [34], and this technique has been used successfully in comatose patients [35]. Its use, however, is confined to a few specialised units. Whether NIV should be attempted in a particular patient must depend on individual circumstances. For instance, if invasive ventilation is not considered appropriate, but NIV would be acceptable, there is nothing to be lost by a trial of NIV, and there are no contraindications in this situation. NIV may not be appropriate in well-documented end-stage disease or when several co-morbidities are present. That the patient can continue to have a say is one potential advantage in this situation.

When NIV can be successfully applied there are clear advantages, particularly a reduction in infectious complications [36, 33, 37, 38] and length of ICU and hospital stay [2], with an attendant reduction in costs [39]. There is no convincing evidence to date that a failed trial of NIV is harmful. However, there is always the danger that, as confidence grows, NIV may be continued for too long in an individual patient to the point of cardiorespiratory arrest. Further data are needed as to when NIV should be abandoned in favour of invasive ventilation. When embarking upon a trial of NIV there should be a clear plan of what will be done should the patient fail and how failure will be recognised.

The study of Conti et al. [18] is a further, perhaps the final, piece in the jigsaw of when NIV is indicated in patients with an acute exacerbation of COPD. It now seems reasonable to suggest a trial of NIV in the vast majority of patients acidotic because of an acute exacerbation of COPD. Early intervention is more likely to be successful [12, 17], but even when patients present later in the natural history of their exacerbation there is still a role for NIV. Being first is often a significant factor when defining a gold standard. Perhaps the time has now come, on the basis of the published evidence, to define NIV as the gold standard mode of ventilatory support for exacerbations of COPD, with ETI and MV regarded as second-line rescue therapy when it fails; as with second-line chemotherapy for cancer this often comes at greater expense and with more risk to the patient.

References

1. Peter JV, Moran JL, Phillips-Hughes J, Warn D (2002) Noninvasive ventilation in acute respiratory failure-a meta-analysis update. Crit Care Med 30:555–562
2. Brochard L, Mancebo J, Wysocki M, Lofaso F, Conti G, Rauss A, Simmoneau G, Benito S, Gasparetto A, Lemaire F, Isabey D, Harf A (1995) Noninvasive ventilation for acute exacerbations of chronic obstructive pulmonary disease. N Engl J Med 333:817–822
3. Kramer N, Meyer TJ, Meharg J, Cece RD, Hill NS (1995) Randomized, prospective trial of noninvasive positive pressure ventilation in acute respiratory failure. Am J Respir Crit Care Med 151:1799–1806
4. Celikel T, Sungur M, Ceyhan B, Karakurt S (1998) Comparison of non-invasive positive pressure ventilation with standard medical therapy in hypercapnic acute respiratory failure. Chest 114:1636–1642
5. Martin TJ, Hovis JD, Costantino JP, Bierman MI, Donahoe MP, Rogers RM, Kreit JW, Sciurba FC, Stiller RA, Sanders MH (2000) A randomized, prospective evaluation of noninvasive ventilation for acute respiratory failure. Am J Respir Crit Care Med 161:807–813
6. Easton C, MacKenzie F (1988) Sensory-perceptual alterations: delirium in the intensive care unit. Heart Lung 17:229–237
7. Bott J, Carroll MP, Conway JH, Keilty SEJ, Ward EM, Brown AM, Paul EA, Elliott MW, Godfrey RC, Wedzicha JA, Moxham J (1993) Randomised controlled trial of nasal ventilation in acute ventilatory failure due to chronic obstructive airways disease. Lancet 341:1555–1557
8. Barbe F, Togores B, Rubi M, Pons S, Maimo A, Agusti AGN (1996) Noninvasive ventilatory support does not facilitate recovery from acute respiratory failure in chronic obstructive pulmonary disease. Eur Respir J 9:1240–1245
9. Wood KA, Lewis L, Von Harz B, Kollef MH (1998) The use of noninvasive positive pressure ventilation in the emergency department. Chest 113:1339–1346
10. Angus RM, Ahmed AA, Fenwick LJ, Peacock AJ (1996) Comparison of the acute effects on gas exchange of nasal ventilation and doxapram in exacerbations of chronic obstructive pulmonary disease. Thorax 51:1048–1050
11. Bardi G, Pierotello R, Desideri M, Valdisseri L, Bottai M, Palla A (2000) Nasal ventilation in COPD exacerbations: early and late results of a prospective, controlled study. Eur Respir J 15:98–104
12. Plant PK, Owen JL, Elliott MW (2000) Early use of non-invasive ventilation for acute exacerbations of chronic obstructive pulmonary disease on general respiratory wards: a multicentre randomised controlled trial. Lancet 355:1931–1935
13. Avdeev SN, Tret'iakov AV, Grigor'iants RA, Kutsenko MA, Chuchalin AG (1998) [Study of the use of noninvasive ventilation of the lungs in acute respiratory insufficiency due exacerbation of chronic obstructive pulmonary disease]. Anesteziol Reanimatol 3:45–51
14. Jeffrey AA, Warren PM, Flenley DC (1992) Acute hypercapnic respiratory failure in patients with chronic obstructive lung disease: risk factors and use of guidelines for management. Thorax 47:34–40
15. Thys F, Roeseler J, Reynaert M, Liistro G, Rodenstein D (2002) Noninvasive ventilation for acute respiratory failure: a prospective randomised placebo-controlled trial. Eur Respir J 20:545–555
16. Ambrosino N, Foglio K, Rubini F, Clini E, Nava S, Vitacca M (1995) Non-invasive mechanical ventilation in acute respiratory failure due to chronic obstructive airways disease: correlates for success. Thorax 50:755–757
17. Plant PK, Owen JL, Elliott MW (2001) Non-invasive ventilation in acute exacerbations of chronic obstructive pulmonary disease: long term survival and predictors of in-hospital outcome. Thorax 56:708–712
18. Conti G, Antonelli M, Navalesi P, Rocco M, Bufi M, Spadetta G, et al Noninvasive versus conventional mechanical ventilation in patients with chronic obstructive pulmonary disease after failure of medical treatment in the ward: a randomized trial. Intensive Care Med (in press)
19. Confalonieri M, Parigi P, Scartabellati A, Aiolfi S, Scorsetti S, Nava S, Gandola L (1996) Noninvasive mechanical ventilation improves the immediate and long-term outcome of COPD patients with acute respiratory failure. Eur Respir J 9:422–430
20. Vitacca M, Clini E, Rubini F, Nava S, Foglio K, Ambrosino N (1996) Non-invasive mechanical ventilation in severe chronic obstructive lung disease and acute respiratory failure: short- and long-term prognosis. Intensive Care Med 22:94–100
21. Shneerson JM (1996) The changing role of mechanical ventilation in COPD. Eur Respir J 9:393–398
22. Coakley JH, Nagendran K, Ormerod IE, Ferguson CN, Hinds CJ (1992) Prolonged neurogenic weakness in patients requiring mechanical ventilation for acute airflow limitation. Chest 101:1413–1416
23. Kollef MH, Levy NT, Ahrens TS, Schaiff R, Prentice D, Sherman G (1998) The use of continuous i.v. sedation is associated with prolongation of mechanical ventilation. Chest 114:541–548
24. Le Bourdelles G, Viires N, Boczkowski J, Seta N, Pavlovic D, Aubier M (1994) Effects of mechanical ventilation on diaphragmatic contractile properties in rats. Am J Respir Crit Care Med 149:1539–1544
25. Berek K, Margreiter J, Willeit J, Berek A, Schmutzhard E, Mutz NJ (1996) Polyneuropathies in critically ill patients: a prospective evaluation. Intensive Care Med 22:849–855

26. Evans TW (2001) International Consensus Conferences in Intensive Care Medicine: non-invasive positive pressure ventilation in acute respiratory failure. Organised jointly by the American Thoracic Society, the European Respiratory Society, the European Society of Intensive Care Medicine, and the Societe de Reanimation de Langue Francaise, and approved by the ATS Board of Directors, December 2000. Intensive Care Med 27:166–178
27. Nava S, Ambrosino N, Clini E, Prato M, Orlando G, Vitacca M, Brigada P, Fracchia C, Rubini F (1998) Noninvasive mechanical ventilation in the weaning of patients with respiratory failure due to chronic obstructive pulmonary disease. A randomized, controlled trial. Ann Intern Med 128:721–728
28. Girault C, Daudenthun I, Chevron V, Tamion F, Leroy J, Bonmarchand G (1999) Noninvasive ventilation as a systematic extubation and weaning technique in acute-on-chronic respiratory failure. A prospective, randomized controlled study. Am J Respir Crit Care Med 160:86–92
29. Hilbert G, Gruson D, Porel L, Gbikpi-Benissan G, Cardinaud JP (1998) Noninvasive pressure support ventilation in COPD patients with post extubation hypercapnic respiratory insufficiency. Eur Respir J 11:1349–1353
30. Soo Hoo GW, Santiago S, Williams AJ (1994) Nasal mechanical ventilation for hypercapnic respiratory failure in chronic obstructive pulmonary disease: determinants of success and failure. Crit Care Med 22:1253–1261
31. Ambrosino N, Nava S, Torbicki A, Riccardi G, Fracchia C, Opasich C, Rampulla C (1993) Haemodynamic effects of pressure support and PEEP ventilation by nasal route in patients with stable chronic obstructive pulmonary disease. Thorax 48:523–528
32. Confalonieri M, Gazzaniga P, Gandola L, Aiolfi S, Della Porta R, Frisinghelli A, Bellone A (1998) Haemodynamic response during initiation of non-invasive positive pressure ventilation in COPD patients with acute ventilatory failure. Respir Med 92:331–337
33. Carlucci A, Richard JC, Wysocki M, Lepage E, Brochard L (2001) Noninvasive versus conventional mechanical ventilation. An epidemiologic survey. Am J Respir Crit Care Med 163:874–880
34. Corrado A, Gorini M (2002) Negative-pressure ventilation: is there still a role? Eur Respir J 20:187–197
35. Corrado A, De Paola E, Gorini M, Messori A, Bruscoli G, Nutini S, Tozzi D, Ginanni R, de Paola (1996) Intermittent negative pressure ventilation in the treatment of hypoxic hypercapnic coma in chronic respiratory insufficiency. Thorax 51:1077–1082
36. Girou E, Schortgen F, Delclaux C, Brun-Buisson C, Blot F, Lefort Y, Lemaire F, Brochard L (2000) Association of noninvasive ventilation with nosocomial infections and survival in critically ill patients. JAMA 284:2361–2367
37. Guerin C, Girard R, Chemorin C, De Varax R, Fournier G (1997) Facial mask noninvasive mechanical ventilation reduces the incidence of nosocomial pneumonia. A prospective epidemiological survey from a single ICU. Intensive Care Med 23:1024–1032
38. Nourdine K, Combes P, Carton M-J, Beuret P, Cannamela A, Ducreux J-C (1999) Does noninvasive ventilation reduce the ICU nosocomial infection risk? A prospective clinical survey. Intensive Care Med 25:567–573
39. Keenan SP, Gregor J, Sibbald WJ, Cook DJ, Gafni A (2000) Noninvasive positive pressure ventilation in the setting of severe, acute exacerbations of chronic obstructive pulmonary disease: more effective and less expensive. Crit Care Med 28:2094–2102

Karl Träger
Peter Radermacher
Xavier Leverve

The adrenergic coin: perfusion and metabolism

The pathologic state of shock is characterized by profound changes in tissue perfusion and metabolism. The main consequence of such pathophysiologic changes clearly affects the hierarchy of priority among the various organs, but which of these changes are adaptive or deleterious is still a question not completely answered. Therefore interfering with some of the main features of shock, such as low blood pressure, may have different consequences according to the flow redistribution and/or to the associated specific metabolic consequences. Vasopressor administration is one of the mainstay treatment approaches for various shock states. Catecholamines are the most widely used vasopressors in this context. In particular during septic shock there are various concepts about the use of adrenergic agents depending on the specific adrenoceptor profile of either endogenous and synthetic catecholamines [1]. The recommendations for the use of catecholamines consider primarily their efficacy in restoring or maintaining adequate systemic hemodynamics but also try to implement effects on regional blood flow and metabolism. Adrenergic agents may also be associated, however, with marked metabolic effects not necessarily linked to their hemodynamic effects [2].

In the treatment of septic shock norepinephrine is the most widely used catecholamine, but in some cases epinephrine may be used as well. For routine clinical use the two catecholamine approaches result in comparable systemic hemodynamics, but differences in receptor subtype specificity may cause discernible redistribution of regional perfusion and organ specific metabolic stimulation, which as a consequence may again lead to a perfusion/metabolism mismatch [3, 4, 5].

Septic shock per se induces profound alterations in cellular energy metabolism [6, 7, 8]. Since additional changes in cellular energetic state are also induced by catecholamines, it is of major interest to investigate during endotoxic shock simultaneously perfusion/oxygenation and metabolic alterations as well as their impact on cellular energy state. Indeed, differences in receptor activation between epinephrine and norepinephrine could be related to different effects, which are linked not only to vasopressor effects but also to the specific metabolic pathways located in various organs explaining thus the heterogeneous effects on cellular energetics.

In their contribution to *Intensive Care Medicine* Levy et al. [9] address the question of the extent to which epinephrine and norepinephrine modulate perfusion, metabolism, and cellular energetics differently in a rodent animal model of acute endotoxemia. They investigated changes in systemic, mesenteric, renal, and femoral blood flow as well as markers of cellular redox and energy state derived both from blood and tissue metabolic determination from heart, muscle, gut, liver, and kidney. The question was: to what extent do epinephrine or norepinephrine alter tissue perfusion and cause additional alterations in endotoxin-induced metabolic disturbances?

First, the authors confirm the well known effect of epinephrine (in contrast to norepinehrine) of increasing glucose and lactate levels in animal models [10, 11, 12, 13] as well as in humans [14, 15, 16] in controls. The endotoxin challenge in the present model was associated with decreased mean arterial pressure and systemic

M.R. Pinsky et al. (eds.), *Applied Physiology in Intensive Care Medicine 2: Physiological Reviews and Editorials*,
DOI 10.1007/978-3-642-28233-1_36, © Springer-Verlag Berlin Heidelberg 2012

blood flow. During endotoxemia lactate levels rose together with increased lactate/pyruvate and decreased ketone body ratios demonstrating disturbances in energy metabolism and tissue energetics. In this condition of endotoxin challenge neither epinephrine nor norepinephrine was associated with increased lactate levels nor did they influence the disturbed lactate/pyruvate and ketone body ratio. Although both catecholamines did restore mean arterial pressure to control values, they failed to restore normal organ blood flow. From this work it is clear that epinephrine and norepinephrine result in different patterns of blood flow during hypodynamic, hypotensive endotoxin shock with particular relevance for mesenteric and for renal perfusion.

However, beyond the effects on perfusion the main interest of this report relies on the simultaneous focus on the metabolic consequences of catecholamines during endotoxemia. Using lactate, pyruvate, lactate/pyruvate, ketone body ratios, and tissue energetic charge in various organs (muscle, heart, gut, liver, kidney) they confirm that high lactate levels are associated with unchanged lactate/pyruvate and ketone body ratios during epinephrine infusion, indicating a metabolic stimulation rather than an energy deficit [17]. During endotoxemic conditions this relationship becomes much more complex, as endotoxin-induced derangements are not further affected by catecholamine treatment with respect to blood derived parameters of cellular and mitochondrial redox state. Interestingly, lactate and the lactate/pyruvate ratio were significantly increased exclusively in the kidney, where catecholamines provoked a dramatic additional reduction in organ blood flow. This was associated with a parallel depletion of tissue ATP levels. Moreover, a decrease in ATP content was also observed in the liver, another highly energy-consuming organ.

These results raise the question of the clinically relevant parameters for measuring cellular energy status. Being readily available under clinical conditions, blood lactate concentration is still one of the most widely used parameters for judging the adequacy of tissue oxygen availability in patients. Although under conditions of severe cardiovascular failure lactate levels have been shown to provide good insight in the effectivity of resuscitation measures [18] and proved to be a prognostic tool [19], there is an ongoing debate about the exclusive use of increased lactate levels in septic patients as an indicator of tissue hypoxia [20, 21, 22, 23, 24, 25, 26, 27]. Additional determination of pyruvate and, hence, calculation of lactate/pyruvate ratio reflecting cytosolic $NAD^+/NADH$ ratio can provide additional information [28, 29]. Increased ketone body ratio for assessing mitochondrial redox state [30] may represent a further indication of uncovering tissue hypoxia as a cause of metabolic derangement. However, ketone body determinations are technically cumbersome for routine practice, and furthermore the ketone body ratio seems to provide measurable effects mainly under severe conditions of irreversible shock [31] or during severe cardiogenic shock [32]. Under clinical conditions of sepsis and septic shock [32, 33] the ketone body ratio seems less sensitive to uncover mitochondrial redox failure. Nevertheless, at least from small series of critically ill patient investigations it has been shown that the ketone body ratio is closely linked with nitrite/nitrate levels as an indicator of sepsis-induced nitric oxide overproduction [34], and therefore the course of the ketone body ratio was suggested as a prognostic measure in patients [35]. This underscores the difficulty of interpreting enhanced lactate levels under clinical situations in terms of its relevance to tissue perfusion.

Disturbances in metabolic parameters are more pronounced in tissues than in blood. This is not surprising since blood values may not necessarily reflect metabolic alterations during clinical observations [29, 36].

Except in the kidney catecholamines have no specific effect on tissue lactate and lactate/pyruvate ratios in the endotoxemic animals, while a decrease in ATP is observed in liver, heart, and mainly kidney. This may highlight a specific feature of endotoxemia and sepsis. Indeed, under experimental [37] and clinical conditions sepsis is associated with hypermetabolism [7, 38], and the metabolically very active organs such as liver and kidney [7, 39] are probably highly vulnerable to endotoxin-induced hypoperfusion. Thus these organs may be endangered by additional stimulation by metabolically active adrenergic agents.

The authors speculate that changes in lactate/pyruvate and ketone body ratios in their model may be due mainly to endotoxin-associated cytopathic mechanisms but not to hypoxic disturbances. The main reasons are thought to be flow-independent alterations in cellular energy metabolism resulting in mitochondrial dysoxia [37, 40]. However, in this model reduced blood flow and impaired oxygen transport could be a main cause of metabolic deterioration. It would be interesting and indeed supportive for the concept of "cytopathic hypoxia" [40] to confirm these data in a model with well preserved organ blood flow.

This endotoxic shock model is characterized by a profound depression of systemic and regional blood flows which is paralleled by metabolic changes possibly related to tissue hypoperfusion [30, 41, 42]. Hence, it is clear that vasoactive treatments are associated with metabolic effects, which may reflect primarily their consequences on blood flow.

Could these observations have an impact on the clinical decision to use epinephrine instead of norepinephrine or vice versa? To our opinion it does. Although epinephrine and norepinephrine have been shown to provide good hemodynamic stabilization in cardiosurgical patients, epinephrine use in contrast to norepinephrine is associated with increased lactate levels, decreased arterial pH and higher blood glucose levels [43] without signs of compromised tissue oxygenation. In septic shock patients, as well, epinephrine may achieve hemodynamic stability [44, 45]. However, under these conditions epinephrine use may be associated not only with compromised regional hepatosplanchnic perfusion [5, 46] but also with profound metabolic alterations as shown by lactic acidosis [47]. Therefore concepts for hemodynamic treatment of septic shock patients should not only aim on hemodynamic parameters, but also limit additional drug-induced metabolic stimulation. Consequently in the case of epinephrine for the treatment of septic shock only a limited use is recommended [1].

The authors addressed the very important question of vasoactive treatment associated effects on organ metabolism during an experimental model of endotoxic shock. As the clinical decision to use specific vasoactive treatment is based mainly on systemic and regional perfusion and oxygen transport, we should keep in mind that metabolic consequences, beyond perfusion effect, may jeopardize organ function by a metabolic overstimulation.

References

1. Vincent JL (2001) Hemodynamic support in septic shock. Intensive Care Med 27 [Suppl 1]:S80–S92
2. Macdonald IA, Bennett T, Fellows EW (1985) Catecholamines and the control of metabolism in man. Clin Sci (Colch) 68:613–619
3. Carpati CM, Astiz ME, Rackow EC (1997) Optimizing gastric mucosal perfusion: all catecholamines may not be created equal. Crit Care Med 25:1624–1625
4. Levy B, Bollaert PE, Lucchelli JP, Sadoune LO, Nace L, Larcan L (1997) Dobutamine improves the adequacy of gastric mucosal perfusion in epinephrine-treated septic shock. Crit Care Med 25:1649–1654
5. Levy B, Bollaert PE, Charpentier C, Nace L, Audibert G, Bauer P, Nabet B, Larcan A (1997) Comparison of norepinephrine and dobutamine to epinephrine for hemodynamics, lactate metabolism, and gastric tonometric variables in septic shock: a prospective randomized study. Intensive Care Med 23:282–287
6. Astiz M, Rackow EC, Weil MH, Schumer W (1988) Early impairment of oxidative metabolism and energy production in severe sepsis. Circ Shock 26:311–320
7. Dahn MS, Mitchell RA, Lange MP, Smith S, Jacobs LA (1995) Hepatic metabolic response to injury and sepsis. Surgery 117:520–530
8. Chioléro R, Revelly JP, Tappy L (1997) Energy metabolism in sepsis and injury. Nutrition 13 [Suppl]:45S–51S
9. Levy B, Mansart A, Bollaert PE, Franck P, Mallie JP (2002) Effects of epinephrine and norepinephrine on hemodynamics, oxidative metabolism and organs energetics in endotoxemic rats. Intensive Care Med DOI 10.1007/s00134-002-1611-0
10. Cori CF, Cori GT (1929) The mechanisms of epinephrine action. I. The influence of epinephrine on the carbohydrate metabolism of fasting rats, with a note on new formation of carbohydrates. J Biol Chem 84:309–319
11. Cori CF, Cori GT (1929) The mechanisms of epinephrine action. IV. The influence of epinephrine on lactic acid production and blood sugar utilization. J Biol Chem 84:683–698
12. Salak N, Pajk W, Knotzer H, Hofstötter H, Schwarz B, Mayr A, Labeck B, Kafka R, Ulmer H, Mutz N, Hasibeder W (2001) Effects of epinephrine on intestinal oxygen supply and mucosal tissue oxygen tension in pigs. Crit Care Med 29:367–373
13. Schwarz B, Hofstötter H, Salak N, Pajk W, Knotzer H, Mayr A, Labeck B, Kafka R, Ulmer H, Hasibeder W (2001) Effects of norepinephrine and phenylephrine on intestinal oxygen supply and mucosal tissue oxygen tension. Intensive Care Med 27:593–601
14. Ensinger H, Träger K, Geisser W, Anhäupl T, Ahnefeld FW, Vogt J, Georgieff M (1994) Glucose and urea production and leucine, ketoisocaproate and alanine fluxes at supraphysiological plasma adrenaline concentrations in volunteers. Intensive Care Med 20:113–118
15. Ensinger H, Träger K (2002) Metabolic effect of vasoactive drugs. In: Vincent JL (ed) Yearbook of intensive care and emergency medicine. Springer, Berlin Heidelberg New York, pp 499–509
16. Ensinger H, Geisser W, Brinkmann A, Wachter U, Vogt J, Radermacher P, Georgieff M, Träger K (2002) Metabolic effects of norepinephrine and dobutamine in healthy volunteers. Shock (in press)
17. James JH, Wagner KR, King JK, Leffler RE, Upputuri RK, Balasubramaniam A, Friend LA, Shelly DA, Paul RJ, Fischer JE (1999) Stimulation of both aerobic glycolysis and Na (+)-K (+)-ATPase activity in skeletal muscle by epinephrine or amylin. Am J Physiol 277:E176–E186
18. Vincent JL, Dufaye P, Berre J, Leeman M, Degaute JP, Kahn RJ (1983) Serial lactate determinations during circulatory shock. Crit Care Med 11:449–451
19. Friedman G, Berlot G, Kahn RJ, Vincent JL (1995) Combined measurements of blood lactate concentrations and gastric intramucosal pH in patients with severe sepsis. Crit Care Med 23: 1184–1193
20. Kirschenbaum LA, Astiz ME, Rackow EC (1998) Interpretation of blood lactate concentrations in patients with sepsis. Lancet 352:921–922
21. Levraut J, Ciebiera JP, Chave S, Rabary O, Jambou P, Carles M, Grimaud D (1998) Mild hyperlactatemia in stable septic patients is due to impaired lactate clearance rather than overproduction. Am J Respir Crit Care Med 157:1021–1026
22. Leverve XM (1999) Energy metabolism in critically ill patients: lactate is a major oxidizable substrate. Curr Opin Clin Nutr Metab Care 2:165–169
23. James JH, Luchette FA, McCarter FD, Fischer JE (1999) Lactate is an unreliable indicator of tissue hypoxia in injury or sepsis. Lancet 354:505–508
24. Bakker J (2001) Lactate: may I have your votes please? Intensive Care Med 27:6–11
25. De Backer D, Creteur J, Silva E, Vincent JL (2001) The hepatosplanchnic area is not a common source of lactate in patients with severe sepsis. Crit Care Med 29:256–261
26. Mizock BA (2001) The hepatosplanchnic area and hyperlactatemia: a tale of two lactates. Crit Care Med 29:447–449
27. Leverve XM, Mustafa I (2002) Lactate: a key metabolite in the intercellular metabolic interplay. Crit Care 6: 284–285
28. Mizock BA, Falk JA (1992) Lactic acidosis in critical illness. Crit Care Med 20:80–93

29. Suistomaa M, Ruokonen E, Kari A, Takala J (2000) Time-pattern of lactate and lactate to pyruvate ratio in the first 24 hours of intensive care emergency admissions. Shock 14:8–12
30. Dishart MK, Schlichtig R, Tønnessen TI, Rozenfeld RA, Simplaceanu E, Williams D, Gayowski TJP (1998) Mitochondrial redox state as a potential detector of liver dysoxia in vivo. J Appl Physiol 84:791–797
31. Kopprasch S, Hörkner U, Orlik H, Kemmer C, Scheuch DW (1989) Energy state, glycolytic intermediates and mitochondrial function in the liver during reversible and irreversible endotoxin shock. Biomed Biochim Acta 48:653–659
32. Levy B, Sadoune LO, Gelot AM, Bollaert PE, Nabet P, Larcan A (2000) Evolution of lactate/pyruvate and arterial ketone body ratios in the early course of catecholamine-treated septic shock. Crit Care Med 28:114–119
33. Gallet D, Goudable J, Vedrinne JM, Viale JP, Annat G (1997) Increased lactate/pyruvate ratio with normal beta-hydroxybutyrate/acetoacetate ratio and lack of oxygen supply dependency in a patient with fatal septic shock. Intensive Care Med 23:114–116
34. Satoi S, Kamiyama Y, Kitade H, Kwon AH, Takahashi K, Wei T, Inoue T, Takahashi H (2000) Nitric oxide production and hepatic dysfunction in patients with postoperative sepsis. Clin Exp Pharmacol Physiol 27:197–201
35. Yassen KA, Galley HF, Lee A, Webster NR (1999) Mitochondrial redox state in the critically ill. Br J Anaesth 83: 325–327
36. Gammaitoni C, Nasraway SA (1994) Normal lactate/pyruvate ratio during overwhelming polymicrobial bacteremia and multiple organ failure. Anesthesiology 80:213–216
37. L'Her E, Sebert P (2001) A global approach to energy metabolism in an experimental model of sepsis. Am J Respir Crit Care Med 164:1444–1447
38. Mizock BA (1995) Alterations in carbohydrate metabolism during stress: a review of the literature. Am J Med 98: 75–84
39. Jungas RL, Halperin ML, Brosnan JT (1992) Quantitative analysis of amino acid oxidation and related gluconeogenesis in humans. Physiol Rev 72: 419–448
40. Fink MP (2002) Cytopathic hypoxia. Is oxygen use impaired in sepsis as a result of an acquired intrinsic derangement in cellular respiration? Crit Care Clin 18:165–175
41. Tenhunen JJ, Jakob SM, Takala JA (2001) Gut luminal lactate release during gradual intestinal ischemia. Intensive Care Med 27:1916–1922
42. Tenhunen JJ, Jakob S, Ruokonen E, Takala J (2002) Jejunal luminal microdialysate lactate in cardiac tamponade-effect of low systemic blood flow on gut mucosa. Intensive Care Med 28: 953–962
43. Totaro RJ, Raper RF (1997) Epinephrine-induced lactic acidosis following cardiopulmonary bypass. Crit Care Med 25:1693–1699
44. Martin C, Saux P, Eon B, Aknin P, Gouin F (1990) Septic shock: a goal-directed therapy using volume loading, dobutamine and/or epinephrine. Acta Anaesthesiol Scand 34:413–417
45. Mackenzie SJ, Kapadia F, Nimmo GR, Armstrong IR, Grant IS (1991) Adrenaline in treatment of septic shock: effects on hemodynamics and oxygen transport. Intensive Care Med 17:36–39
46. Meier-Hellmann A, Reinhart K, Bredle DL, Specht M, Spies CD, Hannemann L (1997) Epinephrine impairs splanchnic perfusion in septic shock. Crit Care Med 25:399–404
47. Day NPJ, Phu NH, Bethell DP, Mai NTH, Chau TTH, Hien TT, White NJ (1996) The effects of dopamine and adrenaline infusions on acid-base balance and systemic haemodynamics in severe infection. Lancet 348:219–223

Paul E. Marik
Michael R. Pinsky

Death by parenteral nutrition

According to the *Merriam-Webster Dictionary* a poison or toxin is "a substance that through its chemical action usually kills, injures or impairs an organism" [1]. Based on this definition, in the critically ill, total parenteral nutrition (TPN) meets all the criteria of a poison/toxin. Furthermore, TPN exhibits other properties common to many toxins, namely, the presence of a dose response curve (the more you give the greater the toxicity), its toxicity is most evident in those with depressed host defense mechanisms (the critically ill) and an antidote exists (enteral nutrition).

Although it is true that no disease is improved by starvation, the route of nutritional support is of fundamental importance in determining outcome from critical illness. It would appear intuitively obvious that the human body is designed to receive nourishment and hydration via the gastrointestinal route. The concept of parenteral nutrition was born in the 1930s with the realization that malnutrition increases the complications associated with many diseases [2]. The origins of "modern" parental nutrition can be traced to the publication in 1937 by Robert Elman [3] of his successful studies in man of intravenous amino acid infusion in the form of protein hydrolysates. Along with other "therapeutic interventions" of the time, TPN was extolled to be the "cure-all" for conditions ranging from heart failure to cancer [4]. However, even at this time there were skeptics who argued that the infusion of amino acids that circumvent the liver is "unphysiological" and probably "toxic to the brain and other organs" [5]. Nonetheless, unlike other treatments that disappeared once their ineffectiveness and toxicity were established by controlled clinical trials [6, 7], TPN in the management of critically ill patients has managed to survive to this day.

The adverse sequelae associated with TPN result from the combined detrimental effects of not directly feeding the bowel, as well as the metabolic, immunological, endocrine, and infective complications associated with infusing a synthetic "nutrient cocktail" into a patients systemic venous system. The gastrointestinal mucosa is metabolically highly active, and enteral nutrition increases mucosal blood flow and provides a direct source of nutrients. Lack of enteral feeding results in gastrointestinal mucosal atrophy, bacterial overgrowth, increased intestinal permeability, and translocation of bacteria and/or bacterial products into the portal circulation [8, 9, 10, 11, 12, 13, 14, 15, 16]. Furthermore, the absence of enteral nutrition causes liver atrophy with rapid depletion of the liver's antioxidant enzyme systems [17]. In addition, TPN is often associated with significant hepatobiliary complications, including hepatosteatosis and hepatocellular injury leading to liver failure [18]. Enteral nutrition has a major effect on the gut-associated lymphoid tissue (GALT), which is the source of most mucosal immunity in humans. Experimental data have demonstrated that the small intestine GALT is preserved by enteral nutrition. However, TPN results in rapid and severe atrophy of GALT [19, 20, 21, 22]. Kundsk et al. [19] demonstrated that GALT atrophy in animals receiving parenteral nutrition is associated with decreased IgA in the secretions of the upper respiratory tract, and that this decreased IgA is associated with a reduced resistance to infection [20, 21]. Enteral feeding during or after parenteral nutrition is associated with rapid repletion of GALT cellularity [20].

TPN is immunosuppressive [23]. In addition to its effects on the GALT, TPN impairs humoral and cellular im-

M.R. Pinsky et al. (eds.), *Applied Physiology in Intensive Care Medicine 2: Physiological Reviews and Editorials*,
DOI 10.1007/978-3-642-28233-1_37, © Springer-Verlag Berlin Heidelberg 2012

munological defenses [23, 24, 25, 26]. TPN is associated with impaired leukocyte chemotaxis, impaired phagocytosis, impaired bacterial and fungal killing, and an attenuated inflammatory response [23, 27, 28, 29, 30]. In a murine intraperitoneal sepsis model, Lin and colleagues [31] have demonstrated that TPN, as compared to enteral nutrition, is associated with decreased mobilization of inflammatory cells and decreased production of tumor necrosis factor-α, interleukin-1β, and interferon-γ, with decreased bacterial clearance. Experimental sepsis models have demonstrated a significantly higher mortality in animals receiving parenteral than enteral nutrition [31, 32, 33, 34]. These data are supported by clinical studies which consistently demonstrate a higher risk of infection in patients receiving TPN than enteral nutrition [6, 7, 35, 36, 37, 38].

In addition to the detrimental effects that TPN has on the gut mucosal function and the immune system, TPN is also associated with an impressive array of metabolic and endocrine complications including hyperglycemia, hypertriglyceridemia, azotemia, metabolic acidosis, an exaggerated stress response, and numerous electrolyte abnormalities [16, 39, 40, 41, 42]. Furthermore, TPN is associated with increased free radical formation [43, 44], a complication that may be of considerable importance in critically ill patients.

The effects of TPN on the gut, the immune system, the liver, and the host's endocrine and metabolic milieu translates into an increased risk of dying during critical illness. Heyland and colleagues [45] performed a meta-analysis of TPN (compared to no nutritional support) in critically ill patients. They demonstrated that in critically ill patients TPN almost doubles the risk of dying (RR 1.78; 95% CI 1.11–2.85). Similarly, using a risk adjusted mortality ratio we have demonstrated that in critically ill ICU patients TPN, as compared to enteral nutrition, doubles the risk of dying [46]. We further showed that the toxicity of TPN can be reduced by the addition of "trickle" enteral nutrition, suggesting that a major cause of TPN-associated increased mortality is atrophy of the gut mucosa and GALT [46, 47].

Several studies in non-critically ill patients have not demonstrated similar increased risk of infectious complications, length of hospital stay, or mortality in patients receiving TPN [48, 49]. Thus TPN should probably be restricted to these patient populations. In critically ill patients, however, the literature strongly supports the view that TPN increases morbidity and mortality. We believe that, based on the evidence, TPN has no place in the management of critically ill patients who can otherwise be fed enterally [4, 5, 50, 51]. Based on clinical trials, enteral nutrition should be initiated upon admission to the ICU. There is no reason for even short periods of starvation even in postoperative gastrointestinal surgery patients [52, 53, 54]. Enteral nutritional support may not be possible in patients with short-gut syndrome. However, these patients are exceedingly rare. In conclusion, for the intensivist the acronym "TPN" may represent "total poisonous nutrition."

References

1. Anonymous (1991) Webster's ninth new collegiate dictionary. Merriam-Webster, Springfield
2. Studely HO (1936) Percentage of weight loss. A basic indicator of surgical risk in patients with chronic peptic ulcer. Nutr Hosp 106 458–60
3. Elman R (1937) Amino acid content of the blood following intravenous injection of hydrolyzed casein. Proc Soc Exp Biol Med 37:437–440
4. McCollum EV (1957) A history of nutrition. Houghton Mifflin, Boston
5. Wretlind A (1992) Recollections of pioneers in nutrition: Landmarks in the development of parenteral nutrition. J Am Coll Nutr 11:366–373
6. Veterans Affairs Total Parenteral Nutrition Cooperative Study Group (1991) Perioperative total parenteral nutrition in surgical patients. N Engl J Med 325:525–532
7. American College of Physicians (1989) Parenteral nutrition in patients receiving cancer chemotherapy. Ann Intern Med 110:734–6
8. Hadfield RJ, Sinclair DG, Houldsworth PE, Evans TW (1995) Effects of enteral and parenteral nutrition on gut mucosal permeability in the critically ill. Am J Respir Crit Care Med 152:1545–1548
9. Nakasaki H, Mitomi T, Tajima T, Ohnishi N, Fujii K (1998) Gut bacterial translocation during total parenteral nutrition in experimental rats and its countermeasure. Am J Surg 175:38–43
10. Shou J, Lappin J, Minnard EA, Daly JM (1994) Total parenteral nutrition, bacterial translocation, and host immune function. Am J Surg 167:145–150
11. Qiu JG, Delany HM, Teh EL, Freundlich L, Gliedman ML, Steinberg JJ, Chang CJ, Levenson SM (1997) Contrasting effects of identical nutrients given parenterally or enterally after 70% hepatectomy: bacterial translocation. Nutrition 13:431–437
12. Levine GM, Deren JJ, Steiger E, Zinno R (1974) Role of oral intake in maintenance of gut mass and disaccharide activity. Gastroenterology 67:975–982
13. Deitch EA (1990) Bacterial translocation of the gut flora. J Trauma 30:S184–S189
14. Langkamp-Henken B, Donovan TB, Pate LM, Maull CD, Kudsk KA (1995) Increased intestinal permeability following blunt and penetrating trauma. Crit Care Med 23:660–664
15. Deitch EA, Winterton J, Li M, Berg R (1987) The gut as a portal of entry for bacteremia. Role of protein malnutrition. Ann Surg 205:681–692
16. Sugiura T, Tashiro T, Yamamori H, Takagi K, Hayashi N, Itabashi T, Toyoda Y, Sano W, Nitta H, Hirano J, Nakajima N, Ito I (1999) Effects of total parenteral nutrition on endotoxin translocation and extent of the stress response in burned rats. Nutrition 15:570–575
17. Strubelt O, Dost-Kempf E, Siegers CP, Younes M, Volpel M, Preuss U, Dreckmann JG (1981) The influence of fasting on the susceptibility of mice to hepatotoxic injury. Toxicol Appl Pharmacol 60:66–77

18. Sandhu IS, Jarvis C, Everson GT (1999) Total parenteral nutrition and cholestasis. Clin Liver Dis 3:489–508
19. Kudsk KA, Li J, Renegar KB (1996) Loss of upper respiratory tract immunity with parenteral feeding. Ann Surg 223:629–635
20. Janu P, Li J, Renegar KB, Kudsk KA (1997) Recovery of gut-associated lymphoid tissue and upper respiratory tract immunity after parenteral nutrition. Ann Surg 225:707–715
21. King BK, Li J, Kudsk KA (1997) A temporal study of TPN-induced changes in gut-associated lymphoid tissue and mucosal immunity. Arch Surg 132:1303–1309
22. Li J, Kudsk KA, Gocinski B, Dent D, Glezer J, Langkamp-Henken B (1995) Effects of parenteral and enteral nutrition on gut-associated lymphoid tissue. J Trauma 39:44–51
23. Alverdy JC, Burke D (1992) Total parenteral nutrition: iatrogenic immunosuppression. Nutrition 8:359–365
24. Gogos CA, Kalfarentzos F (1995) Total parenteral nutrition and immune system activity: a review. Nutrition 11:339–344
25. Gogos CA, Kalfarentzos FE, Zoumbos NC (1990) Effect of different types of total parenteral nutrition on T-lymphocyte subpopulations and NK cells. Am J Clin Nutr 51:119–122
26. Sedman PC, Somers SS, Ramsden CW, Brennan TG, Guillou PJ (1991) Effects of different lipid emulsions on lymphocyte function during total parenteral nutrition. Br J Surg 78:1396–1399
27. Waitzberg DL, Lotierzo PH, Logullo AF, Torrinhas RS, Pereira CC, Meier R (2002) Parenteral lipid emulsions and phagocytic systems. Br J Nutr 87 [Suppl 1]:S49–S57
28. Maderazo EG, Woronick CL, Quercia RA, Hickingbotham N, Drezner AD (1988) The inhibitory effect of parenteral nutrition on recovery of neutrophil locomotory function in blunt trauma. Ann Surg 208:221–226
29. Granato D, Blum S, Rossle C, Le Boucher J, Malnoe A, Dutot G (2000) Effects of parenteral lipid emulsions with different fatty acid composition on immune cell functions in vitro. J Parenter Enteral Nutr JPEN 24:113–118
30. Okada Y, Papp E, Klein NJ, Pierro A (1999) Total parenteral nutrition directly impairs cytokine production after bacterial challenge. J Pediatr Surg 34:277–280
31. Lin MT, Saito H, Fukushima R, Inaba T, Fukatsu K, Inoue T, Furukawa S, Han I, Muto T (1996) Route of nutritional supply influences local, systemic, and remote organ responses to intraperitoneal bacterial challenge. Ann Surg 223:84–93
32. Petersen SR, Kudsk KA, Carpenter G, Sheldon GE (1981) Malnutrition and immunocompetence: increased mortality following an infectious challenge during hyperalimentation. J Trauma 21:528–533
33. Kudsk KA, Carpenter G, Petersen S, Sheldon GF (1981) Effect of enteral and parenteral feeding in malnourished rats with E. coli-hemoglobin adjuvant peritonitis. J Surg Res 31:105–110
34. Kudsk KA, Stone JM, Carpenter G, Sheldon GF (1983) Enteral and parenteral feeding influences mortality after hemoglobin-E. coli peritonitis in normal rats. J Trauma 23:605–609
35. Kudsk KA, Croce MA, Fabian TC, Minard G, Tolley EA, Poret HA, Kuhl MR, Brown RO (1992) Enteral versus parenteral feeding. Effects on septic morbidity after blunt and penetrating abdominal trauma. Ann Surg 215:503–511
36. Moore FA, Feliciano DV, Andrassy RJ, McArdle AH, Booth FV, Morgenstein-Wagner TB, Kellum JM Jr, Welling RE, Moore EE (1992) Early enteral feeding, compared with parenteral, reduces postoperative septic complications. The results of a meta-analysis. Ann Surg 216:172–183
37. Kalfarentzos F, Kehagias J, Mead N, Kokkinis K, Gogos CA (1997) Enteral nutrition is superior to parenteral nutrition in severe acute pancreatitis: results of a randomized prospective trial. Br J Surg 84:1665–1669
38. Abou-Assi S, Craig K, O'Keefe SJ (2002) Hypocaloric jejunal feeding is better than total parenteral nutrition in acute pancreatitis: results of a randomized comparative study. Am J Gastroenterol 97:2255–2262
39. Lyman B (2002) Metabolic complications associated with parenteral nutrition. J Infus Nurs 25:36–44
40. Meadows N (1998) Monitoring and complications of parenteral nutrition. Nutrition 14:806–808
41. Klein CJ, Stanek GS, Wiles CE, III (1998) Overfeeding macronutrients to critically ill adults: metabolic complications. J Am Diet Assoc 98:795–806
42. Lin MT, Saito H, Fukushima R, Inaba T, Fukatsu K, Inoue T, Furukawa S, Han I, Matsuda T, Muto T (1997) Preoperative total parenteral nutrition influences postoperative systemic cytokine responses after colorectal surgery. Nutrition 13:8–12
43. Basu R, Muller DP, Papp E, Merryweather I, Eaton S, Klein N, Pierro A (1999) Free radical formation in infants: the effect of critical illness, parenteral nutrition, and enteral feeding. J Pediatr Surg 34:1091–1095
44. Pitkanen O, Hallman M, Andersson S (1991) Generation of free radicals in lipid emulsion used in parenteral nutrition. Pediatr Res 29:56–59
45. Heyland DK, MacDonald S, Keefe L, Drover JW (1998) Total parenteral nutrition in the critically ill patient: a meta-analysis. JAMA 280:2013–2019
46. Marik PE, Karnack C (2001) The effect of enteral nutrition, parenteral nutrition and parenteral nutrition together with "trickle" feeds on mortality in critically ill ICU patients. Crit Care Med 29 [Suppl]:A126
47. Marik PE, Karnack C, Varon J (2002) The addition of trickle feeds reduces the complications associated with parenteral nutrition. Crit Care Shock 5:165–169
48. Braga M, Gianotti L, Gentilini O, Parisi V, Salis C, Carlo V (2001) Early postoperative enteral nutrition improves gut oxygenation and reduces costs compared with total parenteral nutrition. Crit Care Med 29:242–248
49. Pacelli F, Bossola M, Papa V, Malerba M, Modesti C, Sgadari A, Bellantone R, Doglietto GB, Modesti C, EN-TPN Study Group (2001) Enteral vs parenteral nutrition after major abdominal surgery: an even match. Arch Surg 136:933–936
50. Kennedy BC, Hall GM (2000) Metabolic support of critically ill patients: parenteral nutrition to immunonutrition. Br J Anaesth 85:185–187
51. Spencer CT, Compher C (2001) The development of TPN: an interview with pioneer surgical nutritionist Jonathan E. Rhodes, MD. J Am Diet Assoc 101:747–750
52. Marik PE, Zaloga GP (2001) Early enteral nutrition in acutely ill patients: a systematic review. Crit Care Med 29:2264–2270
53. Silk DB, Gow NM (2001) Postoperative starvation after gastrointestinal surgery. Early feeding is beneficial. BMJ 323:761–762
54. Lewis SJ, Egger M, Sylvester PA, Thomas S (2001) Early enteral feeding versus "nil by mouth" after gastrointestinal surgery: systematic review and meta-analysis of controlled trials. BMJ 323:773–776

Arthur S. Slutsky
Yumiko Imai

Ventilator-induced lung injury, cytokines, PEEP, and mortality: implications for practice and for clinical trials

Introduction

A mainstay in the supportive care of patients with acute lung injury (ALI)/acute respiratory distress syndrome (ARDS) is mechanical ventilation. However, a number of animal and clinical studies have demonstrated that mechanical ventilation itself can worsen preexisting lung injury and produce ventilator-induced lung injury (VILI). Although the most obvious clinical abnormalities of ALI/ARDS are related to lung function, the most common cause of death is dysfunction of other organs, termed multiple organ dysfunction syndrome (MODS) [1], which is commonly accompanied by the systemic inflammatory response syndrome (SIRS). SIRS/MODS is a complex syndrome, often precipitated and intensified by a series of events rather than a single event. Recent clinical trials have demonstrated that in patients with ARDS, protective ventilatory strategies are associated with decreased serum cytokine levels [2, 3], decreased levels of organ dysfunction [3, 4], and decreased mortality [3, 5], perhaps by partially mitigating the development of MODS [6].

There are a number of factors that can precipitate the development of ALI/ARDS, including sepsis, shock, trauma, and aspiration of gastric contents. Among these sepsis is the leading cause and the major contributor to mortality in most ICUs [1, 7, 8]. Thus investigation of the impact of ventilatory strategy in the context of sepsis is of great interest. In their contribution to *Intensive Care Medicine* Herrera and colleagues [9] take a molecular approach to the study of VILI, systemic inflammatory cytokines, and mortality using an in vivo rat sepsis model produced by cecal ligation and perforation. They found that the application of positive end-expiratory pressure (PEEP) above the lower inflection point (LIP) of the respiratory system pressure-volume curve decreased pulmonary and systemic inflammatory cytokines [tumor necrosis factor (TNF) α and interleukin (IL) 6] as well as mortality in septic animals ventilated with low tidal volume (V_T; 6 ml/kg), but when higher PEEP levels were applied with high V_T (20 ml/kg), cytokines and mortality increased. The strengths of the study are the use of a clinically relevant injury model of sepsis and the use of multiple endpoints including mortality. However, it would have been interesting to have had data on the effect of the ventilatory strategies on hemodynamics, especially with large V_T and PEEP. Mechanical ventilation, in particular application of PEEP and use of large V_T, can have detrimental effects on systemic and regional hemodynamics as well as on global oxygen delivery and consumption, as highlighted in many excellent reviews [10, 11, 12]. It is likely that the use of high tidal volumes in conjunction with the high PEEP levels led to significant hemodynamic consequences and contributed to the mortality in this group.

Surrogate endpoints

One of the major problems facing clinical researchers in the context of trials in mechanical ventilation and ARDS is the need to enroll very large numbers of patients if mortality is used as the primary endpoint. The recent ARDSNet trial required over 800 patients to detect a 22% (relative) reduction in mortality in patients with ARDS treated with smaller tidal volumes. As therapies

M.R. Pinsky et al. (eds.), *Applied Physiology in Intensive Care Medicine 2: Physiological Reviews and Editorials*,
DOI 10.1007/978-3-642-28233-1_38, © Springer-Verlag Berlin Heidelberg 2012

improve and as mortality decreases, studies with even more patients will be required to find a similar decrease in mortality. One approach to mitigate this serious problem is to identify appropriate surrogate (also called intermediate) endpoints that can be used instead of mortality. Cytokines/chemokines are reasonable candidates to act as surrogate endpoints since they are continuous variables and hence the sample size required to reach statistical significance would be expected to be substantially less than with a binary variable such as mortality. An important criterion for an intermediate endpoint is that it should have "biological plausibility," i.e., there should be a plausible mechanistic link by which changes in the surrogate endpoint could lead to changes in mortality. There is a growing body of evidence suggesting biological plausibility with respect to the use of cytokines in this regard. In vitro mechanical strain has been shown to cause release of a number of mediators from a variety of lung cells including alveolar epithelial cells, endothelial cells, macrophages, fibroblasts, and smooth muscle cells [13, 14, 15, 16, 17]. Ex vivo, injurious ventilatory strategies in both isolated non-perfused rat lungs and isolated perfused mouse lungs have demonstrated an increase in release of inflammatory mediators [18, 19]. In vivo, Chiumello and colleagues [20] found increases in pulmonary and systemic inflammatory cytokines (TNF-α and macrophage inflammatory protein 2) after injurious mechanical ventilation using an in vivo rat acid aspiration model. There are also human data indicating the potential importance of cytokines. Patients with ARDS randomized to receive a conventional mechanical ventilation strategy had higher levels of a number of BAL and serum cytokines than patients who received a protective ventilatory strategy with PEEP set above the LIP [2], as in the study by Herrera et al.

Recently it has been shown that inflammatory cytokines/chemokines can modulate apoptosis in various cell types [21], and increased apoptosis has been detected in animal models of cecal ligation and perforation [22, 23] as well as in patients dying of sepsis and MODS [24]. We have recently proposed a possible mechanism to explain the decreased MODS observed with a protective ventilatory strategy [25]. Using a rabbit acid aspiration model we found increases in kidney epithelial cell apoptosis in the animals treated with a relatively injurious ventilatory strategy. This increased apoptosis appeared to be related to soluble Fas ligand, a potent pro-apoptotic factor.

The key issue, however, in relation to whether cytokine levels are good surrogate markers in ventilation trials is whether they are correlated with mortality. In this regard the current study is both encouraging and discouraging. The group of patients who had the lowest mortality also had the lowest levels of TNFα and IL-6, but the group that had the highest mortality (large V_T and high PEEP) did not have the highest cytokine levels. This is not surprising. First, animals that died before 3 h did not have cytokine serum cytokine levels measured —if cytokines are important, this would bias the results against finding high levels in the group with the highest mortality. Second, even if cytokines are important in the context of the VILI, they are certainly not the only important factor. It is very likely that the high airway pressure group in the Herrera study had the worst hemodynamics which was likely a major contributing factor to mortality in this group. The use of surrogate markers will have to take into account major physiological derangements which play a major role in outcome. Finally, the current studies were of a short duration, and the major impact of increased cytocine levels would be on a much longer timeframe.

Increased alveolar-capillary permeability

One interesting question is the source of the increased systemic proinflammatory mediators in the study by Herrera. There is evidence that VILI induces cytokine release from epithelial cells in the lung [13, 14, 15, 16, 26], although macrophages and neutrophils are also likely to be quite important. Loss of compartmentalization of local pulmonary inflammatory mediators due to mechanical ventilation has been recently proposed. The alveolar barrier restricts transport of macromolecules of a size similar to that of cytokines (15–20 kDa). After secretion in the lung, cytokines such as TNF-α remain in the alveolar space and leak into the circulation only if there is injury of the alveolar barrier. Several investigators have shown that increased permeability of the alveolar-capillary interface, as a result of lung injury leads to the release of mediators into the circulation that would normally have remained compartmentalized within the alveolar space [27, 28]. Tutor and colleagues [27] employed an isolated perfused rat lung model in which they injected TNF-α into the lung and measured its appearance in the perfusate. They found that the perfusate TNF-α concentrations were increased only when alveolar-capillary permeability was increased and not in normal lung, suggesting that loss of compartmentalization of alveolar TNF-α could occur, but only in the context of damage to the alveolar-capillary membrane. Von Bethmann and colleagues [18] reported that in an isolated perfused murine lung model, ventilation with higher transpulmonary pressure (25 cmH_2O) vs. normal pressure (10 cmH_2O) led to a significant increase in concentration of both TNF-α and IL6 in the perfusate. As compartmentalization of the local pulmonary response is lost, systemic release of inflammatory mediators may promote the massive inflammatory response that underlies MODS.

Recently Stuber and colleagues [29] studied patients with ALI and found that switching to conventional mechanical ventilation (V_T of 12 ml/kg, PEEP of 5 cmH_2O)

from a lung protective strategy (V_T of 5 ml/kg, PEEP of 15 cmH_2O) was associated with a marked increase in plasma cytokine levels within 1 h, while plasma cytokine levels returned to baseline when lung protective settings were reestablished. In contrast, in 39 patients with normal lungs, without ARDS, Wrigge and colleagues [30] found that ventilation with a high V_T (15 ml/kg) and zero PEEP did not affect plasma levels of IL-6, TNF-α, IL-1 receptor antagonist, or IL-10. These data suggest that if the lung is normal, mechanical ventilation even with relatively large V_T is unlikely to increase alveolar capillary permeability and augment the pulmonary inflammatory response, leading to increased production of inflammatory mediators.

Clinical context

Are there any patient care lessons that we can take from the study by Herrera and colleagues? Of course, one cannot extrapolate directly from animal studies to humans, but bearing this caveat in mind it is useful to speculate on the clinical implications of this study. This study demonstrated that PEEP minimizes lung injury, minimizes cytokine levels, and most importantly minimizes mortality, as long as end-inspiratory stretch is minimized. These data are in accord with a large body of experimental and clinical evidence demonstrating the beneficial effects of PEEP on oxygenation, on lung injury, and on cytokine levels in acute lung injury. However, despite these data a recent epidemiological study of ventilator practice demonstrated that 8–16% of patients with ARDS are ventilated with *zero* PEEP [1]. We cannot determine from the Herrera et al. [9] study what the optimal PEEP level should be, but certainly based on this study and many others in the literatures it should not be zero!

The authors used PEEP levels based on the lower inflection point. The underlying physiological rationale underlying the use of PEEP is to try and ensure that the lung is recruited. The choice of PEEP a few cmH_2O higher above the LIP was thought to be reasonable approach to ensure recruitment, but evidence dating back to the middle 1960s [31], recent theoretical studies [32, 33, 34], and recent experimental studies [35, 36] suggest that this approach is not sufficient to ensure full recruitment of the lung. Unfortunately, the optimal approach to setting PEEP is currently not known. Hopefully other studies such as the study by Herrera and colleagues, followed by appropriate clinical studies will help us address this important clinical question.

Reference

1. Esteban A, Anzueto A, Frutos F, Alia I, Brochard L, Stewart TE, Benito S, Epstein SK, Apezteguia C, Nightingale P, Arroliga AC, Tobin MJ (2002) Characteristics and outcomes in adult patients receiving mechanical ventilation: a 28-day international study. JAMA 287:345–355
2. Ranieri VM, Suter PM, Tortorella C, De Tullio R, Dayer JM, Brienza A, Bruno F, Slutsky AS (1999) Effect of mechanical ventilation on inflammatory mediators in patients with acute respiratory distress syndrome: a randomized controlled trial. JAMA 282:54–61
3. Anonymous (2000) Ventilation with lower tidal volumes as compared with traditional tidal volumes for acute lung injury and the acute respiratory distress syndrome. The Acute Respiratory Distress Syndrome Network. N Engl J Med 342:1301–1308
4. Ranieri VM, Giunta F, Suter PM, Slutsky AS (2000) Mechanical ventilation as a mediator of multisystem organ failure in acute respiratory distress syndrome. JAMA 284:43–44
5. Amato MB, Barbas CS, Medeiros DM, Magaldi RB, Schettino GP, Lorenzi-Filho G, Kairalla RA, Deheinzelin D, Munoz C, Oliveira R, Takagaki TY, Carvalho CR (1998) Effect of a protective-ventilation strategy on mortality in the acute respiratory distress syndrome. N Engl J Med 338:347–354
6. Slutsky AS, Tremblay LN (1998) Multiple system organ failure. Is mechanical ventilation a contributing factor? Am J Respir Crit Care Med 157:1721–1725
7. Ware LB, Matthay MA (2000) The acute respiratory distress syndrome. N Engl J Med 342:1334–1349
8. Wyncoll DL, Evans TW (1999) Acute respiratory distress syndrome. Lancet 354:497–501
9. Herrera MT, Toledo C, Valladares F, Muros M, Díaz-Flores L, Flores C, Villar J (2003) Positive end-expiratory pressure modulates local and systemic inflammatory responses in a sepsis-induced lung injury model. Intensive Care Med http://dx.doi.org/10.1007/s00134-003-1756-5
10. De Backer D (2000) The effects of positive end-expiratory pressure on the splanchnic circulation. Intensive Care Med 26:361–363
11. Pinsky MR (2002) Recent advances in the clinical application of heart-lung interactions. Curr Opin Crit Care 8:26–31
12. Russell J A, Phang PT (1994) The oxygen delivery/consumption controversy. Approaches to management of the critically ill. Am J Respir Crit Care Med 149:533–537
13. Grembowicz KP, Sprague D, McNeil PL (1999) Temporary disruption of the plasma membrane is required for c-fos expression in response to mechanical stress. Mol Biol Cell 10:1247–1257
14. Mourgeon E, Isowa N, Keshavjee S, Zhang X, Slutsky AS, Liu M (2000) Mechanical stretch stimulates macrophage inflammatory protein-2 secretion from fetal rat lung cells. Am J Physiol Lung Cell Mol Physiol 279:L699–L706
15. Pugin J, Dunn I, olliet P, Tassaux D, Magnenat JL, Nicod LP, Chevrolet JC (1998) Activation of human macrophages by mechanical ventilation in vitro. Am J Physiol 275:L1040–L1050
16. Quinn D, Tager A, Joseph PM, Bonventre JV, Force T, Hales CA (1999) Stretch-induced mitogen-activated protein kinase activation and interleukin-8 production in type II alveolar cells. Chest 116:89S–90S

17. Vlahakis NE, Schroeder MA, Limper AH, Hubmayr RD (1999) Stretch induces cytokine release by alveolar epithelial cells in vitro. Am J Physiol 277:L167–L173
18. Bethmann AN von, Brasch F, Nusing R, Vogt K, Volk HD, Muller KM, Wendel A, Uhlig S (1998) Hyperventilation induces release of cytokines from perfused mouse lung. Am J Respir Crit Care Med 157:263–272
19. Tremblay L, Valenza F, Ribeiro SP, Li J, Slutsky AS (1997) Injurious ventilatory strategies increase cytokines and c-fos m-RNA expression in an isolated rat lung model. J Clin Invest 99:944–952
20. Chiumello D, Pristine G, Slutsky AS (1999) Mechanical ventilation affects local and systemic cytokines in an animal model of acute respiratory distress syndrome. Am J Respir Crit Care Med 160:109–116
21. Papathanassoglou ED, Moynihan JA, Ackerman MH (2000) Does programmed cell death (apoptosis) play a role in the development of multiple organ dysfunction in critically ill patients? a review and a theoretical framework. Crit Care Med 28:537–549
22. Hiramatsu M, Hotchkiss RS, Karl IE, Buchman TG (1997) Cecal ligation and puncture (CLP) induces apoptosis in thymus, spleen, lung, and gut by an endotoxin and TNF-independent pathway. Shock 7:247–253
23. Hotchkiss RS, Swanson PE, Cobb JP, Jacobson A, Buchman TG, Karl IE (1997) Apoptosis in lymphoid and parenchymal cells during sepsis: findings in normal a. Crit Care Med 25:1298–1307
24. Hotchkiss RS, Swanson PE, Freeman BD, Tinsley KW, Cobb JP, Matuschak GM, Buchman TG, Karl IE (1999) Apoptotic cell death in patients with sepsis, shock, and multiple organ dysfunction. Crit Care Med 27:1230–1251
25. Imai Y, Parodo J, Kajikawa O, de Perrot M, Fischer S, Edwards V, Cutz E, Liu M, Keshavjee S, Martin TR, Marshall JC, Ranieri VM, Slutsky AS (2003) Injurious mechanical ventilation and end-organ epithelial cell apoptosis and organ dysfunction in an experimental model of acute respiratory distress syndrome. JAMA 289:2104–2112
26. Tremblay LN, Miatto D, Hamid Q, Govindarajan A, Slutsky AS (2002) Injurious ventilation induces widespread pulmonary epithelial expression of tumor necrosis factor-alpha and interleukin-6 messenger RNA. Crit Care Med 30:1693–1700
27. Tutor J D, Mason CM, Dobard E, Beckerman RC, Summer WR, Nelson S (1994) Loss of compartmentalization of alveolar tumor necrosis factor after lung injury. Am J Respir Crit Care Med 149:1107–1111
28. Kurahashi K, Kajikawa O, Sawa T, Ohara M, Gropper MA, Frank DS, Martin TR, Wiener-Kronish JP (1999) Pathogenesis of septic shock in Pseudomonas aeruginosa pneumonia. J Clin Invest 104:743–750
29. Stuber F, Wrigge H, Schroeder S, Wetegrove S, Zinserling J, Hoeft A, Putensen C (2002) Kinetic and reversibility of mechanical ventilation-associated pulmonary and systemic inflammatory response in patients with acute lung injury. Intensive Care Med 28:834–841
30. Wrigge H, Zinserling J, Stuber F, von Spiegel T, Hering R, Wetegrove S, Hoeft A, Putensen C (2000) Effects of mechanical ventilation on release of cytokines into systemic circulation in patients with normal pulmonary function. Anesthesiology 93:1413–1417
31. Edward P, Radford JR (1964) Static mechanical properties of mammalian lungs. In: Wallace OF, Hermann R (eds) Handbook of physiology, sect 3, vol I. American Physiological Society, Washington, p 432
32. Hickling KG (2001) Best compliance during a decremental, but not incremental, positive end-expiratory pressure trial is related to open-lung positive end-expiratory pressure: a mathematical model of acute respiratory distress syndrome lungs. Am J Respir Crit Care Med 163:69–78
33. Hickling KG (1998) The pressure-volume curve is greatly modified by recruitment. A mathematical model of ARDS lungs. Am J Respir Crit Care Med 158:194–202
34. Hickling KG (2002) Reinterpreting the pressure-volume curve in patients with acute respiratory distress syndrome. Curr Opin Crit Care 8:32–38
35. Pelosi P, Goldner M, McKibben A, Adams A, Eccher G, Caironi P, Losappio S, Gattinoni L, Marini JJ (2001) Recruitment and derecruitment during acute respiratory failure: an experimental study. Am J Respir Crit Care Med 164:122–130
36. Kloot TE, Blanch L, Melynne YA, Weinert C, Adams AB, Marini JJ, Shapiro RS, Nahum A (2000) Recruitment maneuvers in three experimental models of acute lung injury. Effect on lung volume and gas exchange. Am J Respir Crit Care Med 161:1485–1494

Enrico Calzia
Peter Radermacher

Helium in the treatment of respiratory failure: why not a standard?

The idea of replacing inspired air by helium-oxygen mixtures for treatment of acute respiratory failure is not a new one. In fact, this therapeutic approach has been proposed since the 1930s [1]. According to basic physical laws, airway resistance is dictated by airway geometry as well as by the density and viscosity of the inspired gas mixture, and the physical qualities of inspired gases cannot be dissociated from the resistive properties of the airways. Consequently, when replacing nitrogen with helium airway, resistance is reduced mainly by a substantial decrease of inspired gas density, although viscosity increases slightly. Until now, a huge number of articles has been published reporting beneficial effects of helium-oxygen breathing in patients suffering from asthma or chronic obstructive pulmonary disease (COPD), especially highlighting the improvement in respiratory mechanics [2, 3].

In this issue of *Intensive Care Medicine* a new investigation on helium-oxygen breathing during an experimentally induced acute bronchospasm is presented by Watremez and co-workers [4]. Briefly, their study confirms the benefits with regard to respiratory mechanics, though gas exchange was slightly impaired under helium-oxygen breathing.

In view of this long history of fairly encouraging results, the question must be posed why inspired helium remains an experimental tool until today. First of all, however, a major merit of the authors of the current study needs to be mentioned here. In fact, they were able to improve the animal model of metacholine-induced bronchoconstriction successfully, as presented recently [5], in order to achieve a steady state of sufficient duration. In their case, this was an absolute must, since otherwise gas exchange analysis by means of the MIGET would be unreliable. This experiment, however, also reminds us that the attempt to maintain stable pathologic conditions for prolonged periods artificially is one of the most important properties of experimental models, but also the most difficult to achieve. In this regard, even the induction of bronchospasm by inhaled metacholine is not an easy-to-use experimental tool, even though it is used frequently due to its capacity to simulate such a life-threatening condition. Therefore, even the basic work done by Watremez and co-authors has to be considered as a major step forward. However, a potential limit of the currently presented investigation should also be mentioned: in fact, the porcine lung is well known to differ from the human one in terms of the absence of collateral ventilation. Therefore, gas exchange properties may not be fully comparable between the two species, thus potentially limiting the adequacy of the animal model presented [6].

Apart from these considerations, from a theoretical point of view a decrease in airway resistance during helium-oxygen breathing corresponds well to predictions from theoretical models developed in the 1960s in order to understand better the physical basis of the effects of density and viscosity of inspired gas mixtures on respiratory mechanics [7]. Therefore, the beneficial effects of helium on airway pressures and work of breathing in mechanically ventilated patients is based not only on numerous experimental observations but also on a well understood theory and represents the fundamental scope of this therapeutic approach. In contrast, further effects of helium-oxygen breathing on gas exchange cannot be theoretically predicted due to the complexity of gas trans-

M.R. Pinsky et al. (eds.), *Applied Physiology in Intensive Care Medicine 2: Physiological Reviews and Editorials*,
DOI 10.1007/978-3-642-28233-1_39, © Springer-Verlag Berlin Heidelberg 2012

port within the bronchial tree, which is governed by convection in the upper part, but also by diffusion in the lower segments [8].

Despite this complexity, which may be a major cause of the conflicting results obtained by the research on this topic so far, the literature also suggests that the effects of the physical properties of inhaled gases on pulmonary gas exchange are generally far less impressive when compared to respiratory mechanics. Interestingly, previous experimental data revealed a slightly more homogeneous intrapulmonary gas-mixing during the breathing of high density gases [9]. These results seem fairly surprising at first glance, but they further underscore the complexity of the interplay between convective and diffusive gas transport and gas exchange, suggesting at least partially a potential explanation for why gas exchange may indeed deteriorate when breathing a low density gas like helium and improve with high density gases like sulfur hexafluoride [10].

In summary, there is a large body of evidence that helium breathing may ameliorate severely compromised respiratory functions, mainly by reducing airway resistance. Since these benefits appears to be evident, the question should be posed again: what may be the clinical role of inhaled helium in the future? The first problem is that the currently available data on inhaled helium in severe respiratory disorders like acute asthma or acute exacerbations of chronic obstructive pulmonary disease are not sufficient to prove the benefit of this therapeutic approach clearly, especially with regard to long-term outcome [2, 3, 11]. Exactly for that reason, the widespread therapeutic use of helium-oxygen breathing has been discouraged until now. The second problem is the inspiratory oxygen concentration often required in critical situations: obviously when increasing oxygen concentration the helium fraction must correspondingly be reduced, thus limiting its potential benefits on respiratory mechanics.

The third problem, which is mentioned by most authors but is often considered as a marginal one, may indeed be a major impediment for further definition of the clinical role of inhaled helium: in most emergency or intensive care units the use of helium is not possible at all, since mechanical ventilators do not work properly once standard gas supply is replaced by gas mixtures with altered physical properties. Some relatively simple solutions have been proposed in order to overcome these problems, not only when using helium [12] but also with highly dense gases [13]. Basically, they proved that a sufficiently safe use of mechanical ventilators, even under modified conditions, was possible with the use of appropriate correction factors. Consequently, under experimental conditions helium can be applied safely, as already demonstrated by the authors of the current article themselves [12].

However, it must be strongly recommended that the use of mechanical ventilators under such modified conditions should be restricted to situations where the supervision of adequately experienced personnel is guaranteed. Thus, since inhaled helium has not been at all an easy-to-use tool until now, its use is currently restricted to relatively small clinical or experimental studies. Therefore, even in the future it may remain difficult to gain sufficient experience with inhaled helium in order to define its potential role based on clear evidence. Unfortunately, both the current lack of sufficient clinical evidence as well as the limits imposed by the use of helium with standard ventilators may reciprocally prevent decisive future developments in this field. Exactly for that reason, however, it is important to gain as much experience as possible on the effects of helium inhalation, in order to assess more clearly the possible role of this fairly promising therapeutic approach.

Apart from these problems and limitations, in the near future the role of helium-breathing may be reconsidered in view of the growing popularity of non-invasive ventilation, one of the most recent and promising pulmonary support tools developed over the last years. The clinical data on this topic are still limited, but they have revealed the very encouraging ability of helium-oxygen to reduce inspiratory efforts and improve breathing comfort in spontaneously breathing patients suffering from acute exacerbation of chronic obstructive pulmonary disease [14] or those recovering from prolonged mechanical ventilation during the immediate post-extubation period [15]. Interestingly, from a technical point of view, replacing nitrogen/oxygen by helium/oxygen during non-invasive ventilation may even offer the advantage of decreasing inspiratory efforts without the need of high support pressures, which may be a limitation of the non-invasive technique. Furthermore, once mechanical support and leak compensation has been based on a target pressure, as is usually the case with devices especially designed for non-invasive ventilation, the altered physical properties of the inhaled gas will interfere less with the function of the ventilator [13], thus presumably limiting the technical problems mentioned above.

References

1. Barach AL (1934) Use of helium as a new therapeutic gas. Proc Soc Exp Biol Med 32:462
2. Ho AMH, Lee A, Karmakar MK, Dion PW, Chung DC, Contardi LAH (2003) Heliox vs air-oxygen mixtures for the treatment of patients with acute asthma. A systematic overview. Chest 123: 882–890
3. Rodrigo GJ, Rodrigo C, Pollack CV, Rowe B (2003) Use of helium-oxygen mixtures in the treatment of acute asthma. A systematic review. Chest 123: 891–896

4. Watremez C, Liistro G, deKock M, Roeseler J, Clerbaux T, Detry B, Reynaert M, Gianello P, Jolliet P (2003) Effects of helium-oxygen on respiratory mechanics, gas exchange and ventilation-perfusion relationships in a porcine model of stable methacholine-induced bronchospasm. Intensive Care Med (http://dx.doi.org/10.1007/s00134-003-1779-y)
5. Watremez C, Roeseler J, deKock M, Clerbaux T, Detry B, Reynaert M, Gianello P, Jolliet P, Liistro G (2003) An improved porcine model of stable methacholine-induced bronchospasm. Intensive Care Med 29:119–125
6. Kuriyama T, Latham LP, Horwitz LD, Reeves JT, Wagner WW (1984) Role of collateral ventilation in ventilation-perfusion balance. J Appl Physiol 56: 1500–1506
7. Pedley TJ, Drazen JM (1986) Aerodynamic theory. In: Fishman AP, Macklem PT, Mead J, Geiger SR (eds) Handbook of physiology, Section 3: the respiratory system, Volume III. Williams and Wilkins, Bethesda, pp 41–54
8. Piper J, Scheid P (1986) Diffusion and convection in intrapulmonary gas mixing. In: Fishman AP, Macklem PT, Mead J, Geiger SR (eds) Handbook of physiology, Section 3: the respiratory system, Volume IV. Williams and Wilkins, Bethesda, pp 51–69
9. Schulz H, Schulz A, Eder G, Heyder J (1995) Influence of gas composition on convective and diffusive intrapulmonary gas transport. Exp Lung Res 21: 853–876
10. Gledhill N, Froese AB, Buick FJ, Bryan AC (1978) V_A/Q inhomogeneity and $AaDO_2$ in man during exercise: effects of SF_6 breathing. J Appl Physiol 45:512–515
11. Jolliet Ph, Tassaux D (2003) Usefulness of helium-oxygen mixtures in the treatment of mechanically ventilated patients. Curr Opin Crit Care 9:45–50
12. Tassaux D, Jolliet Ph, Thouret J-M, Roesler J, Dorne R, Chevrolet J-C (1999) Calibration of seven ICU ventilators for mechanical ventilation with helium-oxygen mixtures. Am J Respir Crit Care Med 160:22–32
13. Stahl W, Radermacher P, Calzia E (2000) Functioning of ICU ventilators under hyperbaric conditions – comparison of volume- and pressure-controlled modes. Intensive Care Med 26:442–448
14. Jaber S, Fodil R, Carlucci A, Boussarsar M, Pigeot J, Lemaire F, Harf A, Lofaso F, Isabey D, Brochard L (2000) Noninvasive ventilation with helium-oxygen in acute exacerbations of chronic obstructive pulmonary disease. Am J Respir Crit Care Med 161:1191–1200
15. Jaber S, Carlucci A, Boussarsar M, Fodil R, Pigeot J, Maggiore S, Harf A, Isabey D, Brochard L (2001) Helium-oxygen in the postextubation period decreases inspiratory effort. Am J Respir Crit Care Dis 164:633–637

Peter Varga
Richard Griffiths
René Chiolero
Gérard Nitenberg
Xavier Leverve
Marek Pertkiewicz
Erich Roth
Jan Wernerman
Claude Pichard
Jean-Charles Preiser

Is parenteral nutrition guilty?

Introduction

"Death by parenteral nutrition" was the title of the controversial editorial published in the June issue of *Intensive Care Medicine* by P.E. Marik and M. Pinsky [1]. One might believe that a real event was being described by the authors. Imagine our astonishment, which quickly turned to dismay, when we read the words: "...a poison or toxin is a substance that through its chemical action usually kills, injures or impairs an organism... and by this definition TPN meets all criteria of a poison/toxin, in the critically ill patient receiving parenteral nutrition." We are surprised and perturbed that the authors have missed some important issues regarding the nutrition of patients in intensive care units (ICUs), exchanging sensationalism for sound scientific discussion.

It would appear that the authors believe that the seriously ill patients in ICUs all over the world who due to their condition must receive total parenteral nutrition (TPN) are in fact being poisoned by their professional carers. This frightful accusation, which is a gross generalization and insinuation lacks in our view solid scientific evidence. Furthermore, it can potentially produce a great deal of harm by introducing possible confusion among intensivists and doubt among patients and relatives. Something that has been given safely to patients in ICUs and at home for many years cannot be called a poison. In contrast, anything used incorrectly or in excess may do harm. Exhibiting a dose response and toxicity with excess is a feature of most active therapies, especially in the ICU setting. Even normal food intake has these characteristics, as shown by Western morbidity and mortality changes subsequent to overfeeding. Indeed, overfeeding is easy to achieve with parenteral nutrition (PN), but there is no evidence that PN not given in excess is harmful. What is true with PN is the loss of the benefit related to normal eating, a benefit which cannot be achieved in the patients unable to feed enterally.

Even if we fully agree that enteral feeding should be preferred to PN in critically ill patients whenever possible, we would like to refute many of the arguments of the editorial suggesting that PN is a poison, using a scientific approach.

Proof of the toxicity of PN

No one argues that parenteral feeding is without inherent risks. Naturally over the past decades those working in this field became keenly aware of the potential clinical complications of TPN and established practical guidelines to minimize their impact. Many of the risks of indiscriminate and inappropriate use of PN have been recognized and demonstrated, and there is no doubt that they increase the chance of iatrogenic complications. However, it is possible to avoid such conditions as overfeeding, resulting in hyperglycemia, hypertriglyceridemia, uremia, metabolic acidosis, and electrolyte imbalances by conscientious monitoring and titrating the quality and quantity of nutrients provided. Careful cannulation and maintenance of sterile techniques will prevent or minimize infections or sepsis, immunosuppression can be attenuated by supplementation of glutamine, in

M.R. Pinsky et al. (eds.), *Applied Physiology in Intensive Care Medicine 2: Physiological Reviews and Editorials*,
DOI 10.1007/978-3-642-28233-1_40, © Springer-Verlag Berlin Heidelberg 2012

other words careful respecting guidelines will go a long way to reduce the rate of complication. Not surprisingly, several recent studies on TPN in surgical and critically ill patients report very low rates of metabolic complications. One of the real landmark outcome studies in recent years showed the great benefits of glycemic control in patients receiving early enteral nutrition or PN [2]. The use of closely applied, best evidence nutrition protocols was central to this process and involved enteral nutrition and PN. Such benefits seen in the long-stay patients would not have occurred if PN were a cumulative poison. Outcome was related to the tight glycemic control achieved, but this was established with insulin, and not by underfeeding. Interestingly, although parenterally fed patients required more insulin (+23%) to achieve normoglycemia, quality of glycemia control did not differ in enterally fed patients. We know that underfeeding by omitting lipids and delivering hypocaloric parenteral feeds prevents neither hyperglycemia nor its infectious complications [3], confirming the lack of the dose-related effected implied by the authors of the editorial.

There is a large body of evidence showing that enteral feeding is superior to parenteral feeding in trauma and surgical patients, particularly for septic morbidity. Marik and Pinsky cite the meta-analysis by Heyland et al. [4] on PN vs. no artificial nutrition and state that "in critically ill patients TPN almost doubles the risk of dying." This analysis covered 21 studies with surgical patients and only 6 studies with surgical patients requiring ICU management. Most of these studies had methodological problems: inclusion of non-critically ill surgical patients [5, 6], overfeeding in the PN group [7], combined parenteral and enteral feeding [7, 8], early postoperative parenteral feeding in unstable patients [9], and some probably no longer reflected current practice or were very old studies [9]. This suggests that the strength of evidence of this part of the meta-analysis is low. Similarly, a study of TPN published only as an abstract and quoted in the editorial [10], which seriously limits its impact, showed that the addition of trickle enteral nutrition to PN reduces the toxicity of TPN. This suggests, again, that the problem is not the toxicity of TPN, but that it may be more related to the absence of enteral feeding.

PN is often necessary in critically ill surgical patients

The authors state: "we believe that based on evidence, TPN has no place in the management of the critically ill who can otherwise be fed enterally" and then: "Enteral nutritional support may not be possible in patients with short-bowel syndrome. However, these patients are exceedingly rare." We do not agree with the authors' categorical statement, although it means that the authors accept the existence of patients who cannot be fed enterally. The working group of nutrition and metabolism of the European Society of Intensive Care Medicine (ESICM) has published in this journal a position paper on enteral nutrition describing the limit of enteral nutrition [11]. Also Berger et al. [12] have described the change in TPN and enteral nutrition in their surgical ICU during 10 years: in spite of the authors' conviction that enteral nutrition is the first choice, they found that there are still about 8–10% of the patients who need TPN because enteral nutrition is not possible or not safe. What should we do with them? Let them starve without nutritional support and then die of the complications? Drs. Marik and Pinsky offer little solutions to this problem!

All would agree that there is no place for PN in well nourished patients able to be fed adequately by the enteral route after a reasonable delay. The real problem is encountered when patients do not or can only poorly tolerate enteral feeding. Regrettably a large number of patients can be found in ICUs every day who for various reasons cannot tolerate adequate quantity and quality of nutrients enterally for *many* days. A recent survey by Preiser et al. [13] published in this journal on behalf of the Working Group of Nutrition and Metabolism of the ESICM found that among 2,774 ICU patients 23% were receiving PN! Let us not forget that underfeeding is a debt that must eventually be repaid and, as with all debts, it is made worse when it is compounded [14].

All routes of feeding should be used in ICU patients

We completely agree that all patients are to be fed as close to "normal" as possible, preferably by mouth, nasogastrically or postpylorically. We also agree that TPN should be complemented with enteral feeding when possible. We stand by our established opinion that malnourished patients who for whatever reason are unable to tolerate enteral feeding *must* be fed parenterally. When used wisely TPN can deliver adequate nutrition safely! Depriving the seriously ill of nutrition, underfeeding or starving them, is dangerous and therefore should be avoided. TPN and enteral nutrition are not mutually exclusive. It is our considered opinion that patients requiring nutritional support should be fed accordingly to the adequacy of gastrointestinal function [15].

All artificial nutrition modalities carry risks and this must be balanced with advantages to be gained. Encouraging adequate nutrition by any route is important, but an overzealous or inappropriate promotion of enteral feeding may blind one to its many risks [14]. Enteral feeding also has risks. Many studies show that most of the time enteral feeding provides only partial nutrition [16] for reasons that include setting targets too low, not using protocols [17], slow initiation, and a tendency to stop too readily [18].

It is unclear whether the authors of the editorial believe that the "nutrient cocktail" of amino acids, lipids, carbohydrates, vitamins, and trace elements are poisons or if the lack of intraluminal availability is the problem. The selected evidence that they cite, however, suggests that the nutrients are not to blame, but that the method of delivery is the culprit. The routes do matter and we agree normal is better than abnormal. They cite the elegant work of Li et al. [19] to show us the importance of luminal nutrition in mice. However, the authors fail to mention that the same laboratory demonstrated that the deleterious effects of the standard PN are due in part to its nutrient composition, since many of the features are prevented by the inclusion of glutamine in the amino acid mixture [19]. In addition, there is presently little evidence from clinical studies that TPN causes mucosal atrophy of the gut or bacterial translocation [20].

The central issue is whether there is solid evidence in the literature to support the view that TPN increases morbidity and mortality in the critically ill who cannot be fed enterally. We believe the evidence cited is weak. Indeed, as nearly all the data regarding the risks of TPN come from surgical studies, it is interesting that the authors confirm in the most recent studies that TPN is risk neutral. The authors fail to mention that there is very strong evidence from larger meta-analyses that failing to give PN to a malnourished patient unable to tolerate EN significantly increases mortality [21]. Heyland et al. [4] showed that TPN significantly reduced morbidity in *malnourished* patients. It is difficult to see how TPN could be considered a poison, and it is wiser to consider that this term comes from erroneous interpretations of studies suffering from important methodological biases [20]. It is difficult to see how TPN could be considered a poison! Well controlled studies in similar mixed-fed patients having enteral feed show that there is no evidence of harm but possible benefit from supplemental PN [22]. Drs. Marik and Pinsky, in other situations where good studies are lacking, would you agree with the scientific statement by us... and with a famous Nobel prize that "the absence of evidence is not the evidence of absence"?

Following the paper by Woodcock et al. [23] in which they state: "Indeed, now when correctly applied, the complications of parenteral feeding are less likely to result in death compared with those of enteral nutrition," we expected other editorials and reviews [14, 24], and after the statement "[T]he time has come for the EN vs. TPN to be finally laid to rest. Patients with questionable gastrointestinal function should be fed using a combination of EN and TPN. The enteral feed is increased or decreased according to tolerance of EN and TPN, with the TPN adjusted accordingly" [15]. According to Drs. Marik and Pinsky, it seems that we were wrong.

We are of course ready for further discussion based on sound scientific evidence. We definitely reject their statement: "In conclusion, for the intensivist the acronym 'TPN' may represent 'total poisonous nutrition'." This statement is neither correct nor justified. It has potentially disturbing effects and is unworthy of publication in a highly respected medical journal. It is also unworthy of the authors, whatever their aim was in the first place. We too have looked in a dictionary, namely the *Oxford English Dictionary 2003* and found a definition for poison more applicable to the editorial: wicked, dangerous; hateful, objectionable.

Say no more.

References

1. Marik PE, Pinsky M. Death by parenteral nutrition (2003) Intensive Care Med 29:867–869
2. Van den Berghe G, Wouters P, Weekers F, Verwaest C, Bruyninckx F, Schetz M, Vlasselaers D, Ferdinande P, Lauwers P, Bouillon R (2001) Intensive insulin therapy in the critically patient. N Engl J Med 345:1359–1367
3. McCowen KC, Friel C, Sternberg J, Chan S, Forse RA, Burke PA, Bistrian BR (2000) Hypocaloric total parenteral nutrition: effectiveness in prevention of hypoglycaemia and infectious complications—a randomised clinical trial. Crit Care Med 28:3606–3611
4. Heyland D, MacDonald S, Keefe L, Drover J (1998) Total parenteral nutrition in the critically ill patient. A meta-analysis. JAMA 280:2013–2019
5. Sandstrom R, Drott C, Hyltander A, Arfvidsson B, Schersten T, Wickstrom I, Lundholm K (1993) The effect of postoperative intravenous feeding (TPN) on outcome following major surgery evaluated in a randomized study. Ann Surg 217:185–195
6. Sax HC, Warner BW, Talamini MA, Hamilton FN, Bell RH Jr, Fischer JE, Bower RH (1987) Early total parenteral nutrition in acute pancreatitis: lack of beneficial effects. Am J Surg 153:117–124
7. Herndon DN, Barrow RE, Stein M, Linares H, Rutan TC, Rutan R, Abston S (1989) Increased mortality with intravenous supplemental feeding in severely burned patients. J Burn Care Rehabil 10:309–313
8. Chiarelli AG, Ferrarello S, Piccioli A, Abate A, Chini G, Berioli MB, Peris A, Lippi R (1996) Total enteral nutrition versus mixed enteral and parenteral nutrition in patients at an intensive care unit. Minerva Anestesiol 62:1–7
9. Abel R, Fischer J, Buckley M, Barnett G, Austen W (1976) Malnutrition in cardiac surgical patients: results of a prospective randomized evaluation of early postoperative parenteral nutrition. Arch Surg 111:45–50
10. Marik PE, Karnack C (2001) The effect of enteral nutrition, parenteral nutrition and parenteral nutrition together with "trickle" feeds on mortality in critically ill ICU patients. Crit Care Med 29 [Suppl]:A126

11. Jolliet P, Pichard C, Biolo G, Chiolero R, Grimble G, Leverve X, Nitenberg G, Novak I, Planas M, Preiser JC, Roth E, Schols AM, Wernerman J (1998) Enteral nutrition in intensive care patients: a practical approach. A position paper. Intensive Care Med 24:848–859
12. Berger MM, Chiolero RL, Pannatier A, Cayeux MC, Tappy L (1997) A 10-year survey of nutritional support in a surgical ICU: 1986–1995. Nutrition 13:870–877
13. Preiser JC, Berre J, Carpentier Y, Jolliet P, Pichard C, Van Gossum A, Vincent JL (1999) Management of nutrition in European intensive care units: results of a questionnaire. Intensive Care Med 25:95–101
14. Griffiths RD (2001) Nutrition in intensive care. give enough but choose the route wisely. Nutrition 17:53–55
15. Woodcock N, MacFie J (2002) Optimal nutritional support (and the demise of the enteral versus parenteral controversy). Nutrition 18:523–552
16. Adam S, Batson S (1997) A study of problems associated with the delivery of enteral feed in critically ill patients in five ICU's in UK. Intensive Care Med 23:261–266
17. Spain DA, McClave SA, Sexton LK, Adams JL, Blanford BS, Sullins ME, Owens NA, Snider HL (1999) Infusion protocol improves delivery of enteral tube feeding in the critical care unit. JPEN J Parenter Enteral Nutr 23:288–292
18. McClave SA, Sexton LK, Spain DA, Adams JL, Owens NA, Sullins MB, Blandford BS, Snider HL (1999) Enteral tube feeding in the intensive care unit: Factors impending adequate delivery. Crit Care Med 27:1252–1256
19. Li J, King BK, Janu PG, Renegar KB, Kudsk KA (1998) Glycyl-L-glutamine-enriched total parenteral nutrition maintains small intestine gut-associated lymphoid tissue and upper respiratory tract immunity. JPEN J Parenter Enteral Nutr 22:31–36
20. Nitenberg G (2000) Nutritional support in sepsis: still skeptikal? Curr Opin Crit Care 6:253–266
21. Braunschweig CL, Levy P, Sheean PM, Wang X (2001) Enteral compared with parenteral nutrition: a meta-analysis. Am J Clin Nutr 74:534–542
22. Bauer P, Charpentier C, Bouchet C, Nace L, Raffy F, Gaconnet N (2000) Parenteral with enteral nutrition in the critically ill. Intensive Care Med 26:893–900
23. Woodcock NP, Zeigler D, Palmer MD, Buckley P, Mitchell CJ, MacFie J (2001) Enteral versus parenteral nutrition: a pragmatic study. Nutrition 17:1–12
24. Griffiths RD (2003) Nutritional support in critically ill septic patients. Curr Opin Clin Nutr Metab Care 6:203–210

Michael R. Pinsky

Using ventilation-induced aortic pressure and flow variation to diagnose preload responsiveness

The recent literature has documented that both arterial pulse pressure [1] and left ventricular stroke volume variations [2] induced by positive-pressure ventilation are sensitive and specific markers of preload responsiveness. The greater the degree of flow or pressure variation over the course of the respiratory cycle for a fixed tidal volume, the more likely the subject is to increase their cardiac output in response to a volume challenge and the greater that increase may be. Slama et al. [3] report in this issue that in a rabbit model of graded hemorrhage measures of aortic flow variation during positive-pressure ventilation cardiac output will increase in response to volume expansion. Furthermore, aortic flow variation was more sensitive than aortic pulse pressure variation in describing this effect further into the hemorrhagic state, presumably because arterial tone also increased. Since measures of descending aortic flow, using an esophageal Doppler probe, can be made easily and continuously without the need for complex echocardiographic techniques, this observation is clinically relevant. These concepts have been previously commented upon in this journal [4] and elsewhere [5]; however, the overarching principals of this clinical tool have not been previously described. In retrospect, the above observations may seem intuitively obvious based on simple principles of heart–lung interactions [6] and initial clinical observations [7]. Still, there are several important caveats and limitations to this approach that need to be considered before the clinician proceeds to monitoring arterial pulse pressure or stroke volume variation during ventilation as a routine assessment of preload responsiveness.

Firstly, being preload responsive does not mean that the subject should be given a volume challenge. Normal subjects under general anesthesia without evidence of cardiovascular insufficiency are also preload responsive and do not need a volume challenge. The present author presumes that most of the people reading this article, if sedated and placed on mechanical ventilation, would also display aortic flow variation and be preload responsive; thus, the presence of positive-pressure-induced changes in aortic flow or arterial pulse pressure does not itself define therapy. Independent documentation of cardiovascular insufficiency needs to be sought before the clinician attempts fluid resuscitation based on these measures.

Secondly, these indices that quantify the variation in aortic flow, stroke volume, and arterial systolic and pulse pressures have routinely been demonstrated to outperform more traditional measures of left ventricular preload, such as pulmonary artery occlusion pressure, right atrial pressure, total thoracic blood volume, right ventricular end-diastolic volume, and left ventricular end-diastolic area [1, 2]. In fact, there appears to be little relation between these traditional measures of ventricular preload and preload-responsiveness. This finding also should hardly be surprising. Ventricular filling pressures poorly reflect ventricular volumes [8] and measures of absolute ventricular volumes do not define diastolic compliance [9]. Patients with small left ventricles that are also stiff, as may occur with acute cor pulmonale, tamponade, left ventricular hypertrophy and myocardial fibrosis, will show poor volume responsiveness, whereas patients with large left ventricular volumes, as often occurs with congestive heart failure and afterload reduction, may be quite volume responsive; thus, the second concept is that preload does not equal preload responsiveness. The probable reason why traditional measures of preload have displayed such poor predictive value in defining preload

M.R. Pinsky et al. (eds.), *Applied Physiology in Intensive Care Medicine 2: Physiological Reviews and Editorials*,
DOI 10.1007/978-3-642-28233-1_41, © Springer-Verlag Berlin Heidelberg 2012

responsiveness may be because they are indirect measures of the wrong parameter: left ventricular wall stress.

Thirdly, all the studies reported to date have used positive-pressure ventilation as a cyclic venous return forcing function. They all presume, though not all studies state this clearly, that for a subject to be preload responsive their intrathoracic cardiac performance must be globally responsive to dynamic changes in venous flow. Once again, this is intuitively obvious. If a patient has either severe right or left ventricular failure, then the small changes in venous pressure induced by the pressure forcing function of mechanical ventilation will not alter preload enough to cause changes in output; however, what is often forgotten is that for these aortic pressure and flow measures to detect any variations at all, the input forcing function must be great enough to alter the pressure gradients for right and left ventricular filling [10]. Although controversy exists as to the extent to which positive-pressure ventilation selectively alters either pulmonary venous flow [11] or right ventricular filling [12], all agree that a cyclic change must occur. Accordingly, if the increase in lung volume with each tidal breath is either not great enough to induce changes in pulmonary venous flow [13], or if the positive-pressure breath is associated with spontaneous inspiratory efforts that minimize the changes in venous return [14], then the cyclic perturbations to cardiac filling may not be great enough to induce the cyclic variations in left ventricular filling needed to identify preload responsiveness. Furthermore, one can take a preload-unresponsive patient whose aortic flow variation is <10% and make their flow variation >20% by increasing tidal volume from 8 to 20 ml/kg [7, 8]; thus, the third concept is that the means by which cyclic changes in lung volume and intrathoracic pressure are induced and the consistency of their change over time is a central aspect of the ground-state requirements in the use of cyclic variations in aortic flow and arterial pressure to identify preload responsiveness.

Fourthly, although the primary determinant of arterial pulse pressure variation over a single breath is left ventricular stroke volume variation because changes in aortic impedance and arterial tone cannot change that rapidly (12 of 15), over time this limitation no longer applies. As arterial tone decreases, for example, then for the same aortic flow and stroke volume both mean arterial pressure and pulse pressure will be less. Similarly, if arterial tone were to increase, as often occurs in response to hemorrhage, then for the same aortic flow arterial pressure will be greater. This is the probable reason why Slama et al. [3] observed that flow variation became more sensitive than pulse pressure variation as hemorrhage progressed. Finally, since aortic cross-sectional diameter is not fixed but varies during left ventricular ejection and with changes in aortic input impedance, aortic peak velocity changes do not equate with left ventricular stroke volume or descending aortic flow changes. Although most studies have shown that flow velocity variation thresholds of >15% predict preload responsiveness, and that this threshold is very close to the 13% threshold described for pulse pressure variation, these two measures have never been compared with each other in the same study. Accordingly, the limits of flow or pressure variation needed to identify preload responsiveness will be different if one uses peak aortic flow velocity, mean aortic flow, left ventricular stroke volume, or arterial pulse pressure measures to define preload responsiveness, especially if arterial tone is varying.

Fifthly, like many clinical indices of cardiovascular state, the ventilation-induced changes in left ventricular output and pulse pressure have been analyzed in retrospective studies. No study yet published has prospectively predicted which patients would be preload responsive based on these measures and then shown that their predictions were correct. This procedural limitation should be resolved shortly, as prospective clinical trials of these indices to predict preload responsiveness have recently been completed.

Finally, no monitoring tool, no matter how accurate, by itself has improved patient outcome. It is only with the thoughtful and titrated use of therapies known to improve outcome, but requiring information derived from such monitoring tools, will improved patient outcome realized by the use of these tools. We know that occult tissue hypoperfusion exists in critically ill patients and that appropriate and timely resuscitation improves outcome in all critically ill patients, whereas inappropriate and/or delayed resuscitation increases mortality. Accordingly, this new tool needs to be used in concert with proven therapeutic approaches that utilize its diagnostic power correctly. Thus, we are left with a new and robust, powerful, and clinically relevant diagnostic tool whose thoughtful application in the clinic is gaining acceptance and whose influence on future clinical trials using resuscitation therapies will need to be considered. Clinicians are urged to consider the above physiological limitations when applying these deceivingly simple measures at the bedside to define resuscitation decisions.

References

1. Michard F, Boussat S, Chemla D, Anguel N, Mercat A, Lecarpentier Y, Richard C, Pinsky MR, Teboul JL (2000) Relation between respiratory changes in arterial pulse pressure and fluid responsiveness in septic patients with acute circulatory failure. Am J Respir Crit Care Med 162:134–138
2. Reuter DA, Felbinger TW, Schmidt C, Kilger E, Goedje O, Lamm P, Goetz AE (2002) Stroke volume variation for assessment of cardiac responsiveness to volume loading in mechanically ventilated patients after cardiac surgery. Intensive Care Med 28:392–398
3. Slama M, Masson H, Teboul JL, Arnould ML, Nait-Kaoudjt R, Colas B, Peltier M, Tribouilloy C, Susic D, Frohlich E, Andrejak M (2004) Monitoring of respiratory variations of aortic flow velocity using oesophageal Doppler. Intensive Care Med (http://dx.doi.org/10.1007/s00134-004-2190-z)
4. Pinsky MR (2002) Functional hemodynamic monitoring: asking the right question. Intensive Care Med 28:386–388
5. Pinsky MR (2003) Probing the limits of arterial pulse contour analysis to predict preload-responsiveness. Anes Analg 96:1245–1247
6. Morgan BC, Martin WE, Hornbein TF, Crawford EW, Guntheroth WG (1966) Hemodynamic effects of intermittent positive pressure respiration. Anesthesiology 27:584–590
7. Rooke GA, Schwid HA, Shapira Y (1995) The effect of graded hemorrhage and intravascular volume replacement on systolic pressure variation in humans during mechanical and spontaneous ventilation. Anesth Analg 80:925–932
8. Hansen RM, Viquerat CE, Matthay MA, Wiener-Kronish JP, DeMarco T, Bahtia S, Marks JD, Botvinick EH, Chatterjee K (1986) Poor correlation between pulmonary arterial wedge pressure and left ventricular end-diastolic volume after coronary artery bypass graft surgery. Anesthesiology 64:764–770
9. Pinsky MR (2003) Clinical significance of pulmonary artery occlusion pressure. Intensive Care Med 29:175–178
10. Pinsky MR (1984) Determinants of pulmonary artery flow variation during respiration. J Appl Physiol 56:1237–1245
11. Vieillard-Baron A, Loubieres Y, Schmitt JM, Page B, Dubourg O, Jardin F (1999) Cyclic changes in right ventricular output impedance during mechanical ventilation. J Appl Physiol 87:1644–1650
12. Magder S, Lagonidis D, Erice F (2001) The use of respiratory variations in right atrial pressure to predict the cardiac output response to PEEP. J Crit Care 16:108–114
13. Romand JA, Shi W, Pinsky MR (1995)Cardiopulmonary effects of positive pressure ventilation during acute lung injury. Chest 108:1041–1048
14. Pinsky MR (1984) Instantaneous venous return curves in an intact canine preparation. J Appl Physiol 56:765–771
15. Sylvester JT, Gilbert RD, Traystman RJ, Permutt S (1981) Effects of hypoxia on the closing pressure of the canine systemic arterial circulation. Circ Res 49:980–987

Alain Nitenberg

Evaluation of left ventricular performance: an insolvable problem in human beings? The Graal quest

Evaluation of left ventricular function in human beings and its changes

What is needed to assess ventricular function with special reference to contractility indices from a physiological point of view? First, we have to measure pressures, and for a physiological interpretation of the data, pressures should be recorded with intravascular micromanometers. Second, we need to measure left ventricular volumes and to relate each pressure to the corresponding volume to calculate indices of left ventricular function. Third, as most of the contractility indices are frequency-, preload-, and afterload-dependent, we have to interpret the data taking into account these factors which are also very difficult to assess. All these concerns have been extensively discussed in recent decades and the use of very sophisticated invasive methods such as intracardiac micromanometers and impedance catheters have not totally solved the problems [1, 2, 3, 4]. Thus, when non-invasive methods, such as echocardiography and peripheral arterial pressure, are used the problem seems to be almost insolvable.

Volume loading has been demonstrated to enhance cardiac output by a mechanism called the Frank-Starling law of the heart [5, 6]. Briefly, when an increased quantity of fluid enters the heart, stretching of heart chambers results in an increased contraction of the myocardium that empties the ventricles to a larger extent [7]. In this issue, Kumar et al. report the effects of large volume saline infusion on left ventricular performance indices assessed by echocardiography in normal healthy volunteers. This is a very complicated study that shows that stroke volume and cardiac output are increased significantly because end-diastolic volume is increased and end-systolic volume is reduced. However, it must be pointed out that changes in left ventricular volumes measured by echocardiography (which is not a gold standard method for left ventricular volume measurements) are very small (2.8 ml/m^2 for end-diastolic volume, and 2.1 ml/m^2 for end-systolic volume), which brings into question the physiological relevance of such changes. Because there is a discrepancy between the changes of most of the presumed load-independent indices of contractility—increase in peak-systolic pressure-end-systolic volume index ratio and end-systolic pressure-end-systolic volume index ratio—and no change in end-systolic meridional wall stress/end-systolic volume index ratio, the authors conclude that the initial increase in stroke volume associated with high volume saline infusion is unlikely to represent a true increase in myocardial contractility and that the reduced afterload due to the decrease in blood viscosity might be the main determinant of the increased left ventricular performance. Unfortunately, the absence of blood viscosity and hemoglobin concentration measurements represents an important limitation of the study because it leads to a lot of supposition about changes in blood viscosity and afterload changes when no evaluation of afterload has been made [8, 9]. Indeed, what was the amount of fluid infusion participating in volume loading at the time of measurements? (It could have been of interest to measure diuresis at the time of measurements). Because increase in left ventricular end-diastolic volume and decrease in end-systolic volumes are comparable, the role of the Frank-Starling mechanism cannot be so easily totally excluded because it is well established that the Frank-Starling mechanism increases myocardial

M.R. Pinsky et al. (eds.), *Applied Physiology in Intensive Care Medicine 2: Physiological Reviews and Editorials*,
DOI 10.1007/978-3-642-28233-1_42, © Springer-Verlag Berlin Heidelberg 2012

contractility through two means [10, 11]: 1) when end-diastolic volume is increased, the distance between myofilaments is reduced and the generated force is increased; 2) the number of sarcomeres at the optimal length is increased by volume increase (length-dependent activation of contractile proteins). Moreover, the latest may also occur even when volume is not increased if the shape of the left ventricle is modified (increase in sphericity that can be evaluated by measuring the length/diameter ratio).

Apart from the fact that stroke work, ejection fraction, and fractional shortening are not true indices of contractility (these indices of left ventricular performance are pump function indices which are highly dependent on afterload), and that mean circumferential fractional shortening is not totally preload-independent, there are many limitations to this conclusion due to the way the contractility indices—supposed to be load-independent [12, 13]—were calculated. This is especially the case for end-systolic stress, where end-systolic pressure and end-systolic wall thickness need to be determined simultaneously [13, 14, 15, 16]. End-systolic pressure is very difficult to determine because this pressure is not the aortic pressure at incisura but it is close to peak left ventricular pressure, which may produce great changes in the value of end-systolic stress. On the other hand, although in many publications left ventricular volume is indexed to the body surface area, as suggested by Suga et al. [17], the means used to normalize values is still being discussed (body surface area, lean mass, left ventricular mass, etc.). Moreover, it is not certain that volumes should be indexed for calculation of the ratios used to evaluate left ventricular contractility (end-systolic pressure/end-systolic volume, end-systolic stress/end-systolic volume etc.) [18, 19, 20]. In this study, it must be pointed out that end-systolic stress-to-volume ratio is the only index of contractility that is not enhanced by volume loading, when all the others are increased. More accurate indices could have been calculated to verify that contractility was not involved in enhancement of stroke volume; for example, peak-systolic wall stress and peak-systolic meridional wall stress/end-systolic volume ratio, because end-systolic pressure is closer to peak-systolic pressure than to pressure at the incisura [21, 22, 23]. Another important point is that, as defined by Sagawa et al. [24], end-systole is the point where the left ventricular pressure-volume ratio is maximum when end-ejection occurs when left ventricular volume is minimal, which happens before aortic closure. Last, the end-systolic-derived indices used in this study represent only one coordinate of the end-systolic pressure-volume relationships that do not take into account V_o, the volume at the intercept of the volume axis of the relationship between end-systolic pressure and volume. Thus, small changes in V_o may have a great impact on the slope of the relation which is the true index of contractility: V_o is decreased when contractility is increased and is increased when end-diastolic volume is increased, which makes the conclusion very difficult to uphold in the absence of its determination.

Another point raised by this study which is not discussed by the authors is the potential changes in sympathetic drive that could have been produced by hemodilution and the consecutive decrease in oxygen transport capacity. Apparently, because heart rate did not vary significantly at 3 h, sympathetic stimulation could have been counterbalanced by a parasympathetic stimulation due to stimulation of ventricular mechanoreceptors by end-diastolic volume increase.

In conclusion, when changes in numerous indices are statistically significant but rather moderate and contradictory, the clinical and physiological relevance of the changes should be taken with caution, especially because the accuracy of the non-invasive methods used to achieve the measurements that are involved in calculation of left ventricular function indices are very poor. This could have produced errors that are more important than the changes observed. These results should also be confirmed by using more sophisticated methods, mainly for measurements of left ventricular volume by invasive [25, 26, 27] and non-invasive methods [28, 29, 30], before reaching a definitive conclusion. Whatever the future, we are condemned to obtain information with imperfect tools and to use our brain, especially in patients with unstable hemodynamics in intensive care units.

References

1. Falsetti HL, Mates RE, Grant C, Greene DG, Bunnell IL (1970) Left ventricular wall stress calculated from one plane cineangiography: an approach to force-velocity analysis in man. Circ Res 26:71–83
2. Mehmel HC, Stockins B, Ruffman K, Olshausen K, Schuler G, Kubler W (1981) The linearity of the end-systolic pressure-volume relationship in man and its sensitivity for assessment of left ventricular function. Circulation 63:1216–1222
3. Carabello BA, Spann JF (1984) The uses and limitation of end-systolic indexes of left ventricular function. Circulation 69:1058–1064
4. Asanoi H, Sasayama S, Kameyama T (1989) Ventriculoarterial coupling in normal and failing heart in humans. Circ Res 65:483–493

5. Starling EH (1918) The Linacre lecture of the law of the heart. Longmans, Green, London
6. Guyton AC (1991) Cardiac output, venous return, and their regulation. In: Textbook of medical physiology, 8th edn. Saunders, Philadelphia, pp 321–334
7. Kumar A, Anel R, Bunnell E, Habet K, Neumann A, Wolff D, Rosenson R, Cheang M, Parrillo JE (2004) Effect of large volume infusion on left ventricular volumes, performance, and contractility parameters in normal volunteers. Intensive Care Med (http://dx.doi.org/10.1007/s00134-004-2191-y)
8. Elzinga G, Westerhof N (1973) Pressure and flow generated by the left ventricle against different impedences. Circ Res 32:178–186
9. Saba PS, Roman MJ, Ganau A, Pini R, Jones EC, Pickering TG, Devereux RB (1995) Relationship of effective arterial elastance to demographic and arterial characteristics in normotensive and hypertensive adults. J Hypertens 13:971–977
10. Moss RL, Fitzsimons DP (2002) Frank-Starling relationship. Long on importance, short on mechanism. Circ Res 90:11–13
11. Konhilas JP, Irving TC, de Tombe PP (2002) Myofilament calcium sensitivity in skinned rat cardiac trabeculae: role in interfilament spacing. Circ Res 90:59–65
12. Suga H, Sagawa K, Shoukas AA (1973) Load independence of the instantaneous pressure-volume ratio of the canine left ventricle and effects of epinephrine and heart rate on the ratio. Circ Res 32:314–322
13. Sagawa K, Suga H, Shoukas AA, Bakalar KM (1977) End-systolic pressure-volume ratio: a new index of ventricular contractility. Am J Cardiol 40:748–753
14. Suga H, Sagawa K (1974) Instantaneous pressure-volume relationships and their ratio in the excised supported canine left ventricle. Circ Res 35:117–126
15. Suga H, Igarashi Y, Yamada O, Goto Y (1985) Mechanical efficiency of the left ventricle as a function of preload, afterload, and contractility. Heart Vessels 1:3–8
16. Starling MR, Walsh RA, Dell'Italia IJ, Mancini GBJ, Lasher JC, Lancaster JL (1987) The relationship of various measures of end-systole to left ventricular maximum time-varying elastance in man. Circulation 76:32–43
17. Suga H, Hisano R, Goto Y, Yamada O (1984) Normalization of end-systolic pressure-volume relation and Emax of different sized hearts. Jpn Circ J 48:136–143
18. Belcher P, Boerboom IE, Olinger GN (1985) Standardization of end-systolic pressure-volume relation in the dog. Am J Physiol 249:H547-H553
19. Foult JM, Loiseau A, Nitenberg A (1990) Size dependence of end-systolic stress/volume ratio in humans: implications for evaluation of myocardial contractile performance in pressure and volume overload. J Am Coll Cardiol 16:124–129
20. Nitenberg A, Loiseau A, Antony I (2001) Left ventricular mechanical efficiency in hypertensive patients with and without increased myocardial mass and with normal pump function. Am J Hypertens 14:1231–1238
21. Takahashi M, Sasayama S, Kawai C, Kotoura H (1980) Contractile performance of the hyprtrophied ventricle in patients with systemic hypertension. Circulation 62:116–126
22. de Simone G, Devereux RB, Roman MJ, Ganau A, Saba PS, Alderman MH, Laragh JH (1994) Assessment of left ventricular function by the midwall fractional shortening/end systolic stress relation in human hypertension. J Am Coll Cardiol 23:1444–1451
23. De Simone G, Devereux RB, Koren MJ, Mensah GH, Casale PN, Laragh JH (1996) Midwall left ventricular mechanics. An independent predictor of cardiovascular risk in arterial hypertension. Circulation 93:259–265
24. Sagawa K (1978) The ventricular pressure-volume diagram revisited. Circ Res 43:677–687
25. Lankford EB, Kass DA, Maughan WL, Shoukas AA (1990) Does volume catheter parallel conductance vary during a cardiac cycle? Am J Physiol 258:H1933-H1942
26. Gopakumaran B, Osborn P, Petre JH, Murray PA (1997) A new technique to measure and track blood resistivity in intracardiac impedance volumetry. J Clin Monit 13:363–371
27. Arthur W, Kaye GC (2001) Clinical use of intracardiac impedance: current applications and future perspectives. Pacing Clin Electrophysiol 24:500–506
28. McKay RG, Miller MJ, Ferguson JJ, Momomura S, Sahagian P, Grossman W, Pasternak RC (1986) Assessment of left ventricular end-systolic pressure-volume relations with an impedance catheter and transient use of this system in the evaluation of the cardiotonic effects of dobutamine, milrinone, posicor and epinephrine. J Am Coll Cardiol 8:1152–1160
29. Belardinelli R, Ciampani N, Costantini C, Blandini A, Purcaro A (1996) Comparison of impedance cardiography with thermodilution and direct Fick methods for noninvasive measurement of stroke volume and cardiac output during incremental exercise in patients with ischemic cardiomyopathy. Am J Cardiol 77:1293–1301
30. Staal EM, Steendijk P, Baan J (2003) The trans-cardiac conductance method for on-line measurement of left ventricular volume: assessment of parallel conductance offset volume. Trans Biomed Eng 50:234–240

Philippe Vignon

Evaluation of fluid responsiveness in ventilated septic patients: back to venous return

Introduction

Adequate tissue perfusion and oxygen delivery is the primary goal of the therapeutic management of patients with circulatory failure. Cardiac output—a major determinant of oxygen delivery—is the result of the interaction between the cardiac pump and venous return. Since cardiac output must equal the volume of blood entering the heart, an increase in venous return will increase cardiac output, provided that the venous return curve intersects with the ascending limb of the cardiac function curve [1]. This defines the preload dependence of the heart. In contrast, a further increase in preload when the heart operates on the flat portion of its function curve fails to increase cardiac output and results in increased filling pressure with potential deleterious venous congestion. Importantly, there is no fluid responsiveness of the left ventricle (LV) without right ventricular (RV) preload dependence [2]. A pivotal clinical question frequently raised is, therefore, the evaluation of RV ability to increase its output significantly in response to a fluid challenge. Another clinical question even more challenging to address is to determine if the patient *really* needs a higher cardiac output to improve his current condition.

Venous return and mechanical ventilation

Venous return is determined by the pressure gradient between the mean systemic pressure—the forward pressure that drives back the blood to the heart through the venous resistance—and the right atrial (RA) pressure that represents the back-pressure [3]. Accordingly, blood volume expansion increases the venous return as long as the mean systemic pressure increases more than the RA pressure.

When compared to normal breathing, positive-pressure ventilation increases both the pleural and RA pressures. As a result, decreased pressure gradient for venous return is presumed to participate to the decrease of cardiac output frequently observed under tidal ventilation [1]. In addition, changes in intra-abdominal pressure may also alter venous return, since the rise in pleural pressure induced by positive-pressure ventilation is partially transmitted to the abdomen [4]. The cyclic effect of tidal ventilation on venous return is predominantly influenced by the transmural pressure of both the superior (SVC) and inferior vena cava (IVC). Vena cava transmural pressure is determined by the intravascular pressure—that, in turn, depends on the circulating blood volume and RV function—and by the surrounding pressure (i.e., the intrathoracic pressure for SVC and the intra-abdominal pressure for IVC). Accordingly, echocardiographic assessment of respiratory changes in vena cava caliber promises to yield valuable information on venous return in ventilated patients [5, 6]. In this issue of *Intensive Care Medicine*, three clinical studies convincingly demonstrate that the respiratory variation of SVC [7] and IVC diameters [8, 9], measured using M-mode echocardiography, allow the accurate prediction of fluid responsiveness in septic, ventilated patients.

M.R. Pinsky et al. (eds.), *Applied Physiology in Intensive Care Medicine 2: Physiological Reviews and Editorials*, DOI 10.1007/978-3-642-28233-1_43, © Springer-Verlag Berlin Heidelberg 2012

Respiratory variation of superior vena cava diameter

Due to cyclic variations of pleural pressure induced by tidal ventilation, the SVC diameter is minimal during inspiration and maximal at expiration [5]. In 66 ventilated patients with sepsis and circulatory failure, Vieillard-Baron et al. [7] measured the respiratory variation of SVC diameter expressed as a percentage using transesophageal echocardiography (TEE). Interestingly, a large respiratory variation of SVC diameter (>50%) was predominantly observed in the group of responders to a fluid challenge, whereas SVC collapsibility remained below 30% in most of the non-responders. A threshold value of 36% of SVC collapsibility allowed the separation of responders from non-responders with a sensitivity of 90% and a specificity of 100% [7]. Importantly, in the same study population, six false-positive results of pulse pressure variation to predict fluid responsiveness were equally attributed to a marked inspiratory increase in pulse pressure (rather than a decrease during early expiration) and to the presence of an acute cor pulmonale. This lack of specificity is presumably attributable to the frequency of failing ventricles in septic, ventilated patients [10].

In the presence of a congestive LV failure, tidal ventilation not only increases left-sided preload but also may reduce LV afterload, thereby facilitating stroke output [11]. This may increase the respiratory variation of pulse pressure, especially during inspiration, as noted in three patients in the study by Vieillard-Baron et al. [7]. In ventilated patients with severe RV failure, marked expiratory variation of pulse pressure may reflect an augmented inspiratory decrease of RV stroke volume due to transiently increased outflow impedance [12] rather than hypovolemia, as in the patients described with severe acute cor pulmonale [7]. In complex hemodynamic settings such as septic shock, TEE has the unparalleled advantage over other "blind" techniques of allowing an integrated approach of circulatory failure that includes the evaluation of both RV and LV function, as well as accurate estimation of pulmonary artery pressure. In the presence of failing ventricles and resulting high RA pressure, TEE would presumably disclose a low SVC collapsibility consistent with the absence of cardiac preload dependence, as observed in the current study [7].

Respiratory variations of inferior vena cava diameter

In this issue of *Intensive Care Medicine*, two clinical studies sought to evaluate the ability of respiratory changes in IVC diameter to predict fluid responsiveness in ventilated patients with severe sepsis or septic shock [8, 9]. Both studies showed that a marked inspiratory increase in IVC diameter, measured using M-mode imaging from the subcostal view, was consistent with a preload dependence of the heart. Feissel et al. [8] observed that respiratory variations of IVC diameter of more than 12% allowed differentiation between responders to a fluid challenge and non-responders with positive and negative predictive values of 93% and 92%, respectively. Using a different index of variability, Barbier et al. [9] showed that a threshold value of 18% allowed the prediction of fluid responsiveness with 90% sensitivity and specificity.

The IVC diameter is principally determined by its transmural pressure that, in turn, greatly depends on the level of backward pressure (i.e., RA pressure) and on intra-abdominal pressure [13] rather than pleural pressure, because the intrathoracic segment of this vessel is virtual. Since the cyclic rise in pleural pressure induced by tidal ventilation increases the intramural pressure of both RA and IVC on the one hand, and only a minor proportion of airway pressure is transmitted to the abdomen on the other hand [4], IVC transmural pressure increases at inspiration and the vessel tends to dilate. Although in the current studies respiratory variations of the IVC diameter were amplified in preload-dependent patients [8, 9], they may be reduced, or even abolished, in the presence of elevated RA pressure and fully distended—hence less compliant—IVC as a result of hypervolemia, RV dysfunction or severe pulmonary hypertension. In none of the latter clinical settings, however, would a fluid challenge result in a relevant increase of RV output.

Limitations

The same limitations of the use of respiratory changes in systolic arterial pressure, pulse pressure or LV stroke volume to predict fluid responsiveness [14, 15] apply when measuring the respiratory variation of the vena cava diameter. Firstly, patients must be ventilated in the volume-controlled mode and strictly adapted to the ventilator. Practically, patients should be deeply sedated or paralyzed to preclude any voluntary ventilatory efforts (i.e., inspiratory triggered breaths or active expiratory efforts). Secondly, the volume of tidal breaths influences changes in intrathoracic pressure and associated cyclic hemodynamic variations [16]. One may therefore argue that respiratory variation of the vena cava diameter should be cautiously interpreted when small tidal volumes and high levels of PEEP are used [6]. However, tidal volume also influences fluid responsiveness by shifting the ventricular function curve relative to the venous return curve [1, 17]. In fact, respiratory variation of the vena cava caliber reflects the effects of specific ventilator settings (according to patient condition) on venous return at one point in time. Thirdly, clinical situations associated with increased intra-abdominal pressure (e.g., obesity, abdominal trauma, laparotomized patients) may potentially invalidate the use of respiratory variation in the vena cava (especially IVC) diameter to predict fluid responsiveness. Unfortunately, the intra-abdominal pressure was not measured in all patients of the current studies [8, 9]. Lastly, all three studies published in the current issue of *Intensive Care Medicine* [7, 8, 9] enrolled septic patients who presumably were in sinus rhythm, a crucial criterion of validity for the use of dynamic indices to evaluate fluid responsiveness in ventilated patients [14]. Whether respiratory variation of the vena cava diameter remains valid in predicting RV preload dependence in patients with arrhythmia (e.g., atrial fibrillation) or with cardiopulmonary diseases deserves further studies. All these limitations highlight the fact that respiratory variation of the vena cava diameter will not be a usable marker of venous return in a significant proportion of ventilated critically ill patients.

Clinical relevance

Before embracing respiratory variation of the vena cava diameter as a definite marker of fluid responsiveness, the promising results herein reported should now be validated prospectively in larger cohorts of patients and in other acute conditions than sepsis. Moreover, their clinical impact remains to be determined. In patients with circulatory failure, objective (i.e., quantitative) criteria of fluid responsiveness may help in guiding therapeutic management because the sole clinical judgment fails to identify hypovolemia accurately in a large proportion (59%) of patients [8]. However, as recently emphasized by Magder [15], the potential fluid responsiveness of a given patient does not mean that he *actually* requires blood volume expansion. In patients with shock, the primary goal of acute care should not be to "normalize" a dynamic index of preload dependence, but rather to optimize oxygen delivery and tissue perfusion in order to meet the metabolic demands of the organism, if necessary by increasing cardiac output with volume loading. Accordingly, respiratory variation of the vena cava diameter should be considered as a promising additional tool in the assessment of hemodynamically unstable patients using echocardiography, rather than a quantitative parameter to alter with volume expansion until a target value is reached. We should keep in mind that the (subjective) clinical evaluation of critically ill patients must not be supplanted by the easier access to quantitative (objective) parameters of fluid responsiveness.

Acknowledgements The author gratefully thanks Bernard Cholley, MD, PhD, for his constructive critique of this manuscript.

References

1. Magder S (1993) Shock physiology. In: Pinsky MR, Dhainault JF (eds) Physiological foundations of critical care medicine. Williams and Wilkins, Philadelphia, pp 140–160
2. Magder S (1998) More respect for the CVP. Intensive Care Med 24:651–653
3. Guyton AC, Lindsey AW, Abernathy B, Richardson T (1957) Venous return at various atrial pressures and the normal venous return curve. Am J Physiol 189:609–615
4. Van Den Berg PCM, Jansen JRC, Pinsky MR (2002) Effect of positive pressure on venous return in volume loaded cardiac surgical patients. J Appl Physiol 92:1223–1231
5. Vieillard-Baron A, Augarde R, Prin S, Page B, Beauchet A, Jardin F (2001) Influence of superior vena cava zone condition on cyclic changes in right ventricular outflow during respiratory support. Anesthesiology 95:1083–1088
6. Mitaka C, Nagura T, Sakanishi N, Tsunoda Y, Amaha K (1989) Two-dimensional echocardiographic evaluation of inferior vena cava, right ventricle and left ventricle during positive-pressure ventilation with varying levels of positive end-expiratory pressure. Crit Care Med 17:205–210
7. Vieillard-Baron A, Chergui K, Rabiller A, Peyrouset O, Page B, Beauchet A, Jardin F (2004) Superior vena cava collapsibility as a gauge of volume status in ventilated septic patients. Intensive Care Med (http://dx.doi.org/10.1007/s00134-004-2361-y)
8. Feissel M, Michard F, Faller JP, Teboul JL (2004) The respiratory variation in inferior vena cava diameter as a guide to fluid therapy. Intensive Care Med (http://dx.doi.org/10.1007/s00134-004-2233-5)
9. Barbier C, Loubières Y, Schmit C, Hayon J, Ricôme JL, Jardin F, Vieillard-Baron A (2004) Ability of respiratory changes in inferior vena cava diameter to predict fluid responsiveness in ventilated septic patients. Intensive Care Med (http://dx.doi.org/10.1007/s00134-004-2259-8)
10. Charpentier J, Luyt CE, Fulla Y, Vinsonneau C, Cariou A, Grabar S, Dhainaut JF, Mira JP, Chiche JD (2004) Brain natriuretic peptide: a marker of myocardial dysfunction and prognosis during severe sepsis. Crit Care Med 32:660–665
11. Perel A (1998) Assessing fluid responsiveness by the systolic pressure variation in mechanically ventilated patients. Anesthesiology 89:1309–1310
12. Vieillard-Baron A, Loubières Y, Schmitt JM, Page B, Dubourg O, Jardin F (1999) Cyclic changes in right ventricular output impedance during mechanical ventilation. J Appl Physiol 87:1644–1650
13. Takata M, Wise RA, Robotham JL (1990) Effect of abdominal pressure on venous return: abdominal vascular zone conditions. J Appl Physiol 69:1961–1972
14. Bendjelid K, Romand JA (2003) Fluid responsiveness in mechanically ventilated patients: a review of indices used in intensive care. Intensive Care Med 29:352–360
15. Magder S (2004) Clinical usefulness of respiratory variations in arterial pressure. Am J Respir Crit Care Med 169:151–155
16. Reuter DA, Bayerlein J, Goepfert MSG, Weis FC, Kilger E, Lamm P, Goetz AE (2003) Influence of tidal volume on left ventricular stroke volume variation measured by pulse contour analysis in mechanically ventilated patients. Intensive Care Med 29:476–480
17. Michard F, Teboul JL, Richard C (2003) Influence of tidal volume on stroke volume variations. Does it really matter? Intensive Care Med 29:1613

Sangeeta Mehta
Stefano Nava

Mask ventilation and cardiogenic pulmonary edema: "another brick in the wall"

Current guidelines for the treatment of acute (ACPE) cardiogenic pulmonary edema (CPE) do not include the use of noninvasive ventilation (NIV) [1, 2, 3] as a primary treatment. Nevertheless, both continuous positive airway pressure (CPAP) and pressure support ventilation (nPSV) delivered by mask are commonly employed for the treatment of ACPE [4, 5] because NIV rapidly improves vital signs and reduces the need for endotracheal intubation compared to standard medical therapy [5, 6].

What was known so far?

An early systematic review of three published randomized trials concluded that the evidence supports the use of CPAP in patients with ACPE [7]. In two subsequent prospective randomized studies nPSV more rapidly improved vital signs [8, 9] than usual medical care, and one of these studies found a reduction in intubation rate [8]. Recently Park et al. [10] reported that both CPAP and nPSV are equally effective in reducing intubation rate and 15-day mortality compared with standard care. However, an earlier study [11] conducted in a smaller population demonstrated a better clinical outcome using CPAP. The first study to compare CPAP and nPSV [12] found a higher incidence of myocardial infarction using nPSV; however, this finding has not been confirmed in subsequent studies [8, 9, 10, 11].

Uncontrolled studies [13, 14] have noted that patients who respond to nPSV have a higher baseline carbon dioxide than those who do not respond, suggesting that this strategy is of potential benefit only in patients affected by chronic pulmonary diseases or by disorders in which respiratory muscles are likely to be fatigued. In a recent large prospective randomized trial nPSV resulted in more rapid improvements in dyspnea, respiratory frequency, and PaO_2/FIO_2 ratio than standard medical therapy, and a reduction in intubation rate only in the hypercapnic subgroup [9]. This is in keeping with findings in other forms of respiratory failure, such as community acquired pneumonia [15, 16].

What is new?

It is clear that both CPAP and nPSV effectively treat acute respiratory failure due to CPE [10]. However, the question remains: is one mode of mask ventilation better? To evaluate this question Bellone et al. [17] randomized 36 patients with ACPE and hypercapnia, excluding those with chronic obstructive pulmonary diseases, to nPSV (15/5 cmH_2O) or CPAP (10 cmH_2O). The study was powered to detect a 10-min difference in clinical "resolution of CPE." Both modes rapidly improved the major physiological variables and achieved resolution of CPE, while intubation and mortality rates did not differ between the modes. The rates of intubation and death were similar to previous studies [8, 9, 10, 11]. The authors concluded that nPSV is not superior to CPAP when signs of respiratory pump failure are present.

M.R. Pinsky et al. (eds.), *Applied Physiology in Intensive Care Medicine 2: Physiological Reviews and Editorials*,
DOI 10.1007/978-3-642-28233-1_44, © Springer-Verlag Berlin Heidelberg 2012

Strengths of the study lie in the following. Consecutive eligible patients were enrolled, and randomization was concealed. The groups were well matched at baseline. The study included an aggressive pharmacological protocol for ACPE; however, pharmacological therapy is not reported. The study incorporated nPSV termination criteria and intubation criteria, and there was no cross-over between groups. The authors did not assess patient comfort with the two techniques.

What can we conclude from the study by Bellone et al. [17]? First, at the inspiratory and expiratory pressures applied, nPSV appears to offer no advantage to CPAP in patients with hypercapnic ACPE. Thus unlike patients with hyerpcapnia due to chronic obstructive pulmonary disease, it appears that CPAP alone is sufficient in these patients, along with aggressive medical treatment. Clinically CPAP is simpler to apply and to titrate than nPSV, thus potentially encouraging more clinicians and institutions to utilize NIV in patients with ACPE. Second, given the low intubation rates in both the CPAP and nPSV arms in the current study as well as previous studies, it is no longer acceptable to include an oxygen arm in future studies, and the use of NIV should be considered the "gold standard" treatment for ACPE. Finally, the question of whether nPSV is associated with a lower intubation rate than CPAP remains unresolved, despite the publication of four trials comparing CPAP and nPSV [10, 11, 12, 17], because all the trials have had insufficient power to demonstrate a difference in these objective endpoints.

What remains to be answered?

CPAP is not a "true" ventilator mode because it does not actively assist inspiration; thus its comparison with a ventilatory mode such as nPSV is difficult. In their discussion the authors correctly state that they cannot be sure that inspiratory and expiratory pressures of 15 and 5 cmH_2O respectively are physiologically equivalent to those of 10 cmH_2O of CPAP. In the absence of intrathoracic pressure measurements we cannot be certain that mean airway pressure is similar with the two modes. A more "physiologically correct" titration of nPSV may be to apply a fixed amount of CPAP (e.g., 10 cmH_2O, as is commonly used), with inspiratory assistance either as tolerated or fixed (e.g., 5 cmH_2O) and to compare it with CPAP of 10 cmH_2O.

Finally, to address the question of whether NIV should be considered "first-line" treatment for CPE it is important to know how many patients with CPE actually require ventilatory assistance. In the study by Park et al. [10] only approx. 20% of patients with severe CPE actually met the inclusion criteria. Is this enough to convince the scientific world of the real benefit of the widespread use of mask ventilation, during an episode of CPE?

Bellone et al. [17] have demonstrated that both CPAP and nPSV improve vital signs and improve clinical outcome in patients with hyperapnic ACPE compared to standard medical therapy. However, we still need to identify whether there is a subset of patients who benefit more from nPSV application than from CPAP. Further, are there parameters of disease severity which allow us to better understand which patients really need a form of ventilatory support, and which patients can be successfully treated "only" with standard medical therapy? "Brick by brick" we build our understanding of the role of mask ventilation in the treatment of CPE.

References

1. American College of Cardiology/ American Heart Association Task Force on Practice Guidelines (1995) Guidelines for the evaluation and management of heart failure. J Am Coll Cardiol 26:1376–1398
2. Task Force on the Working group of Heart Failure of the European Society of Cardiology (1997) Guidelines on the treatment of heart failure. Eur Heart J 18:736–753
3. American Heart Association in collaboration with the International Liaison Committee on Resuscitation (2000) Guidelines for cardiopulmonary resuscitation and emergency cardiovascular care. An international consensus on science. Circulation 102 [Suppl I]:I172–I203
4. Carlucci A, Richard JC, Wysocki M, Lepage E, Brochard L (2001) Noninvasive versus conventional mechanical ventilation. An epidemiological survey. Am J Respir Crit Care Med 163:874–880
5. Girou E, Brun-Buisson C, Taille S, Lemaire F, Brochard L (2003) Secular trends in nosocomial infections and mortality associated with noninvasive ventilation in patients with exacerbation of COPD and pulmonary edema. JAMA 290:2985–2991
6. International Consensus Conferences in Intensive Care Medicine (2001) Noninvasive positive pressure ventilation in acute respiratory failure. Intensive Care Med 27:166–178
7. Pang D, Keenan SP, Cook DJ, Sibbald W (1998) The effect of positive pressure airway support on mortality and the need for intubation in cardiogenic pulmonary edema. A systematic review. Chest 114:1185–1192
8. Masip J, Betbese AJ, Paez J, Vecilla F, Canizares R, Padro J, Paz MA, de Otero J, Ballus J (2000) Non-invasive pressure support ventilation versus conventional oxygen therapy in acute cardiogenic pulmonary oedema: a randomised trial. Lancet 356:26–32
9. Nava S, Carbone G, DiBattista N, Bellone A, Baiardi P, Cosentini R, Marenco M, Giostra F, Borasi G, Groff P (2003) Noninvasive ventilation in cardiogenic pulmonary edema: a multicenter randomized trial. Am J Respir Crit Care Med 168:1432–1437

10. Park M, Sangean MC, Volpe Mde S, Feltrim MI, Nozawa E, Leite PF, Amato MB, Lorenzi-Filho G (2004) Randomized, prospective trial of oxygen, continuous positive airway pressure, and bilevel positive airway pressure by face mask in acute cardiogenic pulmonary edema. Crit Care Med 32:2407–2415
11. Crane SD, Elliott MW, Gilligan P, Richards K, Gray AJ (2004) Randomised controlled comparison of continuous positive airways pressure, bilevel non-invasive ventilation, and standard treatment in emergency department patients with acute cardiogenic pulmonary oedema. Emerg Med 21:155–161
12. Mehta S, Jay GD, Woolard RH, Hipona RA, Connolly EM, Cimini DM, Drinkwine JH, Hill NS (1997) Randomized, prospective trial of bilevel versus continuous positive airway pressure in acute pulmonary edema. Crit Care Med 25:620–628
13. Rusterholtz T, Kempf J, Berton C, Gayol S, Tournoud C, Zaehringer M, Jaeger A, Sauder P (1999) Noninvasive pressure support ventilation (NIPSV) with face mask in patients with acute cardiogenic pulmonary edema. Intensive Care Med 25:21–28
14. Hoffmann B, Welte T (1999) The use of noninvasive pressure support ventilation for severe respiratory insufficiency due to pulmonary oedema. Intensive Care Med 25:15–20
15. Wysocki M, Tric L, Wolff MA, Millet H, Herman B (1995) Non-invasive pressure support ventilation in patients with acute respiratory failure: a randomized comparison with conventional therapy. Chest 107:761–768
16. Confalonieri M, Potena A, Carbone G, Della Porta R, Tolley E, Meduri GU (1999) Acute respiratory failure inpatients with severe community acquired pneumonia. A prospective randomised evaluation of non-invasive ventilation. Am J Respir Crit Care Med 160:1585–1591
17. Bellone A. Vettorello M, Monari A, Cortellaro F, Coen D (2005) Noninvasive pressure support ventilation vs. continuous positive airway pressure in acute hypercapnic pulmonary edema. Intensive Care Med (http://dx.doi.org/10.1007/s00134-005-2649-6)

Chiara Bonetto
Pierpaolo Terragni
V. Marco Ranieri

Does high tidal volume generate ALI/ARDS in healthy lungs?

In *Intensive Care Medicine* Gajic and coworkers [1] now report that use for the first 48 h after ICU admission of high tidal volumes (>700 ml) and high peak inspiratory pressures (>30 cmH_2O) is associated with the development of the criteria for acute respiratory distress syndrome (ARDS) in patients requiring mechanical ventilation for surgery, aspiration, sepsis, pneumonia and trauma but who did not have ARDS. Do these results support the concept that stretch due to mechanical ventilation may cause ventilator-induced lung injury (VILI) in healthy lung [2]?

Mechanical ventilation is the main supportive therapy to reestablish sufficient oxygen supply to peripheral organs in all kinds of acute respiratory failure. It was recognized early that, apart from alveolar disruption, mechanical ventilation can increase alveolar-capillary permeability through the overdistension of the lung (volutrauma) and/or worsening lung injury through the tidal recruitment-derecruitment of the collapsed alveoli (atelectrauma) and lead to even more subtle injury manifested by the activation of the inflammatory process (biotrauma) [2].

The theoretical basis of VILI relies on the seminal study of Mead and coworkers [3] who examined the intrapulmonary distribution of pressure in a lung model that included normal and collapsed alveoli. In such model, tidal inflation caused (a) part of the alveoli continuously accessible to ventilation to be hyperinflated and (b) part of the collapsed alveoli to be continuously recruited and derecruited. Under these circumstances when tidal inflation generated an airway opening pressure of 30 cmH_2O, in the area encompassed between the hyperinflated and the normal alveoli and between the continuously recruited-derecruited alveoli and the normally expanded regions, the interstitial pressure was amplified to 140 cmH_2O [3]. This local amplification of pressure may generate mechanical distortion through two mechanisms: shear stress and stress failure [4].

Shear stress is a form of mechanical stress generated when air move across a cell surface, thereby generating a force parallel to the membrane that induces a tangential distortion of the cell. In damaged lungs the development of shear stress is related to the cyclic opening and closing of small airways induced by recruitment-derecruitment of alveolar units. Diseased lungs with a heterogeneous distribution of lesions may be subjected to much greater regional stress than homogeneous lungs. The occlusion of small airways by exudate or apposition of their walls requires high airway pressure to restore airway opening, resulting in shear stress and damage, particularly if the cycle is continuously repeated [4, 5].

Stress failure depends on the development of excessive wall stress, defined as the ratio of alveolar wall tension to thickness. The limited strength of the alveolar-capillary barrier may explain such mechanism of mechanical stress. It is known that high airway pressure between the alveolus and the vascular bed during positive pressure ventilation causes the passage of air across the epithelial surface, along the bronchovascular sheath, and then into the interstitial tissues. The endothelium, so close to the epithelial surface, is subject to stress failure determined by forces

M.R. Pinsky et al. (eds.), *Applied Physiology in Intensive Care Medicine 2: Physiological Reviews and Editorials*,
DOI 10.1007/978-3-642-28233-1_45, © Springer-Verlag Berlin Heidelberg 2012

derived from both transpulmonary and intravascular pressures. The local or regional stress induced by lung inflation may increase microvascular transmural pressures with disruption of capillaries and change the alveolar-capillary barrier. The forces generated by mechanical ventilation may therefore interact with those due to pulmonary vascular perfusion to increase lung injury [4, 6].

These data therefore led to the concept that (a) all the pathophysiological characteristics of ARDS (ventilation-perfusion mismatch and reduced compliance, lung edema, atelectasis, pulmonary inflammation) may be worsened by inappropriate ventilator settings because of the nonhomogeneous distribution of normal lung regions mixed with consolidated, atelectatic regions and regions that can be recruited/de-recruited depending on the particular ventilatory strategy used [7]; (b) normal, homogeneous lungs should not be affected by ventilator settings otherwise injurious for nonhomogeneous lung [4, 8].

Lungs of patients recovering from abdominal surgery are asymmetric along the vertical axis with relatively normal regions located in the nondependent zones, areas of partially collapsed lung and/or alveolar filling located in the middle zones, and area of pulmonary consolidation located in the most dependent regions [9]. Also in these patients mechanical ventilation may hence theoretically induce shear stress and stress failure because of recruitment-derecruitment of atelectatic alveoli and hyperinflation of normal alveoli [4]. However, Wrigge and coworkers [10, 11] found that in patients after minor surgical procedures mechanical ventilation with tidal volumes of 0.8–1.2 l induced no relevant increase in inflammatory mediators.

Similarly to patients following abdominal surgery, the lungs of patients after cardiopulmonary bypass (CPB) for cardiac surgery are asymmetric along the vertical axis with normal regions, areas of partially collapsed lung and/or alveolar filling, and area of pulmonary consolidation located in the nondependent, intermediate, and most dependent regions, respectively [12]. In a recent study in patients requiring CPB for cardiac surgery we found pulmonary and plasmatic concentration of inflammatory mediators to be increase after 6 h of mechanical ventilation only in those patients ventilated with tidal volumes of 10–12 ml/kg (measured body weight) and 2–3 cmH_2O of PEEP, and decreased after 6 h of mechanical ventilation with a tidal volumes of 8 ml/kg (measured body weight) and 10 cmH_2O of PEEP [13].

Two conditions may therefore be required for stress due to mechanical ventilation to induce a relevant inflammatory stimulus: (a) the mechanical conditions determining the activation of mechanical forces such as shear stress and stress failure; (b) the presence of a primary inflammatory stimulus represented by the underlying causes of ARDS [14], by CPB [13] or other ischemia-reperfusion conditions such as lung transplant [15]. Preliminary data from Wrigge and coworkers [16] indicate that after cardiac surgery, ventilation with low tidal volumes decrease pulmonary inflammatory mediators particularly in patients in whom CPB induced a more relevant increase in pulmonary concentration of inflammatory mediators.

Did the lungs of patients included in the Gajic et al. study have both the mechanical conditions and a primary inflammatory stimulus theoretically required to develop VILI? The PaO_2/FIO_2 ratio was lower and the incidence of pneumonia greater in the group that 48 h after ICU admission developed ARDS than in the group that did not develop ARDS. Moreover, acute respiratory failure due to surgery, aspiration, sepsis, pneumonia, and trauma are associated with an overexpression of the inflammatory response [17]. Data from the Gajic et al. study may therefore confirm that mechanical stretch can activate VILI in lungs already injured and inflamed although the observational nature of the study does not provide definitive answers. However, more important than the contribution to the understanding of the basic mechanisms involved with VILI, their study confirms that the use of high tidal volumes is associated with a serious and severe worsening of the clinical prognosis of mechanically ventilated patients. Until future studies become available, clinicians should be extremely cautious in using ventilator settings that lead to plateau pressures higher than 30 cmH_2O in patients without ARDS [1, 18], and the National Institutes of Health protective strategy must be the gold standard ventilatory treatments for patients with ARDS [19, 20].

References

1. Gajic O, Frutos Vivar F, Estaban A, Hubmayr RD, Anzueto A (2005) Ventilators settings as a risk factor for acute respiratory distress syndrome in mechanically ventilated patients. Intensive Care Med (http://dx.doi.org/10.1007/s005-2625-1)
2. Sibilla S, Tredici S, Porro A, Irace M, Guglielmi M, Nicolini G, Tredici G, Valenza F, Gattinoni L (2002) Equal increases in respiratory system elastance reflect similar lung damage in experimental ventilator-induced lung injury. Intensive Care Med 28:196–203
3. Mead J, Takishima T, Leith D (1970) Stress distribuition in lungs: a model of pulmonary elasticity. J Appl Physiol 28:596–608
4. Terragni PP, Rosboch GL, Lisi A, Viale AG, Ranieri VM (2003) How respiratory system mechanics may help in minimizing ventilator-induced lung injury in ARDS patients. Eur Respir J 42:15s–21s

5. Gefen A, Elad D, Shiner RJ (1999) Analysis of stress distribution in the alveolar septa of normal and simulated emphysematic lungs J Biomech 32:891–897
6. West JB, Tsukimoto K, Mathieu-Costello O, Prediletto R (1991) Stress failure in pulmonary capillaries. J Appl Physiol 70:1731–1742
7. Patroniti N, Bellani G, Manfio A, Maggioni E, Giuffrida A, Foti G, Pesenti A (2004) Lung volume in mechanically ventilated patients: measurement by simplified helium dilution compared to quantitative CT scan Intensive Care Med 30:282–289
8. Stüber F, Wrigge H, Schroeder S, Wetegrove S, Zinserling J, Hoeft A, Putensen C (2002) Kinetic and reversibility of mechanical ventilation-associated pulmonary and systemic inflammatory response in patients with acute lung injury Intensive Care Med 28:834–841
9. Hedenstierna G, Santesson J, Baehrendtz S (1984) Variations of regional lung function in acute respiratory failure and during anaesthesia. Intensive Care Med 10:169–177
10. Wrigge H, Zinserling J, Stuber F, von Spiegel T, Hering R, Wetegrove S, Hoeft A, Putensen C (2000) Effects of mechanical ventilation on release of cytokines into systemic circulation in patients with normal pulmonary function. Anesthesiology 93:1413–1417
11. Wrigge H, Uhlig U, Zinserling J, Behrends-Callsen E, Ottersbach G, Fischer M, Uhlig S, Putensen C (2004) The effects of different ventilatory settings on pulmonary and systemic inflammatory responses during major surgery Anesth Analg 98:775–781
12. Hachenberg T, Tenling A, Nystrom SO, Tyden H, Hedenstierna G (1993) Ventilation-perfusion inequality in patients undergoing cardiac surgery Anesthesiology 80:509–519
13. Zupanicich E, Paparella D, Turani F, Munch C, Rossi A, Massaccesi S, Ranieri VM (2005) Mechanical ventilation affects inflammatory mediators in patients undergoing cardiopulmonary bypass for cardiac surgery: a randomized clinical trial. J Thorac Cardiovasc Surg (in press)
14. Ranieri VM, Suter PM, Tortorella C, De Tullio R, Dayer JM, Brienza A, Bruno F, Slutsky AS (1999) Effect of mechanical ventilation on inflammatory mediators in patients with acute respiratory distress syndrome. A randomized controlled trial JAMA 282:54–61
15. Perrot M de, Imai Y, Volgyesi GA, Waddell TK, Liu M, Mullen JB, McRae K, Zhang H, Slutsky AS, Ranieri VM, Keshavjee S (2002) Effect of ventilator-induced lung injury on the development of reperfusion injury in a rat lung transplant model. J Thorac Cardiovasc Surg 124:1137–1144
16. Wrigge H, Uhligh U, Zinserling J, Menzenbach J, Uhligh S, Putensen C (2003) Inflammatory effects of lower tidal volume ventilation after cardiac surgery Intensive Care Med 29: S82
17. Bien MY, Hseu SS, Yien HW, Kuo BI, Lin YT, Wang JH, Kou YR (2004) Breathing pattern variability: a weaning predictor in postoperative patients recovering from systemic inflammatory response syndrome Intensive Care Med 30:241–247
18. Gajic O, Dara SI, Mendez JL, Adesanya AO, Festic E, Caples SM, Rana R, St Sauver JL, Lymp JF, Afessa B, Hubmayr RD (2004) Ventilator-associated lung injury in patients without acute lung injury at the onset of mechanical ventilation Crit Care Med 32:1817–1824
19. Acute Respiratory Distress Syndrome Network (2000) Ventilation with lower tidal volumes as compared with traditional tidal volumes for acute lung injury and the acute respiratory distress syndrome. N Engl J Med 342:1301–1308
20. Sakr Y, Vincent J-L, Reinhart K, Groeneveld J, Michalopoulos A, Sprung CL, Artigas A, Ranieri VM on behalf of the "Sepsis Occurrence in Acutely Ill Patients" investigators (2005) High tidal volume and positive fluid balance are associated with worse outcome in acute lung injury Chest (in press)

Christian Richard
Jean Louis Teboul

Weaning failure from cardiovascular origin

The goal in weaning from mechanical ventilation (MV) is to induce spontaneous breathing (SB) and ultimately extubation. Weaning fails in about 25% of patients meeting weaning criteria and is particularly frequent in patients with chronic obstructive pulmonary disease (COPD) and/or left heart disease [1]. Weaning failure prolongs the duration of MV and increases morbidity and mortality in these critically ill patients [2]. Thus early identification and treatment of the causes of weaning failure is of paramount importance to improve outcome in difficult-to-wean patients.

Although the most frequent cause of weaning failure is respiratory system failure, a possible consequence of the transfer from MV to SB can be acute myocardial ischemia or acute heart dysfunction or failure particularly in patients with prior coronary artery disease or chronic heart disease [3, 4]. Recognition of the cardiac origin of weaning failure is crucial since the use of vasodilators and/or diuretics may result in successful weaning [4, 5]. The clinical signs presented by patients who fail a weaning trial because they develop acute heart failure (e.g., tachypnea, tachycardia, anxiety) are often difficult to distinguish from clinical signs resulting from respiratory system failure. Some preliminary data concerning the time course of B-type natriuretic peptide concentration during an SB trial suggest that this may help the clinician to distinguish between cardiac and respiratory causes of weaning failure [6].

However, as emphasized by Lemaire et al. [5], the use of a pulmonary artery catheter (PAC) remains the "gold standard" to clearly identify the onset of left ventricular dysfunction during SB trial. These authors reported a marked increase in pulmonary artery occluded pressure (PAOP) during a weaning trial in patients suffering from both COPD and left heart disease who failed to wean from MV [5]. It was hypothesized that the rapid development of cardiogenic pulmonary edema is the major cause of weaning failure in these patients. Most of them were successfully weaned after a 10-day period of diuretics administration [5]. This weaning-induced increase in PAOP has been postulated to be related to: (a) the increase in venous return secondary to the abrupt shift from positive to negative intrathoracic pressure and to the increased sympathetic activity, (b) the reduction in left ventricular compliance secondary to weaning-induced myocardial ischemia and/or ventricular interdependence due to increased right ventricular afterload, and (c) the abrupt increase in left ventricular afterload secondary to the negativation of intrathoracic pressure [4, 5, 7, 8]. A marked increase in PAOP during SB was also observed by Jubran et al. [9] in a group of patients who failed to wean. These authors also reported a decrease in mixed venous oxygen saturation (SvO_2) and an increase in oxygen extraction ratio in this group while PAOP, SvO_2, and oxygen extraction ratio did not change, and cardiac index increased in another group of patients who successfully passed the weaning trial [9].

In *Intensive Care Medicine* Zakynthinos et al. [10] now present their detailed analysis of the cardiovascular and metabolic consequences of SB. The presentation of their results may be debatable since they chose to classify their patients according to a calculated variable (i.e., oxygen consumption) which suffers from many limitations rather than based on a measured variable as SvO_2.

M.R. Pinsky et al. (eds.), *Applied Physiology in Intensive Care Medicine 2: Physiological Reviews and Editorials*,
DOI 10.1007/978-3-642-28233-1_46,

However, the authors can be congratulated for reemphasizing the high variability in hemodynamic patterns during weaning and the fact that it is difficult to anticipate their behavior in a given patient without specific measurements of cardiopulmonary variables. Globally, two different cardiovascular behaviors during SB are distinguished by the authors in 18 of the 30 patients who failed to wean from MV. During the SB trial 9 patients exhibited an increase in oxygen consumption (VO_2) and in oxygen extraction ratio and a decrease in SvO_2 despite the increase in cardiac index. A weaning-induced left ventricular dysfunction probably developed in these patients, as also suggested by the increase in PAOP. It can be postulated that these patients had impaired cardiac function, and that the increase in cardiac index was insufficient to increase oxygen transport to meet the increased oxygen demand induced by the weaning process. The decrease in SaO_2 (from 97% to 87%) during SB—probably related to the development of acute pulmonary edema—was partly responsible for the decrease in SvO_2 in this group of patients. In such cases the oxygen extraction ratio rather than SvO_2 must be used as a marker of the VO_2/oxygen supply balance.

The cardiovascular behavior of the other group of patients who failed to wean is less easy to explain. In these patients VO_2 and SvO_2 did not change while cardiac index increased and oxygen extraction decreased. As a result of the increased work of breathing the oxygen demand is expected to increase during a weaning trial [3, 4]. This should result in increased VO_2 and O_2 transport during the weaning trial, as reported in previous clinical studies [5, 11], This was also observed in the study by Zakynthinos et al. in the group of patients who succeeded in weaning (see Electronic Supplementary Material) as well as in one-half of the patients who failed the SB trial [10]. To explain the absence of increase in VO_2 during the SB trial in nine of their patients Zakynthinos et al. hypothesize that respiratory center depression was responsible for the weaning failure [10]. It is difficult to be entirely convinced by this speculative hypothesis since these patients were still able to increase their respiratory rate during the SB trial (from 18 to 31 cycles/min), and there is no reason to postulate that these patients were not normally conscious since their attending physicians decided to attempt to wean them. Therefore an alternate hypothesis would be the inability of these patients to increase their VO_2 in face of weaning-induced increased oxygen demand. This could be the result of limited capacities to extract oxygen and/or a limited cardiac function reserve. In this group of patients blood lactate concentration did not increase during the SB trial, suggesting that VO_2 matched oxygen demand. However, because lactate concentration responds slowly to an acute hypoxic event, and because mechanical ventilation was rapidly reinstituted after the weaning trial, the absence of increase in blood lactate concentration during the SB trial and 2 h later does not exclude the occurrence of global tissue hypoxia during weaning in this category of patients. Unfortunately, it is not possible to give one definitive explanation of the results found in this specific subgroup of patients because of the lack of precise information on the general status (e.g., degree of consciousness, presence of sepsis) and on the cardiovascular status of the studied patients at the time of the SB trial. For example, echocardiographic data were not given and the true incidence of left diastolic or systolic dysfunction was not reported.

Despite some imprecision the merit of the authors is their wish to better understand the causes of weaning failure in patients with COPD and/or cardiac diseases [5, 11, 12]. Two major messages can be drawn from their study: (a) weaning failure can be associated with different cardiovascular patterns and (b) an absence of decrease in SvO_2 during SB may occur in patients who fail to wean. To our opinion, these results justify the need for invasive hemodynamic monitoring during a weaning trial in order to well understand the origin of weaning failure and hence to apply the most adequate therapy.

References

1. Brochard L, Rauss A, Benito S, Conti G, Mancebo J, Rekik N, Gasparetto A, Lemaire F (1994) Comparison of three methods of gradual withdrawal from ventilatory support during weaning from mechanical ventilation. Am J Respir Crit Care Med 150:896–903
2. Ely EW, Baker AM, Dunagan DP, Burke HL, Smith AC, Kelly PT, Johnson MM, Browder RW, Bowton DL, Haponik EF (1996) Effect on the duration of mechanical ventilation of identifying patients capable of breathing spontaneously. N Engl J Med 335:1864–1869
3. Pinsky MR (2000) Breathing as exercise: the cardiovascular response to weaning from mechanical ventilation. Intensive Care Med 26:1164–1166
4. Lamia B, Monnet X, Teboul JL (2005) Weaning-induced cardiac dysfunction. In Vincent JL (ed) Yearbook of intensive care and emergency medicine. Springer, Berlin Heidelberg New York, pp 239–245
5. Lemaire F, Teboul JL, Cinotti L, Giotto G, Abrouk F, Steg G, Macquin-Mavier I, Zapol W (1988) Acute left ventricular dysfunction during unsuccessful weaning from mechanical ventilation. Anesthesiology 69:171–179
6. Mekontso-Dessap A, De Prost N, Braconnier F, Lemaire F, Brun-Buisson C, Brochard L (2004) B type natriuretic peptide and weaning from mechanical ventilation. Intensive Care Med 30: S182

7. Cabello B, Mancebo J (2003) Withdrawal from mechanical ventilation in patients with COPD: the issue of congestive heart failure. In: Vincent JL (ed) Yearbook of intensive care and emergency medicine. Springer, Berlin Heidelberg New York, pp 295–301
8. Hurford WE, Favorito F (1995) Association of myocardial ischemia with failure to wean from mechanical ventilation. Crit Care Med 23:1475–1480
9. Jubran A, Mathru M, Dries D, Tobin M (1998) Continuous recordings of mixed venous oxygen saturation during weaning from mechanical ventilation and the ramifications thereof. Am J Respir Crit Care Med 158:1763–1769
10. Zakynthinos S, Routsi C, Vassilakopoulos T, Kaltsas P, Zakynthinos E, Kazi D, Roussos C (2005) Differential cardio-vascular responses during weaning failure: effects on tissue oxygenation and lactate. Intensive Care Med (DOI: 10.1007/s00134-005-2699-9)
11. De Backer D, El Haddad P, Preiser JC, Vincent JL (2000) Hemodynamic responses to successful weaning from mechanical ventilation after cardiovascular surgery. Intensive Care Med 26:1201–1206
12. Richard C, Teboul JL, Archambaud F, Hebert JL, Michaud P, Auzepy P (1994) Left ventricular function during weaning of patients with chronic obstructive pulmonary disease. Intensive Care Med 20:181–186

Göran Hedenstierna

The hidden pulmonary dysfunction in acute lung injury

In the *Intensive Care Medicine* Aboab and coworkers [1] now show that the use of 100% O_2 in inspired gas at low levels of positive end-expiratory pressure (PEEP 5 cmH_2O) promotes lung collapse and impedes gas exchange in patients with acute lung injury. The collapse could be prevented or at least countered during the 30 min study period by higher levels of PEEP (15 cmH_2O). What do we learn from this?

Firstly, there are two pulmonary causes of impaired oxygenation in acute lung injury. One is the well-known alveolar collapse and/or alveolar flooding that produce shunt [2, 3]. Research and treatment have almost exclusively focused on this cause of dysfunction. The other cause is lung tissue that is still open but poorly ventilated in relation to perfusion, so-called low V_A/Q regions. Low V_A/Q can be caused by bronchoconstriction, airway secretions, reduced lung volume and regional hyperperfusion, to mention some potential mechanisms. Whether a patient with acute lung injury suffers from low V_A/Q in addition to collapse and flooding has been debated [4, 5, 6], but the study by Aboab and coworkers presents further evidence that this is the case. It may not be as important contributor to impaired oxygenation as collapse and flooding but its magnitude should be established. It most likely varies with the cause of acute lung injury and can be expected to be important in obstructive airway disease [7, 8]. Moreover, when attempts are being made to quantify the contributors to impairment of oxygenation, there may already have been a transformation of low V_A/Q regions to collapsed areas with subsequent shunt. It would be interesting to explore this in further detail. However, low V_A/Q regions contribute to impaired oxygenation only at low (e.g., air) and moderate inspired oxygen concentrations whereas at high FIO_2 they oxygenate blood as efficiently as normal V_A/Q regions [9]. Aboab et al. highlight the problem with these regions, i.e., high FIO_2 promotes adsorption atelectasis and increases the shunt.

Low V_A/Q regions can be seen in the healthy subject, and these increase with age [10] presumably by increasing amount of airway closure [11]. A V_A/Q of 0.1 might be seen even in the healthy lung [12], and it causes adsorption atelectasis when breathing gas with high FIO_2! A few minutes of oxygen breathing during induction of anesthesia are a major cause of atelectasis that then remains during the succeeding anesthesia [13]. A modest decrease in FIO_2 to 0.6–0.8 during the induction eliminates or at least reduces the amount of atelectasis [14]. When anesthetized subjects are ventilated with an FIO_2 of 1.0, atelectasis occurs much more rapidly after a recruitment maneuver than if ventilation is provided with a lower FIO_2 of 0.4 [15]. Another observation made in these studies is that when a collapsed lung is opened up by a recruitment maneuver, oxygenation may not always increase to the extent that one might have anticipated. This is because the opened up lung regions may be characterized by a low V_A/Q that still contributes to impeded oxygenation [15]. One may therefore underestimate the amount of recruited lung when looking at the effect on oxygenation.

Secondly, high PEEP levels can keep alveoli recruited even when using high oxygen concentrations. During anesthesia [16] and in the postoperative period after cardiac surgery [17] a recruitment maneuver followed by

M.R. Pinsky et al. (eds.), *Applied Physiology in Intensive Care Medicine 2: Physiological Reviews and Editorials*,
DOI 10.1007/978-3-642-28233-1_47, © Springer-Verlag Berlin Heidelberg 2012

ventilation with PEEP of 10 cmH_2O prevents derecruitment during oxygen breathing. Thus one might say that we do not have a real problem when using high FIO_2 if PEEP is kept at high enough level. However, apart from the well-known potential of baro- and volo-trauma and even biotrauma [18] there may be other consequences of PEEP. Impeded venous return causes a decrease in cardiac output and, if anything, reduces peripheral circulation of potentially vulnerable organs. PEEP increases systemic capillary pressure and may increase capillary leakage. PEEP impedes the lymphatic drainage of lung tissue [19] and of abdominal organs [20]. The latter is because abdominal lymph flow is drained via the thoracic duct that goes through the thoracic cavity and elevated thoracic pressure impedes the lymph flow. Increased capillary leakage and impeded lymph drainage promote edema formation. These new observations may be another reason to avoid high PEEP levels. However, we must await more studies before coming with definite conclusions.

Knowing the relationships between low V_A/Q regions and atelectasis and the influence of the FIO_2 one may ask what oxygenation of blood should be aimed at? Can we avoid excessive use of high FIO_2 and can we avoid use of high PEEP levels? It is interesting to learn that there is no official recommendation what PaO_2 should be the target in the treatment of acute lung injury. In healthy subjects breathing air, a most normal situation, PaO_2 may be 13 kPa (100 mmHg) in a teenager and down to 9 kPa (65–70 mmHg) in a healthy 70-year-old. How often do we accept these levels in an acute respiratory distress syndrome patient but rather want them to be twice as high! High FIO_2 may initiate a vicious cycle with more collapse and more need of oxygen and of PEEP. Despite increasing measures of ventilatory support, the condition may deteriorate, but it may rather be the ventilatory treatment that kills the patient! These thoughts may be considered a little distant from findings of low V_A/Q and oxygen dependence. However, there is certainly good reason now and then to reconsider our ventilatory support of patients with acute lung injury. The study by Aboab and coworkers is a stimulus for such thoughts!

References

1. Aboab J, Jonson B, Kouatchet A, Taille S, Niklason L, Brochard L (2006) Effect of inspired oxygen fraction on alveolar derecruitment in acute respiratory distress syndrome. Intensive Care Med DOI 10.1007/s00134-006-0382-4
2. Gattinoni L, Caironi P, Pelosi P, Goodman LR (2001) What has computed tomography taught us about the acute respiratory distress syndrome? Am J Respir Crit Care 164:1701–1711
3. Hubmayr RD (2002) Perspective on lung injury and recruitment: a skeptical look at the opening and collapse story. Am J Respir Crit Care Med 165:1647–1653
4. Santos C, Ferrer M, Roca J, Torres A, Hernandez C, Rodriguez-Roisin R (2000) Pulmonary gas exchange response to oxygen breathing in acute lung injury. Am J Respir Crit Care Med 161:26–31
5. Suter P, Fairley H, Schlobohm R (1975) Shunt, lung volume and perfusion during short periods of ventilation with oxygen. Anesthesiology 43:617–627
6. Lemaire F, Matamis D, Lampron N, Teisseire B, Harf A (1985) Intrapulmonary shunt is not increased by 100% oxygen ventilation in acute respiratory failure. Bull Eur Physiopathol Respir 21:251–256
7. Barbera JA, Roger N, Roca J, Rovira I, Higenbottam TW, Rodriguez-Roisin R (1996) Worsening of pulmonary gas exchange with nitric oxide inhalation in chronic obstructive pulmonary disease. Lancet 347:436–440
8. Rylander C, Tylen U, Rossi-Norrlund R, Herrmann P, Quintel M, Bake B (2005) Uneven distribution of ventilation in acute respiratory distress syndrome. Crit Care 9:R165–R171
9. West JB (1977) State of the art: Ventilation-perfusion relationships. Am Rev Respir Dis 116:919–943
10. Gunnarsson L, Tokics L, Gustavsson H, Hedenstierna G (1991) Influence of age on atelectasis, formation and gas exchange impairment during general anaesthesia. Br J Anaesth 66:423–432
11. Leblanc P, Ruff F, Milic-Emili J (1970) Effects of age and body position on "airway closure" in man. J Appl Physiol 28:448–451
12. Dantzker DR, Wagner PD, West JB (1975) Instability of lung units with low VA/Q ratios during O2 breathing. J Appl Physiol 38:886–895
13. Rothen HU, Sporre B, Engberg G, Wegenius G, Reber A, Hedenstierna G (1995) Prevention of atelectasis during general anaesthesia. Lancet 345:1387–1391
14. Edmark L, Kostova-Aherdan K, Enlund M, Hedenstierna G (2003) Optimal oxygen concentration during induction of general anesthesia. Anesthesiology 98:28–33
15. Rothen HU, Sporre B, Engberg G, Wegenius G, Högman M, Hedenstierna G (1995) Influence of gas composition on recurrence of atlectasis after a reexpansion maneuver during general anesthesia. Anesthesiology 82:832–842
16. Neumann P, Rothen HU, Berglund JE, Valtysson J, Magnusson L, Hedenstierna G (1999) Positive end-expiratory pressure prevents atelectasis during general anaesthesia even in the presence of a high inspired oxygen concentration. Acta Anaesthesiol Scand 43:295–301
17. Dyhr T, Laursen N, Larsson A (2002) Effects of lung recruitment maneuver and positive end-expiratory pressure on lung volume, respiratory mechanics and alveolar gas mixing in patients ventilated after cardiac surgery. Acta Anaesthesiol Scand 46:717–725
18. Ranieri VM, Suter PM, Tortorella C, De Tullio R, Dayer JM, Brienza A, Bruno F, Slutsky AS (1999) Effect of mechanical ventilation on inflammatory mediators in patients with acute respiratory distress syndrome: a randomized controlled trial. JAMA 282:54–61
19. Frostell C, Blomqvist H, Hedenstierna G, Halbig I, Pieper R (1987) Thoracic and abdominal lymph drainage in relation to mechanical ventilation and PEEP. Acta Anaesthesiol Scand 31:405–411
20. Lattuada M, Hedenstierna G (2006) Abdominal lymph flow in an endotoxin sepsis model: influence of spontaneous breathing and mechanical ventilation. Crit Care Med (in press)

Daniel De Backer
Michael R. Pinsky

Can one predict fluid responsiveness in spontaneously breathing patients?

Prediction of fluid responsiveness has become a topic of intense interest. Although measurements of preload, by whatever technique, are still commonly used to guide fluid therapy [1, 2], these fail to estimate the response to fluids in one-half of the patients [3]. Accordingly, many patients may be subjected to the hazards of fluids [4], without benefiting from hemodynamic improvement.

In patients receiving mechanical ventilatory support predictable heart lung interactions can be used to accurately identify fluid responsiveness by noting the arterial pulse pressure or aortic stroke volume variation over three or more breaths [5]. This is because positive-pressure inspiration induces cyclic increases in right atrial pressure causing in turn inverse changes in venous return, right ventricular filling and ejection and ultimately left ventricular preload. In preload-dependent patients these cyclical changes in ventricular filling induce cyclic changes in stroke volume and arterial pulse pressure, provided that both the right and left ventricles are preload responsive. These cyclic changes in pressure and flow are referred to as pulse pressure variation (Δ PP) and stroke volume variation (Δ SV), respectively. In spontaneously breathing patients the situation is more complex. Spontaneous inspiration induces negative cyclic changes in intrathoracic pressure causing right atrial pressure to also decrease increasing the pressure gradient for venous blood flow. In calves with total artificial hearts spontaneous ventilation induced opposite changes in left ventricular stroke volume than mechanical ventilation [6]. However, unlike artificial hearts whose right and left side filling is independent of each other, in patients with normal hearts Δ PP failed to predict preload response during under either pressure support [7, 8] or spontaneously breathing [8]. Various factors may explain this lack of reliability. Both pressure support ventilation and spontaneous breathing are associated with variability in tidal volume, and both Δ PP and Δ SV are dependent on tidal volume [9, 10]. Similarly, spontaneous inspiratory efforts may increase intra-abdominal pressure because of active compression of abdominal muscles, exaggerating the preload response. Finally, sudden increases in right ventricular end-diastolic volume decrease left ventricular diastolic compliance by the process of ventricular interdependence, which may decrease left ventricular filling and stroke volume independent of preload-responsiveness, because even failing hearts need some end-diastolic volume to generate stroke volume. Soubrier et al. [11] in their contribution to *Intensive Care Medicine* now reason that forced expiratory maneuvers (Valsalva maneuver) may identify preload responsiveness in spontaneously breathing patients when normal spontaneous ventilation do not. Using standardized amplitude of respiratory movements they compared the effects of both a Valsalva maneuver and spontaneous

M.R. Pinsky et al. (eds.), *Applied Physiology in Intensive Care Medicine 2: Physiological Reviews and Editorials*,
DOI 10.1007/978-3-642-28233-1_48, © Springer-Verlag Berlin Heidelberg 2012

breathing on Δ PP to predict preload responsiveness in 32 critically ill patients. During regular spontaneous breathing activity Δ PP was higher in responders to fluid challenge than in nonresponders, but the test performed poorly with a sensitivity of Δ PP greater than 12% of only 63% although specificity was good (92%). The forced maneuver failed to improve the performance of the test, with a decrease in sensitivity to 21% but a maintained specificity (92%). Importantly, the cutoff value of Δ PP increased to 33% during the forced expiratory maneuver, indicating that during this large swing in pleural pressure moderate fluctuations in arterial pressure may not indicate fluid responsiveness. This may be due to several factors. First, applying larger tidal volumes and more negative pleural pressure may transiently shift the patient to preload dependency, which disappears when the patient breaths normally. Second, the Valsalva maneuver may also affect right and left ventricular afterload, which may contribute to respiratory variations in stroke volume [12]. Thus, regrettably, Δ PP and other derived indices cannot be used in spontaneously breathing patients, as slight and sometimes undetected changes in breathing pattern may affect these variables.

Another way to predict fluid responsiveness is to perform an endogenous fluid challenge using passive leg raising. This approach has been used by cardiologists in the cardiac catheterization laboratory for over 50 years. In critically ill patients under mechanical ventilation, with or without spontaneous respiratory movements, an increase in mean aortic flow of more than 10% during passive leg raising reliably predicts the response to fluid challenge [7, 13, 14]. Until now this test has been difficult to apply in conscious and spontaneously breathing patients. Passive leg raising requires the use of a fast response measurement of cardiac output as the increase in cardiac output is transient and may not be maintained when legs are raised for more than a few minutes. Hence esophageal Doppler measures of descending aortic blood flow was used in the three reported studies [7, 13, 14]. Unfortunately, using an esophageal flow probe may be quite uncomfortable in conscious patients. To address this issue both Lamia et al. [15] and Maizel et al. [16] in their contributions to *Intensive Care Medicine* demonstrate that transthoracic echocardiography can be used to measure mean cardiac output during leg raising. They report that an increased change in aortic flow, measured as velocity time interval at the aortic valve (VTIao) by 10–13%, was associated with a positive response to fluid challenge. In both cases the performance of the tests was very good (receiver operating characteristic curve area of 0.96 [15] and 0.90 [16]) with sensitivity and specificity above 80%. Importantly, one-half of the patients in the study by Lamia et al. [15] and all patients in the study by Maizel et al. [16] were spontaneously breathing without any mechanical support.

These studies provide several lessons. First, changes in mean arterial pressure during passive leg raising failed to predict the response to fluid. Similarly, changes in arterial pressure during fluid challenge were only loosely related to changes in cardiac output, again demonstrating that the only way to assess a positive response to fluid in a spontaneously breathing subject is to measure the changes in cardiac output by whatever the technique. Second, changes in left ventricular area or mitral Doppler, reflecting left ventricular preload, were not useful for predicting the response to fluids, indicating again that preload-responsiveness is not the same as preload.

Several limitations of these last two studies should be acknowledged. First, VTIao rather than stroke volume or cardiac output was measured in order to limit errors in calculation. Both studies considered that aortic diameter did not change during passive leg raising and fluid challenge, and thus VTIao reflected stroke volume. However, if passive leg raising induced increased flow and also increased arterial pressure, aortic diameter may also increase, reducing the accuracy of the VTIao to track flow changes [17]. This limitation may not apply to the aortic outflow tract where VTIao is obtained with echocardiography, as this area is somewhat protected by the aortic annulus. Also, although tachycardia is common in hypovolemia, many studies have reported that there is no major change in heart rate during fluid challenge, even in responders, and therefore stroke volume can be used to assess cardiac output changes, which define fluid responsiveness. Second, some patients experienced a significant decrease in cardiac output both during passive leg raising and fluid challenge. This may reflect a stress-induced change in metabolic requirements or reflect vasoconstriction occurring between baseline and subsequent passive leg raising measurements. This underscores the axiom that hemodynamic evaluation should always be performed carefully in conscious patients and that external factors may interfere with the hemodynamic response to an intervention. Finally, although reliable in experts hands (the inter- and intraobserver variability of VTIao were lower than 5% in both studies), investigators less experienced with echocardiographic techniques may not reach this level of accuracy. In particular, small changes in the angle of the echo beam may induce errors in measurements that may be misinterpreted (a 15° angle inducing a 5% error in measurement). More importantly, echocardiography is not always available at any time of the day and cannot be used for continuous monitoring needed for trend analysis. It is likely that other cardiac output measurement techniques, such as pulse contour determinations, would provide similar results and may supplant echocardiography in bedside monitoring of dynamic changes in cardiac output.

Hence the prediction of fluid responsiveness is now feasible in spontaneously breathing patients, but this requires the performance of a passive leg raising test and the dynamic measure of changing cardiac output using fast response measurements techniques. In the hands of the unskilled, much caution needs to be placed on the interpretation of these parameters, but when the data are accurately collected, it represents a new and powerful tool in the critical care diagnostic armamentarium.

References

1. Rivers E, Nguyen B, Havstadt S, Ressler J, Muzzin A, Knoblich B, Peterson E, Tomlanovich M (2001) Early goal-directed therapy in the treatment of severe sepsis and septic shock. N Engl J Med 345:1368–1377
2. Goepfert MS, Reuter DA, Akyol D, Lamm P, Kilger E, Goetz AE (2007) Goal-directed fluid management reduces vasopressor and catecholamine use in cardiac surgery patients. Intensive Care Med 33:96–103
3. Michard F, Teboul JL (2002) Predicting fluid responsiveness in ICU patients: a critical analysis of the evidence. Chest 121:2000–2008
4. Wiedemann HP, Wheeler AP, Bernard GR, Thompson BT, Hayden D, deBoisblanc B, Connors AF Jr, Hite RD, Harabin AL (2006) Comparison of two fluid-management strategies in acute lung injury. N Engl J Med 354:2564–2575
5. Pinsky MR (2004) Using ventilation-induced aortic pressure and flow variation to diagnose preload responsiveness. Intensive Care Med 30:1008–1010
6. Fukamachi K, Irie H, Massiello A, Chen JF, Crouch R, Utoh J, Harasaki H, Golding LA, Kiraly RJ (1992) Effects of mechanical ventilation and spontaneous respiration on hemodynamics in calves with total artificial hearts. ASAIO J 38:M493–M496
7. Monnet X, Rienzo M, Osman D, Anguel N, Richard C, Pinsky MR, Teboul JL (2006) Passive leg raising predicts fluid responsiveness in the critically ill. Crit Care Med 34:1402–1407
8. Heenen S, De Backer D, Vincent JL (2006) How can the response to volume expansion in patients with spontaneous respiratory movements be predicted? Crit Care 10:R102
9. Reuter DA, Bayerlein J, Goepfert MS, Weis FC, Kilger E, Lamm P, Goetz AE (2003) Influence of tidal volume on left ventricular stroke volume variation measured by pulse contour analysis in mechanically ventilated patients. Intensive Care Med 29:476–480
10. De Backer D, Heenen S, Piagnerelli M, Koch M, Vincent JL (2005) Pulse pressure variations to predict fluid responsiveness: influence of tidal volume. Intensive Care Med 31:517–523
11. Soubrier S, Saulnier F, Hubert H, Delour P, Lenci H, Onimus T, Nseir S, Durocher A (2007) Can dynamic indicators help the prediction of fluid responsiveness in spontaneously breathing critically ill patients? Intensive Care Med. DOI 10.1007/s00134-007-0644-9
12. Buda AJ, Pinsky MR, Ingels NB Jr, Daughters GT, Stinson EB, Alderman EL (1979) Effect of intrathoracic pressure on left ventricular performance. N Engl J Med 301:453–459
13. Boulain T, Achard JM, Teboul JL, Richard C, Perrotin D, Ginies G (2002) Changes in BP induced by passive leg raising predict response to fluid loading in critically ill patients. Chest 121:1245–1252
14. Lafanechere A, Pene F, Goulenok C, Delahaye A, Mallet V, Choukroun G, Chiche J, Mira J, Cariou A (2006) Changes in aortic blood flow induced by passive leg raising predict fluid responsiveness in critically ill patients. Crit Care 10:R132
15. Lamia B, Ochagavia A, Monnet X, Chemla D, Richard C, Teboul JL (2007) Echocardiographic prediction of volume responsiveness in critically ill patients with spontaneously breathing activity. Intensive Care Med. DOI 10.1007/s00134-007-0646-7
16. Maizel J, Airapetian N, Lorne E, Tribouilloy C, Massy Z, Slama M (2007) Diagnosis of central hypovolemia by using passive leg raising. Intensive Care Med. DOI 10.1007/s00134-007-0642-y
17. Monnet X, Chemla D, Osman D, Anguel N, Richard C, Pinsky MR, Teboul JL (2007) Measuring aortic diameter improves accuracy of esophageal Doppler in assessing fluid responsiveness. Crit Care Med 35:477–482

John J. Marini

The "open lung" compromise

How best to select positive end-expiratory pressure (PEEP) in acute respiratory distress syndrome (ARDS) remains among the most actively debated questions of critical care practice. Controversy stems partially from imprecision of disease diagnosis, confusion about which objective to prioritize, and uncertainty regarding safe limits for airway pressure. Perhaps the root cause for such indecisiveness, however, involves the mechanical heterogeneity of the acutely diseased lung coupled with the need to set only one PEEP value. In fact, when lung protection is the issue, PEEP selection is always a tradeoff between improving recruitment and increasing tissue stress. The article by Di Rocco and colleagues in this issue [1] offers novel experimental data that address how that compromise is best struck.

How is the optimum PEEP to be recognized at the bedside? Not many years ago, clinicians facing the PEEP selection issue were focused primarily on physiological variables, such as tidal compliance and the efficiency of oxygen exchange. (Some caregivers—perhaps most—still are.) With minimizing shunt the primary objective, high PEEP levels were often selected after relatively long periods of ventilator adjustment. More recently, awareness of the roles of high alveolar pressures and tidal opening and closure cycles in producing ventilator-induced lung injury (VILI) have reshuffled our priorities to emphasize lung protection. Although all are agreed that adverse patterns of ventilation can damage lungs, as yet no firm consensus has emerged as to the hierarchy of factors causative in VILI generation. No doubt remains regarding the importance of maximum tidal stretching pressure—little ventilator-caused injury is likely to result if the plateau pressure *recorded under passive conditions* can be kept low. From that point of general agreement, however, the conceptual waters become murky.

In a fully recruited lung, using sufficient PEEP (and/or associated smaller tidal pressure excursions) dramatically reduces the risk of VILI from any specified plateau pressure. One explanation for PEEP's benefit in this setting is its ability to eliminate high-stress interfaces that exist at the junctions of aerated and atelectatic tissues, to lower shearing stresses, and to prevent repeated recruitment cycles within small airways. Such observations have given rise to the "open lung" approach to the ventilatory management of ARDS and to methods that can be used to accomplish it [2]. Doubters cogently argue that complete lung opening is unnecessary, impossible to accomplish, and requires excessive airway pressure to attain and sustain. This is not an easily settled issue, and although we are slowly making progress, there is still no agreement on the best way to find the "open lung" position.

DiRocco, Carney and Nieman use their novel technique of in vivo video-microscopy and a small animal model of airway instability to address the question of which feature of the static airway pressure–volume (PV) loop correlates best with the lowest "open lung" PEEP [1]. In reporting their experience with directly observed, surfactant-depleted lung tissue, these authors confirm both that alveolar recruitment in this rat model is not completed until the lungs reach total lung capacity (TLC) and that

M.R. Pinsky et al. (eds.), *Applied Physiology in Intensive Care Medicine 2: Physiological Reviews and Editorials*,
DOI 10.1007/978-3-642-28233-1_49, © Springer-Verlag Berlin Heidelberg 2012

the upper inflection point on the deflation limb of the PV curve (UIPd) better indicates the least pressure associated with full recruitment than does the traditionally used lower inflection point (LIP) obtained during inflation. To a point, this makes good sense and resonates with recent theory [3], experimental findings [4] and clinical trial evidence [5]. However, we need to be very careful not to confuse any such *global* measure with certainty regarding *regional* behavior.

Conceptually, there is a "disconnect" between flow, volume, and pressure observations made at the airway opening (which pool information from all lung units) with the events that occur in any specific lung region. The contours of the recordable PV curve—inflation or deflation limb—can only describe the volume or pressure at which tissue overdistension or recruitment *predominates*, not the point at which either no longer occurs. Furthermore, in real-world clinical settings the LIP and UIPd are usually indistinct *zones* that require mathematical curve fitting to estimate, not visually distinct "points" with unequivocal identity features.

We all learned lung physiology from useful but highly oversimplified "balloon on a stick" models that ignore the complexities of diseased anatomy, interdependence and regional behaviors. With that single-compartment healthy lung model in mind, and unintentionally disregarding the mechanical hysteresis of the ARDS lung, easily measured indices of recruitment and overinflation have been popularized that are based on the characteristics of the inspiratory PV curve. Somewhat surprisingly, the LIP, first advocated for the clinical setting by Matamis, Lemaire and colleagues [6], has served reasonably well in at least two "lung protective" clinical trials focused on securing an open lung [7, 8]. Moreover, the ease and speed with which the LIP can be determined at the bedside with automated technology adds to its appeal [9]. By serendipity, the inspiratory pressure associated with the LIP often—but not invariably—approximates the pressure associated with the UIPd. Those two inflections were rather widely separated in the surfactant-depletion model of DiRocco and colleagues, but in other models of injury they may be much closer.

Because a truly open lung—one whose every portion is stable during tidal breathing and without atelectatic units—cannot be achieved without applying tidal pressures that are intolerably elevated, the real questions are: How "open" do we need the lung to be? How high a pressure should we tolerate in pursuit of this elusive goal? If a block of atelectatic tissue has a higher opening pressure than ever experienced during tidal ventilation, is persistent collapse dangerous? Conversely, if it opens readily at low pressure, are the repeated shearing forces tolerable? "Full" recruitment is clearly desirable when this helps prevent VILI in a highly recruitable lung but loses value as the number of units in jeopardy declines. For this reason, open lung strategies should prove more useful earlier than later in the clinical course of ARDS.

Raising PEEP implies an increase in plateau pressure, a reduction in tidal volume (and ventilation), or both. Within already open lung units, raising plateau pressure produces greater tissue stretch, and the strains experienced at the junctions of open and persistently closed units rise disproportionately. Disturbingly, recent analyses can find no safe plateau pressure threshold, even within the ventilating range readily accepted in modern practice [10, 11]. Even though several reassuring explanations can be offered for the correlation between end-tidal pressure and mortality, such observations suggest that PEEP-driven increases of plateau pressure should not be undertaken without concern.

Apart from the very small number of animals investigated, the interesting and carefully collected data of DiRocco and colleagues [1] must be questioned on several methodological levels. As the authors point out, this work cannot be directly extrapolated to the clinical arena. The healthy rats used as the subjects of this study not only had anatomic dimensions an order of magnitude smaller than those of large mammals and humans, but were studied with a highly recruitable, saline lavage preparation—not acute injury that simulates usual clinical causes of lung injury. Hysteresis in this model is quite pronounced and not representative of most clinical conditions. Moreover, PV curves that aptly characterize the lungs of a small animal may not correspond well with those obtained in large animals with gravity-influenced regional mechanics and disproportionate collapse in dependent zones. Even if this "size" reservation is set aside, video-microscopy of alveoli at the pleural surface conducted in a non-dependent region of the open chest under gentle suction may not characterize events occurring deeper within the lungs of closed-chest animals.

One clear lesson emerges from this paper and from others attempting to address the optimal PEEP question: Careful intervention and closely observed feedback are essential when formulating a well-reasoned bedside approach to this common clinical problem. Individual differences in pathology, changeable and heterogeneous mechanics, and serious hazards associated with our therapeutic interventions demand firm grounding in the relevant patho-physiology and preclude easy, formula-driven answers to an innately complex challenge.

References

1. DiRocco J, Carney D, Nieman G (2007) Correlation of alveolar recruitment/derecruitment with inflection points on the pressure–volume curve. Intensive Care Med DOI 10.1007/s00134-007-0629-8 (this issue)
2. Lachmann B (1992) Open up the lung and keep the lung open. Intensive Care Med 18:319–321
3. Hickling KG (2001) Best compliance during a decremental, but not an incremental positive end expiratory pressure trial is related to open lung positive end expratory pressure: a mathematical model of acute respiratory distress syndrome lungs. Am J Respir Crit Care Med 163:69–78
4. Crotti S, Mascheroni D, Caironi P, Pelosi P, Ronzoni G, Mondino M, Marini J, Gattinoni L (2001) Recruitment and de-recruitment during acute respiratory failure: a clinical study. Am J Respir Crit Care Med 164:131–140
5. Girgis K, Hamed H, Khater Y, Kacmarek RM (2006) A decremental PEEP trial identifies the PEEP level that maintains oxygenation after lung recruitment. Respir Care 51:1132–1139
6. Matamis D, Lemaire F, Harf A, Brun-Buisson C, Ansquer JC, Atlan G (1984) Total respiratory pressure–volume curves in the adult respiratory distress syndrome. Chest 86:58–66
7. Amato M, Barbas C, Medeiros D, Magaldi R, Schettino G, Lorenzi-Filho G, Kairalla R, Deheinzelin D, Munoz C, Oliveira R, Takagaki T, Carvalho C (1998) Effect of a protective ventilation strategy on mortality in the acute respiratory distress syndrome. N Engl J Med 338:347–354
8. Villar J, Kacmarek R, Perez-Mendez L, Aguirre-Jaime A (2006) A high positive end-expiratory pressure, low tidal volume ventilatory strategy improves outcome in persistent acute respiratory distress syndrome: a randomized, controlled trial. Crit Care Med 34:1311–1318
9. Servillo G, Svantesson C, Beydon L, Roupie E, Brochard L, Lemaire F, Jonson B (1997) Pressure-volume curves in acute respiratory failure. Automated low flow inflation versus occlusion. Am J Respir Crit Care Med 155:1629–1636
10. Terragni PP, Rosboch G, Tealdi A, Corno E, Menaldo E, Davini O, Gandini G, Herrmann P, Mascia L, Quintel M, Slutsky AS, Gattinoni L, Ranieri V (2007) Tidal hyperinflation during low tidal volume ventilation in acute respiratory distress syndrome. Am J Respir Crit Care Med 175:160–166
11. Hager DN, Krishnan JA, Hayden DL, Brower RG (2005) ARDS Clinical Trials Network. Tidal volume reduction in patients with acute lung injury when plateau pressures are not high. Am J Respir Crit Care Med 172:1241–1245

Christian Mueller

Acute respiratory failure: back to the roots!

Hypoxic respiratory failure is one of the most commonest disorders leading to intensive care unit (ICU) admission and also a common reason for the deterioration of patients already treated in the ICU. It is a very serious condition associated with significant mortality [1, 2]. In recent decades, research and scientific attention has focused nearly exclusively on the pathophysiology and treatment of established causes of hypoxic respiratory failure such as cardiogenic pulmonary edema and the acute respiratory distress syndrome (ARDS) [1, 2]. Therefore, our diagnostic approach to patients with hypoxic respiratory failure has remained both largely unchanged and poorly validated. This is a dilemma because diagnostic uncertainty is very common. The severity of disease and the requirement for immediate ventilatory support often limit our ability to obtain a detailed patient history and physical examination. Chest X-ray is helpful but also associated with important limitations [3].

Lefebvre and colleagues are to be congratulated for shedding light on the diagnostic uncertainty associated with hypoxic respiratory failure in the ICU. In this paper they evaluate a novel approach to diagnose the cause of hypoxic respiratory failure: the measurement of B-type natriuretic peptides, specifically NT-proBNP [4]. B-type natriuretic peptides are quantitative markers of cardiac stress and heart failure (HF) summarizing the extent of systolic and diastolic left ventricular dysfunction, valvular dysfunction, and right ventricular dysfunction [5–7]. B-type natriuretic peptides have been shown to be extremely helpful in the diagnosis and prognosis of HF, particularly in the emergency department (ED). As the diagnostic dilemmas in the ICU are often as challenging as in the ED, recent studies have begun to evaluate whether the use of B-type natriuretic peptides might also be helpful in the ICU [8–12]. Major differences in patient characteristics, disease severity, comorbidity, resources available for the individual patient, and therapies applied between the ICU and the ED require that the potential clinical use of B-type natriuretic peptides in the ICU be defined by specific ICU studies.

Lefebvre and colleagues examined the use of NT-proBNP in 74 cancer patients presenting to the ICU with hypoxic respiratory failure. The rationale for focusing on cancer patients was based on the idea that rapid identification of a cardiac cause of hypoxic respiratory failure could avoid invasive procedures such as bronchoscopy and bronchoalveolar lavage in these patients. They found that NT-proBNP levels were significantly higher in patients with cardiac causes ($n = 16$) than in those with non-cardiac causes ($n = 56$). However, overall the accuracy of NT-proBNP in diagnosing HF was only moderate. NT-proBNP seemed helpful to rule out HF, but not to reliably diagnose HF [4]. The diagnostic uncertainty associated with respiratory failure in the ICU is highlighted by the fact that apparently 24 out of 74 patients received a "furosemide trial". Only 6 of these finally received a gold standard diagnosis of HF. Therefore, furo-

M.R. Pinsky et al. (eds.), *Applied Physiology in Intensive Care Medicine 2: Physiological Reviews and Editorials*,
DOI 10.1007/978-3-642-28233-1_50, © Springer-Verlag Berlin Heidelberg 2012

semide was inappropriately given to 18 patients, and appropriately to only 6 patients. On the other hand, only 6 out of 16 patients with HF received furosemide.

The following considerations might help to put these findings into perspective: First, this cohort of cancer patients differs in many aspects from unselected patients presenting with hypoxic respiratory failure [9, 10]. The patients were roughly 20 years younger and had a very low prevalence of HF as the cause of respiratory failure. Therefore, the findings of this study most likely cannot be transferred to a broader patient population. Second, the ability of an observational study to reliably quantify the diagnostic accuracy of a novel test depends on the accuracy of the gold standard diagnosis. Thus, if the gold standard is incorrect in 25% of patients, a hypothetically perfect novel test with a true accuracy of 100% would result in an accuracy of only 75%. The diagnostic uncertainty associated with hypoxic respiratory failure in the ICU is exemplified by several controversies regarding the gold standard diagnosis used in this study. The diagnosis of cardiac respiratory failure required "the absence of infection or non-infectious pulmonary involvement". This is misleading, as infection is a well-established trigger of acute HF [13]. Also, this definition neglects the clinical reality of two disorders being present and significantly contributing to respiratory failure at the same time. In addition, the gold standard diagnosis in this paper heavily relies on echocardiography. Unfortunately, the echocardiographic diagnosis of left ventricle diastolic dysfunction in critically ill patients is often challenging [14, 15]. We lack systematic studies that have validated, for example, what constitutes normal diastolic function in a 75-year-old woman with non-cardiac respiratory failure receiving positive-pressure ventilation. This limitation is further aggravated by the fact that echocardiography and NT-proBNP testing were performed at different times during ICU stay, as left ventricle diastolic function may change rapidly in response to therapy. Unfortunately, another limitation comes on top of this. As acknowledged by the authors, the detection of a cardiac dysfunction does not imply that the diagnosis of HF is the main cause of respiratory failure. For instance, a patient may have had myocardial infarction 10 years ago: his left ventricular ejection fraction is 40%, which classifies him as having systolic left ventricular dysfunction. If this patient develops respiratory failure due to pneumonia, his echo will be altered at admission but the cause of his respiratory failure is extra-cardiac.

The inherent dilemma of lack of accepted and validated gold standard diagnosis in observational studies can ultimately only be overcome by performing randomized controlled trials that apply objective measures of patient outcome as endpoints. The primary results of a large randomized controlled multicenter study (BASEL II–ICU) will soon become available and help to further elucidate the approach to ICU patients with hypoxic respiratory failure. BASEL II–ICU tests the hypothesis that the use of B-type natriuretic peptide levels in ICU patients with respiratory failure might help to more rapidly and more accurately detect the cause of respiratory failure and ultimately improve patient management and reduce total treatment cost.

References

1. Ware LB, Matthay MA (2000) The acute respiratory distress syndrome. N Engl J Med 342:1334–1339
2. Ware LB, Matthay MA (2005) Acute pulmonary edema. N Engl J Med 353:2788–2796
3. Mueller-Lenke N, Rudez J, Staub D, Laule-Kilian K, Perruchoud AP, Mueller C (2006) Use of chest X-ray in the emergency diagnosis of acute congestive heart failure. Heart 92:695–696
4. Lefebvre A, Kural-Menasche S, Darmon M, Thiery G, Feugeas JP, Schlemmer B, Azoulay E (2008) Use of N-terminal pro-B-type natriuretic peptide to detect cardiac origin in critically ill cancer patients with acute respiratory failure. Intensive Care Med DOI 10.1007/s00134-008-1000-4
5. Mueller C, Breidthardt T, Laule-Kilian K, Christ M, Perruchoud AP (2007) The intergration of BNP and NT-proBNP into clinical medicine. Swiss Med Wkly 137:4–12
6. Yoshitaka Iwanaga Y, Nishi I, Furuichi S, Noguchi T, Sase K, Kihara Y, Goto Y, Nonogi H (2006) B-type natriuretic peptide strongly reflects diastolic wall stress in patients with chronic heart failure. J Am Coll Cardiol 47:742–748
7. Mueller C, Scholer A, Laule-Kilian K, Martina B, Schindler C, Buser P, Pfisterer M, Perruchoud AP (2004) Use of B-type natriuretic peptide in the evaluation and management of acute dyspnea. N Engl J Med 350:647–654
8. McLean AS, Tang B, Nalos M, Huang SJ, Stewart SE (2003) Increased B-type natriuretic peptide (BNP) level is a strong predictor for cardiac dysfunction in intensive care unit patients. Anaesth Intensive Care 31:21–27
9. Karmpaliotis D, Kirtane AJ, Ruisi CP, Polonsky T, Malhotra A, Talmor D, Kosmidou I, Jarolim P, de Lemos JA, Sabatine MS, Gibson CM, Morrow D (2007) Diagnostic and prognostic utility of brain natriuretic peptide in subjects admitted to the ICU with hypoxic respiratory failure due to noncardiogenic and cardiogenic pulmonary edema. Chest 131:964–971
10. Abroug F, Ouanes-Besbes L, Nciri N, Sellami N, Addad F, Hamda KB, Amor AB, Najjar MF, Knani J (2006) Association of left-heart dysfunction with severe exacerbation of chronic obstructive pulmonary disease. Diagnostic performance of biomarkers. Am J Respir Crit Care Med 174:990–996
11. Forfia PR, Watkins SP, Rame JE, Stewart KJ, Shapiro EP (2005) Relationship between B-type natriuretic peptides and pulmonary capillary wedge pressure in the intensive care unit. J Am Coll Cardiol 45:1667–1671

12. Grasso S, Leone A, De Michele M, Anaclerio R, Cafarelli A, Ancona G, Stripoli T, Bruno F, Pugliese P, Dambrosio M, Dalfino L, Di Serio F, Fiore T (2007) Use of N-terminal pro-brain natriuretic peptide to detect acute cardiac dysfunction during weaning failure in difficult-to-wean patients with chronic obstructive pulmonary disease. Crit Care Med 35:96–105
13. The Task Force on Acute Heart Failure of the European Society of Cardiology. Nieminen MS, Böhm M, Cowie MR, Drexler H, Filippatos GS, Jondeau G, Hasin Y, Lopez-Sendon J, Mebazaa A, Metra M, Rhodes A, Swedberg K (2005) Executive summary of the guidelines on the diagnosis and treatment of acute heart failure. Eur Heart J 26:384–416
14. Pirracchio R, Cholley B, De Hert S, Solal AC, Mebazaa A (2007) Diastolic heart failure in anaesthesia and critical care. Br J Anaesth 98:707–721
15. Cholley BP, Vieillard-Baron A, Mebazaa A (2006) Echocardiography in the ICU: time for widespread use! Intensive Care Med 32:9–10

Antoine Vieillard-Baron

Is right ventricular function the one that matters in ARDS patients? Definitely yes

Since the beginning of the 1980s, intensivists have known that acute respiratory distress syndrome (ARDS) is strongly associated with pulmonary hypertension and right ventricular (RV) dysfunction [1, 2]. Three phenomena promote this. First, lung damage per se, which combines alveolar injury with capillary destruction and obstruction by clots. Second, remodeling of the pulmonary circulation, defined as a muscularization of normally nonmuscularized vessels, mediated by hypoxemia and hypercarbia, and finally, positive pressure ventilation, which increases the distending pressure of the lung and thus crushes the pulmonary capillaries. These phenomena are reversible, except for pulmonary capillary destruction, which was especially observed when tidal volume was adjusted to correct the $PaCO_2$, and so the plateau pressure ($P_{plateau}$) is not limited. During this period, RV failure was frequent and associated with high mortality [2–4]. In particular, Jardin et al. found in a series of 23 patients an incidence of acute cor pulmonale (ACP) as high as 61% with 100% mortality in the most severe forms [2]. ACP is considered to reflect RV dysfunction due to an acute increase in RV afterload, as in ARDS. Its definition is echocardiographic: RV dilatation in combination with paradoxical septal motion during systole.

Following the ARDS network study, which demonstrated the beneficial effect of limiting $P_{plateau}$ [5], the question was whether RV dysfunction is a dreaded complication of the past or is still very much with us [6]. This debate is of importance when two very different ventilatory approaches are compared: an "open-lung approach" requiring significant lung-distending pressures in inspiration and also in expiration to "recruit" the lung, but likely to impair the right ventricle [7], and a "RV protective approach," more designed to preserve the right ventricle [8].

In 2001, we reported a series of 75 ARDS patients submitted to low-stretch ventilation, which combines a low positive end-expiratory pressure (PEEP) (mean 7 cm H_2O) and a $P_{plateau}$ below 27 cm H_2O, and in whom we looked for the presence of ACP [9]. We found two main results: first, a 25% incidence of ACP, which is significantly lower than that in older studies, and second, no difference in mortality (32%) in patients with and without ACP [9]. Our results were understood and interpreted by others as indicating that RV dysfunction has now become infrequent and has no impact on prognosis in ARDS patients. This is a terrible error, as well demonstrated by Osman et al. [10]. Using the database of their previous study on the pulmonary artery catheter [11], they demonstrate that RV dysfunction, defined by a central venous pressure (CVP) higher than the pulmonary artery occlusion pressure (PAOP), is a major prognostic factor in ARDS patients [10]. The incidence of this hemodynamic profile was 27%, as

M.R. Pinsky et al. (eds.), *Applied Physiology in Intensive Care Medicine 2: Physiological Reviews and Editorials*,
DOI 10.1007/978-3-642-28233-1_51, © Springer-Verlag Berlin Heidelberg 2012

shown in Table 3 of their study. Although obtained by using a nonoptimal way of diagnosing RV dysfunction, the best one being echocardiography, their results are convincing. But, how to reconcile their results with our 2001 study? Very simple. In our study, we responded to any observation of ACP by immediately making significant adjustments in respiratory management [9]. In particular, $P_{plateau}$ and PEEP were decreased further, if possible, and prone positioning, a maneuver known to have a positive effect on lung mechanics and so on RV function [12], was largely applied (in 63% of patients with ACP but in only 14% of patients without ACP). Conversely, Osman et al. performed a strict observational study, and the definition of RV dysfunction and the statistical analysis are retrospective. Consequently, no recommendation was made for intensivists in the case of RV dysfunction. For instance, we do not know how many and which patients were turned into the prone position in this study. Finally, the comparison of these two studies clearly demonstrates that the impact of RV dysfunction on prognosis can be limited, but providing that the deleterious effects of mechanical ventilation on RV function are strictly controlled. A right ventricle that is already injured because of the lung process is unable to tolerate and adapt to aggressive ventilation. A recent study on a large series of ARDS patients confirms this assertion [13]. It found that the incidence of ACP and its impact on prognosis were strongly related to the range of $P_{plateau}$: in patients with a $P_{plateau}$ below 27 cm H_2O, the incidence of ACP was low—between 10 and 15%—and its impact on mortality was nil, whereas in patients with a $P_{plateau}$ between 27 and 35 cm H_2O the incidence of ACP was close to 35% and had a significant impact on mortality [13]. In the study by Osman et al., it would be interesting to know the prognostic impact of RV dysfunction not only in the whole population but also within different ranges of $P_{plateau}$.

However, the study by Osman et al. is not totally clear. In particular, it is difficult to understand why the combination of a mean pulmonary artery pressure higher than 25 mmHg plus a CVP higher than the PAOP plus a low stroke index did not appear as a prognostic factor [10]. This is more sensitive to greater severity than a CVP higher than PAOP only. This reflects RV failure more than RV dysfunction. One of the explanations, given by the authors, is that when faced with this situation intensivists are more fully alerted to the severity of the disease because of the associated low-flow state and therefore modify the ventilatory and hemodynamic strategies. However, the results presented in the study do not allow a definitive conclusion to be drawn in this regard and a statistical problem is not excluded. Moreover, this may reflect a limitation of pulmonary artery catheterization, which renders difficult the interpretation of a hemodynamic profile with finesse in a real-life situation, where intensivists are mainly focused on cardiac output. Interestingly, and not surprisingly, patients with RV failure had more severely injured lungs with much lower compliance of the respiratory system [10], illustrating once again the impact of the combination lung damage/ positive pressure ventilation on pulmonary circulation and then on RV function.

To conclude, this study and previous studies allow us to claim that daily RV function assessment is mandatory for the management of ARDS patients, especially in the most severe cases. This is now recommended by the French Society of Intensive Care Medicine (SRLF) [14]. Although not really the theme of this editorial, it is important to maintain that the best method for evaluating RV function is echocardiography [15]. Any observation of RV dysfunction, whatever be the cardiac output, should prompt intensivists to adapt their ventilatory management, by decreasing $P_{plateau}$ and limiting PEEP and by using prone positioning.

References

1. Zapol W, Snider M (1977) Pulmonary hypertension in severe acute respiratory failure. N Engl J Med 296:476–480
2. Jardin F, Gueret P, Dubourg O, Farcot JC, Margairaz A, Bourdarias JP (1985) Two-dimensional echocardiographic evaluation of right ventricular size and contractility in acute respiratory failure. Crit Care Med 13:952–956
3. Squara P, Dhainaut JF, Artigas A, Carlet J (1998) Hemodynamic profile in severe ARDS: results of the European Collaborative ARDS study. Intensive Care Med 24:1018–1028
4. Monchi M, Bellenfant F, Cariou A, Joly LM, Thebert D, Laurent I, Dhainaut JF, Brunet F (1998) Early predictive factors of survival in the acute respiratory distress syndrome. A multivariate analysis. Am J Respir Crit Care Med 158:1076–1081
5. The Acute Respiratory Distress Syndrome Network (2000) Ventilation with lower tidal volumes as compared with traditional tidal volumes for acute lung injury and the acute respiratory distress syndrome. N Engl J Med 342:1301–1308
6. Scherrer-Crosbie M, Streckenbach SC, Zapol W (2001) Acute cor pulmonale in acute respiratory distress syndrome: a dreaded complication of the past? Crit Care Med 29:1641–1642
7. Borges J, Okamoto V, Matos G, Caramez M, Arantes P, Barros F, Souza C, Victorino J, Kacmarek R, Barbas C, Carvalho C, Amato M (2006) Reversibility of lung collapse and hypoxemia in early acute respiratory distress syndrome. Am J Respir Crit Care Med 174:268–278

8. Page B, Vieillard-Baron A, Beauchet A, Aegerter P, Prin S, Jardin F (2003) Low stretch ventilation strategy in acute respiratory distress syndrome: eight years of clinical experience in a single center. Crit Care Med 31:765–769
9. Vieillard-Baron A, Schmitt JM, Augarde R, Fellahi JL, Prin S, Page B, Beauchet A, Jardin F (2001) Acute cor pulmonale in acute respiratory distress syndrome submitted to protective ventilation: incidence, clinical implications, and prognosis. Crit Care Med 29:1551–1555
10. Osman D, Monnet X, Castelain V, Anguel N, Warszawski J, Teboul JL, Richard C; for the French Pulmonary Artery Catheter Study Group (2008) Incidence and prognostic value of right ventricular failure in acute respiratory distress syndrome. Intensive Care Med. doi:10.1007/s00134-008-1307-1
11. Richard C, Warszawski J, Anguel N, Deye N, Combes A, Barnoud D, Boulain T, Lefort Y, Fartoukh M, Baud F, Boyer A, Brochard L, Teboul JL (2003) Early use of the pulmonary artery catheter and outcomes in patients with shock and acute respiratory distress syndrome: a randomized controlled trial. JAMA 290:2713–2720
12. Vieillard-Baron A, Charron C, Caille V, Belliard G, Page B, Jardin F (2007) Prone positioning unloads the right ventricle in severe ARDS. Chest 132:1440–1446
13. Jardin F, Vieillard-Baron A (2007) Is there a safe plateau pressure in ARDS? The right heart only knows. Intensive Care Med 33:444–447
14. Richard JC, Girault C, Leteurtre S, Leclerc F, for the experts group of the SRLF (2005) Ventilatory management of acute respiratory distress syndrome in adult patients and children (new-born excepted). Société de réanimation de langue française experts recommendations. Réanimation 14:313–322
15. Vieillard-Baron A, Prin S, Chergui K, Dubourg O, Jardin F (2002) Echo-Doppler demonstration of acute cor pulmonale at the bedside in the medical intensive care unit. Am J Respir Crit Care Med 166:1310–1319

Patrick M. Honore
Olivier Joannes-Boyau
Willem Boer

Strong ion gap and outcome after cardiac arrest: another nail in the coffin of traditional acid–base quantification

The role of unmeasured anions in critical care patients remains a controversial issue. Recent data demonstrate that circulating anions can be quantified and that this might have prognostic value. An alternative approach to acid–base balance, based more squarely on chemical and physical principles, was proposed by Peter Stewart more than 25 years ago [1]. The strong ion difference as later modified by Figge and Fencl [2] corresponds with the net charge balance of all strong ions present in a given solution (the "Fencl–Stewart" approach) [3]. Whilst striving for more accuracy and bedside practicality, Kellum [4] proposed using the strong ion gap (SIG) which corresponds with the difference between the apparent strong ion difference and the effective strong ion difference. In comparison to the traditional anion gap, the SIG is calculated from all charged blood constituents and is now the gold standard for the quantification of unmeasured anions [5]. The origin of these circulating anions remains unclear though clinicians are inclined to believe that those anions are released from ischemic or hypoxic tissue and that quantification of these anions could be more sensitive for prognosis than lactate in these conditions. An elevated SIG has been associated with increased mortality in critically ill children [3] as well in patients undergoing major surgery [6]. No study till now has sought to describe a possible association between outcome after cardiac arrest and SIG. This question is addressed by the study of Funk et al. published in this issue of *Intensive Care Medicine* [7]. For almost two decades, the Stewart approach, though commendable theoretically, seemed to lack usefulness as a tool for the clinician at the bedside. Recognition of the fact that utilization of the traditional anion gap, especially in critically ill patients, was highly unsatisfactory [8], renewed interest for the use of the more accurate SIG, which takes into account all the ions present in a given solution [9]. In this issue, Funk et al. [7] compare SIG versus lactate as a determinant of outcome after cardiac arrest, whereby outcome is described in survivors in terms of neurological performance. An association is indeed demonstrated, independent of time to return of spontaneous circulation, epinephrine dose, age or other acid–base variables. It is asserted that the anions constituting SIG may be surrogates for tissue damage. Additionally, as an association between SIG and cerebral performance category is found, it is postulated that the brain may be a potential source of unmeasured anions after cardiac arrest and arising even before lactate levels increase. While these findings and their exciting explanations remain to be demonstrated in further controlled studies, it is important to point out a number of pitfalls in this study. By far the most important is the retrospective nature of the study design, representing an obvious and serious drawback to

M.R. Pinsky et al. (eds.), *Applied Physiology in Intensive Care Medicine 2: Physiological Reviews and Editorials*,
DOI 10.1007/978-3-642-28233-1_52, © Springer-Verlag Berlin Heidelberg 2012

the validity of the conclusions. Nevertheless, although retrospective, this is a well conducted study, both in terms of methodology and in terms of adjustment for confounding factors. A further drawback of the study is the selective use of bicarbonate in some patients, albeit according to strict criteria, thereby creating, for some at least, a bias in the study. The long period over which the study was conducted is a major concern: it took 12 years to complete the study, a period in which profound changes in treatment of the intensive care patient will have taken place which impacts on the strength of this retrospective study, though the size of the cohort (288 patients in cardiac arrest who were successfully resuscitated) works to the study's advantage. Funk's study highlights the fact that more and more studies are currently evaluating SIG as a possible tool not only for measurement of anions but also as a surrogate marker for tissue damage (sometimes very locally) and as an early and more specific predictor of outcome when compared to traditional acid–base quantification and lactate. Indeed, studies have recently shown that in a general intensive care population, SIG was an independent prognostic factor for mortality even in the presence of a normal acid–base status as traditionally described using the Henderson–Hasselbach equation [10]. The SIG has the theoretical advantage when compared to traditional anion gap (AG) that it remains stable and reliable, even in cases of extremes in PCO_2 and pH, further enhancing its utility in acid–base disturbances in those circumstances [11]. Another potential advantage is the detection of metabolic acidosis that has been offset by a greater metabolic alkalosis especially after liver transplantation [12], thereby facilitating interpretation of complex acid–base changes [12]. The same phenomenon has been described is sepsis too, a situation in which metabolic acidosis maybe offset by concurrent respiratory alkalosis [13]. The relationship between metabolic acidosis, unmeasured anions and mediators released remains unclear [14] especially during special procedures like cardiopulmonary bypass and haemofiltration procedures [14]. In a recently conducted study, an elevated SIG presaged mortality after injury better than admission pH, bicarbonate level and even lactate [15]. Along the same lines, in children after cardiopulmonary bypass, an elevated SIG appears to be superior to lactate as mortality predictor [16]. Nonetheless, controversy persists in particular to what constitutes a normal range of SIG and where abnormal SIG with adverse outcome starts. Indeed, this is reflected in what one could term a transatlantic acid–base debate as American studies describe abnormal values at around 5 mEq/L [17, 18] while studies from Europe and Australasia found far higher values [19]. In this study, the mean SIG from healthy controls was 3.6 mmol/L and an elevated SIG was described when values were above 8.9 mmol/L [7]. Some authors claim that this difference was due to the use of gelatins as an exogenous source of unmeasured anions used in resuscitation [20] but the use of gelatins has diminished in these countries as they can induce hyperoncotic acute kidney injury [21]. Recent work has demonstrated that up to 50% of endogenous low molecular weight anions are sourced from the intermediate metabolism [22]. In conclusion, the study from Funk et al. [7], although retrospective in nature, sheds new light upon the role of SIG after cardiac arrest as a marker of outcome and especially neurological outcome. SIG proved to be a better marker of outcome after cardiac arrest than epinephrine dose, age and other acid–base variables including traditional anion gap and even lactate. They subsequently concluded that the anions constituting SIG may be surrogates of tissue damage that occurred mostly in the brain. However, these conclusions needs to be challenged in further controlled and well-conducted studies. A new era of change in which SIG replaces traditional acid–base quantification is upon us. The speed of this change will remain an area of uncertainty for the near future.

References

1. Stewart PA (1983) Modern quantitative acid–base chemistry: applications in biology and medicine. Can J physiol Pharmacol 61:1444–1461
2. Figge J, Mydosh T, Fencl V (1992) Serum proteins and acid–base equilibria: a follow-up. J Lab clin Med 120:713–719
3. Balasubramanyan N, Havens PL, Hoffman GM (1999) Unmeasured anions identified by the Fencl–Stewart method predict mortality better than base excess, anion gap, and lactate in patients in the pediatric intensive care unit. Crit Care Med 27:1577–1581
4. Kellum JA, Kramer DJ, Pinsky MR (1995) Strong ion gap: a methodology for exploring unexplained anions. J Crit Care 10:51–55
5. Gunnerson KJ (2005) Clinical review: the meaning of acid–base abnormalities in the intensive care unit part 1-epidemiology. Crit Care 9:508–516
6. Kaplan LJ, Kellum JA (2004) Initial pH, base deficit, lactate, anion gap, strong ion difference, and strong ion gap predict outcome from major vascular injury. Crit Care Med 321:1120–1124
7. Funk GC, Doberer D, Richling N, Kneidinger N, Lindner G, Scheeweiss B, Eisenburger P (2008) The strong ion gap and outcome after cardiac arrest in patients treated with therapeutic hypothermia. Intensive Care Med. doi: 10.1007/s00134-008-1315-1
8. Levraut L, Bounatirou T, Ichai C, Ciais JF, Jambou P, Hechema R, Grimaud D (1997) Reliability of anion gap as an indicator of blood lactate in critically ill patients. Intensive Care Med 23:417–422

9. Leblanc M (1999) The acid–base effects of acute hemodialysis. Curr Opin Crit Care 5:468–478
10. Antonini B, Piva S, Paltenghi M, Candiani A, Latronico N (2008) The early phase of critical illness is a progressive aciditic state due to unmeasured anions. Eur J Anaesthesiol 25:566–577
11. Morgan TJ, Cowley DM, Weier SL, Venkatesh B (2007) Stability of the strong ion gap over extremes of PCO_2 and pH. Anaesth Intensive Care 35:370–373
12. Story DA, Vaja R, Poustie SJ, McNicol L (2008) Fencl–Stewart analysis of acid–base changes immediately after liver transplantation. Crit Care Resusc 10:23–26
13. Leisewitz AL, Jacobson LS, de Morais HS, Reyers F (2001) The mixed acid–base disturbances of severe canine babesiosis. J Vet Intern Med 15:445–452
14. Honoré PM, Matson JR (2002) Hemoflitration, adsorption, sieving and the challenge of sepsis therapy design. Crit Care 6:394–396
15. Kaplan LJ, Kellum JA (2008) Comparison of acid base models for prediction of hospital mortality following trauma. Shock 29:662–666
16. Durward A, Tibby SM, Skellet S, Austin C, Anderson D, Murdoch IA (2005) The strong ion gap predicts mortality in children following bypass surgery. Pediatr Crit Care Med 6:281–285
17. Gunnerson KJ, Roberts G, Kellum JA (2003) What is normal strong ion gap (sIG) in healthy subjects and critically ill patients without acid–base abnormalities. Crit Care Med 31:A11
18. Kellum JA (2007) Acid–base disorders and strong ion gap. Contrib Nephrol 156:158–166
19. Cusack RJ, Rhodes A, Lochhead P, Jordan B, Perry S, Ball JA, Grounds RM, Bennett ED (2002) The strong ion gap does not have prognostic value in critically ill patients in a mixed medical/surgical adult ICU. Intensive Care Med 28:864–869
20. Kellum JA (2003) Closing the gap on unmeasured anions. Crit Care 7:219–220
21. Honore PM, Joannes-Boyau O, Boer W (2008) Hyperoncotic colloids in shock and risk of renal injury: enough evidence for a banning order? Intensive Care Med 34 (published online). doi: 10.1007/s00134-008-1225-2
22. Forni LG, McKinnon W, Lord GA, Treacher DF, Peron JM, Hilton PJ (2005) Circulating anions usually associated with the krebs cycle in patients with metabolic acidosis. Crit Care 9:591–595

John J. Marini

Prone positioning for ARDS: defining the target

Although variation of position is innate to healthy subjects, practitioners usually orient critically ill patients in a supine, semirecumbent posture for days to weeks, with only periodic, side-to-side repositioning through a relatively shallow 30–60° arc. Experimental data [1] and clinical observations [2–4] demonstrate physiologic benefit from prone positioning during acute lung injury (ALI), but recent large clinical trials have been unable to confirm survival benefit in diverse populations of patients labeled as having ALI/acute respiratory distress syndrome (ARDS) [5–7]. However, posttrial subgroup analyses hint that certain patient subgroups may indeed benefit from prone orientation. Severely ill patients, those experiencing improved CO_2 exchange, and those ventilated with large tidal volumes appear more likely to benefit than other members of the general cohort [5]. A superb meta-analysis of pooled data appears in this issue, focusing on those relative few with the worst oxygen exchange [8]. This analysis shows convincingly that, while proning cannot be recommended for all patients with acute lung injury, it does hold therapeutic value for some.

With the ascendance of evidence-based approaches to medical practice, clinicians have come to depend on randomized clinical trials (RCTs) to confirm or refute the value of therapeutic options used in medical practice. Although RCTs are of unquestioned benefit when realistic outcome variables and mechanistically sound trial design are applied to an appropriate population, numerous failed trials conducted in critical care settings demonstrate how vulnerable RCTs are to imprecise definitions, loose selection criteria, incomplete physiological understanding, and restricted availability of suitable subjects. In the wake of an RCT that fails to demonstrate outcome benefit, an intervention of life-saving value for a well-selected few may be shelved due to the lack of definitional precision and sufficient numbers.

Prone positioning (PP) provides an illuminating example. There is little question that PP can be expected to redistribute trans-lung forces, reduce the supine gradient of trans-lung pressure [2], recruit and stabilize dorsal lung units, relieve cardiac compression of lung tissue [4], and favor mouthward migration of retained airway secretions [3]. Such actions—on average—reliably improve oxygenation and airway drainage, particularly in the earlier stages of the injury process. However, currently we know neither the optimal daily duration of prone positioning nor when to initiate PP, nor once applied how many days to persist with it.

While many nursing units are now proficient in effecting PP when indicated [9], experience has shown that proning holds the potential for harm as well as good. Stringent precautions must be observed to prevent pressure ulcers and inadvertent misadventures with displaced or kinked tubes and catheters. Such problems are likely to parallel the duration of prone positioning. In theory, mobile and gravity-driven biofluids (infected secretions, inflammatory edema) migrating along the airway have the potential to propagate initially focal injury or infection from dorsal to more ventral zones [10].

Clues from the first large Italian trial of PP suggested that, with mortality reduction as the objective, only

M.R. Pinsky et al. (eds.), *Applied Physiology in Intensive Care Medicine 2: Physiological Reviews and Editorials*,
DOI 10.1007/978-3-642-28233-1_53, © Springer-Verlag Berlin Heidelberg 2012

restricted subsets of patients—those with the most severe disease and those who are recruitable—are good candidates [5, 11]. At first glance, the just published prospective follow-up RCT of PP conducted in ARDS patients with moderate to severe hypoxemia both disappoints in not showing overall benefit and affirms that potential benefits are most likely to accrue in those most severely affected [12]. The signal, while clearly present, is not overwhelmingly strong and would have required enrolment of many more patients for the trend to reach statistical significance. To achieve sufficiently large sample size in such a low-incidence disease state would have required additional years of data collection. Exactly *why* the signal from the severity-targeted study was not stronger is debatable, but one attractive possibility is that ventilator-induced lung injury (VILI) is strongly influenced by tidal volume and plateau pressure, which were more closely regulated in the prospective follow-up study. This lung-protective measure would dampen VILI risk and mask any benefit from proning maneuvers.

The novel contribution of the report by Sud et al. [8], which included studies regardless of proning duration and timing, is that the meta-analysis pools the collective published experience with patients with uncommonly severe disease and thereby helps define the subpopulation likely to benefit from an inconsistently life-saving intervention. Even severe hypoxemia, however, may itself be too inclusive a category to identify those most amenable to PP. The key to survival benefit may not be improved oxygen exchange—which occurs in most proned subjects and can be achieved by redistributing perfusion without increasing the number of functional lung units or relieving stress and strain. As suggested by Gattinoni's earlier analysis [11], recruitment may be the characteristic that determines PP's value, and "recruitable" patients are only a subset of those with severe hypoxemia. Quantitating recruitment at the bedside remains elusive in today's medical practice, but techniques that are just now coming on line, such as electrical impedance tomography (EIT) and gas dilution functional residual capacity (FRC), raise hopes for better precision and logistical feasibility.

Failed RCTs do not invalidate PP as a tool for ARDS management. The work by Sud et al. [8] clearly demonstrates that PP can be life-saving if the patients are well selected and the timing of the intervention is appropriate. How then to best utilize this tool, and in whom? In the absence of unassailable RCT guidance, there are no absolute mandates or prohibitions; the decision to implement PP remains a matter of individual judgment, tempered by empiricism. My own approach is as follows: Unless otherwise contraindicated, an empirical trial of proning should be attempted in those receiving ventilatory support whose severely impaired oxygenation fails to respond to usual measures, including sedation, recruiting maneuvers, and high positive end-expiratory pressure (PEEP). Because misadventures may arise during PP, proning should be limited to those with severe ARDS (as indicated by PaO_2/FiO_2 <100 mmHg) who show convincingly positive recruiting responses within a few hours of being turned. Even when successful, PP is continued no longer than 3–4 days, or until dramatic improvement in the underlying process is documented. Though PaO_2 may adequately classify disease severity, $PaCO_2$ better tracks gas exchange efficiency and perhaps better reflects the recruitment that appears to be central to PP benefit [11]. Recruiting maneuvers are employed after PP, both for their potential to reopen refractory units as well as to set the appropriate level of PEEP. In my view, proning clearly is not to be used in every patient with acute lung injury, but remains a valuable, even life-saving, option for those most likely to succumb to this devastating problem.

References

1. Broccard AF, Shapiro RS, Schmitz LL, Ravenscraft SA, Marini JJ (1997) Influence of prone position on the extent and distribution of lung injury in a high tidal volume oleic acid model of acute respiratory distress syndrome. Crit Care Med 25:16–27
2. Pelosi P, Brazzi L, Gattinoni L (2002) Prone position in acute respiratory distress syndrome. Eur Respir J 20:1017–1028
3. Gillart T, Bazin JE, Guelon D, Constantin JM, Mansoor O, Conio N, Schoeffler P (2000) Effect of bronchial drainage on the improvement in gas exchange observed in ventral decubitus in ARDS. Ann Fr Anesth Reanim 19:156–163
4. Albert RK, Hubmayr RD (2000) The prone position eliminates compression of the lungs by the heart. Am J Respir Crit Care Med 161:1660–1665
5. Gattinoni L, Tognoni G, Pesenti A, Taccone P, Mascheroni D, Labarta V, Malacrida R, Di Giulio P, Fumagalli R, Pelosi P, Brazzi L, Latini R, Prone-Supine Study Group (2001) Effect of prone positioning on the survival of patients with acute respiratory failure. N Engl J Med 345:568–573
6. Guerin C, Gaillard S, Lemasson S, Ayzac L, Girard R, Beuret P, Palmier B, Le QV, Sirodot M, Rosselli S, Cadiergue V, Sainty JM, Barbe P, Combourieu E, Debatty D, Rouffineau J, Ezingeard E, Millet O, Guelon D, Rodriguez L, Martin O, Renault A, Sibille JP, Kaidomar M (2004) Effects of systematic prone positioning in hypoxemic acute respiratory failure: a randomized controlled trial. JAMA 292:2379–2387

7. Mancebo J, Fernández R, Blanch L, Rialp G, Gordo F, Ferrer M, Rodríguez F, Garro P, Ricart P, Vallverdú I, Gich I, Castaño J, Saura P, Domínguez G, Bonet A, Albert RK (2006) A multicenter trial of prolonged prone ventilation in severe acute respiratory distress syndrome. Am J Respir Crit Care Med 173:1233–1239
8. Sud S, Friedrich JO, Taccone P, Polli F, Adhikari NK, Latini R, Pesenti A, Guerin C, Mancebo J, Curley MA, Fernandez R, Chan M-C, Beuret P, Voggenreiter G, Sud M, Tognoni G, Gattinoni L (2010) Prone ventilation reduces mortality in patients with acute respiratory failure and severe hypoxemia: Systematic review and meta-analysis. Intensive Care Med. doi: 10.1007/s00134-009-1748-1
9. Messerole E, Peine P, Wittkopp S, Marini JJ, Albert RK (2002) The pragmatics of prone positioning. Am J Respir Crit Care Med 165:1359–1363
10. Marini JJ, Gattinoni L (2008) Propagation prevention: a complementary mechanism for lung protective ventilation in ARDS. Crit Care Med 36:3252–3258
11. Gattinoni L, Vagginelli F, Carlesso E, Taccone P, Conte V, Chiumello D, Valenza F, Caironi P, Pesenti A, Prone-Supine Study Group (2003) Decrease in $PaCO_2$ with prone position is predictive of improved outcome in acute respiratory distress syndrome. Crit Care Med 31:2727–2733
12. Taccone P, Pesenti A, Latini R, Polli F, Vagginelli F, Mietto C, Caspani L, Raimondi F, Bordone G, Iapichino G, Mancebo J, Guérin C, Ayzac L, Blanch L, Fumagalli R, Tognoni G, Gattinoni L, Prone-Supine II Study Group (2009) Prone positioning in patients with moderate and severe acute respiratory distress syndrome: a randomized controlled trial. JAMA 302:1977–1984

Index

M.R. Pinsky et al. (eds.), *Applied Physiology in Intensive Care Medicine 2: Physiological Reviews and Editorials*,
DOI 10.1007/978-3-642-28233-1, © Springer-Verlag Berlin Heidelberg 2012

V

W

MIX
Papier aus verantwortungsvollen Quellen
Paper from responsible sources
FSC® C105338

If you have any concerns about our products,
you can contact us on
ProductSafety@springernature.com

In case Publisher is established outside the EU,
the EU authorized representative is:
Springer Nature Customer Service Center GmbH
Europaplatz 3, 69115 Heidelberg, Germany

Printed by Libri Plureos GmbH
in Hamburg, Germany